Brian Fleming Research & Learning Library
Ministry of Education
Ministry of Training, Colleges & Universities
900 Bay St. 13th Floor, Mowat Block
Toronto, ON M7A 1L2

D1768772

**Bilingualism and Bilingual Deaf Education**

Perspectives on Deafness

Series Editors
Marc Marschark
Patricia Elizabeth Spencer

*The Gestural Origin of Language*
David F. Armstrong and Sherman E. Wilcox

*Teaching Deaf Learners: Psychological and Developmental Foundations*
Harry Knoors and Marc Marschark

*The People of the Eye: Deaf Ethnicity and Ancestry*
Harlan Lane, Richard C. Pillard, and Ulf Hedberg

*A Lens on Deaf Identities*
Irene W. Leigh

*Deaf Cognition: Foundations and Outcomes*
Edited by Marc Marschark and Peter C. Hauser

*Sign Language Interpreting and Interpreter Education: Directions for Research and Practice*
Edited by Marc Marschark, Rico Peterson, and Elizabeth A. Winston

*The World of Deaf Infants: A Longitudinal Study*
Kathryn P. Meadow-Orlans, Patricia Elizabeth Spencer, and Lynn Sanford Koester

*Advances in the Sign Language Development of Deaf Children*
Edited by Brenda Schick, Marc Marschark, and Patricia Elizabeth Spencer

*Advances in the Spoken Language Development of Deaf and Hard-of-Hearing Children*
Edited by Patricia Elizabeth Spencer and Marc Marschark

# Bilingualism and Bilingual Deaf Education

Edited by
Marc Marschark
Gladys Tang
Harry Knoors

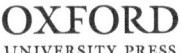

# OXFORD
UNIVERSITY PRESS

Oxford University Press is a department of the University of
Oxford. It furthers the University's objective of excellence in research,
scholarship, and education by publishing worldwide.

Oxford   New York
Auckland   Cape Town   Dar es Salaam   Hong Kong   Karachi
Kuala Lumpur   Madrid   Melbourne   Mexico City   Nairobi
New Delhi   Shanghai   Taipei   Toronto

With offices in
Argentina   Austria   Brazil   Chile   Czech Republic   France   Greece
Guatemala   Hungary   Italy   Japan   Poland   Portugal   Singapore
South Korea   Switzerland   Thailand   Turkey   Ukraine   Vietnam

Oxford is a registered trademark of Oxford University Press
in the UK and certain other countries.

Published in the United States of America by
Oxford University Press
198 Madison Avenue, New York, NY 10016

© Oxford University Press 2014

All rights reserved. No part of this publication may be reproduced, stored in
a retrieval system, or transmitted, in any form or by any means, without the prior
permission in writing of Oxford University Press, or as expressly permitted by law,
by license, or under terms agreed with the appropriate reproduction rights organization.
Inquiries concerning reproduction outside the scope of the above should be sent to the
Rights Department, Oxford University Press, at the address above.

You must not circulate this work in any other form
and you must impose this same condition on any acquirer.

Library of Congress Cataloging-in-Publication Data
Bilingualism and bilingual deaf education / edited by Marc Marschark,
Harry Knoors, Gladys Tang.
   p. cm.
Includes bibliographical references and index.
ISBN 978–0–19–937181–5
1. Deafness—Psychological aspects.   2. Deaf children—Language.
3. Sign language acquisition.   4. Oral communication.   I. Marschark, Marc.
HV2380.B55 2014
371.91'2—dc23
2013050413

9 8 7 6 5 4 3
Printed in the United States of America
on acid-free paper

# Contents

Preface ix
Contributors xiii

1. Bilingualism and Bilingual Deaf Education:
   Time to Take Stock 1
   *Harry Knoors, Gladys Tang, and Marc Marschark*

Part One: Linguistic, Cognitive, and Social Foundations

2. Language Development and Language Interaction in Sign
   Bilingual Language Acquisition 23
   *Carolina Plaza-Pust*

3. Language Acquisition by Bilingual Deaf Preschoolers:
   Theoretical and Methodological Issues and Empirical Data 54
   *Pasquale Rinaldi, Maria Cristina Caselli, Daniela Onofrio,
   and Virginia Volterra*

4. Bimodal Bilingual Cross-Language Interaction:
   Pieces of the Puzzle 74
   *Ellen Ormel and Marcel Giezen*

5. Sign Language and Reading Comprehension:
   No Automatic Transfer 102
   *Daniel Holzinger and Johannes Fellinger*

6. The Influence of Communication Mode on Language
   Development in Children with Cochlear Implants 134
   *Elizabeth A. Walker and J. Bruce Tomblin*

7. Psychosocial Development in Deaf and Hard-of-Hearing
   Children in the Twenty-first Century: Opportunities and
   Challenges 152
   *Manfred Hintermair*

8. Bilingualism and Bimodal Bilingualism in Deaf
   People: A Neurolinguistic Approach 187
   *Ana Mineiro, Maria Vânia Silva Nunes, Mara Moita,
   Sónia Silva, and Alexandre Castro-Caldas*

## Part Two: Education

9. Navigating Two Languages in the Classroom: Goals, Evidence, and Outcomes — 213
   *Marc Marschark and ChongMin Lee*

10. Improving Reading Instruction to Deaf and Hard-of-Hearing Students — 242
    *Loes Wauters and Annet de Klerk*

11. Quality of Instruction in Bilingual Schools for Deaf Children: Through the Children's Eyes and the Camera's Lens — 272
    *Daan Hermans, Loes Wauters, Annet de Klerk, and Harry Knoors*

12. Shifting Contexts and Practices in Sign Bilingual Education in Northern Europe: Implications for Professional Development and Training — 292
    *Ruth Swanwick, Ola Hendar, Jesper Dammeyer, Ann-Elise Kristoffersen, Jackie Salter, and Eva Simonsen*

## Part Three: Bilingual Education in Co-enrollment Settings

13. Language Development of Deaf Children in a Sign Bilingual and Co-enrollment Environment — 313
    *Gladys Tang, Scholastica Lam, and Kun-man Chris Yiu*

14. Social Integration of Deaf and Hard-of-Hearing Students in a Sign Bilingual and Co-enrollment Environment — 342
    *Kun-man Chris Yiu and Gladys Tang*

15. Sign Bilingual and Co-enrollment Education for Children with Cochlear Implants in Madrid, Spain — 368
    *Mar Pérez Martin, Marian Valmaseda Balanzategui, and Gary Morgan*

16. The Twinschool: A Co-enrollment Program in the Netherlands — 396
    *Daan Hermans, Annet de Klerk, Loes Wauters, and Harry Knoors*

17. Co-enrollment in the United States: A Critical Analysis of Benefits and Challenges — 424
    *Shirin Antia and Kelly K. Metz*

**Epilogue**

**18. Perspectives on Bilingualism and Bilingual
    Education for Deaf Learners** 445
*Marc Marschark, Harry Knoors, and Gladys Tang*

**Index** 477

# Preface

At the 2010 International Congress on the Education of the Deaf (ICED), an appeal was made for the return of sign language and Deaf teachers in educating deaf children. The resolution, "A New Era: Deaf Participation and Collaboration," was offered by the ICED 2010 Organizing Committee and the British Columbia Deaf Community in response to accumulating evidence generated by research on signed languages since the 1960s. In fact, even before this global appeal and despite the predominance of oral education in 1970s and 1980s, many countries in Europe, as well as the United States and Australia, already had attempted to incorporate sign language into the education of deaf children in both special and regular school settings.

The surge of interest in bilingual education may be perceived as a reaction against frustrations about the not so impressive outcomes of the oral-only approach in educating and raising many deaf children for decades. Treating sign language as a first language, this bilingual education approach assumes that a stronger first language will support deaf children's acquisition of a written/spoken language, especially with regard to literacy, thus supporting academic attainment more broadly. Other parts of the world have not kept pace with this development. Research on sign language did not reach Asia, for example, until early 1990s, and hence oral education has remained the dominant mode of deaf education in both special and regular settings. Recently, however, there was the establishment of a sign bilingual school for the deaf in Japan (Meisei Gakuen School for the Deaf, 2008) and independent sign bilingual programs in special settings in China (e.g., SigAm Bilingual Education Project for Deaf Children, 2004–2013; UNICEF's Sign Bilingual Program, Tianjin, 2001–2009) and Hong Kong (The Jockey Club Sign Bilingualism and Co-enrollment in Deaf Education Program, 2006). From the perspective of the historical development of bilingual education for the deaf, different countries in the world thus are riding on the concept at different stages of development.

Since its inception, bilingual education in special settings has faced challenges. The language of instruction and communication in the special setting has been a major area of contention. Today, depending on the program, the language of classroom instruction can range from a natural signed language to sign-supported speech to artificial signed communication systems; and use of the vernacular may or may not involve speech. This phenomenon reflects the continuing concerns over the efficacy of language alternatives in educating deaf students. Understandably, parents and educators are looking for evidence indicating that deaf children who are educated bilingually (or via any other method) can eventually perform on par with hearing peers linguistically, cognitively, social-emotionally, and academically. However, with evidence for the bilingual approach being limited, with hearing technology having improved in recent decades, and with the shift in deaf education philosophy from segregation to inclusion, a gradual reduction of bilingual programs in special settings appears imminent.

Trapped in this shifting context of deaf education, experience suggests that reverting to purely oral education for deaf children will not address the large individual differences resulting from the heterogeneity in student characteristics and their diverse backgrounds. One alternative to a reversion to monolingual deaf education is the recent incorporation of sign language into regular school settings within the general rubric of co-enrollment. This new concept of deaf education emerged in response to the call for equal opportunities for accessing the regular curriculum through any language, signed or spoken, and efforts to combine the best qualities of mainstream and special education for deaf and hard-of-hearing (DHH) children.

No one involved in the education of deaf children would disagree that bilingual education is in a constant state of flux, sometimes driven by research findings, sometimes by perceived educational need, and at other times by practical innovations that await verification of their efficacy. If parents, teachers, and schools are to be asked to consider bilingual education, however, we believe that such programs must be constructed on the basis of evidence-based practices, supported by research. We therefore believe that it is high time that we take a broad perspective on the research findings relating to bilingual education and co-enrollment—hence this book.

As different countries in the world have had different paces of developing bilingual education, related empirical findings and evidence from classrooms have been disseminated in diverse settings and publications (or not). We believe it is important for such evidence to be collected and to be made available for reference to those countries, localities, and schools that are considering joining the bilingual movement, so that they can be informed of its latest developments and can choose a mode that best suits their cultural, ideological, and practical needs. In creating this volume to work toward that goal, it is important that the contributors have described a variety of new interdisciplinary studies, ranging from neuro-cognitive aspects of bilingualism and bilingual acquisition to the effects of social-emotional functioning on academic achievement. All of these will enrich the knowledge base of bilingual education. Informed decision-making is necessary when parents or educators are faced with options for educating and raising deaf children, and we offer this volume as a step in supporting all stakeholders involved in deaf education.

As the Table of Contents of this volume reveals, the first section offers discussions about some broader issues of bilingualism with respect to language and linguistics as well as psychosocial development. There are chapters reporting on bilingual acquisition, bimodal bilingual processing, and the neurobiology of bimodal bilingualism. Other chapters focus on relationships between sign language and reading comprehension, as well as sign language and spoken language development of children with cochlear implants. The second section concentrates on educational issues and, specifically, the shifting contexts of the history and philosophy of bilingual education, the effects of using sign languages and spoken language on DHH students' academic outcomes, the quality of instruction in bilingual education, and reading instruction in a bilingual classroom. The last section reports on the evidence with regard to co-enrollment programming for deaf students within regular school settings, a relatively new development in deaf education that has been gaining prominence. Issues discussed with regard to co-enrollment include DHH students' spoken and sign language outcomes, cognitive functioning, and academic attainments, as well as social integration of DHH and hearing students educated within co-enrollment settings.

As bilingual education remains controversial, readers should expect to encounter diverse expectations and research findings in this volume. It is unrealistic at this stage of development to arrive at strong conclusions about bilingual education or to promote a particular form of bilingual education. What we hope to achieve with this volume is to provide readers with sufficient information to be able to place bilingual education in the context of the larger research literature with regard to sign language linguistics, bimodal-bilingual language acquisition, the neuropsychology and psycholinguistics of sign bilingual processing, bilingualism in the context of advanced hearing technologies, and educational philosophy and practice. Such knowledge is necessary not only for informed decision-making but also to help point the way toward modifications in bilingual education or modes of communication that potentially benefit all DHH students and help them to achieve their full potentials.

Gladys Tang, Hong Kong<br>
Harry Knoors, Sint-Michielsgestel, The Netherlands<br>
Marc Marschark, Rochester, New York

# Contributors

**Shirin Antia**
Department of Disability & Psychoeducational Studies
College of Education
University of Arizona
Tucson, Arizona

**Marian Valmaseda Balanzategui**
Equipo Específico de Discapacidad Auditiva
Madrid, Spain

**Alexandre Castro-Caldas**
Institute of Health Sciences
Portuguese Catholic University
Lisboa, Portugal

**Maria Cristina Caselli**
Institute of Cognitive Sciences and Technologies
Italian National Research Council
Rome, Italy

**Jesper Dammeyer**
Department of Psychology
University of Copenhagen
Copenhagen, Denmark

**Johannes Fellinger**
Institut für Sinnes- und Sprachneurologie
Konventhospital Barmherzige Brüder
Linz, Austria

**Annet de Klerk**
Royal Dutch Kentalis
Kentalis Talent
Vught, The Netherlands

**Marcel Giezen**
Laboratory for Language and Cognitive Neuroscience
San Diego State University
San Diego, California

**Ola Hendar**
Department of Psychology
University of Copenhagen
Copenhagen, Denmark

**Daan Hermans**
Royal Dutch Kentalis
Kentalis Academy
Sint-Michielsgestel, The Netherlands

**Manfred Hintermair**
Institut für Sonderpädagogik
Pädagogische Hochschule Heidelberg
Heidelberg, Germany

**Daniel Holzinger**
Institut für Sinnes- und Sprachneurologie
Konventhospital Barmherzige Brüder
Linz, Austria

**Harry Knoors**
Royal Dutch Kentalis
Kentalis Academy
Sint-Michielsgestel, The Netherlands

**Ann-Elise Kristoffersen**
The National Support System for Special Needs Education (Statped)
Oslo, Norway

**Scholastica Lam**
Centre for Sign Linguistics and Deaf Studies
Department of Linguistics and Modern Languages
Chinese University of Hong Kong
Shatin, Hong Kong

**ChongMin Lee**
Center for Education Research Partnerships
National Technical Institute for the Deaf
Rochester Institute of Technology
Rochester, New York

**Marc Marschark**
Center for Education Research Partnerships
National Technical Institute for the Deaf
Rochester Institute of Technology
Rochester, New York

**Kelly K. Metz**
Deptartment of Disability & Psychoeducational Studies
College of Education
University of Arizona
Tucson, Arizona

**Ana Mineiro**
Institute of Health Sciences
Portuguese Catholic University
Lisboa, Portugal

**Gary Morgan**
Deafness, Cognition and Language Research Centre
City University London
London, United Kingdom

**Mar Pérez Martin**
Equipo Específico de Discapacidad Auditiva
Madrid, Spain

**Mara Moita**
Institute of Health Sciences
Portuguese Catholic University
Lisboa, Portugal

**Maria Vânia Silva Nunes**
Institute of Health Sciences
Portuguese Catholic University
Lisboa, Portugal

**Daniela Onofrio**
Institute of Cognitive Sciences and Technologies
Italian National Research Council
Rome, Italy

**Ellen Ormel**
Centre for Language Studies
Department of Linguistics
Radboud University Nijmegen
Nijmegen, The Netherlands

**Carolina Plaza-Pust**
Johann Wolfgang Goethe-Universitaet
Fachbereich Neuere Philologien
Institut für Linguistik
Frankfurt, Germany

**Pasquale Rinaldi**
Institute of Cognitive Sciences and Technologies
Italian National Research Council
Rome, Italy

**Sónia Silva**
Institute of Health Sciences
Portuguese Catholic University
Lisboa, Portugal

**Jackie Salter**
School of Education
University of Leeds
Leeds, United Kingdom

**Eva Simonsen**
The National Support System for Special Needs Education (Statped)
Oslo, Norway

**Ruth Swanwick**
School of Education
University of Leeds
Leeds, United Kingdom

**Gladys Tang**
Centre for Sign Linguistics and Deaf Studies
Department of Linguistics and Modern Languages
Chinese University of Hong Kong
Shatin, Hong Kong

**J. Bruce Tomblin**
Department of Communication Sciences and Disorders
University of Iowa
Iowa City, Iowa

**Virginia Volterra**
Institute of Cognitive Sciences and Technologies
Italian National Research Council
Rome, Italy

**Elizabeth A. Walker**
Department of Communication Sciences and Disorders
University of Iowa
Iowa City, Iowa

**Loes Wauters**
Royal Dutch Kentalis
Kentalis Academy
Sint-Michielsgestel, The Netherlands

**Kun-man Chris Yiu**
Centre for Sign Linguistics and Deaf Studies
Department of Linguistics and Modern Languages
Chinese University of Hong Kong
Shatin, Hong Kong

# 1

# Bilingualism and Bilingual Deaf Education

## *Time to Take Stock*

Harry Knoors, Gladys Tang, and Marc Marschark

Many people in the Deaf community view the 1980s and 1990s as the golden years of deaf education. In that period, linguistic and psychological research into sign language structures, sign language acquisition, and sign language processing in the brain provided the impetus for including sign language in the classroom, whereas previously it had been used mainly in the dormitories and in playgrounds of schools for the deaf, often secretly. Admittedly, this movement had already started in Sweden and Denmark in the 1970s, but it was initially limited to a few small-scale experimental projects. Later, sign bilingual programming gained momentum in countries like the United Kingdom, the United States, Australia, the Netherlands and, more recently, in Spain, Brazil, China, Hong Kong, Taiwan, Japan, Vietnam, and many other countries. Despite these efforts, sign bilingual programming in special settings seems to be on the decline. In some Scandinavian countries, all of the schools for the deaf have closed; in others, only very few sign bilingual programs remain (see Swanwick, Hendar, Dammeyer, Kristoffersen, Salter, & Simonsen, Chapter 12 of this volume). In England in 2012, only 8% of all deaf children were said to use sign language in one form or the other (CRIDE, 2012), and O'Neill and Marschark (2013) found that even among 15- to 27-year-olds, only 15% preferred British Sign Language (BSL) as their primary mode of communication; 75% preferred speech only (8% chose a combination of two).

    The implementation of bilingual deaf education has always been controversial. The lack of firm empirical evidence has made it very difficult to evaluate critically its value in educating deaf students. Since its decline could eventually mean disappearance, it is time to take stock of the development of bilingual deaf education to its present state and to examine how much or in what aspects of deaf education sign language facilitates deaf students in their linguistic, cognitive, and social-emotional development. The synthesis based on current research findings discussed in this volume will enable readers to make suggestions for future directions in deaf education in general and bilingual deaf education in particular.

## CONTEXT AND PHILOSOPHY

The emergence of sign linguistics as a subdiscipline of linguistic research in the 1960s triggered a growing, and continuing, interest in examining the role of natural sign language in raising and educating deaf children. At a broader level, the bilingualism of deaf students in today's society is one that involves the acquisition and use of both a signed language, as a minority language, and at the same time a majority spoken language in its written form and, depending on the country and the students involved, in its spoken or even signed form (Grosjean, 2010). Under these circumstances, students are perceived as bilingual and bicultural; they are thought to capitalize on these facilities in interacting with both worlds. This assumption has encouraged the further development of sign bilingual programming in deaf education over the past three decades.

Bilingual deaf education may be conceptualized in different ways. On one hand, it can be seen as one of various educational options for deaf students, emphasizing the use of both sign language and written (and sometimes spoken) language for educational purposes, because advocates claim that using an accessible, visual language is the way to unlock the curriculum for deaf students (Johnson, Liddell, & Erting, 1989; Knoors & Fortgens, 1995; Marschark, 1993). On the other hand, it is also part of the value system of culturally Deaf people and at least some hearing parents and professionals. In their view, the use of sign language in society in general and education in particular is considered a human right and part of the ultimate "Deaf way" to societal participation (e.g., Skutnabb-Kangas, 1994). As a consequence of this distinction, the goals that one hopes to achieve through bilingual deaf education may differ somewhat—a difference that is certainly reflected in the various bilingual programs around the world (many of which are described in this volume) as well as attempts to evaluate the viability of those programs.

If one opts primarily for the objective of unlocking the curriculum for deaf students, goals would typically focus on students' access to language and to the content of curriculum. These rather instrumental goals typically include promoting first (sign) language acquisition, increasing literacy and numeracy skills, and stimulating cognitive and social skills. An important characteristic of these goals is that they can be evaluated by empirical research. On the other hand, if one conceives of sign language, Deaf culture, and bilingual deaf education as basic elements of the Deaf way of life and sign language use as a human right, evaluation becomes part of a philosophical debate centering on norms and values, and is more related to ethics and morality. This is a rather different form of evaluation, one much less grounded in an empirical research tradition, although an evaluation that involves, for example, looking at quality of life might come close.

In real practice, both of the above conceptions of bilingual education are often intertwined. In discussions about its efficacy and effectiveness, however, the perspective that centers on access to language and curriculum generally dominates. This is the result of various factors. First of all, the prevalent paradigm of evidence-based education ultimately requires evidence by thorough empirical research. Second, since most parents of deaf children are hearing, alien at first to the Deaf community, Deaf culture, and sign language, ethics-related or moral arguments often do not convince them to raise their deaf child bilingually. Instead, real or assumed research evidence is brought into play. In this volume as well, the empirical approach dominates. That is not because we wish to exclude moral and ethical reasoning, but because we believe that, in the end, it is empirical results that will have the greater influence on decision-making about educational options in general and bilingual deaf education in particular.

## FOUNDATIONS

Without sign language research there would be no bilingual deaf education. Emphasizing the importance of linguistic research into signed languages for the subsequent promotion of bilingual deaf education does not mean, however, that other factors did not play an important role. General thoughts about bilingualism and bilingual education, empowerment of Deaf people, and disappointment about the results of exclusively "oral" education all had their share. Nor does the importance of sign language research for the establishment of bilingual deaf education mean that there were no attempts to use sign language in school in earlier years, but they were relatively few and certainly were not within the context of an international movement to make deaf education bilingual.

### Sign Language Research

It was William C. Stokoe who, in the early 1960s, first showed that sign languages such as American Sign Language (ASL) are real languages (e.g., Stokoe, 1960/2005). This triggered the attention of other linguists and psychologists, who began to study various aspects of sign languages, first in the United States, but soon after in the Scandinavian countries and later in various European, Asian, and African countries. These studies revealed the structural richness of sign languages. They brought us insights into the phonological, morphological, syntactic, and pragmatic aspects of sign languages. In general, the architecture of spoken and signed languages in terms of levels of organization is basically the same (Bellugi & Fischer, 1972), but modality differences lead to differences, for example, in the degree of sequential versus simultaneous ordering of lexical elements.

Eventually, research brought to light the existence of many sign languages around the world, including their lexical and grammatical characteristics (see e.g., Wilbur, 1987 for ASL; Kyle & Woll, 1988, for BSL; Baker, Van den Bogaerde, Pfau, & Schermer, 2008, for Sign Language of the Netherlands, SLN; Johnston & Schembri, 2007, for Australian Sign Language, Auslan; and Tang & Yang, 2007, for Hong Kong Sign Language, HKSL). Native acquisition of sign languages by deaf or hearing children of deaf parents proceeds along remarkably similar biological milestones as spoken language acquisition (Lillo-Martin, Koulidobrova, Müller de Quadros, & Chen, 2012; Meier & Newport, 1985; Morgan, Herman, Barriere, & Woll, 2008; Morgan & Woll, 2002; see also Rinaldi, Caselli, Onofrio, & Volterra, Chapter 3 of this volume). Further, processing sign languages in the brain taps basically the same cortical and subcortical areas as spoken languages, provided sign language has been acquired as a native language. This is not to say that modality differences in language do not influence brain organization and functioning, but they do so only to a relatively minor extent (Emmorey, 2002; see also Mineiro, Nunes, Moita, Silva, & Castro-Caldas, Chapter 8 of this volume).

So, the question soon became, given these remarkable parallels in structure, acquisition, and processing, why not use sign language in deaf education?

## Bilingualism and Bilingual Education

For quite some time, scholars were convinced that growing up with two or more languages was harmful for children unless they were very bright (Carrow, 1957). Research in the 1960s and 1970s originating in Canada showed that high scores on intelligence tests were not a requirement for successful bilingual upbringing, but rather a consequence of it (Peal & Lambert, 1962; see also Marschark & Lee, Chapter 9 of this volume). Cognitive advantages, that is, verbal cognitive flexibility, could be the result of being bilingual, provided the conditions at home and in school enabled proficiency in both languages and the transfer of proficiency. It was Cummins who formulated a theory about the interdependence between language proficiency in bilingual learners, summarized in his linguistic interdependence hypothesis: "To the extent that instruction in Lx is effective in promoting proficiency in Lx, transfer of this proficiency to Ly will occur provided there is adequate exposure to Ly (either in school or environment) and adequate motivation to learn Ly" (Cummins, 1981, p. 29).

This hypothesis thus not only states that language proficiency can transfer across languages in bilingual language learners, but also that this only takes place under specific conditions. Cummins's dual iceberg metaphor points to another important aspect of transfer: two languages share, underwater so to speak, a common cognitive academic language proficiency (CALP), but above the water line, the basic interpersonal communication skills (BICS) in the two languages are separate.

Cummins's theory was adopted in many countries, giving way to both transitional and maintenance types of bilingual education, incorporating both majority and minority languages and cultures. Migration in the 1960s and 1970s provided fertile ground for this development, since people came to realize that growing up bilingually was in fact the norm for many children in the world and that acknowledging the minority languages and cultures of immigrants might contribute to their economic and societal participation. In many Western countries there was also a growing appreciation of cultural and linguistic diversity, no doubt one of the spin-offs from the hippie youth culture of the 1960s. Cummins's theory, however, was often misinterpreted, even in the spoken language literature, failing to acknowledge the specific conditions for transfer and the fact that transfer was assumed to be limited to specific aspects of languages. In practice, Cummins's theoretical framework was often taken to mean that learning a second language would automatically, thus without additional efforts, profit from acquiring a first one (see Holzinger & Fellinger, Chapter 5 of this volume).

### Deaf People as a Cultural and Linguistic Minority

In the aftermath of the movement for emancipation of African Americans in the United States and the feminist movement in various Western countries, the emancipation of people with disabilities gained momentum in the Disability Rights Movement. The social theory of disability (e.g., Oliver, 1986) is one reflection of this movement, arguing that society needs to depart from the personal tragedy and medical perspectives on disability and move to a perspective that views disability as a social construct in society. Some deaf people moved this view even further, agreeing with supporters of the social theory on disability that deafness should not be viewed from a minority perspective, but even denying that it is a disability at all. Rather, building on insights from linguistic research into sign languages, deaf people should "regard themselves as a linguistic minority instead of a disability group, as they become more aware of their own mental and physical capacities. They will gradually become more concerned about the preservation and development of their own language. In the future, in every country, I believe, deaf people will be recognized as a cultural variation, instead of a pathological group" (Anderson, 1994, p. 10; see also Lane, 1992; Parasnis, 1998).

Beginning sometime in the 1970s, "deaf" sometimes was written with a capital D, as "Deaf," to indicate membership in this linguistic and cultural community (Woodward, 1972). This view was and is advocated—to various degrees—in many countries. It is reflected in the struggle to have Deaf people appointed in relevant leadership positions (e.g., the Deaf President Now movement, advocating for a Deaf president for Gallaudet University) and in more successful (e.g., Sweden, Finland) and less successful (e.g., the Netherlands) attempts to have sign languages legally recognized by governments. Deaf culture and membership in the Deaf community is celebrated in many ways (e.g., World Deaf Day, the Deaflympics, sign language theater and poetry). Perhaps most impressive were the international Deaf Way conferences in 1989 and 2002 at Gallaudet University in Washington, D.C.

The view of Deaf people as a linguistic and cultural minority group may also be expressed through opposition to any development that is seen to harm the position of Deaf people and their sign languages— for example, cochlear implants and genetic testing (Bauman & Murray, 2010). Sometimes such a view has been fueled by expressions like "genocide of the Deaf community" or "communicative abuse of Deaf children," because these developments can be seen as examples of medical views of deafness or of audism, the real or supposed tendency to view hearing and speaking as superior to watching and signing. Others have expressed their support for the position that Deaf people constitute a linguistic and cultural minority in milder ways, sometimes even allowing for a mixed view, seeing Deaf people as a linguistic minority but at the same time also as people with a disability, at least in a world dominated by hearing people.

## Results of Oral Deaf Education

The fact that bilingual deaf education became an appealing concept not only to Deaf adults but also to many hearing parents and hearing teachers in deaf education no doubt was also fueled by disappointment about the results of "oral" deaf education, involving only spoken and written language. This disappointment grew in the 1960s and rose even further after the publication of the seminal work by Robert Conrad in 1979, *The Deaf Schoolchild: Language and Cognitive Functioning*. Conrad's nationwide study in the United Kingdom made clear that many orally educated deaf children left their school with extremely low reading levels, despite many years of education and a normal learning potential. Parents and teachers began to acknowledge that oral programs failed to educate many deaf children adequately (Bergmann, 1994, p. 84). A renewed interest in manual communication was first reflected in the adoption of the Total Communication philosophy during the 1970s (see Marschark, Knoors & Tang, Chapter 18 of this volume). Soon, however, the idea arose—although it was not well supported by research, to say the least—that Total Communication did not result in any significant improvement of literacy levels of deaf children either. The call for bilingual deaf education was out.

Sweden was first to adopt this new concept. At the end of the 1970s and in the early 1980s, deaf education in that country changed from predominantly oral to bilingual. According to one of its most prominent supporters in the early years, the linguist Inger Ahlgren (1994), "One important impetus for this change was a small research project carried out by two deaf colleagues and myself between 1975 and 1979. The main question for that project can, in retrospect, be formulated as: Could sign language be a first language or mother tongue for deaf children with hearing parents in a way similar to how it works for deaf children with deaf parents?" (p. 55). Ahlgren reported that they studied four families with young deaf children, varying in age between 8 months and 20 months at first contact. Two families had deaf parents, two had hearing parents. After a relatively modest intervention that included two one-week courses of sign language instruction within a one-year period and meetings between hearing parents, their deaf children, and deaf adults every six weeks for half a day (a total of 240 hours of sign language exposure for the deaf children with hearing parents), Ahlgren and her colleagues concluded from videotaped evaluations that the sign language acquisition of both deaf children with hearing parents progressed very fast and that they reached an age-adequate level of proficiency. "That both these children reached an age-adequate level of language development with this relatively meagre exposure sheds light on the strong capacity for language acquisition that humans are born with" (Ahlgren, 1994, p. 60).

The promises of age-adequate language levels, of major increases in literacy levels, and of considerable improvement in social and emotional functioning, compared to oral only or Total Communication programs (Barnum, 1984; Bouvet, 1990; Mahshie, 1995), became driving forces behind the initiation of bilingual deaf education in more European countries, in several schools for the deaf in the United Kingdom, the United States, and Australia and to a varying extent in other countries around the globe. According to Livingston (1997), deaf students should be taught in the same way as hearing students, and to accomplish this both ASL and English need to coexist in the classroom.

## OBJECTIVES AND PROGRAMMING

Most bilingual deaf programs have as their main objective the promotion of first language acquisition and learning through the provision of the accessible sign language. A second objective of many programs is that incorporation of sign language, Deaf culture, and deaf professionals in education will enhance deaf children's social and emotional development in general and their identity development in particular. A third objective of many, but not all, programs is improvement of proficiency in the second (i.e., majority or vernacular) language through reading and writing, building on a sign language base. And, finally, the promotion of academic achievement is one of the objectives of bilingual programs.

Thus a common feature of bilingual deaf programs is that they build on the acquisition of sign language. In fact, within schools and programs for deaf students, the use of sign language in social interactions has long been reported, partly due to the presence of deaf children born to deaf parents who serve as sign language models for linguistic input within the school community. Because of its accessibility, it seems natural that this language is seen as the first or dominant language of deaf children, even if they are born into hearing families. The spoken/written language of their parents thus is seen as a second language. At this point, the similarities between bilingual programs stop and diversity starts. Some of the diversity relates to the point in time at which the second language is used in education (from the start or later), the modality in which this second language is offered (written only or also spoken), and the amount of input and instruction in both languages (the second language as a subject or in use during 50% of the time).

Many of the original bilingual programs in Scandinavian countries opted for a successive model of bilingual education, establishing a firm base in sign language in the first 5 to 6 years of life and having deaf children learn the country's majority language, mainly in its written form, after the age of 6. This approach was motivated by the assumption that spoken language is not accessible for deaf children. Svartholm (1994, p. 64), for example, stated, "That speech and lip-reading are unsuitable as vehicles for full communication is clear; otherwise oral education should have had a better outcome in general. The fragments perceived by the child via vision and the auditory sense, if any, can simply not be said to represent language to the child." According to Svartholm, following earlier views of Inger Ahlgren, learning a second language from print is possible through comparisons and contrastive explanations of differences and similarities between signed and written language, but requires so much cognitive effort that it cannot be expected from children under 6 years of age.

Others have opted for a different form of bilingual programming, providing input of the second language not only in written but also in spoken language from the start of education onward (e.g., Pickersgill, 1998). So, instead of successive bilingual education, parallel bilingual education is advocated, sometimes emphasizing that both languages should be equally represented in the input. This equality of the languages in bilingual education is the case for co-enrollment programming, as discussed in several chapters in this volume, and also in schools for the deaf, particularly in countries where speech and spoken language training is considered a standard rehabilitation procedure for deaf children from early childhood. In the case of the Netherlands, for example, Knoors and Fortgens (1995) opted for a different model, because they considered it important that deaf children will learn the language that dominates Dutch society, so spoken Dutch, to the largest extent possible. Although in learning Dutch the written form ultimately will be very important, Knoors and Fortgens considered it appropriate to offer deaf toddlers an input of spoken Dutch, often with speech supporting signs. They did so, not only because there saw many objections to very early introduction of large amounts of written language, but also they wanted to avoid every risk that late input of spoken language may hinder mental processing because some cortical brain areas have lost their function.

## SCHOOL SETTING

For interpersonal transfer of language, a community of language users is necessary. In the case of sign languages, this community is constituted only to a limited extent by families of native sign language users, that is, Deaf parents and their deaf and hearing offspring. Because over 95% of deaf children are born into hearing families, schools for the deaf in general, and residential schools in particular, have always been at the heart of the transmission of sign language and Deaf culture. It therefore should not come as a surprise that the first bilingual programs for deaf children typically were based in schools for the deaf. Initially, these were residential schools, but with the growth of day schools for the deaf, many of these became bilingual as well. Only later, after educational philosophy began to put more and more emphasis on mainstreaming and, somewhat later, inclusion, did some bilingual programs become based in regular schools. The introduction of sign bilingualism and co-enrollment programs was the result (Kirchner, 1994; Kreimeyer, Crooke, Drye, Egbert, & Klein, 2000; see also, in this volume: Tang, Lam & Yiu, Chapter 13; and Yiu & Tang, Chapter 14; Pérez Martin, Valmaseda Balanzategui, & Morgan, Chapter 15; Hermans, De Klerk, Wauters, & Knoors, Chapter 16; and Antia & Metz, Chapter 17). These programs maintain the important role played by sign language in supporting deaf students' overall development and education. Equally important in the co-enrollment environment, they argue, are the development of spoken language and the students' access to a regular curriculum and a majority community.

## BILINGUAL DEAF EDUCATION: ISSUES AT STAKE

During the early years of bilingual deaf education the foundational assumption, quite simplistically, was that if access to sign language was provided, deaf children would learn on par with their hearing peers (e.g., Marschark, 1993). In fact, very little research evidence has been put forward to indicate that this is the case (Knoors & Marschark, 2012, 2014; Spencer & Marschark, 2010). The implementation of bilingual deaf education thus often took place based on limited, if any, research. Of course, some in the field warned that establishing bilingual deaf education would be quite a challenge (Pickersgill & Gregory, 1998), but in the sheer optimism accompanying the new bilingual concept, these warnings were, if not neglected, simply put aside for the time being. All energy was needed to build the system and to convince teachers, parents, and politicians of the potential benefits of bilingual deaf education. The theoretical foundations of bilingual deaf education were strong, and it was expected that soon evidence would show its benefits.

But reality proved much harder over the past 30-odd years. Bilingual deaf education was challenged in various ways; it even came under pressure within the region of its birth, Scandinavia (see Swanwick, Hendar, Dammeyer, Kristoffersen, Salter, & Simonsen, Chapter 12 of this volume). Various factors played a role in this shift. One, of course, was the advent of cochlear implantation, providing many deaf children with considerably more access to (and possibly the ability to acquire) spoken language than before. In addition, as bilingualism and bilingual education in general were discussed, the theoretical foundations of bilingual deaf education were challenged, and more research about deaf learners became available. And, finally, the relative lack of empirical support for many of the optimistic claims made by advocates of bilingual deaf education became a matter for concern as well (Spencer & Marschark, 2010).

At the same time, many countries, particularly those that had undergone a period of colonization, such as Singapore and Hong Kong, adopted bilingual policies, often in the absence of scientific research into linguistics and language acquisition, but for internal political or educational reasons. To date, this global trend of bilingualism or multilingualism has been supported, as we know now much more about bilingualism than we did a few decades ago. We know now, for instance, that most people in this world live in circumstances where multilingualism is the rule rather than the exception. Research points to distinct cognitive advantages of growing up bilingually, provided that learning conditions are optimal (Bialystok & Craik, 2010). These advantages counterbalance the apparent disadvantage of bilingualism, namely that the proficiency of a bilingual person in each language separately is less than the language proficiency of a monolingual person. Deaf bilinguals seem no exception in these conclusions (see Ormel & Giezen, Chapter 4 of this volume).

One would assume that results from scientific research, added to the acknowledgment that all of us live in a global world, would have led to an increase of bilingual education programs in general, and in some areas this has been the case, for example, in the increase of Dutch-English programs in education in the Netherlands. In some countries, this increase has almost always been limited to "high-status" languages, in which proficiency pays an economic profit. But educational inclusion of minority languages has been far less successful, for example, as reflected in the end of teaching minority languages in primary schools in the Netherlands and the change of the Bilingual Education Act into the English Language Acquisition, Language Enhancement, and Academic Achievement Act in the United States (e.g., Johnson, 2010).

In many Western countries, the growing trend of globalization has been accompanied by a desire for clearly structured educational and social environments emphasizing indigenous national and cultural characteristics. At the same time, the original enthusiasm about appreciating cultural and linguistic diversity in many Western countries has been exchanged for bitter debates about the failure of multicultural society. In this context, it is not easy to argue that appreciating Deaf culture and sign language will pay off for many deaf children and their future children. This is most evident in an era when early cochlear implantation provides considerable progress in access to and proficiency in spoken language and promises even more, rightfully or not.

But the theoretical foundations of bilingual deaf education already had been challenged before this current sociopolitical shift. Specifically, the applicability of Cummins's Linguistic Interdependence model initially was questioned by Mayer and Wells (1996; Mayer & Akamatsu, 1999). The assumption that transfer could occur between a sign language and a written/spoken language was called into question because the conditions in Cummins's interdependency hypothesis—shared foundational proficiencies—could not be fulfilled. At the same time, however, various studies have indicated that sign language proficiency correlates with reading proficiency (e.g., Hermans, Knoors, Ormel, & Verhoeven, 2008; Prinz & Strong, 1998; Strong & Prinz, 1997), suggesting transfer even if Cummins's framework does not apply. Such findings notwithstanding, there are indications that spoken language proficiency correlates more highly than sign language with reading proficiency in bilingual deaf children (Niederberger, 2008) and that transfer between sign and written language may only occur after a certain threshold proficiency in sign language has been reached (Hermans, Ormel & Knoors, 2010; see also Holzinger & Fellinger, Chapter 5 of this volume). Still unclear is whether the cognitive advantages shown to occur in unimodal bilingualism in hearing children and adults translate to hearing and deaf children and adults being or becoming bimodal bilinguals (see Ormel & Giezen, Chapter 4 of this volume; Plaza-Pust, Chapter 2 of this volume).

Coincidentally, the timing of the introduction of pediatric cochlear implantation co-occurred with the enthusiastic and energetic advent of bilingual deaf education in many countries. No wonder that many Deaf and some hearing proponents of bilingual deaf education at first denied or played down the benefits of implantation. Opposition and resistance characterized many of the actions on the bilingualism side, while not acknowledging the benefits of early cochlear implantation for many (though not all) deaf children. Those opponents definitely miscalculated the feelings of most (hearing) parents who were not so much opposed to signing, but wanted their deaf children to hear and speak their family language as well as possible.[1]

From the perspective that Deaf people finally had experienced recognition of their sign languages, Deaf culture, Deaf community, and thus of their Deaf identity, the opposition to medical solutions such as cochlear implantation is understandable. Nevertheless, it certainly was not academically sound to ignore the many positive results from cochlear implantation research or to neglect the perspective of hearing parents of deaf children and the limited evidence for the benefits of bilingual deaf education. Do programs that utilize only spoken language offer deaf children with cochlear implants advantages in language learning and academic achievement over bilingual programs? There are research results that point in that direction, even if the advantages are not large (e.g., Spencer & Marschark, 2010; Walker & Tomblin, Chapter 6 of this volume). However, there are also pitfalls in interpreting many of the relevant studies. Comparability of participant samples is one, because the placement of deaf students in oral versus bilingual programs is not randomized, but rather is characterized by selection bias. In reality, deaf children from advantaged backgrounds and with better learning potential have a greater likelihood of ending up in oral programs compared to deaf children from less affluent backgrounds or those with learning problems, who more frequently tend to be placed in sign-oriented (bilingual) programs. Further, in studies comparing the language proficiencies of deaf children in monolingual as compared to bilingual programs, the spoken or written language proficiency of bilingual deaf children usually is compared with that of monolingual hearing children (i.e., rather than bilingual children) in order to justify the effectiveness of oral approaches to deaf education. One may question whether this is a fair comparison.

On the other hand, one needs to admit that one of the major challenges of bilingual deaf education is the creation of a rich bilingual learning environment. The key problem is the fact that most parents and teachers are hearing, and to create such an environment they first have to learn sign language. That this is not an easy task, requiring a tremendous effort from those involved, has been acknowledged by proponents of bilingual deaf education. In reflecting on her observations on bilingual deaf education in Sweden and Denmark, Mahshie (1995, p. 139) wrote: "Although parents seem to learn [sign language] well under these circumstances, I also noticed among parents and professionals a degree of realism—a recognition that these parents are adult learners of a second language who have jobs, lives, and often have other children in addition to their Deaf child. Nevertheless, according to the preschool and first grade teachers I interviewed, a high percentage of parents in these countries DO learn enough of the language of the Deaf community to communicate high-level concepts to their children well before those children enter first grade." Still, one also gets the feeling that the challenge of hearing parents and teachers learning to sign was sometimes underestimated. In Denmark, according to Bergmann (1994), teachers of the deaf were required to devote 510 to 580 hours to learn Danish Sign Language, but a sign language training course of only 170 hours was created for them. We now know from studies of foreign (spoken) language learning that in order to achieve the advanced levels of proficiency necessary to teach in a second language, a minimum of 750 hours is needed for languages such as English, whereas 1,320 to 2,760 hours are needed for languages such as German, Greek, Arabic, Mandarin Chinese, and Malayan (Tschirner, 2005). Often, these advanced levels can only be achieved if learners of a second language live for an extended time in countries where they are immersed in this language. Given that sign languages are so different from spoken languages, it seems reasonable to assume that far more hours in sign language instruction than 170 to 580 are needed in order to have hearing teachers (and parents) achieve advanced levels. Not surprisingly, Mahshie (1995) argued that Deaf teachers are absolutely crucial for the success of any bilingual program. It seems fair to state that of all countries implementing bilingual deaf education, the Scandinavian countries have put most efforts into achieving this goal. Still, Mahshie noted that in Sweden in 1988, only about 40 qualified Deaf teachers worked in educational programs from preschool through university levels. A school like the Manilla school for the deaf in Stockholm succeeded in employing 10 Deaf teachers out of 55, nearly 20%.

The point of this discussion is not to downplay the serious efforts that have been undertaken to provide good sign language models to deaf children and to train hearing parents and teachers accordingly. Rather, the point is that there is every reason to think that the challenges involved in accomplishing this are enormous. And there is no research available yet to show the extent to which such rich bilingual environments actually were successfully created for deaf children (Knoors, 2007; Knoors & Marschark, 2012). Equally disappointing is the relative lack of studies into the quality of instruction in (bilingual) classrooms with deaf students (but see Hermans, Wauters, De Klerk, & Knoors, Chapter 11 of this volume).

Perhaps at the early stages of implementing bilingual deaf education the above issues did not seem too much of a problem; after all, deaf children in these programs were said to achieve far better than they had before, in oral programs. According to Britta Hansen of Denmark (cited in Mahshie, 1995, p. 17), for example, "The reading skills of the children have improved tremendously compared to what we used to see in the education of the Deaf generally. Whereas 10–15% of deaf children used to learn to read for meaning, we now see 55% of them being able to do this at the age of 12. That means 55% read Danish at an age-appropriate level." These results, almost miraculously good, of course raised expectations. Unfortunately, there was no empirical research to substantiate this type of statement, with the notable exception of Heiling (1998; see also Wauters & De Klerk, Chapter 10 of this volume), who obtained findings that she later was unable to replicate (see Bagga-Gupta, 2004).

Bagga-Gupta (2004) sought an explanation for the rise of bilingual deaf education without a solid evidence base in the exemplary political recognition of sign language in Sweden. She concluded that "[at] a time when researchers in other nations in the world were arguing for the acknowledgement of their SL's in their school systems, SSL had been accorded political recognition in Sweden and work to incorporate this into the existent Deaf educational settings was initiated. This perhaps explains why the Swedish bilingual model was seen as an exemplary system by scholars and professionals..." (p. 27).

Knoors (1997, p. 54) was among the first to criticize the lack of empirical research on the effects of bilingual deaf education: "Bilingual education for deaf children [. . .] is simply taken for granted, being seen as an almost miraculous concept in which teaching theorists, teachers, parents, psychologists and linguists simply believe, a concept that will solve all problems in education of the deaf, a concept that does not need to be made fully operational through good research into effects and good practices. It would not be the first time that ideology and emotion have confounded the issues that are really at stake in deaf education."

Only a few studies have tried to evaluate directly the outcomes of bilingual programs for deaf children (see also Marschark & Lee, Chapter 9 of this volume). Nover, Andrews, Baker, Everart, and Bradford (2002) reported reading comprehension scores of deaf students, aged 8–12 years, of one bilingual program in the United States. Although the researchers noted that the scores were significantly above the national norms (medians) for deaf children (Traxler, 2000), in fact the effect is only small, showing modest differences of about 5–25 points, a less than 1% difference. Lange, Lane-Outlaw, Lange and Sherwood (2013) studied sign language proficiency and reading and math achievement in deaf students in a bilingual program in the United States that uses the same language-planning curriculum as in the study by Nover et al. (2002). They compared academic achievement growth among those students with those of hearing students in a norming sample who had comparable initial achievement levels. After four years of bilingual education, reading scores indicated that 41% of the deaf students showed growth scores at or above the level of the comparison group, whereas the percentage for math scores was 55. However, deaf students in the school who were achieving at the lowest levels were excluded from their study (and it is unclear what proportion of students that was).

Large-scale studies in academic achievement and reading comprehension in countries where bilingual deaf education dominates (Sweden, Denmark, the Netherlands) have failed to show significant progress (Coppens, Tellings, Van der Veld, Schreuder, & Verhoeven, 2012; Hendar, 2009; Rydberg, Gellerstedt, & Danermark, 2009; Wauters, Van Bon, & Tellings, 2006). It should therefore come as no surprise that researchers have concluded that bilingual deaf education may have a strong theoretical foundation, but simply lacks empirical evidence (Knoors & Marschark, 2012, 2014; Mayer & Leigh, 2010; Spencer & Marschark, 2010).

Taken together, the combined effects of the positive results of digital hearing aids and cochlear implantation for many deaf children, the lack of empirical evidence for positive results from bilingual deaf education, and the efforts it takes to establish qualitative good bilingual education and bilingual home environments easily lead to a picture in which it makes sense to abandon the once promising concept of bilingual deaf education. Developments in Norway, Sweden, Denmark, and the United Kingdom definitely point in that direction (Swanwick, Hendar, Dammeyer, Kristoffersen, Salter, & Simonsen, Chapter 12 of this volume). The history of deaf education, however, is marked with adopting and abandoning approaches without sufficient evidence, sometimes giving the impression that it is fashion more than reason that controls developments in the field—often to the detriment of deaf children. There are still good reasons to assume that bilingual deaf education is a sound educational option for at least some, and potentially many, deaf children, for enhancing their social-emotional development (see Hintermair, Chapter 7 of this volume; Yiu & Tang, Chapter 14 of this volume). True, the rapid changes in deaf education as a consequence of universal newborn hearing screening, hearing aid technologies, and cochlear implantation may result in more fluid identities of deaf children and adults and in flexible language profiles, instead of distinctly separate first and second languages. But fluid identities and flexible profiles leave considerable space for Deaf culture and sign language to play a significant role, perhaps in more flexible ways than was envisaged in the first few decades of bilingual deaf education (Knoors & Marschark, 2012). Insofar as not all deaf children profit equally from their cochlear implants, to some extent it makes sense to argue that bilingual education can reduce potential harm to deaf children (Humphries et al., 2012). But in order to make that case, the evidence base for the benefits of bilingual deaf education must become stronger.

With the preceding as our backdrop, the primary purpose of this edited volume has been to bring together diverse issues and evidence concerning bilingualism among deaf individuals, examined in the context of language acquisition, bilingual processing, and deaf education. Bilingual deaf education is set in the current conceptions of sign bilingualism and co-enrollment models, examining the effectiveness of incorporating sign language into regular classrooms with pedagogical procedures that will nurture bilingualism and biculturalism in educating not only deaf but also hearing students. It is hoped that the volume will provide readers with a better picture of how these issues might impact areas of linguistic skills, psychological and interpersonal functioning, and related academic and social outcomes of deaf individuals, among others. Ultimately, we expect that this volume at least will establish some shared understandings of what are meant by "bilingualism," "bilingual education," and "co-enrollment programming," and hopefully will chart directions for future research in this broadly defined but all-important area.

## NOTE

[1] The steadily increasing popularity of cochlear implantation for the children of Deaf parents is an interesting story as well, but one better told by others.

## REFERENCES

Ahlgren, I. (1994). Sign language as the first language. In I. Ahlgren & K. Hyltenstam (Eds.), *Bilingualism in deaf education* (pp. 55–60). Hamburg, Germany: Signum Verlag.

Anderson, Y. (1994). Deaf people as a linguistic minority. In I. Ahlgren & K. Hyltenstam (Eds.), *Bilingualism in deaf education* (pp. 9–14). Hamburg, Germany: Signum Verlag.

Bagga-Gupta, S. (2004). *Literacies and deaf education: A theoretical analysis of the international and Swedish literature*. Forskning i Fokus No. 23. Stockholm, Sweden: The Swedish National Agency for School Improvement.

Baker, A., Van den Bogaerde, B., Pfau, R., & Schermer, T. (2008). *Gebarentaalwetenschap: Een inleiding*. [Sign language studies: An introduction]. Deventer, Netherlands: Van Tricht.

Barnum, M. (1984). In support of bilingual/bicultural education for deaf children. *American Annals of the Deaf, 129*(5), 404–408.

Bauman, H-D. L., & Murray, J. J. (2010). Deaf studies in the 21st century: "Deaf-gain" and the future of human diversity. In M. Marschark & P. E. Spencer (Eds.), *The Oxford handbook of deaf studies, language, and education* (vol. 2, pp. 210–225). New York, NY: Oxford University Press.

Bellugi, U., & Fischer, S. (1972). A comparison of sign language and spoken language. *Cognition, 1*, 173–200.

Bergmann, R. (1994). Teaching sign language as a mother tongue in the education of deaf children in Denmark. In I. Ahlgren & K. Hyltenstam (Eds.), *Bilingualism in deaf education* (pp. 83–90). Hamburg, Germany: Signum Verlag.

Bialystok, E., & Craik, F. I. M. (2010). Cognitive and linguistic processing in the bilingual mind. *Current Directions in Psychological Science, 19*, 19–23.

Bouvet, D. (1990). *The path to language: Toward bilingual education for deaf children.* Bristol, UK: Multilingual Matters Ltd.

Carrow, S. M. A. (1957). Linguistic functioning of bilingual and monolingual children. *Journal of Speech and Hearing Disorders, 22*(3), 371–380.

Coppens, K., Tellings, A., van der Veld, W., Schreuder, R., & Verhoeven, L. (2012). Vocabulary development in children with hearing loss: The role of child, family, and educational variables. *Research in Developmental Disabilities, 33*, 119–128.

CRIDE (2012). CRIDE report on 2012 survey on educational provision for deaf children in England. Consortium for Research into Deaf Education. Retrieved on April 21, 2013, from www.ndcs.org.uk/professional_support/national_data/uk_education_.html

Cummins, J. (1981). *Bilingualism and minority language children.* Ontario, Canada: Ontario Institute for Studies in Education.

Emmorey, K. (2002). *Language, cognition, and the brain: Insights from sign language research.* Mahwah, NJ: Lawrence Erlbaum Associates.

Grosjean, François (2010). Bilingualism, biculturalism, and deafness. *International Journal of Bilingual Education and Bilingualism, 13*(2), 133–145.

Heiling, K. (1998). Bilingual vs. oral education. In A. Weisel (Ed.), *Issues unresolved: New perspectives on language and deaf education* (pp. 141–147). Washington, DC: Gallaudet University Press.

Hendar, O. (2009). *Goal fulfillment in school for the deaf and hearing impaired.* Härnösand, Sweden: National Agency for Special Needs Education and Schools.

Hermans, D., Knoors, H., Ormel, E., & Verhoeven, L. (2008). The relationship between the reading and signing skills of deaf children in bilingual education programs. *Journal of Deaf Studies and Deaf Education, 13*, 518–530.

Hermans, D., Ormel, E., & Knoors, H. (2010). On the relation between the signing and reading skills of deaf bilinguals. *International Journal of Bilingual Education and Bilingualism, 13*, 187–199.

Humphries, T., Kushalnagar, P., Mathur, G., Napoli, D. J., Padden, C., Rathmann, C., & Smith, C. R. (2012). Language acquisition for deaf children: Reducing the harms of zero tolerance to the use of alternative approaches. *Harm Reduction Journal, 2012*, 9–16.

Johnson, D. C. (2010). The relationship between applied linguistic research and language policy for bilingual education. *Applied Linguistics, 31*(1), 72–93.

Johnson, R. E., Liddell, S. K., & Erting, C. J. (1989). *Unlocking the curriculum: Principles for achieving access in deaf education.* Washington, DC: Gallaudet University.

Johnston, T., & Schembri, A. (2007). *Australian Sign Language: An introduction to sign language linguistics.* Cambridge, UK: Cambridge University Press.

Kirchner, C. J. (1994). Co-enrollment as an inclusion model. *American Annals of the Deaf, 139*, 163–164.

Knoors, H. (1997). Book review, "Bilingualism in deaf education, edited by Inger Ahlgren and Kenneth Hyltenstam." *Deafness and Education International 21*(3), 53–54.

Knoors, H. (2007). Educational responses to varying objectives of parents of deaf children: A Dutch perspective. *Journal of Deaf Studies and Deaf Education, 12,* 243–253.

Knoors, H., & Fortgens, C. (1995). Het Rotterdams tweetaligheidsproject: Twee talen voor dove kleuters. [The Rotterdam bilingual project: Two languages for deaf toddlers]. *Van Horen Zeggen, 35*(1), 4–11.

Knoors, H., & Marschark, M. (2012). Language planning for the 21st century: Revisiting bilingual language policy for deaf children. *Journal of Deaf Studies and Deaf Education, 17,* 291–305.

Knoors, H., & Marschark, M. (2012). *Teaching deaf learners: Psychological and developmental foundations.* New York, NY: Oxford University Press.

Kreimeyer, K. H., Crooke, P., Drye, C., Egbert, V., & Klein, B. (2000). Academic and social benefits of a co-enrollment model of inclusive education for deaf and hard-of-hearing children. *Journal of Deaf Studies and Deaf Education, 5,* 174–185.

Kyle, J. G., & Woll, B. (1988). *Sign Language: The study of deaf people and their language.* Cambridge, UK: Cambridge University Press.

Lane, H. L. (1992). *The mask of benevolence: Disabling the deaf community.* New York, NY: Knopf.

Lange, C. M., Lane-Outlaw, S., Lange, W. E., & Sherwood, D. L. (2013). American Sign Language/English bilingual model: A longitudinal study of academic growth. *Journal of Deaf Studies and Deaf Education, 18,* 532–544.

Lillo-Martin, D., Koulidobrova, H., Müller de Quadros, R., Chen Pichler, D. (2012). Bilingual language synthesis: Evidence from WH-questions in bimodal bilinguals. In Biller, A.K., Chung, E.Y., Kimball, A. E. (Eds.), *Proceedings of the 36th Annual Boston University Conference on Language Development* (pp. 302–314). Somerville, MA: Cascadilla Press.

Livingston, S. (1997). *Rethinking the education of deaf students: Theory and practice from a teacher's perspective.* Portsmouth, NH: Heinemann.

Marschark, M. (1993). *Psychological development of deaf children.* New York, NY: Oxford University Press.

Mahshie, S. N. (1995). *Educating deaf children bilingually: With insights and applications from Sweden and Denmark.* Washington, DC: Gallaudet University Press.

Mayer, C., & Wells, G. (1996). Can the linguistic interdependence theory support a bilingual-bicultural model of literacy education for deaf students? *Journal of Deaf Studies and Deaf Education, 1,* 93–107.

Mayer, C., & Akamatsu, C. (1999). Bilingual-bicultural models of literacy education for deaf students: Considering the claims. *Journal of Deaf Studies and Deaf Education, 4*(1), 1–8.

Mayer, C., & Leigh, G. (2010). The changing context for sign bilingual education programs: Issues in language and the development of literacy. *International Journal of Bilingual Education and Bilingualism, 13*(2), 175–186.

Morgan, G., & Woll, B. (Eds.) (2002). *Directions in sign language acquisition.* Amsterdam, Netherlands: John Benjamins.

Morgan, G., Herman, R., Barriere, I. & Woll, B. (2008). The onset and mastery of spatial language in children acquiring British Sign Language. *Cognitive Development, 23,* 1–9.

Newport, E. L., & Meier, R. P. (1985). The acquisition of American Sign Language. In D. I. Slobin (Ed.), *The cross linguistic study of language acquisition, Vol. 1: The data* (pp. 881–938). Hillsdale, NJ: Lawrence Erlbaum Associates.

Niederberger, N. (2008). Does the knowledge of a natural sign language facilitate deaf children's learning to read and write? Insights from French Sign Language and written French data. In C. P. Plaza-Pust & E. M. López, (Eds.), *Sign bilingualism: Language development, interaction and maintenance in sign language contact situations* (pp. 51–72). Amsterdam, Netherlands: John Benjamins.

Nover, S., Andrews, J., Baker, S., Everhart, V., & Bradford, M. (2002). *ASL/English bilingual instruction for deaf students: Evaluation and impact study*. Final report 1997–2002. Retrieved April 2, 2013, from http://www.gallaudet.edu/Documents/year5.pdf.

Oliver, M. (1986). Social policy and disability: Some theoretical issues. *Disability, Handicap & Society, 1*(1), 5–17.

O'Neill, R. & Marschark, M. (2013). Evaluating the views of deaf young people on their school experience and transition to adult life. Nuffield Foundation Project Report. Retrieved on September 19, 2013, from http://www.blendedlearning.me/DASS/site/.

Parasnis, I. (Ed.). (1998). *Cultural and language diversity and the deaf experience*. Cambridge, UK: Cambridge University Press.

Peal, E., & Lambert, W. E. (1962). The relation of bilingualism to intelligence. *Psychological Monographs: General and applied, 76*(27), 1–23.

Pickersgill, M. (1998). Bilingualism—current policy and practice. In S. Gregory, P. Knight, W. McCracken, S. Powers, & L. Watson (Eds.), *Issues in deaf education* (pp. 98–97). Oxon, UK: David Fulton Publishers.

Pickersgill M, and Gregory S. (1998). *Sign bilingualism: A model*. Wembley, UK: LASER.

Prinz, P. M., & Strong, M. (1998). ASL proficiency and English literacy within a bilingual deaf education model of instruction. *Topics in Language Disorders, 18*(4), 47–60.

Rydberg, E., Gellerstedt, L. C., & Danermark, B. (2009). Toward an equal level of educational attainment between deaf and hearing people in Sweden? *Journal of Deaf Studies and Deaf Education, 14*, 312–323.

Svartholm, K. (1994). Second language learning in the deaf. In I. Ahlgren & K. Hyltenstam (Eds.), *Bilingualism in deaf education* (pp. 61–70). Hamburg, Germany: Signum Verlag.

Skutnabb-Kangas, T. (1994). Linguistic human rights: A prerequisite for bilingualism. In I. Ahlgren & K. Hyltenstam (Eds.), *Bilingualism in deaf education* (pp. 139–159). Hamburg, Germany: Signum Verlag.

Spencer, P. E., & Marschark, M. (2010). *Evidence-based practice in educating deaf and hard-of-hearing students*. New York, NY: Oxford University Press.

Stokoe, W. C. (1960/2005). Sign language structure: An outline of the visual communication system of the American deaf. *Studies in Linguistics, Occasional Papers 8*. Buffalo, NY: Department of Anthropology and Linguistics, University of Buffalo. Reprinted in *Journal of Deaf Studies and Deaf Education, 10*, 3–37.

Strong, M., & Prinz, P. (1997). A study of the relationship between American Sign Language and English literacy. *Journal of Deaf Studies and Deaf Education, 2*, 37–46.

Tang, G., & Yang, G. (2007). Events of motion and causation in Hong Kong Sign Language. *Lingua, 117*(7), 1216–1257.

Traxler, C. (2000). The Stanford Achievement Test, 9th Edition: National norming and performance standards for deaf and hard-of-hearing students. *Journal of Deaf Studies and Deaf Education, 5*, 337–348.

Tschirner, E. (2005). Das ACTFL OPI und der Europäische Referenzrahmen. *Babylonia 2*, 50–55.

Wauters, L. N., Van Bon, W. H. J., & Tellings, A. E. J. M. (2006). Reading comprehension of Dutch deaf children. *Reading and Writing, 19*, 49–76.

Wilbur, R. B. (1987). *American Sign Language: Linguistic and applied dimensions.* New York, NY: Little, Brown.

Woodward, J. (1972). Implications for Sociolinguistic Research among the Deaf. *Sign Language Studies, 1*(1), 1–7.

# Part One

## Linguistic, Cognitive, and Social Foundations

# 2

# Language Development and Language Interaction in Sign Bilingual Language Acquisition

Carolina Plaza-Pust

Bilingual language acquisition in deaf learners offers a rich field of research into the complex interrelation of external and internal factors that shape the outcomes of language contact situations. Bilingualism involving a sign language and an oral language (henceforth *sign bilingualism*) is neither territorially determined nor does it typically emerge as a result of migration or a specific family language policy related to the linguistic background of deaf individuals. For the majority of deaf children not born to signing parents, the path to bilingualism depends on appropriate supportive measures.

Sign bilingual education programs implemented as of the late twentieth century in several countries have opened a new perspective in research on language acquisition in deaf learners, hitherto determined by a pathological view of deafness that regarded language development in this population as an idiosyncratic phenomenon. Padden (1998, p. 103), for example, emphasized the relevance of viewing "language acquisition as the development of interacting systems, each of which has specific social uses." This view not only implies that sign bilinguals marshal their linguistic resources in their everyday lives (p. 100), but also that sign bilingual learners will skillfully exploit their linguistic competences in the course of their bilingual development. Bilingual deaf learners are exposed to a variety of languages and codes, including sign language, spoken language, written language, signed systems, and fingerspelling. How do they react to this diversity in their environments? What does their linguistic behavior reveal about their bilingual language development?

In recent years, scholars have sought to obtain a better understanding of the impact of bilingualism on language development in deaf learners. A review of the available literature makes apparent that research on bilingual deaf learners has been conducted from various theoretical perspectives. From an educational linguistics perspective, for example, scholars have been concerned with language skills attained by bilingual deaf learners in order to determine whether bilingual education benefits deaf students. In particular, they have sought to obtain further insights into the nature of the relationship between the two languages in the light of Cummins's interdependence hypothesis (1981) in order to determine whether the promotion of sign language as a first language (L1) has a facilitating effect on the attainment of literacy skills in the oral language as a second language (L2) (see Holzinger & Fellinger, Chapter 5 of this volume; Tang, Lam, & Yiu, Chapter 13 of this volume).

Other researchers have looked at bilingual deaf learners' bilingual language acquisition in the light of current hypotheses in the field of developmental linguistics. Given the specific circumstances that determine exposure to and access of the two languages in this particular type of bilingualism, scholars have been concerned with critical period effects deriving from a delay in the exposure to a fully accessible first language. Further, they have sought to identify commonalities and differences between bilingual deaf learners and other types of learners (Ormel & Giezen, Chapter 4 of this volume). Finally, the role of language contact phenomena in the course of bilingual development has not only been investigated in relation to developing language systems but also in relation to the pragmatic skills developed by deaf learners as bilingual communicators.

A review of the available literature also reveals that different types of measures have been used to assess bilingual deaf learners' language knowledge in the domains of the lexicon, morphosyntax, and discourse. Different types of data have been collected in longitudinal and cross-sectional studies, ranging from spontaneous data to data elicited in standardized tests.

Another issue concerns the population investigated. Unlike in research on hearing children's bilingual development, longitudinal studies of family bilingualism continue to be rare. This comes as no surprise given the sociolinguistic situation of deaf learners, for whom the family is rarely the socializing unit for their bilingualism. By contrast, several cohorts of bilingually educated deaf students, most of them children of hearing non-signing parents, have been investigated in the context of research concomitant to bilingual education programs.

Taken on the whole, the studies undertaken provide important insights into the bilingualism of deaf learners. To date, however, there is a lack of convergence of the different lines of research sketched previously. The ongoing debate in a field that is marked by the fundamental question of whether or not bilingualism benefits deaf learners underscores the relevance of integrating the knowledge that can be gleaned from the available research about the development of deaf children and youth as bilingual language learners and bilingual communicators. The present chapter aims to contribute to this endeavor by providing a critical appraisal of the main hypotheses put forward and the main findings obtained regarding language development and language interaction in sign bilingual language acquisition. The chapter is divided into three main sections. The first section, dedicated to the research conducted in the light of the interdependence hypothesis, is followed by a section in which the main findings obtained about bilingual language acquisition in deaf learners are discussed. The third section focuses on language contact phenomena. The chapter closes with a section summarizing the relevance of the research undertaken and highlighting some of the main challenges that must be confronted in future research.

## SIGN BILINGUALISM AND THE INTERDEPENDENCE HYPOTHESIS

Commonly, the assumption that deaf students benefit from a promotion of L1 sign language in the educational context is elaborated along the lines of Cummins's (1979) interdependence hypothesis, originally developed in relation to linguistic minority students. Cummins's hypothesis targets functional distinctions in language use and the relevance of their mastery for academic achievement in acquisition situations in which the home language (L1) differs from the language used in school (L2). While children confronted with features of literary discourse at home can be assumed to profit from the knowledge attained at home for their mastery of literacy-related tasks in school, when such an "alignment" is not given, compensatory measures need to be taken.

Following Cummins's hypothesis, L1 teaching will be necessary to foster an adequate development of academic language while children progressively acquire their L2. With respect to the acquisition of academic skills in the latter, the assumption is that children can draw on the knowledge developed in their L1, as academic skills in the L1 and the L2, unlike conversational skills, are assumed to develop interdependently and to make up what is referred to as the "common underlying proficiency" (Cummins, 1981, p. 24). According to Cummins (1991, p. 86), correlations between L1 and L2 academic language skills "reflect underlying cognitive attributes of the individual that manifest themselves in both languages."

The interdependence hypothesis has been widely used for the justification of a bilingual approach in the education of deaf students. Basically, it is argued that because the role of the spoken language is limited in the linguistic and academic development of deaf children, sign language promotion as a base or primary language is fundamental for their cognitive and communicative development, even though it is seldom the home language for these children (Kuntze, 1998; Strong & Prinz, 2000). Another difference between the acquisition scenarios of deaf and hearing children pertains to the circumstance that sign languages have no written form that would be used in literacy-related activities. Because of this circumstance, some authors argue that sign language cannot facilitate the acquisition of L2 literacy. As Mayer and Leigh (2010, p. 181) put it, "there are not specific text-based proficiencies to transfer from a signed L1 to a spoken L2."

Other scholars, by contrast, have argued that the positive correlations of spoken/written language and sign language skills documented for ASL-English (Hoffmeister, 2000; Strong & Prinz, 2000) and other language pairs (Dubuisson, Parisot, & Vercaingne-Ménard, 2008, for Quebec Sign Language [LSQ]-French; Niederberger, 2008, for French Sign Language [LSF]-French) provide support for the assumption that good performances in both languages are linked. As for the specific sign language skills that might be associated with literacy skills, some authors claim that interaction mainly operates at the level of story grammar and other narrative skills (Wilbur, 2000). Other researchers, in contrast, maintain that the interaction involves specific linguistic skills manifested in the comprehension and production of sign language and written language (Chamberlain & Mayberry, 2000; Hoffmeister, 2000; Strong & Prinz, 2000). In their studies, higher correlations were obtained between narrative comprehension and production levels in ASL and English reading and writing levels than between ASL morphosyntactic measures and English reading and writing. Niederberger (2008) reports a significant correlation of global scores in LSF and French and observes that correlations between narrative skills in both languages were higher than those relating to morphosyntactic skills. Additionally, sign language comprehension skills were found to be highly correlated with French writing skills. Sign language production skills, in turn, highly correlated with French reading skills. Given that LSF narrative skills also correlated with French morphosyntactic skills, Niederberger concluded that the interaction of both languages involves more than global narrative skills.

Dubuisson and colleagues' (2008) study shows a relationship between improvement in children's use of spatial markers in LSQ (taken as an indicator of global proficiency in LSQ) and their ability to infer information when reading French. With respect to global ability in the use of space in LSQ and global reading comprehension, the authors report a highly significant correlation in the first year of the study. More specifically, a correlation was found between the ability to assign loci in LSQ and the ability to infer information in reading. In a two-year follow-up, they observe a correlation between locus assignment in LSQ and locating information expressed in the text in reading, and global LSQ scores and locating information in reading.

The results obtained indicating positive correlations of sign language and oral language skills have been used to argue that "deaf children benefit from early exposure to a natural sign language for their literacy development" (Niederberger, 2008, p. 45). However, as has been pointed out by some scholars, correlations documented do not provide any direct information about a causal relationship between skills attained in the two languages (Marschark & Lee, Chapter 9 of this volume; Plaza-Pust & Morales-López, 2008). As remarked upon by Verhoeven (1994, p. 388), "[a] correlation only indicates a relationship between two variables without providing information about the causal direction, if any." Moreover, some of the relations identified remain unaccounted for at a theoretical level, in particular, those that concern grammatical properties of the languages and higher level processes involved in reading and writing.

Mayer and Leigh (2010, p. 177) went a step further in their critique by calling into question the "applicability of the linguistic interdependence theory to the situation of deaf learners, particularly as it pertains to the development of language and text-based literacy." Mayer and Leigh's critique rests on the assumption that deaf learners cannot attain the oral language through interactions with print only. They go on to argue that deaf learners cannot reach a sufficient level of L2 proficiency ("threshold level" in Cummins's terms) "necessary [. . .] for mediating the L2 literacy learning process" (2010, p. 181). As a way out of the dilemma, they speculate on the benefit of the simultaneous use of signs and speech "as a viable option for providing access to a primary form of the L2" (Mayer & Leigh, 2010, p. 181). Although the authors refer to the contact language used in the Deaf community (so-called contact signing), what they have in mind (a simultaneous use of all elements in both modalities of expression) is rather reminiscent of the artificial type of mode mixing developed in the tradition of Total Communication (TC) programs. Interestingly, Mayer and Leigh's argumentation does not only disregard that the lack of success of TC programs was one of the factors that led to a reorientation in the field of education and the implementation of bilingual programs (for detailed discussions, see Plaza-Pust, in press; Spencer & Tomblin, 2006; among others). What is also overlooked is that bimodal communication is commonly used in many bilingual education programs not only as a tool in the teaching of the oral language, but also as a means to secure communication between the hearing teacher and the deaf students (Plaza-Pust, 2004).

Mayer and Leigh (2010, p. 177) do not question the interdependence model as such, but rather its applicability "in a context that involves signed and spoken language where learners do not have access to the target L2 as it is typically used." From a developmental perspective, however, the use of this model to explain the linguistic behavior of bilingual learners must be called into question. Cummins's hypothesis about the relevance of the promotion of the L1 and the related demand of bilingual education needs to be understood in the context of a controversy about whether compensatory measures for linguistic minority students should involve the promotion of the L1 at all (Paradis, Genesee, & Crago, 2011). Cummins's hypothesis has the merit of drawing attention to the circumstance that learning content matter while learning the language is to the disadvantage of the learners. However, the interdependence model is mistaken where it implies that successful bilingual education is bound to an additive type of bilingualism (Romaine, 1996; cf. also Tang, Lam, & Yiu, Chapter 13 of this volume, for a discussion).

Cummins's model is by no means a comprehensive model of bilingual language development. Neither does it account for how multilingual knowledge is organized. Whether languages develop separately or in an interconnected manner in bilingual language acquisition can only be determined on the basis of a sound theory of language. Different levels of linguistic analysis need to be distinguished in order to identify the dimensions of interaction in the organization of multilingual knowledge. Language used for academic purposes does not constitute a monolithic skill, but rather involves the choice of particular registers, syntactic structures, and discursive means, all of which are specific to a given language. These language-specific characteristics must all be learned (Gogolin, 2009; Paradis et al., 2011; Schleppengrell & O'Hallaron, 2011). Hence, it comes as no surprise that the development of literacy skills represents a protracted development, even in L1 acquisition.

What the preceding observations make apparent is that educational models of bilingualism involve a global picture of the linguistic and educational needs of bilingual learners. Consequently, global measures of linguistic ability conducted in this tradition aim at maximum scope (Pienemann & Keßler, 2007, p. 263). The goal is to provide a global assessment of the level of linguistic proficiency attained. Global notions of proficiency, as remarked upon by Pienemann and Keßler (2007, p. 266), represent constructs that are fundamentally different from "the construct of developing linguistic systems used in language acquisition research."

From a developmental linguistics perspective, scholars are interested in obtaining further insights into the evolution of learner systems by looking at developmental trajectories in either language and the role of language contact in the development of multilingual competence. The following sections are dedicated to a summary of the main hypotheses put forward and empirical findings obtained about bilingual language development in deaf learners.

### Bilingual Language Acquisition in Deaf Learners

Over the last decades, bilingualism research has sought to contribute to a better understanding of the organization of multilingual competence.

Issues that have been addressed concern the impact of bilingualism on the development of the languages involved. Apart from the question of whether developmental trajectories are similar to those observed in monolingual language acquisition, scholars have been concerned with the potential interaction of the languages attained in the course of bilingual development.

In bilingualism research on hearing learners, the age of exposure is commonly used as a criterion to distinguish three different types of acquisition situations: bilingual first language acquisition (learners are exposed to two languages from birth), child second language acquisition (learners are exposed to a second language (L2) after age 3), and adult second language acquisition (learners are exposed to an L2 in adolescence/adulthood) (Paradis et al., 2011). Based on this differentiation, researchers have sought to obtain further insights into the impact of age and previously available language knowledge on language development. Implicit to the differentiation of acquisition scenarios is the attribution of the status of first language (L1) to the language(s) acquired from birth, whereby full access to the language(s) is assumed.

Turning to bilingual deaf learners, a review of the available literature makes apparent that *accessibility* is commonly considered the defining criterion of the language assigned the L1 label, that is, sign language (Grosjean, 2008; Leuninger, 2000; Plaza-Pust, 2008; among others), even though the oral language in its spoken form might be the first language they are exposed to (particularly in the case of children of non-signing parents). Because deaf learners have no or only limited access to the spoken language used in their environment, it is generally assumed that they learn it effectively in its written form as a second language (L2) only at a later age (in school).

For the majority of deaf children born to hearing non-signing parents, however, the age of exposure to sign language seldom occurs from birth. Whether and when they are exposed to the language depends on multiple factors, including parents' choices about language, medical advice, early intervention, and the availability of sign bilingual education programs (Plaza-Pust, 2004).

## Critical Period Effects

Variation in the age of exposure to a fully accessible L1 marks a crucial difference between deaf bilingual learners and hearing bilingual learners for whom exposure to the L2 majority language might vary, but for whom exposure to a fully accessible L1 from birth can be taken for granted. Consequently, questions concerning the impact of bilingualism on deaf children's language development are intimately tied to the more fundamental issue of "[h]ow early linguistic experience affect[s] the trajectory of language acquisition over the life span" (Mayberry, 2007).

The results obtained in several studies undertaken by Mayberry and her colleagues (see Mayberry, 2007, for a summary) point to the relevance of the age factor (age of exposure) in sign bilingualism. Crucially, a lack of fully accessible language during the sensitive period for language acquisition affects deaf learners' L1 and L2 competences.

In the studies conducted by Mayberry and colleagues, L2 learners of English who differed in their age of exposure to L1 were found to perform equally well on measures of their syntactic L2 knowledge when their age of exposure to the L2 was the same and their exposure to L1 had occurred early on, irrespective of the modality of expression of the L1. However, the performance of those learners who had no exposure to an accessible first language early on was found to be poorer, and at near-chance level for complex syntactic structures, which can be taken as an indication of the relevance of accessible input during the sensitive period for language acquisition (Mayberry & Lock, 2003).

In addition, the available research indicates that late learners of L1 sign language (at age 5–10 years) may not ever become fully fluent in the language. Based on the evidence obtained, Mayberry (2007, p. 537) concluded that "the effects of age of L1 acquisition on both L1 and L2 outcome are apparent across levels of linguistic structure, namely, syntax, phonology, and the lexicon." Hence, there is a fundamental sense in which "L1 and L2 acquisition are clearly interdependent" (Mayberry 2007, p. 543).

**Sign Language Development**

Sign language development has been primarily investigated in native learners of the language. Although these learners grow up in a situation of intense language contact, their bilingualism has seldom been taken into consideration in studies that focus on their acquisition of sign language. However, the insights obtained into sign language development in this population are of relevance for an appropriate evaluation of sign language acquisition in bilingual deaf learners born to non-signing parents, who are typically exposed to the language at a later age.

The developmental trajectories of L1 sign language and L1 spoken language have been found to be similar in that after the transition from the babbling stage to the one-word stage, L1 sign language learners, like L1 spoken language learners, also go through a two-word stage before they produce more complex utterances (Baker et al., 2005). This evidence indicates that "the child's discovery of the units and rules of grammar is an abstract process that transcends sensory-motor modality" (Mayberry & Squires, 2006, p. 291).

Recent research also has provided further insights into specific challenges faced by sign language learners related to typological characteristics of languages that use the visuo-gestural modality of expression, and whose organization is characterized by a high degree of simultaneity. Crucially, the research undertaken indicates that full mastery of the linguistic use of sign space is the result of a prolonged learning process. This is reflected in the protracted development documented for grammatical phenomena that involve the syntax-discourse interface. A characteristic feature of sign languages is the association of referents with a specific location (locus) in the sign space, a process referred to as *referential establishment* (Bellugi et al., 1990). Loci picked out by pronouns or agreement verbs encode information at the levels of syntax and discourse. The modulation of agreement verbs, for example, expresses person and number features shared between the verb and its arguments. This information is relevant at the level of morphosyntax. Picking out the same loci, in turn, is used to mark referential identity. This information is relevant at the level of discourse.

The appropriate use of agreement verbs, spatial verbs, and classifier constructions involves a consistent and contrastive use of referential loci to indicate referential identity in discourse. Studies on both ASL and BSL conclude that it takes several years before learners fully master these linguistic devices and the pragmatic constraints on their appropriate usage in discourse (cf. Lillo-Martin, 1999; Mayberry & Squires, 2006; Morgan, 2006; Slobin, 2008). For example, agreement verbs have been found to appear first in their citation form, at times in combination with overt lexical arguments. While learners mark agreement verbs for present and non-present referents only several months later (Hänel, 2005; Lillo-Martin, 1999), it takes them several years before they use referential loci consistently. Earlier, they fail to distinguish different loci for different referents or do not use the same loci for the same referents. These errors reflect remaining shortcomings at the level of discourse (Plaza-Pust, in press).

Turning to bilingually educated deaf learners born to hearing non-signing parents, little is known about the early stages of sign language development in this population, and whether their development is characterized by the milestones identified for native learners of the language. Typically, the studies undertaken involve students attending bilingual programs at a later age. In general, the results obtained corroborate the findings sketched previously for native learners of the language (Niederberger, 2004; Plaza-Pust, in press; Tuller, Blondel, & Niederberger, 2007; Vercaingne-Ménard et al., 2001).

In a cross-sectional study, Niederberger (2004) investigated the morphosyntactic and narrative skills of bilingually (LSF-French) educated deaf children in the French-speaking part of Switzerland (39 participants, age 8–17 years) on the basis of the TELSF (Test de LSF). The study focused on the comprehension and the production of classifier constructions and narratives. The appropriate use of classifier constructions was found to be subject to a high degree of individual variation (Niederberger, 2004; Tuller et al., 2007, p. 361). At the narrative level, participants were found to introduce characters appropriately, whereas they did not yet fully master reference maintenance. Tuller and colleagues (2007, p. 362) remark on the protracted development in these areas and relate it to the learning situation of these children who are exposed to non-native input at home and later in school. On a critical note, however, assumptions about a developmental delay remain tentative where no comparative native learner data are available, as is the case of LSF (and many other sign languages).

Further insights into sign language competences of bilingual deaf learners were obtained by Plaza-Pust (in press) in the context of a longitudinal investigation of the acquisition of DGS (*Deutsche Gebärdensprache*, German Sign Language) and German in deaf students attending the bilingual education program established at a deaf school in Berlin (the main findings about written language acquisition are discussed later in this chapter). The participants of the study (n = 6) were all children of hearing parents. Their age of exposure to DGS ranged from 2 to 4 years. All had attended a preschool at which DGS was used as a vehicular language. The students' age at the beginning of the bilingual program (first year primary school) ranged from 6 to 7 years.

Signed narratives were elicited on the basis of the picture storybook *Frog, Where Are You?* (Mayer, 1969). Diagnostic criteria used in the qualitative analysis of the data collected were defined on the basis of a descriptive framework of DGS and a working proposal about the main developmental milestones in the acquisition of the language. The descriptive framework of DGS elaborated within the theoretical framework of the generative paradigm was based on the available literature about the morphological and syntactic characteristics of DGS (Hänel, 2005; Happ & Vorköper, 2006). The working proposal about the acquisition of DGS was elaborated on the basis of the structure-building hypothesis (Fritzenschaft et al., 1991, for child L1 acquisition; Siebert-Ott, 2011, for child L2 acquisition; Plaza-Pust, 2000, and Vainikka & Young-Scholten, 1996, for adult L2 acquisition). This hypothesis maintains that learners expand their learner grammars progressively. The gradual expansion of the available structure is assumed to be the result of a complex interplay between language-specific knowledge and the information available in the linguistic environment. Grammatical processes, such as verb agreement, become operative once the syntactic structures they are associated with are in place. The working proposal about the main developmental milestones in the acquisition of DGS was based on the findings obtained by Hänel (2005) in a study of the acquisition of agreement verbs in two deaf children of native DGS signers, and a critical review of the major findings documented in the literature about the main developmental milestones in the acquisition of other sign languages.

The participants, who were of a rather advanced age at the onset of the study (age 8–10 years), were found to have full competence of the target syntactic structure. Grammatical processes such as verb inflection, the signaling and marking of referential shift, subordination and question formation were found to be operative. While all participants had a command of the target structure, the analyses of the data revealed that they differed regarding their command of discourse constraints on the use of linguistic devices, including referential loci, reference forms, and spatial relations. While some learners use linguistic devices at a local, sentential level, other learners pay attention to a consistent use of linguistic devices for the purpose of creating cohesion and coherence. The different strategies used by two participants in the study, Muhammed and Hamida, to mark reference in the retelling of the frog story is illustrative of the individual variation observed.

Muhammed's examples in 1–3 illustrate the consistent use of loci to mark referential identity.[1] The locus established via $DET_{LOK}$ in 1 is picked out by the agreement verb SEH ("see") and $DET_{EXISTENZ}$ in 2, and also by the classifier verb NEHM ("take") in 3.

(1) VIELLEICHT   FROSCH   $[DET_{LOK}]_E$         (Muhammed, file 1)
    perhaps         frog        there
    "Perhaps the frog is there."

(2) DANN SEH$_1$: $[DET_{EXISTENZ}]_E$  FROSCH   (Muhammed, file 1)
    then   see      there-is           frog
    "Then (he) sees there is a frog."

(3) DANN   $[NEHM_{CL:\mu}]_1$                    (Muhammed, file 1)
    then    take
    "Then (he = the boy) takes the frog."

Muhammed uses referential loci not only consistently but also contrastively, so that reference to different characters is unambiguously marked throughout the narrative. His consistent and contrastive use of referential loci contrasts with Hamida's use of the sign space. Hamida marks shifted referential frameworks (SRFs), which she uses fairly frequently, non-manually via a change in body orientation and eye gaze direction. In sign language linguistics the notion of *referential framework* is used to designate the set of referential loci used in a particular discourse situation (Bellugi et al., 1990, p. 18). Two types of referential frameworks are distinguished: (a) the *fixed* referential framework (FRF) and (b) the *shifted* referential framework (SRF) (Morgan 2006). In a narrative, FRFs are commonly used to express the narrator's perspective, while SRFs are used to express the character's perspective.

Hamida clearly distinguishes FRFs from SRFs via non-manual marking; however, she does not pick out referential loci contrastively (in fact, the loci were all picked out in the space in front of her), with the effect that different protagonists are associated with the same locus. Narrative passages in Hamida's narrative are difficult to understand, in particular, where protagonists are not introduced or are reintroduced via other (lexical) means.

The participants' narratives produced one and a half years after the onset of the study reveal further progress in the command of DGS, not only regarding the appropriate use of linguistic devices involving the syntax-discourse interface, but also concerning the functions that linguistic means might serve. At this stage, participants express temporal and causal relations of story events, they use complex clauses to recount the protagonists' emotions and thoughts, and they demonstrate an advanced mastery of the linguistic use of the sign space for narrative purposes. Examples 4–5, produced by the participant Christa, are provided for further illustration. Through the sequence in 4 the audience learns that the boy and the dog are tired and that they wish to go to bed. In 4-a, the adverbial PLÖTZLICH ("suddenly") constitutes a stylistic means used to highlight the temporal relation between this and previous narrative events. Example 5, in turn, involving a complex construction with the modal verb KANN ("can"), which is in turn selected by the verb REALISIER ("realize"), provides information on the dog's reflection about his situation after having stuck his head into the jar.

(4) a. PLÖTZLICH    BEIDE    MÜDE              (Christa, file 3)
       *suddenly*      *both*   *tired*
       "Suddenly (they) are both tired."
    b. WUNSCH:    BETT    SCHLAFEN
       *wish*       *bed*    *sleep*
       "(They) wish to go to bed, sleep."
(5) HUND    REALISIER:    KANN$_{NEG}$    GUT    SEH    (Christa, file 3)
    *dog*    *realise*      *cannot*        *good*  *see*
    "The dog realizes he can't see well."

The findings obtained by Plaza-Pust regarding a protracted development of the use of linguistic devices needed to mark cohesion are in line with other studies focusing on the development of story grammar and narrative discourse in sign language (cf. Vercaingne-Ménard, Godard, & Labelle, 2001, for a study of narrative production in LSQ in deaf children of hearing parents, and Becker, 2009, for a study of narrative productions of deaf learners with different degrees of proficiency in DGS). However, sign language competence in bilingually educated deaf students has seldom been subjected to qualitative analyses that would provide a detailed picture of the structural knowledge attained by learners in this acquisition situation. The theoretically founded approach elaborated in Plaza-Pust (in press) allows for the scrutiny of empirical data with a view to determining what it really means to have a command of the grammatical properties of a language and to track down the origin of potentially remaining gaps. An analysis along these lines is required where the evaluation of deaf learners' bilingual language acquisition is at stake. Crucially, the scope of a potential developmental asynchrony between both languages can only be determined with precision where the competences attained in both languages are analyzed with equal scrutiny.

**Written Language Development**

Deaf learners exposed to sign language from birth or in early childhood approach the task of learning the oral language in a bilingual acquisition situation. What is the impact of bilingualism on their acquisition of the language of the environment? A review of the available literature makes apparent that the ongoing debate about this central issue is not only determined by different views about the relation between L2 written language and L1 sign language. The ongoing controversy is also marked by the more fundamental question of how deaf learners, monolingual and bilingual, attain the written language with limited or no access to speech.

*Attaining the Writing System*

Two main views can be distinguished with respect to the impact of hearing loss on written language acquisition. Some scholars argue that the written language can be directly acquired by bilingual deaf children as an L2 (Günther, 2003; Leuninger, 2000; Mayberry, 2007; Plaza-Pust, 2008; Vercaingne-Ménard, Parisot, & Dubuisson, 2005). Implicit in this hypothesis is the assumption that the two modalities of expression of oral languages—that is, the auditory-oral (spoken language) and the visuo-graphemic (written language)—have an equal status in that neither is more directly related to underlying language knowledge (cf. Neef & Primus, 2001). Consequently, it is argued that deaf learners, for whom the visuo-graphemic modality of the language is fully accessible, can acquire the target grammar directly *via* written language. According to Günther (2003), for example, written language represents an autonomous semiotic system, albeit one that is related to spoken language.

Other scholars have expressed their skepticism regarding this position and have pointed to the cascading effects they assume to follow from a lack of access to the spoken language on the attainment of the written language. Roughly, learners are believed to face problems in learning the notational system, which in turn would affect the language knowledge attained. Further, limitations in the acquisition of the language would go along with difficulties in the learning of content matter, which would be ultimately reflected in a lack of academic achievement.

This line of argumentation rests on the assumption that phonological awareness represents a requisite for a successful attainment of writing systems (in particular, alphabetical systems) (Mayer, 2007; Musselman,

2000). Other authors, by contrast, maintain that the speech-print relation is not unidirectional, and that deaf and hearing learners might take different pathways in the endeavor of attaining the written language. This view is in line with current assumptions about the bidirectional nature of the relationship between written language attainment and phonological awareness, whereby phonological awareness, facilitating early written language acquisition, is further expanded as a result of literacy development (Riches & Genesee, 2006, p. 73). Studies on reading skills in deaf learners indicate that rather than a precursor of literacy, phonological awareness develops as a consequence of learning to read (Kyle & Harris, 2011, p. 291).

The assumption that learners differ with respect to preferred processing routes (phonemic, graphemic, or both) is supported by the observation that deaf and hearing learners differ in the distribution of types of spelling errors in their written productions. Typically, deaf writers' errors involve letter inversions, omissions, or substitutions, rather than errors related to sound-letter correspondences that are characteristic of early hearing learners' productions.

Deaf students attending the Berlin bilingual education program were found to mainly use a graphemic writing strategy in their second year of primary school (Günther & Hennies, 2011). Günther and Hennies (2011, p. 22f.) remark that the participants produced only few word writing errors. The study also included a comparison of the written productions of bilingually educated deaf students with those of hard-of-hearing students enrolled at deaf schools, and written productions of low to moderate hard-of-hearing students mainstreamed with additional support from itinerant teachers for the deaf. The analysis of the errors produced by the hard-of-hearing students enrolled at deaf schools revealed an orientation toward the spoken language. However, the authors remarked that the deviances observed could not only be explained by the use of a phonemic writing strategy, as they often consisted of what the authors refer to as "word ruins" (Günther & Hennies, 2011, p. 36). Because such written forms have no apparent structure, the authors speculated that the auditory perception of these learners is too weak for them to be able to structure words phonemically (ibid.). By contrast, hard-of-hearing students mainstreamed with additional support were found to produce fewer errors, and their deviances were found to be more similar to those observed in hearing students of the same grade.

*Attaining the Target L2 Grammar*

The question of whether developmental trajectories in bilingual deaf learners' attainment of the written language are similar to those documented for learners of the language in other acquisition situations remains largely unexplored. Some authors have remarked on the rule-based character of some errors, which would suggest that they are developmentally constrained (Wilbur, 2000). However, only a few scholars have been concerned with the progress that learners make in their attainment of the written language.

Schäfke (2005) provided the first insights into the attainment of German syntax by deaf students attending the first bilingual education program established in Germany at a deaf school in Hamburg. Although Schäfke's investigation primarily concerned the development of narrative skills, the study also included a part dedicated to the participants' attainment of German sentence structure. All participants (n = 8) had attained DGS and LBG skills before enrollment in the bilingual education program (during early intervention programs and/or at preschool). Schäfke's longitudinal study comprised three samples of written narratives. The first, collected toward the end of primary school, was elicited on the basis of a short picture storybook. The second sample, collected five years later, and the third sample, collected two years after that, were elicited on the basis of two different video clips.

Based on the analysis of the data collected, Schäfke proposed a developmental model of the learners' progressive mastery of the "overall organisation of sentences" (2005, p. 269f.) that comprises four stages: at stage 0, words are strung together without any apparent organizational principle; at stage 1, learners recognize relations between sentence elements that go together; at stage 2, they organize word order in main clauses according to a fixed sentence schema; and at stage 3, they eventually master the structure for subordinated clauses. Schäfke assumed that the attainment of further specific properties of the target grammar, such as the distribution of finite and non-finite verb forms in a sentence (so-called German verb bracket), results from a progressive "fine-tuning" (2005, p. 269), a notion that she adopts from the whole language approach. Basically, the idea is that learners first attain a broad concept of grammatical phenomena (such as the distinction of sentence parts, or the differentiation between main and embedded clauses) before they go on to attain the respective language-specific properties in terms of a progressive fine-tuning.

Schäfke's (2005) study was the first of its kind in Germany to document bilingual deaf learners' acquisition of German sentence structure. However, her descriptive account of the learners' development remains idiosyncratic to the field of language acquisition of deaf students. The developmental model proposed was not based on a theoretically sound description of the target German grammar, nor did it take into consideration what is known about the development of German grammar in other acquisition situations.

With respect to the nature of the learning mechanisms that would underlie deaf learners' acquisition of German, Schäfke's position remains ambivalent. Schäfke acknowledges differences between deaf and hearing learners, in particular, concerning age of exposure and quality of input. However, her uncertainty about whether deaf learners also draw on language-specific learning mechanisms, like hearing learners of the language, is reflected in her considerations about an early promotion of written language. According to the author, the relevance of such measures would have to be emphasized if it turned out that deaf learners, too, draw on language-specific knowledge.

The question about commonalities and differences between bilingual deaf learners' and hearing learners' acquisition of German grammar is addressed in Plaza-Pust's (in press) longitudinal study of bilingual DGS-German deaf learners mentioned previously. That study covered five samples of written narratives collected during the first two years of the longitudinal study (sessions were scheduled every 5–6 months). The written narratives were elicited on the basis of the same picture storybook used for the assessment of the participants' command of DGS (that is, the so-called frog story). The qualitative analysis of the data was based on diagnostic criteria established on the basis of current hypotheses about the structural properties of German developed within the generative paradigm, and the developmental sequence documented in numerous studies on the acquisition of this language in monolingual and bilingual learners.

The main developmental milestones identified in the acquisition of German morphosyntax reflect the progressive expansion of elementary structures (cf. Plaza-Pust, 2008, for a detailed discussion). Learners of German are confronted with several challenges in their acquisition of the target grammar, notably the so-called verb-second constraint, and the verb placement asymmetry that characterizes German word order in main and embedded clauses. In main clauses (cf. example 6), finite verbs obligatorily appear in sentence-second position (hence the notion of V2 constraint), preceded by subjects or non-subjects (for example, adverbs or direct objects). Non-finite elements of the verbal complex, such as participles, infinitives, and separable prefixes, obligatorily appear in sentence-final position, whereby adverbs, negators, and verb complements appear inside the so-called "verb bracket". In complementizer-introduced embedded clauses (cf. example 7), by contrast, the verb appears in sentence-final position.

(6) Den   Hut   kann   die   Frau    nicht   aufsetzen
    *the   hat   can    the   woman   not     on-put*
    "The woman cannot put on the hat."

(7) Ich weiß, dass die Frau   den Hut  nicht   aufgesetzt hat
    *I know that the woman the hat    not     on-put     has*
    "I know that the woman has not put on the hat."

Based on the qualitative analysis of the data, individual profiles were established for each participant. In addition, the data were subjected to quantitative analyses to obtain a better picture of selected phenomena, such as verb inflection and verb placement. The individual developmental profiles that were established document the spectrum of individual variation at the onset of the study. While learners like Simon produce only elementary sentential structures (cf. example 8), Maria stands out as the only learner who has a command of the full sentential structure (cf. example 9). Regarding subsequent progress, the data reveal that the development of the target morphosyntax represents a protracted development for some learners. For one learner, Simon, no progress was observed regarding the expansion of the elementary sentential structure available at the beginning of the study.

(8) Timo    gehen    ein    Loch                          (Simon, file 1)
    *Timo    go        one    hole*
    "Timo goes to the hole."

(9) ... weil    Max    und    Bello    mag    nicht    allei    schlafen.
                                                              (Maria, file 1)
    *... because    Max    and    Bello    like    not    alone    sleep*
    "...because Max and Bello do not like to sleep alone."

A comparison of bilingual deaf learners' productions with those of other learners of German reveals similarities and differences in their attainment of the language. One major difference pertains to early elementary structures produced by the deaf participants in the study and L1 learners of German. The frequent use of a subject-verb-complement (SVX) format by the former contrasts with L1 learners' preference for a sentence-final verb placement. This tendency to place the verb in the final position has been argued to be of advantage in building up the target structure (from right to left), including the different positions in which verbs might appear (Tracy, 2002). Because DGS is a verb-final (SOV) language, the use of the SVX pattern cannot be the result of an influence from this language. This marks a difference from other L2 learners of the language who have been found to initially make use of their L1 SOV pattern (Vainikka & Young-Scholten, 1996). According to Plaza-Pust (2008), the participants' use of the SVX schema is likely to result from teaching practices oriented toward the learning of a basic sentential format (indeed, in personal communications with the author, teachers reported focusing initially on the mastery of a basic SVX pattern). What is overlooked in this practice is that learners who adhere to the SVX pattern are confronted with the task of restructuring their learner grammar in a way that is similar to L2 learners of German with an SVO L1 (e.g., L1 Romance learners), to accommodate the verb bracket, and later verb final placement in embedded clauses. As remarked upon by Plaza-Pust (in press), several errors produced by the participants concerning verb placement corroborate this assumption.

A second major finding of the study concerns the nature of changes in learner grammars. In this respect, commonalities between deaf learners and other learners of German become apparent. Typically, the transition from one stage to the next does not occur instantaneously but rather is characterized by the alternative production of target-like and target-deviant patterns. For example, after the initial use of elementary structures, learners make use of an expanded structure (the so-called inflection phrase) to accommodate constructions with periphrastic and/or separable verb forms. The distribution of finite and non-finite elements reflects the availability of different positions in which verbs might appear (cf. example 10). However, the available structure is not fully exploited, as word order in constructions with lexical verbs continues to be target-deviant (cf. example 11). In particular, adverbs or negators appear before the main verb in these constructions, which indicates that the relevant grammatical processes are not applied. Interestingly, the discrepancy between constructions with periphrastic verb forms and lexical verbs is well documented for adult second language learners of German (Plaza-Pust, 2000).

(10) Jason hat auf Peter geschimpft.          (Fuad, file 4)
*Jason has on Peter told.him.off*
"Jason told Peter off."

(11) Peter schnell läuft weil Bienen sauer auf Peter.
                                              (Fuad, file 4)
*Peter fast runs because bees angry on Peter*
"Peter runs fast because the bees are angry with him."

Variation also occurs with respect to the implementation of the verb second property. Typically, target-deviant V3 constructions alternate with target-like V2 constructions (cf. examples 12–13), before the V2 constraint is applied across the board.

(12) Am Morgen wacht Tim und Tom auf.         (Maria, file 2)
*at.the morning wakes Tim and Tom up*
"In the morning Tim and Tom wake up."

(13) Am Nacht Pia wünscht weg läuft.          (Maria, file 2)
*at.the night Pia wishes away runs*
"In the evening Pia wants to go away."

This variation, too, has been observed in the data of other L2 learners of German. Interestingly, some L1 learners of German have also been found to grapple with the different verb positions available in the German sentence structure (cf. examples 14–16 from Fritzenschaft et al., 1991, p. 89, our translation).

(14) hab ich großen traktor\
*have I big tractor*
"I have a big tractor."

(15) du    hast    eine    schere    dabei\
     *you   have    a       scissors  with-you*
     "You got some scissors with you."
(16) hier   ich    des     mal    holen
     *here  I      that    ptl.   fetch*
     "I (will) get this one here."

According to Plaza-Pust (in press), the evidence obtained indicates that the dynamics that characterize the organization of multilingual knowledge in bilingual deaf learners is similar to the one observed in other types of bilingual learners, although the development of the L2 proceeds at a much lower pace in some of the deaf learners participating in the study. With the exception of one participant, Maria, for whom the command of the L2 German structure was documented at the onset of the study, all other participants were found to be dealing with the attainment of the target L2 sentence structure throughout the time span covered by the study.

Furthermore, the comparison of the developmental profiles established for German and DGS reveals not only that individual variation is more pronounced in the attainment of written German than in the acquisition of DGS. The observation that none of participants but one had accomplished the task of attaining the target German structure by the end of the study, whereas they all had a command of the full DGS structure from the beginning of the investigation, is indicative of the scope of the developmental asymmetry between the two languages in their bilingual development.

### Cross-Modal Language Contact Phenomena

Over the last decades, research on bilingual hearing learners has sought to clarify the role of language contact phenomena in bilingual language development. The dynamics of bilingual communication, including the combinations of elements of both languages (language mixing), has been found to provide valuable insights not only into the competences attained in either language at the grammatical level but also into the pragmatic and discourse skills developed (Lanza, 1997).

### Language Choice

Important insights into the input-output relationship in bilingual language acquisition have been obtained in research dedicated to children's language choice in relation to their interlocutors and the reactions of these to their language choice (de Houwer, 2007; Lanza, 1997). As de Houwer (2007, p. 42) remarked, "[y]oung bilingual children are in general very responsive vis-à-vis the sociolinguistic norms that exist in their environment regarding language choice."

The complexity and intensity of language contact that characterizes interactions of deaf mothers (n = 4) with their deaf and hearing children (n = 6; 3d, 3h) from age 1 to 6 are documented in Baker and Van den Bogaerde's studies (2008). The analysis of the longitudinal data with a focus on rate and types of sign-speech mixes documented different mixing patterns and rates in the deaf mothers' productions in relation to the hearing status of the children. This relation was, in turn, mirrored in the productions of the children. While all children were exposed to a fair amount of simultaneous language mixing (code-blending), the deaf mothers used more NGT with their deaf children, whereas they used more Dutch with the hearing children. The children in turn differ regarding their choice of code-blending and NGT. While the deaf children use predominantly NGT with their mothers, hearing children use code-blending more frequently than the deaf children (although their use of mixing increases over time), and they use more Dutch. These findings are also indicative of the changing dynamics of the sign-speech contact situation in a family environment, determined by the competences of the bilingual learners, which change over time.

**Cross-Modal Language Borrowing**

From a developmental perspective, language contact phenomena have also been found to provide important insights into how bilingual deaf learners creatively pool their linguistic resources in their attainment of the target grammars. Günther (1999) attributed a crucial role to sign language in the bilingual development of deaf learners, not only at the general level of knowledge (general world knowledge, and knowledge about story grammar), but also in the attainment of the L2 written language structure in terms of a structural gap-filling strategy: learners compensate gaps in their written language grammar by borrowing structures from sign language. Günther, Schäfke, Koppitz, and Matthei's (2004) analysis (cf. also Schäfke, 2005) of written productions produced by bilingual students attending the Hamburg program revealed that this type of borrowing is temporarily delimited, as borrowing decreases with the learners' attainment of L2 written German. Further, the longitudinal study revealed that learners differ with respect to whether or not they make use of DGS borrowings. Apart from translations of DGS expressions, the authors mentioned borrowings involving word order (for example, the verb-final order characteristic of DGS, which is ungrammatical in German main clauses), and subject drop.

Günther and colleagues' (2004) study provided only a global picture of language mixing at the grammatical level without further details about the structures affected and how they might relate to the development in the two languages. However, the general assumptions about the learners' creative use of the linguistic resources available to them are well in line with current assumptions in the field of bilingualism research.

A more detailed analysis is provided in Plaza-Pust (2008, in press). She observed that cross-modal language mixing changes over time in the bilingual development of the bilingual DGS-German participants in the longitudinal study introduced previously. Although the incidence of language mixing was found to be low in this study, the analysis of the language contact phenomena identified reveals that language mixing is developmentally constrained. Plaza-Pust further remarked that some candidates of mixing need to be interpreted with caution. The recurrent production of combinations of elements that lack a verb form but have a propositional meaning in the participants' early written productions (cf. example 17) are a case in point. Verb drop in these constructions that would require a copula could be assumed to be the result of a mixing of DGS given that DGS has no copula verbs. However, because similar verbless patterns have been observed also in monolingual and child L2 acquisition of German (cf. example 18 from Tracy, 1991, p. 300, and example 19 from Diehl, Christen, Leuenberger, Pelvat, & Studer, 2000, p. 75), copula drop seems to be a developmentally constrained phenomenon at this stage. What this example makes apparent is that knowledge about learner errors in other acquisition situations avoids jumping to conclusions about the nature of deaf learner errors. Particularly bilingual (deaf and hearing) learners' errors are often too readily interpreted in relation to their bilingualism.

(17) Da    ein    veil    Frosch.                         (Fuad, file 1)
     there  a      many    frog
     "There are many frogs."

(18) da     nase\                                          (Stephanie, 1;10.1)
     there  nose

(19) Das    Wasser    kalt.                                (Caroline C4/5, 4)
     the    water     cold

Other verbless constructions consisting of hypotactic combinations of several sequences with verb drop, such as example 20, which also contains the complementizer *weil* ("because"), mark a difference in verbless constructions produced by L2 and L1 learners, respectively. These examples illustrate how second language learners more advanced in their narrative development than young infants tend to concatenate elementary structures to express complex meanings, despite the remaining gaps in the L2 at the structural and lexical levels. Furthermore, the example also documents how deaf learners of L2 German, like other L2 learners of the language (cf. Klein, 2000), use L2 functional elements (in this case, the conjunction *weil*) despite the lack of the target structural properties associated with these items.

(20) Der    Junge    weg      weil      da       Eule.    (Hamida, file 1)
     the    boy      away     because   there    owl
     "The boy (goes) away because there is an owl."

Other types of language contact phenomena involve relexifications of DGS structural formats (e.g., figure-ground, SOV). Example 21 illustrates the arrangement of elements following the figure-ground principle (deer = "ground", Paul = "figure") whereby the repetition of the full NP referring to the ground (that is, the deer) reflects the learner's lack of the German pronominal system at the time. Example 22 is an example of a loan translation of a DGS proposition. What looks like a random combination of words (lacking a verb, and with a rather unusual placement of a preposition in sentence-final position) turns out to represent an instance of a cross-modal translation of a DGS classifier construction. Meaning units that would be simultaneously expressed in DGS are mapped onto German lexical items that are arranged *sequentially* in German. Crucially, such cross-modal translations involve lexical and structural adaptations of the expressions borrowed, which are determined by the properties of the recipient language (in this case, German) (cf. Winford, 2003, p. 42f., for a discussion of spoken language contact phenomena). Where this type of mixing is produced by a learner of the language, the elements used reflect the lexical and structural means available in the L2.

(21) der ein Hirsch Paul liegen mit Hirsch.    (Muhammed, file 1)
     the  a  deer   Paul  lies   with deer
     "Paul lies on the deer."

(22) Der Hund Glas den Kopfen in.    (Simon, file 3)
     the dog glass the head   in
     "The dog puts his head into a glass."

Finally, example 23 is illustrative of the type of language mixing observed at the time when learners are dealing with the expansion of their early elementary syntactic structure so as to accommodate complex verb constructions and other grammatical phenomena. During this phase there is a remarkable increase of constructions with the preposition *auf* ("on"). The examples illustrate that *auf* is not only correctly used to case mark the object with verbs that subcategorize for this preposition (cf. example 24), but also erroneously with verbs that do not (cf. example 23).

According to Plaza-Pust (2008), the erroneous use of *auf* as a free morpheme to express the grammatical relation between transitive verbs and their objects is the result of three conspiring phenomena: (a) the remaining gaps regarding the German case-marking and determiner systems, (b) the borrowing of DGS PAM (*personal agreement marker*), commonly translated as AUF ("on"), and (c) the analysis of the morphological components of agreement verbs in DGS and the subsequent translation into German through the use of the German case-marking preposition *auf*.

(23) Tom   mag   auf   Frosch und        auch Paul.    (Fuad, file 3)
     Tom   likes  on    frog    and   also  Paul
     "Tom likes the frog and Paul, too."
(24) Paul  fällt  auf   dem   Boden               (Fuad, file 3)
     Paul  falls  on    the   floor
     "Paul falls on the floor."

In summary, the findings obtained regarding cross-modal language mixing in the course of sign bilingual development are well in line with current assumptions in the broader domain of bilingualism research. Based on the evidence obtained in numerous studies on learners of different language pairs, including hearing learners of a sign language and a spoken language (Petitto et al., 2001), there is agreement that bilingual learners develop two separate but interconnected systems (Paradis et al., 2011). Language contact phenomena in the productions of bilingual learners involving lexical and structural borrowings of one language into the other have been found to represent systematic phenomena that are developmentally constrained. The preceding discussion of cross-modal language contact phenomena in bilingual deaf learners' productions suggests that this observation holds equally for this particular type of bilingual language acquisition. Crucially, the sophisticated combinations of two distinct grammars in mixed utterances indicate that learners know, by virtue of their language endowment, that grammars share certain properties in fundamental ways, irrespective of the modality of expression. This knowledge represents the basis for bilingual learners' pooling of resources (Plaza-Pust, in press).

## Code-Switching in the Classroom

In the course of their development, children learn the functional and pragmatic dimensions of language use and develop the capacity to reflect upon and think about language, commonly referred to as metalinguistic awareness. It is important to note that metalinguistic awareness is not attained spontaneously but is acquired through reflection on structural and communicative characteristics of the target language(s) in academic settings (Ravid & Tolchinsky, 2002).

Research into communication practices in the sign bilingual classroom has been concerned with the roles attributed to the languages and codes used and how bilingual students develop communicative and metalinguistic skills in this acquisition situation. The promotion of associations between the languages at a metalinguistic level commonly includes the use of teaching techniques referred to as *chaining* (Humphries & MacDougall, 2000; Padden & Ramsey, 1998) or *sandwiching*, where written, finger spelled, and spoken/mouthed items with the same referent follow each other.

Contrastive properties of the two languages might not always be pointed out explicitly. As remarked upon by Hennies and Stein (2011), they might also be inferred through the presence of deaf and hearing teachers in the classroom, in particular when it comes to pragmatic or discourse aspects of the languages involved. Unfortunately, this type of "implicit" contrast not only remains largely unexplored, it also remains a component restricted to bilingual education programs that include team teaching.

Another important issue that deserves further attention concerns the linguistic behavior of deaf and hearing teachers in their interactions with bilingual deaf students. Mugnier (2006a, b) reported on the results obtained in a qualitative study of the dynamics of bilingual communication in LSF and French during text comprehension activities in a class of deaf students enrolled at an integration school in France. The corpus comprises recordings of interactions between deaf students (n = 8) and their teachers in two different situations. In their interactions with the hearing teacher, the language used was French. During the text comprehension activities with the deaf teacher, the language used was LSF. The qualitative analysis aimed to determine how language contact in the classroom might promote the linguistic potentials of the students (Mugnier, 2006a, p. 154).

According to Mugnier, the data collected during the sessions conducted by the hearing teacher in French reveal how the students, who cannot display their knowledge in French only, develop bilingual practices as they use both languages in their interaction with the teacher (ibid.). However, their responses in LSF are not taken up by the hearing teacher, who only reacts to the spoken parts of the response (Mugnier, 2006a, p. 156). Following Mugnier (2006b, p. 416) the teacher and the students engage in two parallel discourses, conducted in two languages (LSF and French), which renders the interaction "bi-monolingual" rather than bilingual (Mugnier, 2006b, p. 427). The deaf teacher, by contrast, was found to promote bilingual interactions, connecting LSF and written French. Typically, the alternation of the languages in these bilingual interactions would follow the use of the pattern "written French > LSF > spoken French/LSF > LSF > written French" (Mugnier, 2006a, p. 156). In these interactions the use of the two languages serves to "co-construct" a teacher/student discourse that is characterized by the metalinguistic dimension of the vocabulary activity during the text comprehension task (Mugnier 2006b, 419). At the same time, the author remarks on difficulties that still remain in these co-construction activities, resulting from the developmental asynchrony between the two languages, which make it necessary, at the didactic level, to explicitly establish "bridges" between the two languages (Mugnier, 2006b, p. 423).

## CONCLUSIONS

The portrait of bilingual deaf learners that emerges from the studies reviewed throughout the preceding sections contrasts sharply with attributions of confusion or delay that are commonly assigned to sign bilingualism by opponents of the promotion of bilingualism in deaf education. Typically, advocates of a monolingual (oral) education maintain that the use of sign language will not only reduce the motivation in the child to learn the oral language but also the time that can be spent for its teaching. Further, they believe that the use of sign language would alienate deaf children from the surrounding (hearing) society. To date, however, there is a lack of evidence of the negative effects attributed to the use of sign language in deaf education.

Quite to the contrary, the research undertaken over the last years indicates that bilingual deaf learners pool their linguistic resources in multiple ways. In the course of their bilingual development they acquire two separate but interconnected language systems; they also learn to use the languages appropriately in diverse communicative situations, and they attain metalinguistic knowledge about the languages they acquire.

The review of the research offered in this chapter is certainly not a comprehensive one. However, the discussion of the different lines of research and the summary of the main findings obtained is indicative of what is currently known about bilingual deaf learners. The critical appraisal of the studies conducted also allows for the identification of challenges that remain to be tackled in the future with a view to obtaining a better understanding of sign bilingualism.

Crucially, the review of the research reveals that although the bilingual promotion of deaf learners marked a change in their perception as bilingual learners, their bilingualism continues to be largely regarded in isolation. Current assumptions in the broader field of bilingualism research about bilingual language acquisition regarding developmental trajectories and the role of language contact in the course of bilingual development are seldom taken into consideration. The specific circumstances that determine language development in deaf learners, though different in many respects from the (idealized) typical language learner, do not justify its study as an isolated phenomenon. Commonalities and differences between deaf learners' bilingual development and other types of bilingual language acquisition can only be identified by embedding research on deaf learners into the broader context of bilingualism research. The assumption implies that the investigation of deaf learners' language acquisition, the challenges they face in the course of their development, and their errors and their achievements needs to be footed on a well-defined theoretical framework. Only when this requirement is fulfilled will it be possible to obtain further insights into the nature of the knowledge attained and the way it is acquired, allowing also for a differentiation of the factors (internal and external) that might affect the developmental process.

At the empirical level, more research is needed about the development of deaf learners in both languages. Thus far, only a few studies are available that would provide further insights into the developmental asynchrony between the two languages. The sophisticated knowledge of sign language that becomes apparent in the signed productions of bilingual learners often goes unnoticed when the focus is put on literacy skills in the oral language. The interest in clarifying the question about the impact of bilingualism on bilingual deaf learners' literacy skills is understandable against the backdrop of the ongoing debate in the field about whether or not bilingualism is for the benefit of deaf learners. However, it is precisely where bilingualism is considered as a variable that it needs to be assessed appropriately.

Qualitative developmental studies have provided intriguing evidence about the scope of individual variation regarding the attainment of specific language properties. The spectrum of individual variation documented is indicative of the circumstance that sign bilingualism is not a monolithic phenomenon. Certainly, current studies are providing a more differentiated picture of deaf learners' competences in both languages. The dynamics of the language contact situation in which these learners grow up represents one of the major challenges that will have to be tackled in future research. Indeed, the increasing heterogeneity of deaf learners' profiles related to changes in (a) demographics (migration), (b) hearing aid technology (cochlear implantation), and (c) education (diversification of options, mainstreaming) calls for a more flexible concept of bilingualism that would not only consider variation in the attribution of L1 and L2 labels to the two languages, but also the possibility that what is considered to be their dominant language might change over time.

Certainly, these developments represent a challenge not only for the investigation of bilingual competences of deaf learners. Professionals in the field of deaf education, too, are confronted with the task of adapting didactic conceptions of bilingual education to the abilities and needs of an increasingly heterogeneous population. It seems clear that a successful mastery of the tasks that lie ahead will depend on the exchange and collaboration of experts in both fields.

**NOTE**

[1] The transcription conventions used for sign language examples are as follows: German glosses of signs appear in upper case. The subscript NEG is used to indicate negation through derivation. DET is used for determiners, pronouns, and locatives, distinguished by subscripts (e.g., EXISTENZ is used for existential determiners, LOK for locatives). Agreement marking

is represented by subscripts. Numbers indicate person agreement, letters from the Latin alphabet locations. CL is used as an abbreviation for classifier; Greek letters (λ, μ, θ) indicate agreement with arguments. Clauses in complex sentence constructions are separated by a colon.

## REFERENCES

Bellugi, U., Lillo-Martin, D., O'Grady, L., & van Hoek, K. (1990). The development of spatialized syntactic mechanisms in American Sign Language. In W. Edmondson, & F. Karlsson (Eds.), *SLR '87. Papers from the Fourth International Symposium on Sign Language Research* (pp. 16–25). Hamburg: Signum.

Baker, A., & Van den Bogaerde, B. (2008). Code-mixing in signs and words in input to and output from children. In C. Plaza Pust & E. Morales-López (Eds.), *Sign bilingualism: Language development, interaction, and maintenance in sign language contact situations* (pp. 1–28). Amsterdam: Benjamins.

Baker, A., Van den Bogaerde, B., & Woll, B. (2005). Methods and procedures in sign language acquisition studies. *Sign Language and Linguistics, 8,* 7–58.

Becker, C. (2009). Narrative competences of deaf children in German Sign Language. *Sign Language & Linguistics, 2,* 113–160.

Chamberlain, C., & Mayberry, R. I. (2000). Theorizing about the relation between American Sign Language and reading. In J. P. Morford & R. I. Mayberry (Eds.), *Language Acquisition by Eye* (pp. 221–260). Mahwah, NJ: Erlbaum.

Cummins, J. (1979). Linguistic interdependence and the educational development of bilingual children. *Review of Educational Research, 49,* 222–251.

Cummins, J. (1981). The role of primary language development in promoting educational success for language minority students. In California State Department of Education (Ed.), *Schooling and language minority students: A theoretical framework* (pp. 3–49). Los Angeles: Evaluation, Dissemination and Assessment Center California State University.

Cummins, J. (1991). Interdependence of first- and second-language proficiency in bilingual children. In E. Bialystok (Ed.), *Language processing in bilingual children* (pp. 70–89). Cambridge, UK: Cambridge University Press.

De Houwer, A. (2007). Parental language input patterns and children's bilingual use. *Applied Psycholinguistics, 28,* 411–424.

Diehl, E., Christen, H., Leuenberger, S., Pelvat, I., & Studer, T. (2000). *Grammatikunterricht: Alles für die Katz? Untersuchungen zum Zweitspracherwerb Deutsch.* Tübingen: Niemeyer.

Dubuisson, C., Parisot, A.-M. & Vercaingne-Ménard, A. (2008). Bilingualism and deafness: Correlations between deaf students' ability to use space in Quebec Sign Language and their reading comprehension in French. In C. Plaza-Pust & E. Morales-López (Eds.), *Sign bilingualism: Language development, interaction, and maintenance in sign language contact situations* (pp. 51–71). Amsterdam: John Benjamins.

Fritzenschaft, A., Gawlitzek-Maiwald, I., Tracy, R., & Winkler, S. (1991). Wege zur komplexen Syntax. *Zeitschrift für Sprachwissenschaft, 9,* 52–134.

Gogolin, I. (2009). Zweisprachigkeit und die Entwicklung bildungssprachlicher Fähigkeiten. In I. Gogolin & U. Neumann (Eds.), *Streitfall Zweisprachigkeit— The bilingualism controversy* (pp. 263–280). Springer online.

Grosjean, Francois (2008). *Studying bilinguals*. Oxford: Oxford University Press.
Günther, K.-B. (1999). Schulversuch Bilingualer Unterricht an der Hamburger Gehörlosenschule—konzeptuelle Grundlagen und vorläufige Zwischenbilanz. In T. Kaul & A. Becker (Eds.), *Gebärdensprache in Erziehung und Unterricht* (pp. 21–47). Hamburg: hörgeschädigte kinder.
Günther, K.-B. (2003). Entwicklung des Wortschreibens bei gehörlosen und schwerhörigen Kindern. *forum, 11*, 35–70.
Günther, K.-B & Hennies, J. (2011). Schriftsprachliche Kompetenzentwicklung (1): Schreiben. In K.-B. Günther & J. Hennies (Eds.), *Bilingualer Unterricht in Gebärden-, Schrift- und Lautsprache mit hörgeschädigten SchülerInnen in der Primarstufe: Zwischenbericht zum Berliner bilingualen Schulversuch* (pp. 15–58). Hamburg: Signum.
Günther, K.-B., Schäfke, I., Koppitz, Mv. K. & Matthei, M. (2004). Vergleichende Untersuchungen zur Entwicklung der Textproduktionskompetenz und Erzählkompetenz. In K.-B. Günther & I. Schäfke (Eds.), *Bilinguale Erziehung als Förderkonzept für gehörlose SchülerInnen: Abschlussbericht zum Hamburger Bilingualen Schulversuch* (pp. 189–267). Hamburg: Signum.
Hänel, B. (2005). *Der Erwerb der Deutschen Gebärdensprache als Erstsprache: Die frühkindliche Sprachentwicklung von Subjekt- und Objektverbkongruenz in DGS*. Tübingen: Gunter Narr.
Happ, D., & Vorköper, M.-O. (2006). *Deutsche Gebärdensprache: Ein Lehr- und Arbeitsbuch*. Frankfurt am Main: Fachhochschulverlag.
Hennies, J. & Stein, M. (2011). Unterrichtsbeispiele aus dem kontrastiven Anfangsunterricht. In K.-B. Günther & J. Hennies (Eds.), *Bilingualer Unterricht in Gebärden-, Schrift- und Lautsprache mit hörgeschädigten SchülerInnen in der Primarstufe: Zwischenbericht zum Berliner bilingualen Schulversuch* (pp. 185–190). Hamburg: Signum.
Hoffmeister, R. J. (2000). A piece of the puzzle: ASL and reading comprehension in deaf children. In C. Chamberlain, J. P. Morford, & R. I. Mayberry (Eds.), *Language acquisition by eye* (pp. 143–163). Mahwah, NJ: Erlbaum.
Humphries, T., & MacDougall, F. (2000). "Chaining" and other links making connections between American Sign Language and English in two types of school. *Visual Anthropology Review, 15*, 84–94.
Klein, W. (2000). Prozesse des Zweitspracherwerbs. In H. Grimm (Ed.), *Enzyklopädie der Psychologie. Vol. 3: Sprachentwicklung* (pp. 537–570). Göttingen: Hogrefe.
Kuntze, M. (1998). Codeswitching in ASL and written English language contact. In K. Emmorey & H. Lane (Eds.), *The signs of language revisited: An anthology to honor Ursula Bellugi and Edward Klima* (pp. 287–302). Mahwah, NJ: Erlbaum.
Kyle, F. E., & Harris, M. (2011). Longitudinal patterns of emerging literacy in beginning deaf and hearing readers. *Journal of Deaf Studies and Deaf Education, 16*, 289–304.
Lanza, E. (1997). *Language mixing in infant bilingualism: A sociolinguistic perspective*. Oxford, UK: Clarendon.
Leuninger, H. (2000). Mit den Augen lernen: Gebärdenspracherwerb. In H. Grimm (Ed.), *Enzyklopädie der Psychologie. Bd. IV: Sprachentwicklung* (pp. 229–270). Göttingen: Hogrefe.
Lillo-Martin, D. (1999). Modality effects and modularity in language acquisition: The acquisition of American Sign Language. In W. T. Ritchie &

T. K. Bhatia (Eds.), *Handbook of language acquisition* (pp. 531–567). San Diego, CA: Academic Press.

Mayberry, R. I. (2007). When timing is everything: Age of first-language acquisition effects on second-language learning. *Applied Psycholinguistics, 28,* 537–549.

Mayberry, R. I., & Lock, E. (2003). Age constraints on first versus second language acquisition: Evidence for linguistic plasticity and epigenesis. *Brain and Language, 87,* 369–384.

Mayberry, R. I., & Squires, B. (2006). Sign language acquisition. In K. Brown (Ed.), *Encyclopedia of language and linguistics,* 2nd ed., vol. 11 (pp. 291–296). Oxford, UK: Elsevier.

Mayer, C. (2007). What really matters in the early literacy development of deaf children. *Journal of Deaf Studies and Deaf Education, 12,* 411–431.

Mayer, C., & Leigh, G. (2010). The changing context for sign bilingual education programs: Issues in language and the development of literacy. *International Journal of Bilingual Education and Bilingualism, 13,* 175–186.

Morgan, G. (2006). The development of narrative skills in British Sign Language. In B. Schick, M. Marschark, & P. E. Spencer (Eds.), *Advances in the sign-language development of deaf children* (pp. 314–343). New York, NY: Oxford University Press.

Mugnier, S. (2006a). Le bilinguisme des enfants sourds: De quelques freins aux possibles moteurs. *GLOTTOPOL Revue de sociolinguistique en ligne.* Retrieved from http://www.univ-rouen.fr/dyalang/glottopol.

Mugnier, S. (2006b). Surdités, plurilinguisme et Ecole: Approches sociolinguistiques et sociodidactiques des bilinguismes d'enfants sourds de CE2. Ph thesis, Université Stendhal–Grenoble 3, France.

Musselman, C. (2000). How do children who can't hear learn to read an alphabetic script? A review of the literature on reading and deafness. *Journal of Deaf Studies and Deaf Education, 5,* 9–31.

Neef, M., & Primus, B. (2001). Stumme Zeugen der Autonomie—Eine Replik auf Ossner. *Linguistische Berichte, 187,* 353–378.

Niederberger, N. (2004). Capacités langagières en langue des signes française et en français écrit chez l'enfant sourd bilingue: Quelles relations? PhD dissertation, University of Geneva, Switzerland.

Niederberger, N. (2008). Does the knowledge of a natural sign language facilitate deaf children's learning to read and write? Insights from French Sign Language and written French data. In C. Plaza-Pust & E. Morales-López (Eds.), *Sign bilingualism: Language development, interaction, and maintenance in sign language contact situations* (pp. 29–50). Amsterdam: John Benjamins.

Padden, C. (1998). Early bilingual lives of deaf children. In I. Parasnis (Ed.), *Cultural and language diversity and the deaf experience* (pp. 79–116). Cambridge, UK: Cambridge University Press.

Padden, C., & Ramsey, C. (1998). Reading ability in signing deaf children. *Topics in Language Disorders, 18,* 30–46.

Paradis, J., Genesee, F., & Crago, M. B. (2011). *Dual language development and disorders.* Baltimore, MD: Brookes.

Pienemann, M., & Keßler, J. U. (2007). Measuring bilingualism. In P. Auer & L. Wei (Eds.), *Handbook of multilingualism and multilingual communication* (pp. 247–274). Berlin: Mouton de Gruyter.

Plaza-Pust, C. (2000). *Linguistic theory and adult second language acquisition: On the relation between the lexicon and the syntax.* Frankfurt am Main: Peter Lang.

Plaza-Pust, C. (2004). The path toward bilingualism: Problems and perspectives with regard to the inclusion of sign language in deaf education. In M. Van Herreweghe, & M. Vermeerbergen (Eds.), *To the lexicon and beyond: Sociolinguistics in European deaf communities* (pp. 141–170). Washington, DC: Gallaudet University Press.

Plaza-Pust, C. (2008). Why variation matters: On language contact in the development of L2 written German. In C. Plaza-Pust & E. Morales-López (Eds.), *Sign bilingualism: Language development, interaction, and maintenance in sign language contact situations* (pp. 73–135). Amsterdam: John Benjamins.

Plaza Pust, C. (in press). Bilingualism and deafness: On language contact in the bilingual acquisition of sign language and written language. Berlin: Mouton de Gruyter.

Plaza-Pust, C. & E. Morales-López (2008). Sign bilingualism: Language development, interaction, and maintenance in sign language contact situations. In C. Plaza-Pust & E. Morales-López (Eds.), *Sign bilingualism: Language development, interaction, and maintenance in sign language contact situations* (pp. 333–379). Amsterdam: John Benjamins.

Ravid, D., & Tolchinsky, L. (2002). Developing linguistic literacy: A comprehensive model. *Journal of Child Language, 29,* 417–447.

Riches, C. & Genesee, F. (2006). Literacy: Crosslinguistic and crossmodal issues. In F. Genesee, K. Lindholm-Leary, W. M. Saunders, & C. Donna (Eds.), *Educating English language learners: A synthesis of research evidence* (pp. 64–108). Cambridge, UK: Cambridge University Press.

Romaine, S. (1996). Bilingualism. In W. C. Ritchie & T. K. Bhatia (Eds.), *Handbook of Second Language Acquisition* (pp. 571–601). San Diego: Academic Press.

Schäfke, I. (2005). *Untersuchungen zum Erwerb der Textproduktionskompetenz bei hörgeschädigten Schülern.* Hamburg: Signum.

Schleppengrell, M. J., & O'Hallaron, C. L. (2011). Teaching academic language in L2 secondary settings. *Annual Review of Applied Linguistics, 31,* 3–18.

Siebert-Ott, G. M. (2001). *Frühe Mehrsprachigkeit: Probleme des Grammatikerwerbs in multilingualen und multikulturellen Kontexten.* Tübigen: Niemeyer.

Slobin, D. I. (2008). Breaking the moulds: Signed languages and the nature of human language. *Sign Language Studies, 8,* 114–130.

Spencer, P. E., & Tomblin, J. B. (2006). Speech production and spoken language development of children using "Total Communication." In P. E. Spencer & M. Marschark (Eds.), *Advances in the spoken language development of deaf and hard-of-hearing children* (pp. 166–192). New York, NY: Oxford University Press.

Strong, M., & Prinz, P. (2000). Is American Sign Language skill related to English literacy? In C. Chamberlain, J. P. Morford, & R. I. Mayberry (Eds.), *Language acquisition by eye* (pp. 131–142). Mahwah, NJ: Lawrence Erlbaum.

Tracy, R. (1991). *Sprachliche Strukturentwicklung: Linguistische und kognitionspsychologische Aspekte einer Theorie des Erstspracherwerbs.* Tübingen: Narr.

Tracy, R. (2002). Growing (clausal) roots: All children start out (and may remain) multilingual. *Linguistics, 40,* 653–686.

Tuller, L., Blondel, M. & Niederberger, N. (2007). Growing up bilingual in French and French Sign Language. In D. Ayoun (Ed.), *French applied linguistics* (pp. 334–376). Amsterdam: John Benjamins.

Vainikka, A., & Young-Scholten, M. (1996). Gradual development of L2 phrase structure. *Second Language Research, 12,* 7–39.

Vercaingne-Ménard, A., Godard, L., & Labelle, M. (2001). The emergence of narrative discourse in three young deaf children. In V. Dively, M. Metzger, S. Taub, & A. M. Baer (Eds.), *Signed languages: Discoveries from international research* (pp. 120–133). Washington, DC: Gallaudet University Press.

Vercaingne-Ménard, A., Parisot, A.-M., & Dubuisson, C. (2005). *L'approche bilingue à l'école Gadbois: Six années d'expérimentation. Bilan et recommandations.* Rapport déposé au ministère de l'Éducation du Québec. Montréal: Université du Québec à Montréal.

Verhoeven, L. T. (1994). Transfer in bilingual development: The linguistic Interdependence Hypothesis revisited. *Language Learning, 44,* 381–415.

Wilbur, R. (2000). The use of ASL to support the development of English and literacy. *Journal of Deaf Studies and Deaf Education, 5,* 81–104.

Winford, D. (2003). *An introduction to contact linguistics.* Oxford, UK: Blackwell.

# 3

# Language Acquisition by Bilingual Deaf Preschoolers

## *Theoretical and Methodological Issues and Empirical Data*

Pasquale Rinaldi, Maria Cristina Caselli, Daniela Onofrio, and Virginia Volterra

### THEORETICAL ISSUES AND THE ITALIAN SITUATION

In comparison to hearing children exposed to two spoken languages (*unimodal* bilinguals), *bimodal* bilingual deaf children learning a spoken and a signed language constitute not one but many different populations. This variety reflects a wide range of factors, such as the time of onset of bilingualism, the amount of exposure to each language, and the settings in which each language is acquired and used. In Italy, as in many other countries, only 5–10% of deaf children acquire a sign language natively from deaf signing parents (Caselli, Maragna, & Volterra, 2006). Native signing children benefit from a more homogeneous language experience than non-native signers, but even within deaf signing families, large individual differences can be found between children who are first generation native signers (i.e., whose grandparents are hearing) and second/third generation signers. Furthermore, not all Italian deaf parents use Italian Sign Language (LIS) with their children. This may be because the deaf parents had not acquired LIS themselves and use only Italian. Another reason may be that some parents, although they do sign themselves, are afraid to use LIS with their children (Caselli et al., 2006). The strong opposition toward sign language imposed by the Milan Congress of 1880 has had a strong and lasting influence on the educational environment of the following generations of deaf persons. Even today, some deaf parents have been raised with the false impression that the use of signs may prevent the acquisition and mastery of spoken language.

The bimodal bilingual population includes not only deaf and hearing individuals from deaf signing families, but also deaf persons from hearing families. Deaf children (with deaf or hearing parents) who are exposed to sign language from birth or early in life acquire this language in the same manner, following similar maturational milestones to those of hearing children acquiring their native spoken language (Caselli, 1994; Cormier, Schembri, Vinson, & Orfanidou, 2012; Newport & Meier, 1985; Petitto et al., 2001; Pizzuto, 2002; Pizzuto, Ardito, Caselli, & Volterra, 2001). According to Grosjean (2010), the bilingualism found in Deaf communities can be defined as a form of *minority language bilingualism*, in which the members of the community acquire and use both the minority language (sign language) and the majority language in its written form and sometimes in its spoken or even a signed form (signed Italian). In Italy, all deaf people learn and use the spoken and written form of Italian (the majority language), and most of them also acquire and use LIS in their everyday life. Importantly, however, there is a large individual variability in the proficiency in each language, a factor that will be discussed throughout this chapter in more detail.

It is important to note that LIS as a minority language has not yet received full official recognition by the Italian government. Therefore the bilingual status of Deaf Italians also has not yet been officially recognized. Research on sign language began in Italy about 30 years ago. Previously, signed communication was used primarily in informal settings among deaf people and did not even have a name. Since 1981, the fingerspelled sign L-I-S, based on manual alphabet initials for *Lingua dei Segni Italiana*, was gradually introduced to Italian Deaf people as a name sign for the language (Volterra, 1987). In the following years, research projects were developed to describe this language and its acquisition processes, as well as related historical factors. Interest in LIS also began to grow in the fields of rehabilitation and education, and training programs for hearing and deaf professionals were created.

In 1988, the European Parliament initiated the path toward recognition of all national sign languages and encouraged the publication of dictionaries and the establishment of courses and interpreting services, as well as television programs for the Deaf. In 1992 a special Italian law on the rights of disabled persons was adopted, which supported students and families by offering the possibility of obtaining signing teaching assistants in schools and LIS interpreters in universities (see Maragna & Marziale, 2012, for further information on this law and its modifications). Thanks to this law, LIS courses, bilingual educational programs, and interpreting services often were funded and supported by local governments or at the national level (Geraci, 2012).

**Unimodal and Bimodal Bilingualism: Similarities and Differences**

Italian deaf bilinguals share many similarities with hearing bilinguals, in particular with children from migrant parents who usually acquire the minority language at home and the majority language in other environments (Pearson, 2007). It is widely accepted that for both hearing and deaf persons the acquisition and use of minority languages, even those of lower status, are fundamental for the building of self-identity and the construction of cultural and linguistic values. However, as is often the case with minority languages, LIS is used by a restricted number of people and is often felt to be a low-status communicative code compared to Italian, which is regarded as the majority language. LIS is thus rarely considered for use within larger and public settings or by the media. This is one of the ways in which the lower status of a minority language in the community can hamper the development of that language.

Several studies have shown that children in a bilingual environment learn the majority language quite easily in the course of everyday living, but acquisition of a minority language requires special attention and safeguarding in order to compensate for differences in input level (de Houwer, 2007; Gathercole & Thomas, 2009; Morgan & Woll, 2002; Pearson, Fernandez, Lewedag, & Oller, 1997). When a minority language is involved, both deaf bimodal bilinguals and hearing unimodal bilinguals have a tendency to evaluate their language competencies as inadequate, not perceiving themselves as being bilingual even though they use two (or more) languages regularly (Grosjean, 1985; 2010). In the case of the deaf, they feel that they do not fully master either the Italian language or LIS. A further similarity between deaf and hearing bilinguals is that they both use their languages for different purposes, in different contexts, with different people. Even if some contexts are covered by both languages, others are specific to only one language, though contacts between the two languages often occur in all situations of bilingualism.

Bimodal bilingualism does, however, also present some interesting differences from unimodal bilingualism. In bimodal bilingualism, one language (the spoken language) is mainly perceived and expressed by the auditory-vocal modality, while the other language (sign) is mainly perceived and expressed by the visual-gestural modality (Emmorey, Petrich, & Gollan, 2012; Pinto & Volterra, 2008).

In LIS, as in all sign languages, face-to-face interaction is essential. A consequence of this is that the amount of language input available to a deaf child is less than the language input to which a hearing child has access from his or her hearing parents and from the broader speaking environment. Furthermore, if the conversational partner is signing, but the child is not looking, no actual input can occur (Harris, Clibbens, Chasin, & Tibbitts, 1989; Kyle, Ackerman, & Woll, 1987; Swisher, 2000; van den Bogaerde, 2000). Harris (1992) defines *uptake* as the input that is actually attended to by the deaf child, and this must be carefully measured. Deaf mothers, but not all hearing mothers, often spontaneously adopt specific strategies to ensure better communicative exchanges with their deaf children (Capirci, Pirchio, & Soldani, 2007).

Another interesting difference is related to the fact that one of the languages (i.e., the spoken language) requires auditory perception but that residual hearing capacities are very different among deaf people. All deaf children exposed to LIS also are exposed to spoken and written Italian in speech therapy sessions, in the school environment, and at home. Spoken Italian development in both monolingual and bimodal bilingual deaf children is often significantly delayed, at least in the first stages of language acquisition, as compared to hearing children. The large individual variability in Italian language skills may be partially accounted for by considering specific factors, such as age at diagnosis of hearing loss, age at which language rehabilitation started, nonverbal cognitive abilities, as well as use of hearing aids or cochlear implants (Caselli et al., 2012; Pizzuto et al., 2001; Rinaldi & Caselli, 2009; see Swanwick, Hendar, Dammeyer, Kristoffersen, Salter, & Simonsen, Chapter 12 of this volume). All of these factors affect the amount and quality of spoken Italian input that the deaf child may uptake.

A further difference is that, unlike the process that occurs in cases of unimodal bilingualism, in which both languages are produced by a single output channel, in bimodal bilingualism there are two output channels. As a consequence, bimodal bilinguals rarely switch languages sequentially as unimodal bilinguals usually do, but instead more frequently use *code-blends*, producing signs and spoken words at the same time (Baker & van der Bogaerde, 2008; Donati & Branchini, 2013; Emmorey, Borinstein, & Thompson, 2005; Emmorey et al., 2012; Pizzuto, 2002).

Finally, another difference is that hearing children exposed at home to a minority language naturally become bilingual, as they will be exposed to the majority language in everyday life outside their home. In the case of deaf children of deaf parents, the spoken majority language is not naturally acquired, but has to be learned in formal contexts (i.e., speech therapy). For most deaf children of hearing families whose native language is the spoken majority language, "natural" contexts of acquisition must be provided also for the minority language because sign language is not naturally acquired at home.

**Differing Educational Contexts for Bimodal Bilingualism**

Since 1990, some Italian hearing families have offered their deaf children the opportunity to be exposed to LIS early in life at home (e.g., through the presence of a signing babysitter), in day-care centers, and in schools where bimodal bilingual education programs are used (Caselli & Corazza, 1997). Deaf children in Italy are provided with different types of schooling. At the present time, the great majority of deaf children attend mainstream public schools along with hearing children. In most of these schools, Italian (spoken and written) is the only language used, both for providing instruction and for communication purposes (see Caselli et al., 2006; Meristo et al., 2007). There are no sign language interpreters, the support teacher in the classroom does not use sign language, and teachers and students in the classroom communicate in spoken Italian.

Since 1992, children's families have the right to request the presence in the classroom of a teaching assistant competent in LIS, or they may find a school with a bilingual curriculum using LIS and Italian for both deaf and hearing pupils. In the situation where a teaching assistant competent in LIS is available, the deaf child can be provided with individual explanations in LIS, in Signed Italian (SI) or in Sign-Supported Italian (SSI),[1] for a maximum of 20 hours a week. For the rest of the school curriculum, teaching is provided only through spoken Italian. In most cases, there is only one deaf child in a class of hearing children.

Very few public schools offer a bilingual curriculum that involves a consistent use of Italian and LIS within the classroom. In these schools, teachers either use LIS, SI, or SSI, or there is an LIS interpreter who simultaneously translates the teacher's and students' messages from Italian to LIS and vice versa. In these schools, LIS is also taught as a subject to deaf and hearing pupils for a minimum of 1 hour per week up to a maximum of 6 hours per week. Usually two or more deaf children are present in the same classroom (Ardito, Caselli, Vecchietti, & Volterra, 2008; Russo Cardona & Volterra, 2007; Teruggi, 2003).

In recent years, in Italy as in other countries, the growing number of deaf children who have received cochlear implantation (CI) in their early years has resulted in hampered access to a bimodal bilingual school curriculum. Clinicians still consider sign language as an obstacle to—or at best a useless tool for—the acquisition of spoken language. They unfortunately continue to advise or even to insist that parents keep their cochlear implanted child away from sign language (Percy-Smith, Cayé-Thomasen, Breinegaard, & Jensen, 2010; for a recent debate on this topic, see Humphries et al., 2012; Knoors & Marschark, 2012; Rinaldi & Caselli, 2014; see also Walker & Tomblin, Chapter 6 of this volume; Marschark & Lee, Chapter 9 of this volume). Some of these children are later exposed to LIS because they do not experience success with their CIs. Other children with CIs express curiosity about the Deaf community and learn sign language in adolescence or when they meet other signers, whether in school or even much later, after having left school.

We believe that early bimodal bilingualism is crucial for the development of deaf children, but the study of the acquisition of sign language and spoken/written language, as well as the interrelationship of these languages, poses several methodological challenges both for research and practice that will be discussed in the next section.

## EVALUATION OF LINGUISTIC SKILLS: METHODOLOGICAL QUESTIONS

Assessment is the process of gathering and interpreting data relevant for understanding and describing language acquisition processes. In the case of bilingualism, assessment is an especially complex task.

For children learning two languages, developmental changes in language acquisition are characterized by changes in the acquisition of each language, which do not, however, always occur in parallel: Which language is strongest, or *dominant,* may fluctuate across age and learning opportunities. Furthermore, at any given point in time, a single language may not be completely dominant or stronger across all measures, topics, settings, or subcomponents of language proficiency. The result, if tested on the full range of tasks that comprise language proficiency at any point during the very dynamic period characterizing language development, is that bilingual children may perform better on some tasks in one language but better on other tasks in the other language (Kohnert, 2010; Kohnert & Bates, 2002). Uneven performance across tasks, settings, and languages is most evident in developing bilinguals who use each of their languages with different partners (e.g., parents, teachers, siblings, peers), in different settings (e.g., home, school, Internet, playground environments) and for different purposes (e.g., telling stories, solving math problems). From a practical standpoint, evidence of uneven performance across language tasks and distributed skills within linguistic domains indicate that single language scores may not adequately capture the total language ability of dual-language learners.

Several studies on bilingualism have shown that fully evaluating both languages might help in providing a better estimate of bilinguals' linguistic competencies, thereby accounting for similarities and differences between languages (Person, Fernandez, & Oller, 1993; Pettenati, Vacchini, Stefanini, & Caselli, 2011). The assessment of competencies in each of the languages that the child is acquiring must also be integrated with the observation of the relationship between the two languages. Contacts that frequently occur between the two languages are referred to as *code-mixing phenomena*. Languages can interact in a sequential manner, as in *code-switching*, commonly documented for unimodal bilingualism, or in a simultaneous manner, as in *code-blending*, a phenomenon that is unique to bimodal bilingualism. Bimodal bilinguals do not always stop speaking to sign or stop signing to speak. Often they produce sign and speech simultaneously, and the resulting code-blends are generally semantically equivalent. For a code-blend, two lexical representations must be selected, whereas for a code-switch, only one lexical item is selected and production of the translation equivalent must be suppressed (Emmorey et al., 2012).

These code-mixing phenomena are relevant to the strategies adopted by the child trying to produce efficient communication. The form of language mixing used by children may often change to accommodate the specific language of their interlocutors. Moreover, the code-mixing that occurs may also depend on how the child is able to express ideas and concepts regardless of the language in which the communicative interaction occurs.

Some researchers argue that language mixing does not reflect confusion but rather demonstrates the bilingual child's distinct representation of his or her two input languages from an early age (Genesee, Nicoladis, & Paradis, 1995; Petitto et al., 2001; Rinaldi, 2008). This theoretical hypothesis requires an integrated language form of assessment. However, the extraordinary heterogeneity of experiences and proficiency of bilingual children present some formidable challenges for those who wish to develop procedures and standardized norms-referenced measures appropriate for any particular group of dual-language learners, especially when the bilingualism involves a minority language, as in the case of sign languages.

For both unimodal and bimodal bilingual children exposed to a minority language, a valid assessment can be achieved by using a combination of methods and procedures to evaluate the linguistic environment and the linguistic competence of the child in both languages. Among the sources of information relevant to the assessment are interviews with family members. In accordance with other studies (Gutierrez-Clellen & Kreiter, 2003; Kanto, Huttunen, & Laakso, 2013; Paradis, Emmerzael, & Duncan, 2010), we consider it crucial also to collect information on the child's linguistic environment, specifically the following: the age at which the child was first exposed to each language, the amount of input and nature of linguistic exposure, as well as the parents' educational level and their beliefs, goals, and concerns related to the child's linguistic development. It is also important to acknowledge any other cultures to which the child has been frequently exposed (Kohnert, 2008). All these data relate to the linguistic competence achieved by the child to be evaluated through direct or indirect assessment tools.

In assessing the language skills of bimodal bilingual deaf children, it is crucial to use reliable and valid evaluation procedures for testing and monitoring both sign language and spoken language development. Although many valid reliable assessment tools exist to evaluate spoken and written language, the assessment of sign language abilities is often conducted through informal descriptive evaluation. There are still few sign-based tests for deaf children whose validity has been clearly established (Miller, 2008).

In designing a sign language test, it is important to identify the acquisition processes related to the specific sign language assessed and which target structures are acquired at a specific developmental stage. However, there are very few studies on the acquisition of sign languages, thus rendering difficult the development of appropriate tests (Haug, 2011). Some existing tests that were developed to assess sign language abilities in one specific sign language have been adapted to other sign languages. (i.e., the Test for American Sign Language and the British Sign Language Receptive Skills Tests have been adapted in order to be used in other linguistic contexts). However, the effectiveness of these adaptations has not always been straightforward, and differences in linguistic structures and cultural factors have resulted in complicating the adaptation (Haug & Mann, 2008). In other cases, researchers have attempted to translate and/or adapt tests developed for spoken language assessment. For example, the MacArthur-Bates Communicative Development Inventories (MB-CDI, Fenson et al., 2007), an internationally and widely used test that has proven to be a reliable and valid tool to assess children's early spoken language development, has been adapted to measure development in some sign languages (e.g. American Sign Language by Anderson & Reilly, 2002, and British Sign Language by Woolfe, Herman, Roy, & Woll, 2010).

In Italy, as well as in many other countries, very few tests for sign language assessment have been developed and/or adapted. Where testing materials exist, they have been used with small samples of deaf children from both deaf signing parents and hearing parents who have chosen a bimodal bilingual educational approach for their children (Pizzuto, 2002; Pizzuto et al., 2001; Rinaldi, 2008; Rinaldi & Caselli, 2009; Rinaldi, Caselli, Di Renzo, Gulli & Volterra, 2014; Tomasuolo, Fellini, Di Renzo, & Volterra, 2010). In the following section we will briefly review three studies conducted on Italian bimodal bilingual children, which address some of these methodological issues.

## ITALIAN SIGN LANGUAGE AND SPOKEN ITALIAN IN DEAF PRESCHOOLERS: EMPIRICAL DATA

Most studies on language acquisition and development in Italian deaf children have focused either on spoken and written abilities or on the signed modality (Fabbretti & Tomasuolo, 2006; Pizzuto, 2002; Rinaldi & Caselli, 2009; Tomasuolo et al., 2010, 2013). Only a very few studies have analyzed both modalities (i.e., LIS and spoken Italian) in bilingual bimodal Italian deaf preschoolers. In this section we will report on three such studies, which all share some important methodological characteristics. In all three studies, reliable assessment tools that have been validated for the evaluation of spoken Italian were adapted for LIS evaluation in collaboration with deaf signing experts. The deaf children were assessed in spoken Italian by hearing examiners proficient in LIS and were assessed in LIS by bimodal bilingual deaf examiners.

### Study 1: Cognitive and Linguistic Skills of Deaf Preschoolers from Deaf and Hearing Families

The first study was part of a larger project aimed at evaluating several aspects of deaf children's cognitive, communicative, and linguistic development. This research included an investigation of some of the major factors that notoriously interact in complex ways to determine a deaf child's developmental outcome, including family environment (i.e., deaf vs. hearing parents), language used at home (i.e., sign vs. speech, or combinations of both), presence and type of speech therapy intervention, and parents' educational background. Parent interviews were conducted to explore educational choices and other crucial aspects such as emotional/relational patterns within the family (including parents' acceptance of and adjustment to the child's deafness) and parental attitudes with respect to bimodal bilingualism and toward the Deaf community.

Eleven deaf Italian preschoolers (aged from 3 years and 11 months to 5 years and 11 months) attending the same class participated in the study: five with deaf parents and six with hearing parents (for further details, see Caselli & Volterra, 2003; Pizzuto, et al., 1998, 2001; Volterra, Caselli & Pizzuto, 2000). The children's receptive and expressive language skills were evaluated by adopting, as much as possible, comparable assessment procedures for examining signed and spoken language and for comparing deaf children's performance with that of their hearing peers. Here we will report only data pertaining to nonverbal cognitive development and on lexical and grammar comprehension. Cognitive development was assessed using the Test of Visual Motor Integration (Berry & Buktenica, 1997) and the Leiter International Performance Scale (Roid & Miller, 1997). Lexical and grammatical comprehension was assessed using the Peabody Picture Vocabulary Test (Dunn & Dunn, 1981) and the Test for Grammatical Comprehension in Children (Chilosi & Cipriani, 1995), respectively.

Results showed that children's nonverbal cognitive abilities were within or above the normal limits of hearing peers. Children's performance in language tasks revealed large individual variability. However, children from deaf families and those from hearing families exhibited comparable performance patterns not only in the two tasks presented in spoken Italian, but also in the LIS version of the lexical comprehension task. Among the five children who exhibited lower performance, three children (all from deaf families) had either withdrawn from speech therapy or had never received any structured spoken language education. Spoken language education and participation in bilingual school with hearing and deaf children seemed to play a positive role.

With regard to the tests administered in LIS, no clear differences in lexical tasks emerged between deaf children of deaf parents and deaf children of hearing parents, although better comprehension was found for most children of deaf parents in the grammatical task. These data indicate that full exposure to LIS seems to be necessary for developing good receptive skills, not only in the lexicon but also particularly in the grammar. In other words, a partial exposure to LIS does not appear to be sufficient for the development of grammatical comprehension for which a complete LIS input is needed (Pizzuto et al., 2001).

Finally, most children exhibiting greater linguistic performance had parents who, regardless of their hearing or deaf status, were well adjusted to their child's deafness. These parents actively participated in the child's education, promoting the child's autonomy and an awareness of the culture and language of both the Deaf and the hearing communities. In short, these families had chosen to acculturate their deaf children into both the Deaf and the hearing worlds.

## Study 2: Lexical Production Assessment and Total Conceptual Vocabulary (TCV)

The aim of the research study by Rinaldi (2008) was to analyze lexical production in deaf bimodal bilingual Italian preschoolers, taking into account chronological age (CA) as well as language age (LA), which here refers to the time elapsed since wearing a hearing aid and beginning speech therapy. Language mixing phenomena were considered with regard to the language (spoken Italian vs. LIS) in which the test was administered. A total of 14 deaf preschoolers with hearing parents participated in the study. All of the children regularly used hearing aids and none of them had a cochlear implant. All attended speech therapy sessions and were exposed to spoken Italian and LIS at home and attended a bilingual preschool with hearing children. A picture-naming task (Picture Naming Game, *PiNG*), designed to assess lexical comprehension and production, was used (Bello et al., 2012).

On the basis of the preference shown toward one or the other language in two brief preliminary interactions with a deaf and a hearing interlocutor, respectively, the children were divided into two subgroups. Half of the participants received the test in spoken Italian by a bilingual hearing experimenter who gave the instructions and maintained communicative interaction in spoken Italian. The other half received the test given in LIS by a bilingual deaf experimenter who gave the instructions and maintained communicative interaction in LIS. The expectation was that the children would answer in the language in which the test was administered, but answers provided in either of the two languages were scored. If the child provided a correct answer to an item, but expressed the answer in the other language (e.g., correctly answering only in LIS when spoken Italian was being assessed or vice versa), the item was scored as correct (the total conceptual vocabulary, TCV), and the language in which the answer was given was noted.

This procedure was taken from Pearson and colleages (1993), who used this scoring procedure for the evaluation of lexical abilities in unimodal bilingual children. The number of "concepts" that the child is reported to produce (i.e., the *conceptual score*) was calculated regardless of the language used, counting correct code-blending answers only once (i.e., if the child, while viewing the picture of a dog, correctly answered by stating "dog" while also producing the LIS sign for "dog," the answer was coded as correct only once), but these instances were also recorded as occurrences of code-blending.

Children who received the test in spoken Italian had a mean CA of 52 months (range: 36–68 months) and a mean LA of 27 months (range: 12–43 months). These children showed a delay in lexical production when compared with hearing peers, but their skills were similar to those of hearing children with the same LA. Notwithstanding the fact that the test was administered in spoken Italian, deaf children provided 24% of the total correct answers in LIS. Thus in terms of TCV, their lexical skills may be considered no different from their hearing peers and higher with respect to hearing children matched for LA.

Children who received the test in LIS had a mean CA of 55 months (range: 38–69 months) and a mean LA of 33 months (range: 18–42 months). These children showed similar lexical production skills when compared with hearing peers and slightly higher skills with respect to children with the same LA. Similar to the children who received the test in spoken Italian, the children who received the test in LIS produced some correct answers in spoken Italian (representing 3% of overall correct answers). We can assume that a code-switching strategy from spoken Italian to LIS and vice versa could help children to find the meaning they want to express. In relation to occurrences of code-blending, both groups of children produced more than one-third of correct answers simultaneously in both languages (37% for the group who received the test in spoken Italian, 34% for the group who received the test in LIS).

These results show that whether deaf bimodal bilingual children are evaluated taking into account both languages, in terms of their total conceptual vocabulary, their lexical skills are within normal limits with respect to monolingual hearing peers. Furthermore, these data indicate that the deaf bimodal bilinguals who participated in this study do not show a definite preference for one or the other language in responding to test materials. Correct answers often involved both signs and words (i.e., more than 30% of correct answers were code-blends). Overall results showed that children tended to shift from one language to the other in a very flexible way, regardless of the language in which they were being assessed. These data support the idea that lexical competencies and communicative modalities of deaf bimodal bilingual children reflect the flexibility that their own parents, educators, and peers show in everyday communication by continuously alternating and combining spoken Italian and Italian Sign Language, sometimes in the form of code-blends (Emmorey et al., 2012; Pizzuto, 2002).

### Study 3: Bimodal Bilingualism and Cochlear Implants: A Longitudinal Study

The relationship between LIS and spoken Italian was also investigated in a recent study on early phases of language development in one deaf child of hearing parents who had received a cochlear implant at the age of 2 years and 6 months (Rinaldi & Caselli, 2014; Rinaldi, Di Renzo, Massoni, & Caselli, 2012). Since the diagnosis of hearing loss at 1 year of age, the child was exposed to both LIS and spoken Italian in a bilingual environment. The child was followed longitudinally from age 2 years and 6 months to 5 years and 1 month.

This study focused on lexical comprehension and production and also on morphosyntactic comprehension, something that is particularly difficult for deaf children, even those who have a CI (Caselli et al., 2012). Different tests were used according to the chronological age of the child. Lexical comprehension and production were assessed using the Italian version of the MacArthur-Bates CDI (Rinaldi & Caselli, 2009), Picture Naming Game (Bello et al., 2012), Boston Naming Test (Riva, Nichelli, & Devoti, 2000); and Peabody Picture Vocabulary Test (Stella, Pizzoli, & Tressoldi, 2000). Morphosyntactic comprehension was assessed using the Morphosyntactic Comprehension Test (Rustioni, Metz, & Lancaster, 2007). The scoring of lexical production considered both languages (i.e., spoken Italian and LIS) and the resulting total conceptual vocabularies (TCVs) were similar to the results of Study 1, described previously. Under special consideration in this study were the rate of vocabulary growth (in relation to spoken Italian) and the relationship between the two languages/modalities (in regard to time elapsed from CI activation).

Results showed that when both languages (TCV) were considered, the child's lexical skills were within normal limits with respect to his monolingual hearing peers. For the period of time covered by this data, growth in lexical comprehension and production of language in comparison with spoken Italian was very similar to that showed by the child's hearing peers. Nevertheless, although the child's pace in development was close to that of his hearing peers, a developmental gap remained. The child's skills in lexical comprehension were at the lower limit of the normal range, while in morphosyntactic comprehension and in lexical production his skills were at the same level in comparison to monolingual hearing peers.

A sign language dominance was evident before CI activation but later (i.e., 5–10 months after CI activation), the child began to increase the lexical repertoire in spoken Italian even if the words were always produced together with the corresponding signs. Finally, after about 18 months of CI use, the child began to differentiate more effectively between the two languages and their contexts of use, with words being produced without the corresponding signs. It is worthy of note that bimodal productions were, however, still frequently present, particularly when test difficulty increased. At this developmental stage, sign language may play an important role in allowing the child to talk about ideas and concepts that he is not yet able to express clearly in spoken

Italian, opening a window on new landscapes of learning in spoken language. In sum, not only did early acquisition of sign language not hinder the acquisition of spoken language for this child with a CI, but also the former provided a scaffolded acquisition of the latter (Walker & Tomblin, Chapter 6 of this volume).

## CONCLUDING REMARKS AND FUTURE CHALLENGES

In this chapter we have discussed theoretical and methodological issues that need to be addressed in the study of bimodal bilingualism in deaf children, particularly in the Italian context. The acquisition and use of both spoken Italian and LIS by deaf Italian children is fundamental for building their self-identity, as members of both the Deaf community and of the larger Italian community. This kind of bilingualism could allow deaf children and adults to move between one culture and language and the other, depending on the different contexts and the different people involved.

In recent years, the maintenance of bimodal bilingualism among Italian deaf children has become increasingly difficult. The families of the majority of deaf children receiving a CI early in life are discouraged from exposing their children to LIS and are dissuaded from pursuing a bimodal bilingual form of education. The research discussed here indicates that, on the contrary, early bimodal bilingualism is crucial for deaf children for a scaffolded development of their cognitive and communicative skills, and for promoting language acquisition processes across modalities. A recent study on Italian deaf children between 6 and 14 years of age has shown that the school environment influences linguistic and cognitive skills more than do other factors such as the hearing status of parents and/or the age of first exposure to LIS. In fact, deaf children attending a school with a bimodal bilingual curriculum for both the deaf and hearing pupils performed significantly better in several tasks assessing linguistic abilities in LIS, compared to a group of signing deaf children attending other types of schools (Tomasuolo et al., 2013). In this study, deaf children attending the bilingual school also performed better in some linguistic tasks assessing LIS in comparison to hearing peers performing the same tasks in spoken Italian.

Unfortunately, research on the long-term outcome of bimodal bilingual education received by Italian children is still scarce (Marschark & Lee, Chapter 9 of this volume). In the previous section, we reviewed the few existing studies conducted on early stages of language acquisition in both languages (spoken Italian and LIS), but no studies to date have been conducted on older Italian children or adolescents who have been exposed to both languages early in life, taking into account their linguistic competence in both languages. What the existing studies have shown is that reliable assessment of the child's sign language and spoken/written linguistic abilities, as well as of the relationship between the two languages, poses several methodological challenges for both research and practice. Studies of the structures, acquisition, and use of sign language are very few, and normative data are not widely available; thus the development of tests is very difficult. To the best of our knowledge, standardized tools to evaluate bimodal bilingual deaf children's development do not currently exist. Importantly, methodologies that allow consideration of very specific linguistic factors, which also have been poorly or not at all explored in previous studies, must be defined. In particular, we believe that adequate direct and indirect tools to evaluate comprehension abilities are needed, as these assessment tools are still scarce for both sign language and spoken/written language.

Another relevant methodological issue is the limited possibility for analysis of linguistic structures of sign languages and of their acquisition and mastery. The absence of a reliable means for representing linguistic forms of sign languages could also lead to improper analysis, in particular in relation to issues such as segmentation and relevance of features (Petitta, Di Renzo, Chiari & Rossini, 2013). Furthermore, the linguistic assessment of the bimodal bilingual deaf child must be integrated with information, collected through interviews with family members, about the child's linguistic environment. Linguistic environment information, such as parents' beliefs about bilingualism, the contexts in which each language is used, together with the age at which the child was first exposed to each language and the amount of input received in each language, may aid in understanding processes underlying the acquisition and development of sign languages.

We believe that this type of integrated language assessment in which each language is evaluated and linguistic background is investigated may be conducted only by building an effective working team that includes both deaf and hearing researchers as well as parents. Deaf professionals are absolutely necessary not only for data collection and transcription, but also in all research phases, from the development of tools, which take into account sign language acquisition processes, to the interpretation of results.

Finally, the presence of deaf professionals during the child's evaluation may have a positive impact on the attitudes of both deaf and hearing parents. Working together with a team that includes deaf and hearing professionals could offer parents a direct experience of integration in which deaf adults are recognized and respected as having an important and specific professional role. Indeed, their participation in the assessment may allow the parents to consider not only their child's weaknesses (as a consequence of the hearing loss), but also their child's strengths and potentialities. This experience may improve parents' acceptance of and adjustment to the child's deafness, as well as their future expectations regarding their child's achievement. As a result, parents may be willing to provide their deaf children with the opportunity to acquire two languages and to learn about two cultures, thus allowing them to become bilingual and bicultural adults (Grosjean, 2010). This opportunity becomes feasible, however, only if adequate educational and social services are provided. Italian deaf students have only recently had the opportunity to attend university and/or professional courses with an interpreting service in LIS and to receive degrees as psychologists, teachers, or teacher assistants. On the positive side, the Italian Deaf community, during the past two years, has requested official recognition for Italian Sign Language and bimodal bilingual education (http://www.lissubito.com)—a testimony to an increasing and important empowerment.

## ACKNOWLEDGMENTS

This work was partially funded by the Nando Peretti Foundation under the grant agreement no. 2012/34 to Maria Cristina Caselli, by the Education, Audiovisual and Culture Executive Agency, "SignMET" (543264-LLP-1-2013-1-IT-KA2-KA2MP) to Pasquale Rinaldi and by Fondazione Cassa di Risparmio di Trento e Rovereto. We wish to thank Laura Sparaci and Penny Boyes Braem for their insightful comments.

## NOTE

[1] SI and SSI both rely on spoken Italian words simultaneously accompanied by the corresponding LIS signs. In addition, SSI uses fingerspelling for Italian function words.

## REFERENCES

Anderson, D., & Reilly, J. (2002). The MacArthur Communicative Development Inventory: Normative data for American Sign Language. *Journal of Deaf Studies and Deaf Education, 7*, 83–119.

Ardito, B., Caselli, M. C., Vecchietti, A., & Volterra, V. (2008). Deaf and hearing children: Reading together in Preschool. In C. Plaza-Pust, & E. Morales-López (Eds.), *Sign Bilingualism: Language development, interaction, and maintenance in sign language contact situations* (pp. 137–164). Amsterdam; Philadelphia: John Benjamins Publishing.

Baker A., & van den Bogaerde B. (2008). Code-mixing in signs and words in input to and output from children. In C. Plaza-Pust, & E. Morales-López (Eds.), *Sign Bilingualism: Language development, interaction, and maintenance in sign language contact situations*, (pp. 1–27). Amsterdam; Philadelphia: John Benjamins Publishing.

Bello, A., Giannantoni, P., Pettenati, P., Stefanini, S., & Caselli, M. C. (2012). Assessing lexicon: Validation and developmental data of the Picture Naming Game (PiNG), a new picture naming task for toddlers. *International Journal of Language and Communication Disorders, 47*, 589–602.

Capirci, O., Pirchio, S., & Soldani, R. (2007). Interazione tra genitori e figli sordi in una situazione di gioco: analisi delle modalità e delle funzioni comunicative [Parents-deaf child interactions during play: Analysis of modalities and of communicative functions]. *Psicologia Clinica dello Sviluppo, 11*, 407–428.

Caselli, M. C. (1994). Communicative gestures and first words. In V. Volterra, & C. Ertings (Eds.), *From gesture to language in hearing and deaf children* (pp. 56–68). Washington, DC: Gallaudet University Press.

Caselli, M. C., & Corazza, S. (Eds.) (1997). *LIS: Studi, esperienze e ricerche sulla lingua dei segni in Italia* [LIS: Studies, practices and research on Sign Language in Italy]. Pisa, Italy: Edizioni del Cerro.

Caselli, M. C., Maragna, S., & Volterra, V. (2006). *Linguaggio e sordità: Gesti, segni e parole nello sviluppo e nell'educazione* [Language and deafness: Gestures, signs and words in development and education]. Bologna, Italy: Il Mulino.

Caselli, M. C., Rinaldi, P., Varuzza, C., Giuliani, A., & Burdo, S. (2012). Cochlear implant in the second year of life: Lexical and grammatical outcomes. *Journal of Speech Language and Hearing Research, 55*, 382–394.

Caselli, M. C., & Volterra, V. (2003). Linguaggio e Cognizione: Uno studio su bambini sordi di età prescolare [Cognition and language: A study of deaf preschoolers]. In P. Corsano (a cura di), *Processi di Sviluppo nel ciclo di vita: Saggi in onore di Marta Montanini Manfredi* [Developmental processes in the lifespan: Essay in honor of Marta Montanini Manfredi] (pp. 487–525). Milan, Italy: Edizioni Unicopli.

Chilosi, A. M., & Cipriani, P. (1995). TCGB. *Test di comprensione grammaticale per bambini* [Grammar Comprehension Test for Children]. Tirrenia, Italy: Edizioni del Cerro.

Cormier, K., Schembri, A., Vinson, D., & Orfanidou, E. (2012). First language acquisition differs from second language acquisition in prelingually deaf signers: Evidence from sensitivity to grammaticality judgment in British Sign Language. *Cognition, 124*, 50–65.

de Houwer, A. (2007). Parental language input patterns and children's bilingual use. *Applied Psycholinguistics, 28*, 411–424.

Donati, C., & Branchini, C. (2013). Challenging linearization: Simultaneous mixing in the production of bimodal bilinguals. In T. Biberauer & I. Roberts (Eds.), *Challenges to linearization* (pp. 93–128). Berlin, Germany: Mouton de Gruyter.

Dunn, L. M., & Dunn, L. M. (1981). *Peabody Picture Vocabulary Test-Revised.* Circle Pines, MN: American Guidance Service.

Emmorey, K., Borinstein, H. B., & Thompson, R. (2005). Bimodal bilingualism: Code-blending between spoken English and American Sign Language. In J. Cohen, K. McAlister, K. Rolstad, & J. MacSwan (Eds.), *Proceedings of the 4th International Symposium on Bilingualism* (pp. 663–673). Somerville, MA: Cascadilla Press.

Emmorey, K., Petrich, J. A. F., & Gollan, T. H. (2012). Bilingual processing of ASL-English code-blends: The consequence of accessing two lexical representations simultaneously. *Journal of Memory and Language, 67*, 199–210.

Fabbretti, D., & Tomasuolo, E. (2006). *Scrittura e sordità* [Written language and deafness]. Rome: Carocci.

Fenson, L., Marchman, V., Thal, D., Dale, P., Reznick, J. S., & Bates, E. (2007). *MacArthur Communicative Development Inventories: User's guide and technical manual second edition*. Baltimore, MD: Brookes.

Gathercole, V. C. M., & Thomas, E. M. (2009). Bilingual first-language development: Dominant language takeover, threatened minority language take-up. *Bilingualism: Language and Cognition, 12,* 213–237.

Genesee, F., Nicoladis, E., & Paradis, J. (1995). Language differentiation in early bilingual development. *Journal of Child Language, 22,* 611–631.

Geraci, C. (2012). Language policy and planning: The case of Italian Sign Language. *Sign Language Studies, 12,* 494–518.

Grosjean, F. (1985). The bilingual as a competent but specific speaker-hearer. *Journal of Multilingual and Multicultural Development, 6,* 467–477.

Grosjean, F. (2010). Bilingualism, biculturalism, and deafness. *International Journal of Bilingual Education and Bilingualism, 13,* 133–145.

Gutierrez-Clellen, F. V., & Kreiter, J. (2003). Understanding child bilingual acquisition using parent and teacher reports. *Applied Psycholinguistics, 24,* 267–288.

Harris, M. (1992). *Language experience and early language development: From input to uptake.* Hove, UK: Lawrence Erlbaum.

Harris, M., Clibbens, J., Chasin, J., & Tibbitts, R. (1989). The social context of early sign language development. *First Language, 9,* 81–97.

Haug, T. (2011). Approaching sign language test construction: Adaptation of the German Sign Language Receptive Skills Test. *Journal of Deaf Studies and Deaf Education, 16,* 343–361.

Haug, T., & Mann, W. (2008). Adapting tests of sign language assessment for other sign languages: A review of linguistic, cultural, and psychometric problems. *Journal of Deaf Studies and Deaf Education, 13,* 138–147.

Humphries, T., Kushalnagar, P., Mathur, G., Napoli, D. J., Padden, C., Rathmann, C., & Smith, S. (2012). Language acquisition for deaf children: Reducing the harms of zero tolerance to the use of alternative approaches. *Harm Reduction Journal, 9,* 16.

Kanto, L., Huttunen, K., & Laakso, M. L. (2013). Relationship between the linguistic environments and early bilingual language development of hearing children in Deaf-parented families. *Journal of Deaf Studies and Deaf Education, 18,* 242–260.

Knoors, H., & Marschark, M. (2012). Language planning for the 21st century: Revisiting bilingual language policy for deaf children. *Journal of Deaf Studies and Deaf Education, 17,* 291–305.

Kohnert, K. (2008). *Language disorders in bilingual children and adults.* San Diego, CA: Plural.

Kohnert, K. (2010). Bilingual children with primary language impairment: Issues, evidence and implications for clinical actions. *Journal of Communication Disorders, 43,* 465–474.

Kohnert, K., & Bates, E. (2002). Balancing bilinguals II: Lexical comprehension and cognitive processing in children learning Spanish and English. *Journal of Speech, Language, and Hearing Research, 45,* 347–359.

Kyle, J., Ackerman, J., & Woll, B. (1987). Early motherinfant interactions: Language and prelanguage in deaf families. In P. Griffiths, A. Mills, & J. Local (Eds.), *Proceedings of the Child Language Seminar.* York, UK: University of York.

Maragna, S., & Marziale, B. (2012). *I diritti dei sordi. Uno strumento di orientamento per la famiglia e gli operatori: Educazione, integrazione e servizi* [The right of the Deaf: A tool for families and professionals: Education, inclusion and services]. Milan, Italy: Franco Angeli.

Meristo, M., Falkman, K. W., Hjelmquist, E., Tedoldi, M., Surian, L., & Siegal, M. (2007). Language access and theory of mind reasoning: Evidence from deaf children in bilingual and oralist environments. *Developmental Psychology, 43,* 1156–1169.

Miller, M. (2008). Sign iconicity and receptive vocabulary testing. *American Annals of the Deaf, 152,* 441–449.

Morgan, G., & Woll, B. (2002). Introduction. In G. Morgan, & B. Woll (Eds.), *Directions in sign language acquisition* (pp. xi–xx). Amsterdam; Philadelphia: John Benjamins Publishing.

Newport, E. L., & Meier, R. P. (1985). The acquisition of American Sign Language. In D. I. Slobin (Eds.), *The cross-linguistic study of language acquisition.* Hillsdale, NJ: Erlbaum.

Paradis, J., Emmerzael, K., & Duncan, T. S. (2010). Assessment of English language learners: Using parent report on first language development. *Journal of Communication Disorders, 43,* 474–497.

Pearson, B. (2007). Social factors in childhood bilingualism in the United States. *Applied Psycholinguistics, 28,* 399–410.

Pearson, B. Z., Fernandez, S. C., Lewedeg, V., & Oller, D. K (1997). The relation of input factors to lexical learning by bilingual toddlers. *Applied Psycholinguistics, 18,* 41–58.

Pearson, B. Z., Fernandez, S. C., & Oller, D. K. (1993). Lexical development in bilingual infants and toddlers: Comparison to monolingual norms. *Language Learning, 43,* 93–120.

Percy-Smith, L., Cayé-Thomasen, P., Breinegaard, N., & Jensen, J. H. (2010). Parental mode of communication is essential for speech and language outcomes in cochlear implanted children. *Acta Otolaryngology, 130,* 708–715.

Petitta, G., Di Renzo, A., Chiari, I., & Rossini, P. (2013). Sign language representation: New approaches to the study of Italian Sign Language (LIS). In L. Meurant, A. Sinte, M. Van Herreweghe, & M. Vermeerbergen (Eds.), *Sign language research, uses and practices: Crossing views on theoretical and applied sign language linguistics* (pp. 137–158). Berlin; New York: Mouton De Gruyter-Ishara Press.

Petitto, L. A., Katerelos, M., Levy, B., Gauna, K., Tétrault, K., & Ferraro, V. (2001). Bilingual signed and spoken language acquisition from birth: Implications for mechanisms underlying early bilingual language acquisition. *Journal of Child Language, 28,* 453–496.

Pettenati, P., Vacchini, D., Stefanini, S., & Caselli, M. C. (2011). Parole e Frasi nel primo vocabolario di bambini bilingui Italiano-Spagnolo [Words and sentences in early vocabulary of Italian-Spanish bilingual children]. *Rivista di Psicolinguistica Applicata [Journal of Applied Psicholinguistics], 11,* 49–67.

Pinto, M. A., & Volterra, V. (2008). Editoriale [Editorial]. In M. A. Pinto, & V. Volterra (Eds.), Bilinguismo lingue dei segni/Lingue vocali: Aspetti educativi e psicolinguistici [Sign languages/spoken languages bilingualism: Educational and psycholinguistic issues]. *Rivista di Psicolinguistica Applicata [Journal of Applied Psycholinguistics], 8,* 9–19.

Pizzuto, E. (2002). The development of Italian Sign Language (LIS) in deaf preschoolers. In G. Morgan, & B. Woll (Eds.), *Directions in sign language acquisition* (pp. 77–114). Amsterdam; Philadelphia: John Benjamins Publishing.

Pizzuto, E., Ardito, B., Caselli, M. C., & Volterra, V. (2001). Cognition and language in Italian deaf preschoolers of deaf and hearing families. In M. D. Clark,

M. Marschark, & M. Karchmer (Eds.), *Cognition, context and deafness* (pp. 49–70). Washington, DC: Gallaudet University Press.

Pizzuto, E., Caselli, M. C., Ardito, B., Osella, T. Albertoni, A., Santarelli, B., & Cafasso, R. (1998). Assessing cognitive, relational, and language abilities of deaf preschoolers in italy. In A. Weisel (Ed.), *Issues unresolved: New perspectives on language and deaf education* (pp. 41–52). Washington, DC: Gallaudet University Press.

Rinaldi, P. (2008). Competenze lessicali di bambini sordi bilingui in età prescolare [Lexical competencies of deaf bilingual preschoolers]. *Rivista di Psicolinguistica Applicata [Journal of Applied Psycholinguistics], 8*, 93–107.

Rinaldi, P., & Caselli, M. C. (2009). Lexical and grammatical abilities in deaf Italian preschoolers: The role of duration of formal language experience. *Journal of Deaf Studies and Deaf Education, 14*, 63–75.

Rinaldi, P., & Caselli, M. C. (2014). Language development in a bimodal bilingual child with cochlear implant: A longitudinal study. *Bilingualism: Language and Cognition.* doi:10.1017/S1366728913000849

Rinaldi, P., Caselli, M. C., Di Renzo, A., Gulli, T., & Volterra, V. (2014). Sign vocabulary in deaf toddlers exposed to Sign Language since birth. *Journal of Deaf Studies and Deaf Education.* doi: 10.1093/deafed/enu007

Rinaldi, P., Di Renzo, A., Massoni, P., & Caselli, M. C. (2012). Lingua dei segni e impianto cocleare: Un incontro possibile [Sign language and cochlear implant: Finding harmony] *Rivista di Psicolinguistica Applicata [Journal of Applied Psycholinguistics], 12*, 47–64.

Riva, D., Nichelli, F., & Devoti, M. (2000). Developmental aspects of verbal fluency and confrontation naming in children. *Brain and Language, 7*, 267–284.

Roid, G. H., & Miller, L. J. (1997). *Leiter International Performance Scale—Revised.* Florence, Italy: Giunti Organizzazioni Speciali.

Russo Cardona, T., & Volterra, V. (2007). *Le lingue dei segni: Storia e Semiotica* [Sign languages: History and semiotics]. Rome, Italy: Carocci.

Rustioni Metz Lancaster, D. (2007). *Test di Comprensione Morfosintattica* [Grammar Comprehension Test]. Florence, Italy: Giunti Organizzazioni Speciali.

Stella, G., Pizzoli, C., & Tressoldi, P. E. (2000). *Peabody—R. Test di vocabolario recettivo* [Peabody-R. Receptive vocabulary test]. Turin, Italy: Omega.

Swisher, V. (2000). Learning to converse: How deaf mothers support the development of attention and conversational skills in their young deaf children. In P. Spencer, C. J. Erting, & M. Marschark (Eds.), *The deaf child in the family and at school* (pp. 21–40). Mahwah, NJ: Lawrence Erlbaum Associates.

Teruggi, L. A. (Eds.) (2003). *Una Scuola, due lingue: L'esperienza di bilinguismo della scuola dell'Infanzia ed Elementare di Cossato* [One school, two languages: Bilingual experience in Cossato's kindergarten and primary school]. Milan, Italy: Franco Angeli.

Tomasuolo, E., Fellini, L., Di Renzo, A., & Volterra, V. (2010). Assessing lexical production in deaf signing children with the Boston naming test. *Language, Interaction and Acquisition, 1*, 110–128.

Tomasuolo, E., Valeri, G., Di Renzo, A., Pasqualetti, P., & Volterra, V. (2013). Deaf children attending different school environments: Sign Language abilities and theory of mind. *Journal of Deaf Studies and Deaf Education, 18*, 12–29.

van den Bogaerde, B. (2000). *Input and interaction in deaf families.* Unpublished doctoral dissertation, University of Amsterdam. Utrecht: LOT. http://dare.uva.nl/record/86454.

Volterra, V. (Eds.) (1987). *La lingua italiana dei segni* [Italian Sign Language]. Bologna, Italy: Il Mulino.

Volterra, V., Caselli, M. C., & Pizzuto, E. (2000). Language, cognition and deafness. *Seminars in Hearing, 21*, 343–358.

Woolfe, T., Herman, R., Roy, P., & Woll, B. (2010). Early vocabulary development in deaf native signers: A British Sign Language adaptation of the communicative development inventories. *Journal of Child Psychology and Psychiatry, 51*, 322–331.

# 4

# Bimodal Bilingual Cross-Language Interaction

## *Pieces of the Puzzle*

Ellen Ormel and Marcel Giezen

It has been well established that persons with two or more spoken languages[1] activate the various languages they are familiar with when producing or comprehending one of them. In other words, language processing by spoken language bilinguals seems to be always influenced by the different languages they know. This cross-language interaction, also referred to as cross-language activation or language co-activation, is observed for bilinguals who learned both languages from birth as well as bilinguals who learned one of the languages at a later age, and for both adults and children.

Recently, researchers have started to investigate whether similar patterns of cross-language interaction occur for bilinguals fluent in a sign language and a spoken language—languages that use different articulatory and perceptual mechanisms and have non-overlapping phonological systems. The term *bimodal bilingualism* has been introduced for this unique type of bilingualism. Similar to bilinguals in two spoken languages, or *unimodal* bilinguals,[2] bimodal bilinguals may be exposed to both languages from birth or, alternatively, they become familiar with one of the languages at a later age (e.g., to become an interpreter).

Bimodal bilingual language users may either be deaf or hearing. In contrast to many deaf children, hearing children who grow up in deaf families often become skilled in both a sign language and a spoken language from an early age. Although sign language is often the primary language acquired at home, the child usually picks up the spoken language from the environment, for example, at day care and from other family members. For deaf children, the linguistic environment is more complex, especially for those with hearing parents. Deaf children with hearing parents show a more variable range of skills in both languages compared to deaf children with deaf parents, largely depending on the language(s) that parents prefer to adopt in raising their deaf child, their own language use, and the degree of access the child has to the speech signal. In families with hearing parents, spoken language is generally used on a regular basis, at least to some extent among parents and hearing siblings. Most hearing parents acquire signing skills only after discovering the hearing loss of their child. As a consequence, large variation can be observed in their signing proficiency and thus also in the degree of sign exposure available to deaf children. Moreover, for an increasing number of deaf children with cochlear implants, sign language is introduced only later in their lives, or perhaps not at all. For deaf children from deaf families, by contrast, sign language is usually the primary language at home. Spoken language may to varying degrees also be present in the child's immediate environment.

For each of these examples of bimodal bilinguals, who differ in onsets of acquisition and degrees of fluencies in each of their languages, it is important to know whether they experience cross-language interaction. One of the main reasons that this is important is that bilingual language use in spoken language bilinguals affects not only language processing, but also processing in non-linguistic domains. A growing body of research has suggested that bilingualism functions as a form of brain exercise and can result in selective advantages in cognitive functioning, for example, in inhibitory control, goal monitoring, and task-switching abilities. Although the exact nature and scope of "bilingual advantages" in cognitive control are still unclear, it is often assumed that the cross-language activation and language selection that comes with being bilingual are responsible for these advantages. In the past couple of years, several studies have investigated cross-language interaction for bimodal bilinguals. Their various results suggest that cross-language activation is not unique to unimodal bilinguals, but also characterizes bimodal bilingual language processing. Research on possible bilingual advantages in cognitive control for bimodal bilinguals has started only recently.

In this chapter, a comprehensive overview is provided of past and ongoing research in bimodal bilingual language processing, and some of its missing pieces are identified. In the first section of the chapter, studies of cross-language interaction with bimodal bilingual adults and children are reviewed; in the second section, effects of bimodal bilingualism on non-linguistic cognitive control abilities are discussed; in the third section, effects of age of acquisition and language proficiency on patterns of cross-language interaction in bimodal bilinguals are addressed. A discussion of some of the educational implications of the reviewed research concludes the chapter.

## BILINGUAL CROSS-LANGUAGE INTERACTION

Before studies of *cross-language activation* are discussed, it is important to briefly mention the other ways in which two languages can interact. For instance, studies of *code-mixing* and *code-blending*, the mixing of elements from two languages together in the production of one utterance, are not reviewed in this chapter. Although code-mixing and code-blending are very explicit and visible forms of interaction between two languages, they are rather different from cross-language activation, where one language affects the processing of another language in a more implicit and less visible manner.

Studies on cross-linguistic *transfer* are also not discussed. Cross-linguistic transfer is often defined as the structural influence of one language on another, typically influence from the first language (L1) on production in the second language (L2) at the level of phonology, morphology, or syntax (for a review, see, e.g., Meisel, 2004). For studies on code-mixing, code-blending, and transfer between a spoken and a sign language by bimodal bilingual children and adults, readers are referred to other sources (e.g., Baker & Van den Bogaerde, 2008; Emmorey, Borinstein, Thompson, & Gollan, 2008; Petitto et al., 2001; de Quadros, Lillo-Martin, & Chen Pichler, 2010; Van den Bogaerde & Baker, 2006; see also Plaza-Pust, Chapter 2 of this volume). Finally, studies on cross-language associations are not included. These studies examine, for instance, correlations between L1 and L2 proficiency in different language domains (e.g., Melby-Lervåg & Lervåg, 2011), or correlations between lexical-grammatical development in both languages in simultaneous bilingual children (e.g., Parra, Hoff, & Core, 2011). Comparable research with deaf children has mainly focused on the role of signing proficiency in reading acquisition (e.g., Hermans, Knoors, Ormel, & Verhoeven, 2008; Hermans, Ormel, Knoors, & Verhoeven, 2008; Hermans, Ormel, & Knoors, 2010; Hoffmeister, 2000; Strong & Prinz, 1997), although a few recent studies have investigated cross-language associations in phonological and lexical development in children with cochlear implants (Giezen, Baker, & Escudero, 2014; Müller de Quadros, Cruz, Pizzio, Chen-Pichler, & Lillo-Martin, 2013; Seal et al., 2011; see also Rinaldi, Caselli, Onofrio, and Volterra, Chapter 3 of this volume, and Pérez Martin, Valmaseda Balanzategui, and Morgan, Chapter 15 of this volume).

**Cross-Language Interaction in Unimodal Bilingual Adults**

Cross-language activation, the activation of one language during production or comprehension of the other language, is a very robust characteristic of unimodal bilingual language processing. The language user is usually not aware of this co-activation. Cross-language activation between two spoken languages is often assumed to result from similar sounding words between the two languages. For example, for a Spanish-English bilingual, hearing the English word *pear* initially not only automatically activates similar sounding English words such as *pencil*, but also similar sounding Spanish words, such as *perro* ("dog"). In one of the first studies on lexical activation across different languages, Dutch-English bilinguals named pictures in English while they were presented with auditory English distractor words (Hermans, Bongaerts, De Bot, & Schreuder, 1998). Compared to unrelated distractor words, participants were slower to respond when the distractor word was phonologically related to the Dutch translation of the English word they had to produce (e.g., a picture of a mountain presented with the distractor word *bench*, which is phonologically related to the Dutch translation of "mountain", *berg*), compared to unrelated distractor words. The authors interpreted this result as evidence that the participants co-activated the Dutch names of the pictures.

In another seminal study, Marian and Spivey (2003) found that cross-language activation also occurs during language comprehension. In this study, Russian-English bilinguals listened to English words while looking at a display with four pictures and their eye movements were monitored. In addition to a picture of the English target word, some of the displays contained a picture of a cross-language phonological competitor (e.g., a picture of a *stamp*, which translates as *marka* in Russian, when the English target word was *marker*). The bilingual participants looked relatively more at the picture of the cross-language phonological competitor than at unrelated pictures, suggesting that they co-activated the Russian names of the pictures during the task. Other studies have, for instance, shown that spoken language bilinguals process cognate words (similar in form and meaning across the two languages) differently from non-cognate words (different in form and meaning across the two languages), which has also been used as evidence for cross-language activation (e.g., Yudes, Macizo, & Bajo, 2010).

Cross-language activation is exhibited not only by bilinguals who grew up in families where more than one language was spoken on a regular basis, that is, simultaneous bilinguals, but also by bilinguals who learned a second spoken language later in life, that is, sequential bilinguals (for reviews, see e.g., Dijkstra & Van Heuven, 2002; Kroll, Bogulski, & McClain, 2012). In fact, it has been found that adult learners co-activate their L1 when processing words or sentences in their L2 during the initial stages of L2 acquisition. Cross-language activation in the opposite direction, that is, activation of the L2 during L1 processing, is only observed with increased proficiency in the L2 (Van Hell & Tanner, 2012). Simply stated, the stronger language interferes more with the weaker language than the other way around. In simultaneous bilinguals, similarly, processing in the weaker, non-dominant language (e.g., a minority language) is more affected by the stronger, dominant language (e.g., the majority language spoken by the surrounding community) than the other way around.

## Cross-Language Interaction in Bimodal Bilingual Adults

In recent years, several studies have provided evidence for cross-language activation in diverse groups of bimodal bilingual adults, both deaf and hearing, and both simultaneous and sequential learners. First of all, Grote and Linz (2003) found, to their surprise, that hearing bimodal bilingual adults showed effects of activation of sign iconicity while comprehending written words. In their study, participants had to decide whether pairs of pictures and written words were semantically related or not. Crucially, while participants were instructed to respond to pictures and written words, their responses indicated that iconic information of the corresponding sign translation equivalents affected their decision-making. More recently, Morford, Wilkinson, Villwock, Piñar, and Kroll (2011) observed that phonological overlap between sign translation equivalents affected semantic judgments to written English word pairs by deaf American Sign Language (ASL)-English bilingual adults (see also Kubus, Villwock, Morford, & Rathmann, 2014). For example, participants were quicker to decide that two English words were semantically related (e.g., *apple* and *onion*) when their ASL sign translation equivalents overlapped in sign phonology (the ASL signs APPLE and ONION differ in location features, but overlap in all other phonological features). Similar to the results by Grote and Linz, the finding by Morford and colleagues that responses to written words are affected by form relationships between their sign translation equivalents provides evidence that deaf bimodal bilinguals co-activate signs during written word processing.

In a related study, Shook and Marian (2012) examined co-activation of signs during *spoken* word comprehension instead of written word comprehension in an eye-tracking study with simultaneous and sequential hearing ASL-English bilingual adults. Participants were presented with spoken words while looking at displays with four pictures, which consisted of the target picture (that matched the spoken word) and three distractor pictures, while their eye movements were monitored. Some of the displays included a picture of a cross-language phonological competitor, for example a picture of "paper" in a trial with the English target word *cheese*. Although *cheese* and *paper* are phonologically unrelated in English, the ASL signs for CHEESE and PAPER share the same location and handshape features and differ only in movement features. When they heard the word *cheese*, ASL-English bilinguals looked relatively more at the picture of "paper" than the other two distractor pictures, suggesting that they were co-activating ASL signs during the experiment.

Giezen and Emmorey (2013) similarly investigated cross-language activation during spoken word recognition using a picture-naming task. Simultaneous and sequential hearing ASL-English bilingual adults named pictures in ASL while English auditory distractor words were presented, some of which had sign translations that were phonologically related to the target sign they had to produce (e.g., a picture of "chair" with the distractor word *train*; the ASL signs for TRAIN and CHAIR overlap in handshape and location features, but differ in movement features). Compared to unrelated distractor words, participants were faster in naming pictures in ASL when the distractor word was phonologically related in ASL to the target sign (the sign that matched the picture). This study thus shows that co-activation of sign translations when listening to spoken words affects sign production.

All the studies of cross-language activation in bimodal bilinguals discussed so far investigated sign activation during written or spoken word processing. Ormel and colleagues (Ormel, Hermans, Van der Loop, Hermes, & Van Hell, in preparation; Van Hell, Ormel, Van der Loop, & Hermans, 2009) have provided the first piece of evidence of co-activation in the reverse direction, that is, spoken word activation during sign processing. In their study, Dutch sign language interpreters in training were shown NGT (*Nederlandse Gebarentaal*, Sign Language of the Netherlands) signs in a sign-picture verification task and were asked to indicate whether the sign and picture referred to the same concept or not. Phonological overlap in the rhymes of the Dutch translation equivalents of the NGT signs affected the time needed to make verification judgments, showing that participants co-activated spoken Dutch translations when processing the signs in the experiment. Importantly, the researchers controlled for the information about the Dutch words that might be extracted from the mouthings in the signs by having the participants complete one set of stimuli with display of the mouthings and one set without. Both stimuli sets revealed similar co-activation patterns. Hosemann, Altvater-Mackensen, Hermann, and Mani (2013) obtained similar preliminary results in a recent neurophysiological study with German deaf bimodal bilingual adults, in which sign sentences (as opposed to sign pairs) were presented and Event Related Potentials (ERP) were measured.

In summary, most studies thus far that have investigated cross-language activation between a spoken or written language and a sign language in deaf and hearing bimodal bilingual adults found evidence of co-activation (but see Hanson & Feldman, 1989, for an early study with deaf ASL-English bilinguals that failed to find such evidence). Despite these apparent similarities in cross-language interaction between unimodal and bimodal bilinguals adults, it nevertheless is very well possible that the underlying mechanisms of co-activation are different. For unimodal bilinguals, at least co-activation during language comprehension is generally assumed to result from segmental bottom-up activation of similar-sounding words across the two languages, which requires (partly) shared phonological systems between the two languages. Given that there is little to no shared phonological system between spoken and sign languages, cross-language activation in bimodal bilinguals cannot easily be explained through segmental bottom-up activation, and instead may rely more on top-down activation from the semantic or conceptual level (see Shook & Marian, 2009, for discussion).[3]

Furthermore, it is possible that the mechanisms for cross-language activation also partly differ between *hearing* and *deaf* bimodal bilinguals. Deaf bimodal bilinguals may have established strong direct connections between signs and orthographic information in their mental lexicon, for instance, if they (at least partly) learned to read through sign (see also Morford et al., 2011). Because of their full access to spoken language phonology, hearing bimodal bilinguals are unlikely to have established similar connections, and co-activation might therefore rely more strongly on semantic mediation (see also Shook & Marian, 2009). Only a handful of studies on cross-language activation in bimodal bilinguals adults have been published thus far. More studies are therefore clearly needed, especially studies that use different experimental paradigms to confirm the findings thus far. At the same time, studies that use the same experimental paradigm but with both deaf and hearing bimodal bilingual adults would be very welcome, in order to gain insight into similarities and differences in the underlying mechanisms of co-activation.

Finally, it is possible that cross-language interaction might develop differently in deaf and/or hearing bimodal bilingual children when compared to unimodal bilingual children, for instance, because of their more variable language acquisition context. This will be discussed in the next section.

**Cross-Language Interaction from a Developmental Perspective**

This section on cross-language interaction in bilingual children begins with an outline of what is known about the emergence of cross-language activation for unimodal bilingual children. Next, the only study thus far that has investigated cross-language activation for bimodal bilingual children will be discussed in some detail.

*Cross-Language Interaction in Children Learning Two Spoken Languages*

Similar to bilingual adults, an important distinction that needs to be made for bilingual children is between bilingual first language acquisition and (early) second language acquisition, that is, simultaneous and sequential bilingualism. For children who acquire two languages from birth, both languages develop relatively independently (for a review, see De Houwer, 2009). Children who are only exposed to the second language later in childhood already have the native language system in place and can therefore use their L1 knowledge in acquiring the L2. Although researchers once thought that the bilingual language system was undifferentiated in the early stages of language acquisition, it is now clear that children separate different languages in the input from very early on (Curtin, Byers-Heinlein, & Werker, 2011; De Houwer, 2005; Nicoladis & Genesee, 1997). In fact, Gervain and Werker (2013) recently showed that infants in bilingual environments use prosodic cues associated with different word orders to separate the two languages in the input as young as 7 months of age.

Given the abundance of studies on cross-language activation in bilingual adults, it is quite surprising that there are only a handful of studies with bilingual children, all relatively recent (e.g., Brenders, Van Hell, & Dijkstra, 2011; Jared, Cormier, Levy, & Wade-Wooley, 2012). Most of these studies looked at differences in how bilingual children process words that are similar in form and meaning between the two languages (cognates), compared to words that are different in form and meaning between the two languages (non-cognates). The findings from these studies have clearly shown that beginning and intermediate child L2 learners, as well as early simultaneous bilingual learners, show robust cross-language activation in the developing bilingual system, even as early as 2–3 years of age (Von Holzen & Mani, 2012). However, because of the children's relatively low levels of proficiency in the L2 in these studies, cross-language activation was found to be asymmetrical, that is, reliable in the direction from L1 to L2, but weaker or absent in the direction from L2 to L1. This parallels the findings for adult second language learners with relatively low levels of L2 proficiency (see the section on cross-language interaction in unimodal bilingual adults).

*Cross-Language Interaction in Children Learning a Spoken Language and a Sign Language*

As far as we know, only one study has specifically investigated cross-language activation in deaf children (Ormel, Hermans, Knoors, & Verhoeven, 2012), and no studies have yet been published on cross-language activation in hearing bimodal bilingual children. Ormel et al. (2012) used a word-picture verification paradigm and manipulated the phonological overlap between the sign translation equivalents of the written words and the pictures. The children in this study were 9- to 13-year-old deaf Dutch children who were learning spoken Dutch and NGT. Their task was to decide whether a written word and picture referred to the same concept or not by pressing one of two buttons. For instance, children read the printed word *dog* ("hond") and saw a picture of a *chair* ("stoel") and then had to press "no" (not the same concept). The signs DOG and CHAIR are phonologically related in NGT (i.e., they share location, orientation, and movement features, but differ in handshape features), but are not phonologically related in spoken Dutch. The children took longer and made more errors when deciding that the written word and picture did not refer to the same concept when the word and the picture were phonologically related through their sign translations (as in the *dog-chair* example), than when the word and picture were unrelated in either spoken Dutch or NGT, indicating co-activation of NGT signs during the experiment.

Ormel and colleagues (2012) proposed the model illustrated in Figure 4.1 to represent the process of written word recognition and co-activation of sign phonology in deaf children. In this model, once lexical orthography is activated for the purpose of written word recognition (e.g., recognizing the letter string d-o-g as the orthographical lexical representation *dog*), the sign translation equivalent of the activated written word is also automatically activated (i.e., the sign DOG), either through direct links between the sign and the lexical orthographical representation or through their shared semantic representation. Once the lexical sign is activated, activation feeds down to the composing sub-lexical sign elements (i.e., the specific handshape, movement, location, and orientation features). When this occurs, not only are the sub-lexical sign elements for the sign DOG activated, but other lexical signs that share one or more of those sub-lexical sign elements (i.e., its lexical neighbors) are activated as well (including the sign CHAIR, which shares location, movement, and orientation features with the sign DOG).

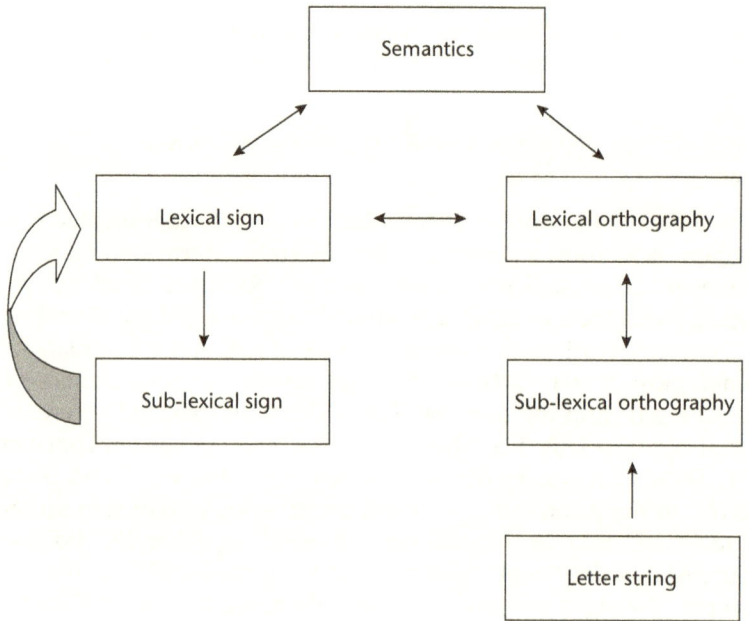

**Figure 4.1 Sign activation during visual word recognition by bilingual deaf children.**

Such lexical neighbors in the visual modality compete for recognition, similar to the lexical competition of phonologically similar words (e.g., *chair* and *champion*) during spoken word recognition (e.g., Magnuson, Dixon, Tanenhaus, & Aslin, 2007).

Although not too many generalizations can be made on the basis of just one study, the results appear to show that, similar to bimodal bilingual adults and unimodal bilingual children, deaf bimodal bilingual children co-activate their two languages. Nevertheless, a few important questions remain unanswered. For instance, like most studies on cross-language activation in adult bimodal bilinguals, this study looked at co-activation of signs during written word recognition, that is, activation of the stronger language during processing of the weaker language (see also Ormel, 2008). As we explained in the previous section on cross-language interaction in unimodal bilingual children, this is the direction for which the strongest effects are to be expected (i.e., co-activation of the stronger language during processing of the weaker language). It remains to be seen whether cross-language activation in the opposite direction, that is, spoken or written language activation during sign processing, can also be observed for deaf children.

Perhaps more important, the children in this study were 9 years of age and older and had been exposed to both spoken Dutch and NGT for several years. For unimodal bilingual children, there is evidence for cross-language activation at much younger ages, but we do not know whether this is also true for younger deaf children. Furthermore, NGT was considered the more dominant language for the children in this study and (written) Dutch the less dominant language. Formal exposure to both NGT and written Dutch started at the age of 4 years for these children, but many had attended preschools for deaf children where NGT was used. Potentially crucial factors for predicting cross-language activation for deaf children, such as age of acquisition, length of exposure, and relative proficiency in the sign language and written/spoken language, are unexplored as yet. This large gap in the bimodal bilingual literature will be addressed in more detail in the third section of this chapter. First, another important line of research in the study of (bimodal) bilingualism will be discussed, namely, the effects of bilingual language use on non-linguistic cognitive functioning.

## BEYOND LEARNING AND USING TWO LANGUAGES: EFFECTS OF BILINGUALISM ON COGNITIVE CONTROL

Over the past few years, a growing body of research has shown that bilingualism of spoken languages seems to function as a form of brain exercise (for reviews, see e.g., Bialystok, Craik, Green, & Gollan, 2009; Bialystok, Craik, & Luk, 2012). Peal and Lambert (1963) were among the first to show that bilingualism has positive effects on cognitive functioning, in sharp contrast to former beliefs that bilingualism might be damaging and might cause severe confusion for children. In their influential work, monolingual and bilingual children in Montreal were compared on a series of intelligence tests. The outcomes showed that the bilingual children outperformed their monolingual peers, and the authors concluded that bilingual children have enhanced mental flexibility. More recent research has confirmed these earlier findings and has particularly shown that (unimodal) bilingualism can lead to enhanced performance in specific domains of executive functioning. In this section of the chapter, we succinctly review existing research on the effects of bilingualism on cognitive functioning by unimodal bilingual adults and children and discuss how the findings may or may not apply to bimodal bilinguals.

### Cognitive Control in Unimodal Bilingual Adults

As we have seen, bilingual language users constantly co-activate the various languages they are familiar with. As a consequence, they must inhibit access to the non-relevant language while maintaining attention on the language that is being processed on-line (Bialystok et al., 2009). In this way, the use of two spoken languages is assumed to benefit bilinguals' attention control network and to result in enhanced executive control (e.g., Costa, Hernández, Costa-Faidella, & Sebastiàn-Gallés, 2009; Garbin et al., 2010). This translates to better performance compared to monolinguals on tasks that involve, for instance, interference suppression, set maintenance, goal monitoring, and task switching (Bialystok et al., 2009). It should be noted, however, that a bilingual advantage in cognitive control is not found in all studies, and that some studies have found advantages only for specific tasks or for specific subsets of bilingual participants (for discussion, see Hilchey & Klein, 2011; Paap & Greenberg, 2013). That these bilingual benefits nevertheless really matter has been aptly demonstrated by several studies with elderly people that showed that the diagnosis of Alzheimer's disease for bilinguals is postponed by around five years, presumably because bilingualism affords a certain degree of "cognitive reserve" in the face of age-related decline in cognitive functioning (e.g., Craik, Bialystok, & Freedman, 2010).

Several recent studies have tried to directly link bilingual language processing to non-linguistic cognitive control mechanisms to provide an explanation for how bilingualism might enhance executive control. These studies have, for instance, shown that more experienced language switchers are better task switchers than less experienced language switchers (e.g., Prior & Gollan, 2011; Soveri, Rodriguez-Fornells, & Laine, 2011), and that better interference suppression is associated with reduced cognate facilitation during picture naming (Linck, Hoshino, & Kroll, 2008), reduced processing costs when switching between languages (Linck, Schwieter, & Sunderman, 2012), and reduced cross-language activation during spoken word comprehension (Blumenfeld & Marian, 2013; Mercier, Pivneva, & Titone, 2014). Finally, a recent Event Related Potential study found evidence for an ERN (Error-Related Negativity)-like response when bilinguals produced cognate words in a picture-naming task (Acheson, Ganushchak, Christoffels, & Hagoort, 2012). This ERN component has been associated with monitoring response conflict and is also found during conflict situations in non-linguistic cognitive control tasks. The observation of a similar response during the production of cognates suggests that the activation of cognate words results in a conflict between overlapping representations in the two languages and leads to an increase in monitoring demands. All these studies provide important indications as to how bilingual language use may require a specific kind of monitoring or conflict resolution and how bilingual experience may lead to enhanced (non-linguistic) cognitive control abilities.

**Cognitive Control in Children Learning Two Spoken Languages**

As we have seen in the first part of this chapter, cross-language interaction is not only characteristic of language processing by bilingual adults, but also of language processing by bilingual children who are still developing their respective languages. Therefore, bilingual children develop not only two languages, but also the control mechanisms responsible for language selection. As a result, bilingual children might already be expected to show enhanced cognitive control compared to their monolingual peers. Indeed, several studies have found bilingual advantages for children on tasks that require inhibition and conflict resolution (e.g., Bialystok, Martin, & Viswanathan, 2005; Carlson & Melzoff, 2008; Martin-Rhee & Bialystok, 2008; Morton & Harper, 2007; Poarch & Van Hell, 2012; Yang, Yang, & Lust, 2011), although some studies have suggested that the advantages are broader and more likely involve the ability to *coordinate* multiple executive control components (Bialystok, 2010, 2011). While these studies involved children who were generally between 4 and 12 years old, another study by Kovács and Mehler (2009) has suggested that a bilingual advantage in cognitive control might have much earlier roots. In their study, 7-month-old bilingual and monolingual infants learned to respond to a speech or visual cue to anticipate a visual reward on one side of a screen. When the cue was changed to predict the reward on the other side of the screen, only the bilingual infants successfully redirected their anticipatory looks, which the authors interpreted as evidence that they had better cognitive control than the monolingual infants.

A study by Poarch and Van Hell (2012) is particularly informative because bilingual children (5- to 8-year-olds) were compared who were either native in both languages, second language learners, trilingual children with native exposure to the first two languages, and monolingual children. Their results showed enhanced conflict resolution for the trilingual and simultaneous bilingual children compared to the sequential bilingual children. Moreover, they found a clear advantage compared to monolingual children only for the trilingual and simultaneous bilingual children, but not (yet) for the sequential bilingual children. Thus, the degree of experience with two or more languages seems to be crucial in predicting enhancements in cognitive control in children.

Furthermore, the specific nature of the bilingual experience might also influence whether or not advantages in cognitive control are developed. To address this possibility, Barac and Bialystok (2012) compared the performance of Spanish-English, French-English, and Chinese-English bilingual children and English monolingual children on several language tasks and a non-linguistic executive control task. The three bilingual groups differed in similarity of the two spoken languages, the language of schooling, and cultural background. Although structural similarity and language of schooling did affect performance on the language tasks, the three bilingual groups did not differ on the executive control task, and all groups outperformed the monolingual children. These results suggest that cognitive control advantages in bilingual children are quite general and are not restricted to children learning structurally similar languages or children from certain cultural backgrounds (see also Engel de Abreu, Cruz-Santos, Tourinho, & Bialystok, 2011). However, any two spoken languages, regardless of how structurally different they are, share the same articulatory and perceptual mechanisms and are arguably more similar than a spoken language and a sign language. It therefore cannot be automatically assumed that bimodal bilinguals should experience the same advantages in cognitive control.

## Cognitive Control in Bimodal Bilinguals

The first study to look at cognitive control in bimodal bilinguals compared the performance of hearing simultaneous ASL-English bimodal bilingual adults, unimodal bilingual adults from different L1 backgrounds, and English monolingual adults on a non-linguistic conflict resolution task (Emmorey, Luk, Pyers, & Bialystok, 2008). The unimodal bilinguals were faster than the other two groups, and the bimodal bilinguals did not differ from the monolinguals, suggesting that (hearing) bimodal bilinguals do not experience the same advantages in cognitive control as unimodal bilinguals. The researchers argued that bimodal bilingualism places lower demands on language control than unimodal bilingualism because, in contrast to words from two spoken languages, signs and spoken words can be produced concurrently, which requires less monitoring to ensure that the correct language is being selected. Furthermore, they suggested that, in contrast to unimodal bilinguals, who need to attend to and perceptually discriminate between two spoken languages, perceptual cues to language membership are unambiguous for bimodal bilinguals.

In another study on cognitive control in bimodal bilinguals, Kushalnagar, Hannay, and Hernández (2010) compared the performance of balanced and unbalanced deaf ASL-English bilingual adults on a (low-level) selective attention task and a (high-level) attention-switching task. Whereas the two groups performed similarly on the selective attention task, the balanced bilinguals performed better than the unbalanced bilinguals on the attention-switching task, suggesting that there might be enhancements in cognitive flexibility for bimodal bilinguals who are highly proficient in both languages. However, this study did not include comparison samples of unimodal bilinguals or monolinguals.

Taking a different approach, Giezen, Blumenfeld, Shook, Marian, and Emmorey (submitted) looked for evidence that bimodal bilinguals actually engage non-linguistic cognitive control mechanisms for language control. They correlated co-activation of ASL during English spoken word comprehension with non-linguistic inhibitory control in a group of hearing simultaneous and sequential ASL-English bilingual adults. This study was modeled after work by Blumenfeld and Marian (2013), who found associations between non-linguistic inhibitory control and the degree and time course of cross-language activation in Spanish-English unimodal bilinguals. Using the same eye-tracking paradigm as Shook and Marian (2012), Giezen and colleagues found that better performance on the inhibitory control task was associated with reduced co-activation of ASL during English spoken word recognition, indicating that, similar to unimodal bilinguals, bimodal bilinguals engage non-linguistic inhibition mechanisms to control cross-language activation.

In addition to these studies with proficient signers, it is worth mentioning that several studies are currently in progress or have just been completed that investigate improvements in cognitive control for hearing L2 learners enrolled in sign language programs or teacher/interpreter programs (Macnamara and Conway, 2013, for ASL; Ng, Ormel, Giezen, & Van Zuilen, in preparation, for NGT; Stone & Vinson, 2013, for BSL). For instance, Macnamara and Conway (2013) tested ASL interpreter students on a battery of cognitive tests at the beginning of their program and two years later. They found that the students improved on measures of task switching, mental flexibility, psychomotor speed, and on two working memory tasks. These studies will hopefully contribute to a better understanding of the development of potential advantages in cognitive control for bimodal bilinguals.

Finally, in our own work in progress (Ormel, Giezen, & Van Zuilen, in preparation; Ormel, Giezen, & Van Zuilen, 2013), we hypothesize that bimodal bilingualism might very well lead to enhancements in selective cognitive functions, but perhaps not in the same way as for unimodal bilinguals (see also Van Dijk, Christoffels, Postma, & Hermans, 2012). It is well known that experience with a visuospatial language can enhance specific non-linguistic visuospatial abilities, such as mental rotation, image generation, face processing, motion categorization, and memory for spatial locations (for discussion, see e.g., Emmorey, 2002, Chapter 8). Similarly, it is likely that mentally juggling a spoken language and a sign language places different demands on the bilingual monitoring system than juggling two or more spoken languages. For instance, whereas unimodal bilinguals coordinate information from visual and auditory resources to a limited degree during language processing, bimodal bilingual language processing requires strong and specific coordination of multiple modalities. This is not only the case during language production (Emmorey, Petrich, & Gollan, 2012; Kovelman et al., 2009; Vinson, Thompson, Skinner, Fox, & Vigliocco, 2010), but arguably also during language comprehension (Shook & Marian, 2009). Moreover, the nature of the bimodal bilingual experience and any associated bimodal bilingual advantages may differ between deaf and hearing bimodal bilinguals, given their distinct sensory experiences. One of the possibilities we are therefore currently exploring is whether various groups of bimodal bilinguals might develop selective cognitive advantages in the ability to monitor and coordinate information *across* modalities (i.e., visual, auditory, and motor), instead of, or in addition to, the ability to inhibit or monitor information *within* one modality.

In summary, whether bimodal bilingual adults exhibit enhanced cognitive control abilities and, if so, whether they are of the same nature as for unimodal bilinguals, are unfortunately unclear at this point. Only two studies have been published on the topic thus far, with conflicting findings, but other studies are currently under way. Finally, although a few studies have investigated executive functioning in deaf bimodal bilingual children (see e.g., Hauser, Lukomski, & Hillman, 2008 for discussion), these did not look at cognitive control specifically and also not from the perspective of possible bilingual advantages. Whether any bimodal bilingual advantages for adults might therefore also apply to deaf or hearing children is again an open question, and will probably heavily depend on the age of acquisition of each language, as well as the relative proficiency in each language. As will be discussed in the next section, insight into these two important factors in bimodal bilingual language acquisition is arguably the largest missing piece in the bimodal bilingual puzzle.

## THE ROLE OF AGE OF ACQUISITION AND LANGUAGE PROFICIENCY

Bilinguals, whether unimodal or bimodal, can acquire their two languages simultaneously or can acquire one language as a native language and the other at a later age. Evidently, "at a later age" is a rather broad description, and the actual age of acquisition may be crucial to the effort that is needed to reach a certain level of language fluency (Hyltenstam & Abrahamsson, 2003). Moreover, as we have seen, the age of acquisition of the second language and, related to this, children's relative proficiency in each language are important factors in predicting specific patterns of cross-language activation and in predicting "bilingual advantages" in cognitive control for unimodal bilinguals.

As we already have discussed in the introduction, for most deaf children the language acquisition context is more complex than a clear distinction based on native and non-native languages. Given that many deaf children do not get full exposure to a sign language and/or a spoken language immediately from birth, their languages may develop less optimally compared to deaf native bilinguals as well as to deaf native users of at least one language, that is, sign language. Deaf children's exposure to sign language depends on parents' (sign) language usage, but also on whether they have contact with other deaf signers who could serve as parental or educational role models/advisors and who can encourage the use of signs (Benedict & Bodner-Johnson, 2012). Deaf children's exposure to spoken language largely depends on the degree of access to the speech signal. However, even for children who had cochlear implantation at a young age, there is substantial inter-individual variation in speech-processing abilities (e.g., Peterson, Pisoni & Miyamoto, 2010), and only a relatively small proportion of deaf children will develop spoken language in a native and age-adequate manner when compared to hearing peers (e.g., Geers et al., 2008, 2009; Niparko et al., 2010). These considerations underline the complexity of determining age of acquisition and degree of nativeness of the different languages for many deaf children.

In spoken language studies, much attention has been given to the question of whether there is a "critical" or "sensitive" period' for language acquisition, that is, a period of increased language-learning opportunities (Johnson & Newport, 1989; Lenneberg, 1967; Singleton, 2005). For example, studies of speech learning have shown that children learn phonological contrasts in a second language faster than adults do (e.g., Aoyama, Flege, Guion, Akahane-Yamada, & Yamada, 2004). Similarly, Kovelman, Baker, and Petitto (2008) found that the age of L2 acquisition had a strong impact on reading performance in the second language; the earlier the better. Other studies have investigated age-related effects on language processing and ultimate attainment in the L2, typically showing advantages for earlier ages of acquisition, although it is not always clear whether the observed effects are really due to differences in age of acquisition or other, uncontrolled factors such as length of L2 exposure or the setting in which the L2 is acquired (for discussion, see e.g., Birdsong, 2006; Muñoz & Singleton, 2011). Researchers have also shown a growing interest in studying individual differences that may contribute to the learning curve for second language learners, such as learning strategies and motivation (Dörnyei, 2005).

Strong effects of age of acquisition have also been observed for sign languages, not only when acquired as a second language, but also as a first language (Cormier, Schembri, Orfanidou, & Vinson, 2013; Mayberry, Chen, Witcher, & Klein, 2011; Morford, Grieve-Smith, MacFarlane, Staley, & Waters, 2008). When sign language is acquired at a later age as a first language (e.g., during adolescence and in the rare case of little to no language acquisition and schooling before that time), the initial stages of language acquisition resemble acquisition from birth, but lexical and syntactic acquisition starts to slow down after two years of sign language exposure (Ferjan Ramírez, Lieberman, & Mayberry, 2013a, 2013b; the teens in this study were first exposed to ASL at the age of 14 years). Furthermore, ultimate signing proficiency of late first language learners of a sign language seems to be limited at all levels of linguistic structure compared to native signers (e.g., Mayberry & Eichen, 1991). Importantly, late acquisition of a first language also negatively impacts subsequent acquisition of a second language, independent of language modality (Mayberry, 2002, 2007; Mayberry & Lock, 2003).

As yet, we are uninformed as to how precisely a sign language and a spoken language integrate into an interactive language system as well as how the integration process depends on the varying degrees of exposure in the first years. Thus far, only a handful of studies on cross-language activation in bimodal bilingual adults and children have been published, and none of these studies explicitly addressed the issue of age of acquisition and (bilingual) language exposure. However, given that the age of acquisition of a sign language is crucial for ultimate language attainment, and given that many deaf children lack sufficient exposure to linguistic input until they manage to grasp the spoken language sufficiently, we expect that the dynamic interaction between the two languages will similarly be affected by the age of acquisition of both languages.

Studies with unimodal bilinguals have shown that sequential bilingual children and adults co-activate their L1 when processing in the L2, but not necessarily the other way around. The more proficient a child or adult is in the L2, the more likely it is to influence L1 processing. Simultaneous balanced bilingual children and adults likely co-activate consistently in both directions (see e.g., Dimitropoulou, Dunabeitia, & Carreiras, 2011). There is no immediately apparent reason to expect that language processing by sequential and simultaneous bimodal bilingual adults would exhibit different (a)symmetries when compared to unimodal bilinguals, and studies with bimodal bilingual adults have found evidence for cross-language activation in both directions (although not in the same study). However, as far as we know, no study has yet directly compared cross-language activation between simultaneous and sequential bimodal bilingual adults, or between sequential bimodal bilingual adults with early and later ages of L2 acquisition, or lower and higher L2 proficiency. Similarly, no study has yet looked at the role of age of acquisition and language proficiency in predicting cross-language activation for bimodal bilingual children. Given the important educational implications of bilingualism and potential benefits in cognitive control for deaf children, and at the same time the apparent difficulty of providing sufficient (bilingual) language exposure to deaf children, it is crucial to investigate the effects of age of acquisition and language proficiency in future research with bimodal bilingual children. It would seem especially important to compare cross-language activation for deaf bimodal bilingual children with and without early sign language exposure to investigate any consequences for the dynamics of the bilingual language system when neither of the two languages is acquired as early as from birth.

## IMPLICATIONS FOR EDUCATIONAL PRACTICE

Research on cross-language interaction in bimodal bilinguals has only just started; developmental studies in particular are few and far between. Nevertheless, there appear to be important parallels between what years of research have revealed about cross-language interaction for unimodal bilingual adults and what has thus far been found for bimodal bilingual adults. These parallels lead to important expectations regarding bilingual language development in hearing and deaf bimodal bilingual children, especially when they are compared to monolingual children.

Although the focus in this chapter is on experimental studies investigating cross-language interaction in bilinguals and the possible benefits of language co-activation for non-linguistic cognitive control abilities, the interactive nature of bilingual language processing also has other consequences, some of which might be interpreted as bilingual *dis*advantages. For instance, unimodal bilingual children and adults have repeatedly been found to have lower vocabularies in each of their languages than their monolingual counterparts, and also show slower reaction times or lower scores on tasks that require rapid lexical access, such as picture naming, lexical decision, or verbal fluency (for discussion, see Bialystok, 2009). Importantly, these so-called "disadvantages" of being bilingual are often attributed to the same co-activation processes that are argued to be responsible for the bilingual "advantages" in cognitive control.

Assuming that cross-language interaction for bimodal bilingual children to a large extent parallels what has been found for unimodal bilingual children, then the spoken and signed vocabulary of bimodal bilingual children (hearing or deaf) might similarly be expected to be smaller for each modality than for monolingual children, but equal or even larger when both modalities are taken into consideration. It is therefore important to consider the total conceptual vocabulary of a bilingual child, and to be aware that both languages will contribute to that total vocabulary (see Hermans, Wauters, De Klerk, & Knoors, Chapter 11 of this volume; Tang, Lam, & Yiu, Chapter 13 of this volume). Along the same line of reasoning, there is absolutely no need to become alarmed by slightly slower response times or more errors on specific language processing tasks for bimodal bilingual children. This is a phenomenon typical of most bilingual children, and it does not deter the development of each language. These considerations seem particularly relevant for studies that compare written or spoken word processing in bimodal bilingual deaf children to (monolingual) children with normal hearing, or studies that compare language processing by children with cochlear implants with and without a sign language in their linguistic environment (e.g., Schwartz, Steinman, Ying, Ying Mistal, & Houston, 2013).

At the same time, although the necessary scientific evidence is not yet available, significant parallels in cross-language interaction between unimodal and bimodal bilingual children open up the possibility that bimodal bilingual children may similarly profit from enhanced cognitive control abilities. Therefore, instead of tallying disadvantages and advantages, it seems to make more sense to embrace the fact that the acquisition of any two or more languages results in a different and unique language-processing system that is characterized by dynamic interactions at all levels. This unique feature of the bilingual language system nevertheless allows for both languages to develop, to gain knowledge about the linguistic structure of multiple languages, and to have the benefit of being able to communicate with a wider range of language users.

In recent years, educational institutions are confronted with changing technological opportunities for deaf children, with associated changes of language policies. The introduction of the cochlear implant has resulted in increased access to spoken language for many children (Walker & Tomblin, Chapter 6 of this volume). One consequence has been the reduced access to sign language and thus also a reduced possibility for bimodal bilingual language learning. Instead of rising in popularity, as had been the case in many countries in the past few decades, bilingual education is currently on the decline again in many of those same countries, and is disappearing altogether in some others (see Swanwick, Hendar, Dammeyer, Kristoffersen, Salter, & Simonsen, Chapter 12 of this volume). This concerns not only primary and secondary education, but also early day-care programs.

On the surface, changing language policies seem a logical result of increased access to sound and accompanying improvement in speech abilities and spoken language development. Without a question, deaf children are likely to benefit from a good grasp of the surrounding spoken language. However, is a "rather good grasp of a spoken language" sufficient for a deaf child? Who decides what is sufficient, and is sufficient really sufficient? In other words, should the focus be on seemingly sufficient language levels, or instead on a maximally stimulating linguistic and communicative environment for deaf children? After all, sign language is the only language that is fully accessible to the deaf child (with or without an implant).

Furthermore, is it recommendable to wait for insufficient achievements in spoken language abilities before deciding that exposure to sign language may need to be provided? Although it is the hope that the speech production and comprehension of children with a cochlear implant will take off smoothly, the reality is that spoken language development often trails behind that of hearing peers, and many deaf children rely heavily on visual information. This "wait-and-see" attitude implicitly seems to consider sign languages solely as a support system in order to gain sufficient skills in the spoken language, as opposed to a language that has a wide range of advantages in terms of cognitive, linguistic, and emotional development for deaf children.

Finally, as discussed in the previous section, the age of acquisition is not only an important factor in spoken language acquisition, but also in sign language acquisition. Simply put: the earlier the better. Evidently, the day-to-day practicalities are not always easy, and theoretical linguistic arguments may not always match up nicely with the challenging task of providing sign language to a deaf child who is born in a hearing family. Still, parents, researchers, educators, and other professionals should strive for maximal language learning opportunities in any given family. It is important to remember that a deaf child remains a deaf child, regardless of increased access to the spoken language through, for instance, a cochlear implant. As such, we need to be cautious of excluding irreversible learning opportunities that early language exposure can provide (e.g., Humphries et al., 2012; Kushalnagar et al., 2010).

For instance, it would seem beneficial to provide fast-track sign language and communication (crash) courses to parents, as well as to create a network of support around the family in which the child and his or her family are exposed to sign language and advice on a wide range of topics by deaf parents and educators. The presence of a broadly stimulating communicative environment would, of course, need to be continued in day-care settings and in (primary) education. In order to provide such an enhancement in the communicative environment, close collaboration is required between different expert parties involved in the first few years of the deaf child, including early family support services and medical professionals, who are the main source of information for parents. Currently, a wide gap remains between these parties. On the one hand, many linguists and developmental psychologists realize the importance of early language exposure and bimodal bilingualism for deaf children, regardless of the technological developments. On the other hand, many medical professionals strictly focus on encouraging maximal exposure to sound and speech. This ambivalence in information from professionals can be highly confusing for parents, and clearly does not benefit the deaf child.

Overall, it can be concluded that the unique dynamics of bimodal bilingual language processing are far from clear and promise to attract an extensive amount of intriguing research in the next few years. At the moment, the field is in particular need of studies on the effects of early language exposure for bimodal bilingual language processing. As we hope to have made clear in this chapter, the study of cross-language interaction in bimodal bilinguals and its associations with, for instance, enhancements in cognitive control abilities for bimodal bilinguals has important implications for the bilingual education of deaf children.

## ACKNOWLEDGMENTS

Preparation of this chapter was supported in part by NWO Veni grant 275-89-019 (EO) and NWO Rubicon grant 446-10-022 (MG).

## NOTES

[1] It is important to note that we use the term "bilingualism" throughout this chapter to refer to fluency in two or more languages. The findings and considerations we discuss often apply to bilinguals as well as multilinguals.

[2] Although bilinguals in two different sign languages are also unimodal bilinguals, the term is used in this chapter strictly to refer to bilinguals in two (or more) spoken languages.

[3] It has been proposed that, during the initial stages of L2 acquisition, semantic access to L2 words occurs only indirectly through L1 mediation (e.g., Kroll, Michael, Tokowicz, & Dufour, 2002). Although this might provide an alternative explanation for co-activation of signs during written word recognition in bimodal bilinguals, it should be noted that all the bimodal bilingual participants in the studies reviewed here were quite proficient in both languages.

## REFERENCES

Acheson, D. J. Ganushchak, L. Y., Christoffels, I. K., & Hagoort, P. (2012). Conflict monitoring in speech production: Physiological evidence from bilingual picture naming. *Brain and Language, 123*(2), 131–136.

Aoyama, K., Flege, E. J., Guion, S. G., Akahane-Yamada, R., & Yamada, T. (2004). Perceived phonetic dissimilarity and L2 speech learning: The case of Japanese /r/ and English /l/ and /r/. *Journal of Phonetics, 32*(2), 233–250.

Baker, A., & Van den Bogaerde, B. (2008). Codemixing in signs and words in input to and output from children. In C. Plaza-Pust & E. Morales Lopéz (Eds.),

*Sign bilingualism: Language development, interaction, and maintenance in sign language contact situations*. Studies in Bilingualism 38 (pp. 1–27). Amsterdam, Netherlands: John Benjamins Publishing.

Benedict, B. S., & Bodner-Johnson, B. (2012). *Bilingual deaf and hearing families: Narrative interviews*. Washington, DC: Gallaudet University Press.

Bialystok, E. (2009). Bilingualism: The good, the bad, and the indifferent. *Bilingualism: Language and Cognition, 12*(1), 3–11.

Bialystok, E. (2010). Global-local and trial-making tasks by monolingual and bilingual children: Beyond inhibition. *Developmental Psychology, 46*(1), 93–105.

Bialystok, E. (2011). Coordination of executive functions in monolingual and bilingual children. *Journal of Experimental Child Psychology, 110*(3), 461–468.

Bialystok, E., Graig, F. I. M., Green, D., & Gollan, T. (2009). Bilingual minds. *Psychological Science in the Public Interest, 10*(3), 89–129.

Bialystok, E., Craik, F. I. M., & Luk, G. (2012). Bilingualism: Consequences for mind and brain. *Trends in Cognitive Sciences, 16*(4), 240–250.

Bialystok, E., Martin, M. M., & Viswanathan, M. (2005). Bilingualism across the lifespan: The rise and fall of inhibitory control. *International Journal of Bilingualism, 9*(1), 103–119.

Birdsong, D. (2006). Age and second language acquisition and processing: A selective overview. *Language Learning, 56*(S1), 9–49.

Blumenfeld, H. K., & Marian, V. (2013). Parallel language activation and cognitive control during spoken word recognition in bilinguals. *Journal of Cognitive Psychology, 25*(5), 547–567.

Brenders, P., Van Hell, J., & Dijkstra, T. (2011). Word recognition in child second language learners: Evidence from cognates and false friends. *Journal of Experimental Child Psychology, 109*(4), 383–396.

Carlson, S., & Melzhoff, A. N. (2008). Bilingual experience and executive functioning in young children. *Developmental Science, 11*(2), 282–298.

Cormier, K., Schembri, A., Vinson, D., & Orfanidou, E. (2013). First language acquisition differs from second language acquisition in prelingually deaf signers: Evidence from sensitivity to grammaticality judgment in British Sign Language. *Cognition, 124*(1), 50–65.

Costa, A., Hernández, M., Costa-Faidella, J., & Sebastiàn-Gallés, N. (2009). On the bilingual advantage in conflict processing: Now you see it and now you don't. *Cognition, 113*(2), 135–149.

Craik, F. I. M., Bialystok, E., & Freedman, M. (2010). Delaying the onset of Alzheimer's disease: Bilingualism as a form of cognitive reserve. *Neurology, 75*(19), 1726–1729.

Curtin, S., Byers-Heinlein, K., & Werker, J. F. (2011). Bilingual beginnings as a lens for theory development: PRIMIR in focus. *Journal of Phonetics, 39*(4), 492–504.

De Houwer, A. (2005). Early bilingual acquisition: Focus on morphosyntax and the separate development hypothesis. In J. F. Kroll & A. de Groot (Eds.), *Handbook of bilingualism: psycholinguistic approaches* (pp. 30–48). New York, NY: Oxford University Press.

De Houwer, A. (2009). *Bilingual first language acquisition*. Clevedon, UK: Multilingual Matters.

De Quadros, R., Lillo-Martin, D., & Chen Pichler, D. (2010). Two languages but one computation: Code-blending in bimodal bilingual development. Paper presented at the *10th Theoretical Issues in Sign Language Research Conference*, West Lafayette, IN, September 29–October 2.

Dijkstra, A. F. J., & Van Heuven, W. J. B. (2002). Modeling bilingual word recognition: Past, present and future. *Bilingualism: Language and Cognition, 5*(3), 219–225.

Dimitropoulou, M., Duñabeitia, J. A., & Carreiras, M. (2011). Two words, one meaning: Evidence of automatic co-activation of translation equivalents. *Frontiers in Psychology, 2*(188), 1–20.

Dörnyei, Z. (2005). *The psychology of the language learner: Individual differences in second language acquisition*. Mahwah, NJ: Lawrence Erlbaum Associates.

Emmorey, K. (2002). *Language, cognition and the brain: Insights from sign language research*. Mahwah, NJ: Lawrence Erlbaum Associates.

Emmorey, K., Borinstein, H. B., Thompson, R., & Gollan, T. H. (2008). Bimodal bilingualism. *Bilingualism: Language and Cognition, 11*(1), 43–61.

Emmorey, K., Luk, G., Pyers, J. E., & Bialystok, E. (2008). The source of enhanced cognitive control in bilinguals. *Psychological Science, 19*(2), 1201–1206.

Emmorey, K., Petrich, J. A. F., & Gollan, T. H. (2012). Bilingual processing of ASL–English code-blends: The consequences of accessing two lexical representations simultaneously. *Journal of Memory and Language, 67*(1), 199–210.

Engel de Abreu, P. M. J., Cruz-Santos, A., Tourinho, C. J., Martin, R., & Bialystok, E. (2012). Bilingualism enriches the poor: Enhanced cognitive control in low-income minority children. *Psychological Science, 23*(11), 1364–1371.

Ferjan Ramírez, N., Lieberman, A. M., & Mayberry, R. I. (2013a). The initial stages of first-language acquisition begun in adolescence: When late looks early. *Journal of Child Language, 40*(2), 391–414.

Ferjan Ramírez, N., Lieberman, A. M., & Mayberry, R. I. (2013b). How far and how fast: A longitudinal study on ASL acquisition in adolescent home signers. Paper presented at the *11th Theoretical Issues in Sign Language Research Conference*, London, United Kingdom, July 10–13.

Garbin, G., Sanjuan, A., Forn, C., Bustamante, J. C., Rodriguez-Pujadas, A., Belloch, V., Hernández, M., et al. (2010). Bridging language and attention: Brain basis of the impact of bilingualism on cognitive control. *NeuroImage, 53*(4), 1272–1278.

Geers, A. E., Tobey, E. A., Moog, J. S., & Brenner, C. (2008). Long-term outcomes of cochlear implantation in the preschool years: From elementary grades to high school. *International Journal of Audiology, 47*(S2), 21–30.

Geers, A. E., Moog, J. S., Biedenstein, J., Brenner, C., & Hayes, H. (2009). Spoken language scores of children using cochlear implants compared to hearing age-mates at school entry. *Journal of Deaf Studies and Deaf Education, 14*(3), 371–385.

Gervain, J., & Werker, J. F. (2013). Prosody cues word order in 7-month-old bilingual infants. *Nature Communications, 4*, 1490.

Giezen, M. R., Baker, A. E., & Escudero, P. (2014). Relationships between spoken word and sign processing in children with cochlear implants. *Journal of Deaf Studies and Deaf Education, 19*(1), 107–125.

Giezen, M. R., Emmorey, K. (2013). Lexical selection and language co-activation in bimodal bilinguals. Poster presented at the *2013 Psychonomics Society Annual Meeting*, Toronto, Canada, November 14–17.

Giezen, M. R., Blumenfeld, H. K., Shook, A., Marian, V., & Emmorey, K. (submitted). Parallel language activation and inhibitory control in bimodal bilinguals.

Grote, K., & Linz, E. (2003). The influence of sign language iconicity on semantic conceptualization. In W. G. Muller & O. Fisher (Eds.), *From sign to signing: iconicity in language and literature 3* (pp. 23–40). Amsterdam, The Netherlands: John Benjamins Publishing.

Hanson, V., & Feldman, L. (1989). Language specificity in lexical organization: Evidence from deaf signers' lexical organization of American sign language and English. *Memory & Cognition, 17*(3), 292–301.

Hauser, P. C., Lukomski, J., & Hillman, T. (2008). Development of deaf and hard-of-hearing students' executive functioning. In M. Marschark & P. C. Hauser (Eds.), *Deaf cognition: foundations and outcomes* (pp. 286–308). Oxford, NY: Oxford University Press.

Hermans, D., Bongaerts, T., De Bot, K., & Schreuder, R. (1998). Producing words in a foreign language: Can speakers prevent interference from their first language? *Bilingualism: Language and Cognition, 1*(3), 213–229.

Hermans, D., Ormel, E., Knoors, H., & Verhoeven, L. (2008). The relation between the reading and signing skills of deaf children: The role of vocabulary. *Journal of Deaf Studies and Deaf Education, 13*(4), 518–530.

Hermans, D., Knoors, H., Ormel, E., & Verhoeven, L. (2008). A model of reading vocabulary acquisition for deaf children in bilingual education programs. *Journal of Deaf Studies and Deaf Education, 13*(2), 155–174.

Hermans, D., Ormel, E., & Knoors, H. (2010). On the relationship between the signing and reading skills of deaf bilinguals. *International Journal of Bilingual Education and Bilingualism, 13*(2), 187–199.

Hilchey, M., & Klein, R. M. (2011). Are there bilingual advantages on nonlinguistic interference tasks? Implications for the plasticity of executive control processes. *Psychonomic Bulletin & Review, 18*(4), 625–658.

Hoffmeister, R. (2000). A piece of the puzzle: ASL and reading comprehension in deaf children. In C. Chamberlain, J. Morford, & R. Mayberry (Eds.), *Language acquisition by eye* (pp. 143–163). Hillsdale, NJ: Lawrence Erlbaum Associates.

Hosemann, J., Altvater-Mackensen, N., Herrman, A., & Mani, N. (2013). Cross-modal language activation. Does processing a sign (L1) also activate its corresponding written translations (L2)? Poster presented at the *11th Theoretical Issues in Sign Language Research Conference*, London, United Kingdom, July 10–13.

Humphries, T., Kushalnagar, P., Marthur, G., Napoli, D. J., Padden, C., Rathmann, C., & Smith, S. (2012). Cochlear implants and the right to language: Ethical considerations, the ideal situation, and practical measures toward reaching the ideal. In C. Umat, & R. A. Tange (Eds.), *Cochlear implant research updates*. InTech. Available from: http://www.intechopen.com/books/cochlear-implant-research-updates/the-right-to-language-ethical-considerations-ideal-situation-and-practical-measures-toward-reachi.

Hyltenstam, K., & Abrahamsson, N. (2003). Maturational constraints in SLA. In C. J. Doughty, H. Long (Eds.), *The handbook of second language acquisition* (pp. 539–588). Oxford, UK: Blackwell Publishing Ltd.

Jared, D., Cormier, P., Levy, B. A., & Wade-Woolley, L. (2012). Cross-language activation of phonology in young bilingual readers. *Reading and Writing*, 25(6), 1327–1343.

Johnson, J. S., & Newport, E. L. (1989). Critical period effects in second language learning: The influence of maturational state on the acquisition of English as a second language, *Cognitive Psychology*, 21(1), 60–99.

Kovács, A. M., & Mehler, J. (2009). Cognitive gains in 7-month-old bilingual infants. *Proceedings of the National Academy of Sciences of the United States of America*, 106(16), 6556–6560.

Kovelman, I., Baker, S. A., & Petitto, L. A. (2008). Age of first bilingual language exposure as a new window into bilingual reading development. *Bilingualism: Language and Cognition*, 11(2), 203–223.

Kovelman, I., Shalinsky, M. H., White, K. S., Schmitt, S. N., Berens, M. S., Paymer, N., & Petitto, L. A. (2009). Dual language use in sign-speech bimodal binguals: fNIRS brain-imaging evidence. *Brain and Language*, 109(2–3), 112–123.

Kroll, J. F., Michael, E., Tokowicz, N., & Dufour, R. (2002). The development of lexical fluency in a second language. *Second Language Research*, 18(2), 137–171.

Kroll, J., Bogulsky, C. A., & McClain, R. (2012). Psycholinguistic perspectives on second language learning and bilingualism: The course of cross-language competition. *Linguistic Approaches to Bilingualism*, 2(1), 1–24.

Kubus, O., Villwock, A., Morford, J. P., & Rathmann, C. (2014). Word recognition in deaf readers: Cross-language activation of German Sign Language and German. *Applied Psycholinguistics*. Published online: 27 January 2014, doi:10.1017/S0142716413000520.

Kushalnagar, P., Hannay, H. J., & Hernandez, A. E. (2010). Bilingualism and attention: A study of balanced and unbalanced bilingual deaf users of American Sign Language and English. *Journal of Deaf Studies and Deaf Education*, 15(3), 263–273.

Kushalnagar, P., Mathur, G., Moreland, C. J., Napoli, D. J., Osterling, W., Padden, C., & Rathmann, C. (2010). Infants and children with hearing loss need early language access. *Journal of Clinical Ethics*, 21(2), 143–154.

Lenneberg, E. H. (1967). *Biological foundations of language*. New York, NY: Wiley.

Linck, J., Hoshino, N., & Kroll, J. F. (2008). Cross-language lexical processes and inhibitory control. *The Mental Lexicon*, 3(3), 349–374.

Linck, J. A., Schwieter, J. W., & Sunderman, G. (2012). Inhibitory control predicts language switching performance in trilingual speech production. *Bilingualism: Language and Cognition*, 15(3), 651–662.

MacNamara, B. N., & Conway, A. R. A. (2013). Novel evidence in support of the bilingual advantage: Influences of task demands and experience on cognitive control and working memory. *Psychonomic Bulletin & Review*. Published online: 4 October 2013, doi:10.3758/s13423-013-0524-y.

Magnuson, J. S., J. A. Dixon, M. K. Tanenhaus, & R. N. Aslin (2007). The dynamics of lexical competition during spoken word recognition. *Cognitive Psychology*, 31(1), 133–156.

Marian, V., & Spivey, M. J. (2003). Competing activation in bilingual language processing: Within- and between-language competition. *Bilingualism: Language and Cognition*, 6(2), 97–115.

Martin-Rhee, M. M., & Bialystok, E. (2008). The development of two types of inhibitory control in monolingual and bilingual children. *Bilingualism: Language and Cognition*, *11*(1), 81–93.

Mayberry, R. (2002). Cognitive development in deaf children: The interface of language and perception in neuropsychology. In S. J. Segalowitz and I. Rapin (Eds.), *Handbook of neuropsychology*, 2nd ed., vol. 8, part II (pp. 71–107). Amsterdam, Netherlands: Elsevier.

Mayberry, R. I. (2007). When timing is everything: Age of first-language acquisition effects on second-language learning. *Applied Psycholinguistics*, *28*(3), 537–549.

Mayberry, R. I., Chen, J.-K., Witcher, P., & Klein, D. (2011). Age of acquisition effects on the functional organization of language in the adult brain. *Brain and Language*, *119*(1), 16–29.

Mayberry, R. & Eichen, E. B. (1991). The long-lasting advantage of learning sign language in childhood: Another look at the critical period for language acquisition. *Journal of Memory and Language*, *30*(4), 486–512.

Mayberry, R. I., & Lock, E. (2003). Age constraints on first versus second language acquisition: Evidence for linguistic plasticity and epigenesis. *Brain and Language*, *87*(3), 369–384.

Meisel, J. (2004). The bilingual child. In T. K. Bhatia & W. C. Ritchie (Eds.), *The handbook of bilingualism* (pp. 91–113). Malden, MA: Blackwell Publishers.

Melby-Lervåg, M., & Lervåg, A. (2011). Cross-linguistic transfer of oral language, decoding, phonological awareness and reading comprehension: A meta-analysis of the correlational evidence. *Journal of Research in Reading*, *34*(1), 114–135.

Mercier, J., Pivneva, I., & Titone, D. (2014). Individual differences in inhibitory control relate to bilingual spoken word processing. *Bilingualism: Language and Cognition*, *17*(1), 89–117.

Morford, J. P., Grieve-Smith, A. B., MacFarlane, J., Staley, J., & Waters, G. (2008). Effects of language experience on the perception of American Sign Language, *Cognition*, *109*(1), 41–53.

Morford, J., Wilkinson, E., Villwock, A., Piñar, P., & Kroll, J. F. (2011). When deaf signers read English: Do written words activate their sign translations? *Cognition*, *118*(2), 286–292.

Morton, J. B., & Harper, S. N. (2007). What did Simon say? Revisiting the bilingual advantage. *Developmental Science*, *10*(6), 719–726.

Müller de Quadros, R., Cruz, C. R., Pizzio, A. L., Chen-Pichler, D., & Lillo Martin, D. (2013). More than the sum of the parts: Bimodal bilingual language acquisition—phonological aspects. *First Conference on Sign Language Acquisition*, Lisbon, Portugal, March 21–23.

Muñoz, C., & Singleton, D. (2011). A critical review of age-related research on L2 ultimate attainment. *Language Teaching*, *44*(1), 1–35.

Ng, Z. Y., Ormel, E., Giezen, M. R., & Van Zuilen, M. (in preparation). Consequences of bimodality for cognitive functioning: Evidence from the early stages of late bimodal bilingual language learners.

Nicoladis, E., & Genesee, F. (1997). Language development in preschool bilingual children. *Journal of Speech-Language Pathology and Audiology*, *21*(4), 258–270.

Niparko, J. K., Tobey, E. A., Thal, D. J., Eisenberg, L. S., Wang, N.-Y., Quittner, A. L., & Fink, N. E. (2010). Spoken language development in children following cochlear implantation. *Journal of the American Medical Association, 303*(15), 1498–1506.

Ormel, E. (2008). *Visual word recognition in bilingual deaf children.* Unpublished PhD dissertation, Radboud University, Nijmegen.

Ormel, E., Hermans, D., Knoors, H., & Verhoeven, L. (2012). Cross-language effects in written word recognition: The case of bilingual deaf children. *Bilingualism: Language and Cognition, 15*(2), 280–303.

Ormel, E., Giezen, M. R., & Van Zuilen, M. (2013). Bimodal bilinguals; cognitive advantages in multimodal coordination? Linking unique bimodal language processes to cognitive control in speech-sign bilinguals. Poster presented at the *International Workshop on Bilingualism and Cognitive control*, Cracow, Poland, May 15–17.

Ormel, E., Giezen, M. R., & Van Zuilen, M. (in preparation). Disentangling the consequences of bimodal cognitive language processing in terms of cognitive control in deaf and hearing sign-speech bilinguals.

Ormel, E., Hermans, D., Van der Loop, J., Hermes, E., & Van Hell, J. G. (in preparation). Cross-language interaction in unimodal and bimodal bilinguals.

Paap, K. R., & Greenberg, Z. I. (2013). There is no coherent evidence for a bilingual advantage in executive processing. *Cognitive Psychology, 66*(2), 232–258.

Parra, M., Hoff, E., & Core, C. (2011). Relations among language exposure, phonological memory, and language development in Spanish-English bilingually developing 2-year-olds. *Journal of Experimental Child Psychology, 108*(1), 113–125.

Peal, E., & Lambert, W. (1963). The relation of bilingualism to intelligence. *Psychological Monographs: General and Applied, 76*, 1–23.

Peterson, N. R., Pisoni, D. B., & Miyamoto, R. T. (2010). Cochlear implants and spoken language processing abilities: Review and assessment of the literature. *Restorative Neurology and Neuroscience, 28*(2), 237–250.

Petitto, L. A., Katerelos, M., Levy, B. G., Gauna, K., Tétreault, K., & Ferraro, V. (2001). Bilingual signed and spoken language acquisition from birth: Implications for the mechanisms underlying early bilingual language acquisition. *Journal of Child Language, 28*(2), 453–496.

Poarch, G. J., & Van Hell, J. G. (2012). Executive functions and inhibitory control in multilingual children: Evidence from second-language learners, bilinguals, and trilinguals. *Journal of Experimental Child Psychology, 113*(4), 535–551.

Prior, A., & Gollan, T. H. (2011). Good language-switchers are good task-switchers: evidence from Spanish-English and Mandarin-English bilinguals. *Journal of the International Neuropsychological Society, 17*(4), 682–691.

Schwartz, R. G., Steinman, S. S., Ying, E., Ying Mystal, E., & Houston, D. M. (2013). Language processing in children with cochlear implants: A preliminary report on lexical access for production and comprehension. *Clinical Linguistics and Phonetics, 27*(4), 264–277.

Seal, B. C., Nussbaum, D. B., Belzner, K. A., Scott, S., & Waddy-Smith, B. (2011). Consonant and sign phoneme acquisition in signing children following cochlear implantation. *Cochlear Implants International, 12*(1), 34–43.

Shook, A., & Marian, V. (2009). Language processing in bimodal bilinguals. In E. Caldwell (Ed.), *Bilinguals: Cognition, education and language processing* (pp. 35–64). Hauppage, NY: Nova Science Publishers.

Shook, A., & Marian, V. (2012). Bimodal bilinguals co-activate both languages during spoken comprehension. *Cognition*, *124*(3), 314–324.

Singleton, D. (2005). The critical period hypothesis: A coat of many colours. *International Review of Applied Linguistics in Language Teaching*, *43*(4), 269–285.

Soveri, A., Rodriguez-Fornells, A., & Laine, M. (2011). Is there a relationship between language switching and executive functions in bilingualism? Introducing a within group analysis approach. *Frontiers in Psychology*, *2*(183), 1–8.

Stone, C., & Vinson, D. (2013). Enhanced cognition from L2 BSL acquisition. Paper presented at the *11th Theoretical Issues in Sign Language Research Conference*, London, UK, July 10–13.

Strong, M., & Prinz, P. M. (1997). A study of the relationship between ASL and English literacy. *Journal of Deaf Studies and Deaf Education*, *2*(1), 37–46.

Van den Bogaerde, B., & Baker, A. E. (2006). Code-mixing in mother-child interactions in deaf families. *Sign Language and Linguistics*, *8*(1/2), 155–178.

Van Dijk, R., Christoffels, I., Postma, A., & Hermans, D. (2012). The relation between the working memory skills of Sign Language interpreters and the quality of their interpretations. *Bilingualism: Language and Cognition*, *15*(3), 340–350.

Van Hell, J. G., Ormel, E., Van der Loop, J., & Hermans, D. (2009). Cross-language interaction in unimodal and bimodal bilinguals. Paper presented at the *16th Conference of the European Society for Cognitive Psychology*. Cracow, Poland, September 2–5.

Van Hell, J. G., & Tanner, D. (2012). Second language proficiency and cross-language lexical activation. *Language Learning*, *62*(S2), 148–171.

Vinson, D. P., Thompson, R. L., Skinner, R., Fox, R., & Vigliocco, G. (2010). The hands and the mouth do not always slip together in British Sign Language: Dissociating articulatory channels in the lexicons. *Psychological Science*, *21*(8), 1158–1167.

Von Holzen, K., & Mani, N. (2012). Language nonselective lexical access in bilingual toddlers. *Journal of Experimental Child Psychology*, *113*(4), 569–586.

Yang, S., Yang, H., & Lust, B. (2011). Early childhood bilingualism leads to advances in executive attention: Dissociating culture and language. *Bilingualism: Language and Cognition*, *14*(3), 412–422.

Yudes, C., Macizo, P., & Bajo, T. (2010). Cognate effects in bilingual language comprehension tasks. *NeuroReport*, *21*(7), 507–512.

# 5

# Sign Language and Reading Comprehension

## *No Automatic Transfer*

Daniel Holzinger and Johannes Fellinger

### RELATIONSHIPS BETWEEN FIRST LANGUAGE SKILLS AND SECOND LANGUAGE LITERACY

Cummins's "linguistic interdependence" principle (1978, 1979) is often cited as the theoretical framework underlying approaches to the bilingual education of deaf students (Israelite, Ewoldt, & Hoffmeister, 1992; Rodda, Cumming & Fewer, 1993; see Wauters & De Klerk, Chapter 10 of this volume). This principle suggests that proficiency in a first language (L1) will positively support the learning of a second language (L2), if there is adequate exposure to L2 and motivation to learn. Furthermore, Cummins (1989) proposed that a certain threshold level of proficiency in L1 might be necessary to facilitate linguistic competence in L2. He distinguished between basic interpersonal communicative language skills and general cognitive/academic language skills, such as linguistic skills beyond a surface level (e.g., range of vocabulary, complex syntax), language-related problem-solving skills, and literacy skills. According to the interdependence hypothesis, this underlying cognitive/academic proficiency is common across languages and facilitates the transfer of general higher level language and literacy-related skills across languages. Therefore, as elaborated later by Cummins (1981, 1986), the hypothesis not only predicts skills transfer from L1 to L2, but also from L2 to L1.

Adapted to bilingual models of education for deaf students, this hypothesis suggests that if sign language serves as L1, then a high proficiency in sign language will lead to a generally deeper conceptual and linguistic proficiency, and thus a quasi-automatic transfer to literacy in the majority language (L2). However, the applicability of Cummins's model to bilingual deaf education has been questioned for a number of reasons (Mayer & Akamatsu, 2011). Above all, a signed L1 and a written/spoken L2 do not share a common mode. Some studies have found evidence for a very limited transfer of morphosyntatic and lexical/semantic spoken language skills from L1 to L2 (Castilla, Pérez-Leroux, & Restrepo, 2009; Verhoeven, 2001, 2007). There is more consistent evidence for interdependence among L2 children's literacy abilities than for their spoken language abilities (Cummins, 2000, 1991; López & Greenfield, 2004; Oller & Eilers, 2002; Riches & Genesee, 2006). In other words, higher levels of L1 literacy have been correlated with the development of L2 literacy (Canale, Frenette, & Belanger, 1987; Cumming, 1989). However, there is no widely accepted practical written form of any sign language that could serve as basis for L1 literacy that could be transferred to a spoken L2. Therefore, a direct application of Cummins's model to bilingual deaf education might not be possible. In addition, the difference in modality between spoken and signed languages, reflected in significant structural differences at the sublexical and morphosyntactic levels, makes a direct transfer from sign language to spoken language literacy unlikely (Mayer & Wells, 1996). In short, there is no clear evidence that elaborate sign language skills can lead to a general deeper conceptual and linguistic proficiency that will support the acquisition of literacy skills in L2.

There is much evidence from studies of hearing learners that L2 face-to-face comprehension and expressive proficiency in spoken language are essential to the development of L2 reading comprehension and writing ability (Hoover & Gough, 1990; Hornberger, 1989; Reese, Garnier, Gallimore, & Goldenberg, 2000). Even well-developed literacy skills in L1, however, are not sufficient to develop literacy in a second language when there is a lack of fluency in the spoken language. For students who are deaf or hard of hearing, access to the spoken form of L2 and participation in the rich variety of social communication situations that promotes complex language acquisition is severely restricted. As a consequence, deaf children typically demonstrate deficits in vocabulary (Kelly, 1996; Marschark, Lang, & Albertini, 2002; Paul, 1998), morphosyntax (Kelly, 1996; King & Quigley, 1985), pragmatics (Goberis et al., 2012), and general knowledge (Jackson, Paul, & Smith, 1997), all of which are correlated with problems in reading comprehension. In addition, word identification problems in reading comprehension can be associated with a limited access to the phonological code of L2, which is a consequence of the limited speech discrimination and speech production skills of deaf and hard-of-hearing students (Holzinger, 2010; Kyle & Harris, 2006). Finally, limited spoken language proficiency is often associated with deficits in working memory, which is required for reading comprehension and word decoding in both hearing and deaf individuals (Gathercole, 2006; Pisoni et al., 2008).

Previous studies of bilingualism that have focused on two spoken languages do not suggest that there is any reason to delay a child's exposure to L2 until a certain level of L1 has been attained. According to most proponents of bilingual programs for deaf students, neither a spoken language nor a signed form thereof plays an integral role in literacy acquisition (Livingston, 1997; Lucas & Valli, 1992). Usually, spoken language instruction in bilingual programs for deaf students is only offered (if at all) after a basic knowledge in L2 print has been acquired, which is usually at school age (Swanwick, Hendar, Dammeyer, Kristoffersen, Salter, & Simonsen, Chapter 12 of this volume). At a preschool age, L2 in its written modality is usually introduced only at a sublexical (and lexical) level through the use of fingerspelling. Many neurolinguistic (Weber-Fox & Neville, 1996, 1999) and psycholinguistic (Haznedar, 2006; Möhring, 2001; Rothweiler, 2006) studies have shown that early access to L2, rather than the level of L1, is related to L2 outcomes at school age. Furthermore, this early access goes hand in hand with academic success in general (Hopf, 2005; Kovelman, Baker, & Pettito, 2008).

## USE OF SIGN LANGUAGE AND READING COMPREHENSION

A number of studies, particularly early research, focused on how the use of sign language in the education of profoundly deaf students influenced L2 literacy. In these studies, the students were usually grouped by whether they used sign language as their primary mode of communication in their families and/or schools, and this was assessed according to the hearing status of their parents or their attendance at a school for the deaf, rather than by their sign language skills as assessed by standardized instruments.

The often-replicated observation that deaf children of deaf parents outperform deaf children of hearing parents in academic achievement and reading comprehension was one of the motivations for developing signed bilingual programs (Kusché, Greenberg, & Garfield, 1983; Meadow, 1968; Stuckless & Birch, 1966; Vernon & Koh, 1970; but see Marschark & Lee, chapter 9 of this volume). The use of sign language in the family was thought to positively affect the academic outcomes of deaf students. For example, Kampfe and Turechek (1987) demonstrated that deaf children's reading comprehension was positively correlated with their mothers' sign language proficiency. Kusché, Greenberg, and Garfield (1983) found better reading comprehension outcomes in deaf children with deaf siblings. However, sign language use in the family (and consequently fluency in sign language as L1 before children come to school and start to learn written English) might not be the only key factor that explains reading and academic outcomes. Other alternative explanations include genetic etiologies of hearing loss that are associated with a lower percentage of additional handicaps, parental acceptance of deafness, earlier detection of deafness, and natural and highly functional early parent-child interactions (Mayer & Akamatsu, 2011, p. 17).

A Dutch study of a group of 87 children with a hearing loss of more than 80 dB (mean age 10 years and 11 months) in bilingual education programs (Hermans, Knoors, Ormel, & Verhoeven, 2008) found no correlation between the level of reading comprehension and children's preferred mode of communication at school: sign language, sign supported speech, spoken Dutch, or any combination (see Hermans, Wauters, De Klerk, & Knoors, Chapter 11 of this volume). Children who exclusively preferred sign language did not score higher on Dutch story comprehension tasks. Interestingly, deaf children of deaf parents scored significantly higher than those of hearing parents. This finding can be interpreted to support the hypothesis that the deaf children of deaf parents have an advantage beyond the role of sign language as L1. However, even children of deaf parents achieved a mean reading level far below that of their hearing peers.

In a very early study, Brasel and Quigley (1977) found a positive correlation between the parental use of manual English rather than sign language or spoken language and academic achievement (English syntactic abilities) in four groups of deaf students between the ages of 10 and 18 years and 11 months. Similarly, Connor and Zwolan (2004) analyzed factors affecting reading comprehension in a sample of 91 cochlear-implanted children (mean age 11 years) with profound prelingual hearing loss. The children were assigned to one of two groups according to their primary communication method before cochlear implantation. The total communication group used sign systems based on English (Signed English and Signing Exact English), whereas the second group used only spoken language. Classification in the total communication group was correlated with a higher pre-implant vocabulary, but did not significantly predict stronger reading comprehension. In another study of children with cochlear implants, Connor, Hieber, Arts, and Zwolan (2000) found that total communication approaches had moderately positive effects on English vocabulary acquisition. However, Robbins, Bollard, and Green (1999) found that 6 months after cochlear implantation, there was no difference in the English language performance of children who used spoken English only versus those in total communication programs.

In a group of 81 cochlear-implanted students in the Netherlands, Vermeulen (2007) failed to find a direct effect of an exclusion of sign language on receptive vocabulary, which is strongly associated with reading outcomes. However, better outcomes in receptive vocabulary were associated with better auditory speech discrimination, which in turn was associated with mainstream education that excluded sign language. These results demonstrate the necessity of assessing deaf children's speech perception and spoken language ability when the relationship between sign language use and reading comprehension is investigated. Geers and colleagues (2002) studied language development in a group of 136 children after cochlear implantation. They found the spoken communication mode positively explained a variance of only 7% of reading outcomes.

In summary, the use of sign language may be positively related to reading comprehension; however, the results of various studies are contradictory. The variations in outcomes may not be directly related to sign language, but to other factors related to growing up in a deaf family. Such factors include early access to a functional language and efficient communication that influences reading comprehension. There are indications that the use of manually coded English, which is a visualization of (parts of) English morphosyntax, can be an advantage for the development of reading comprehension. Furthermore, spoken language abilities need to be taken into account in the investigation of correlates of reading comprehension. Furthermore, due to a lack of standardized instruments, data on sign language proficiency were not included in the early studies of sign language use and reading comprehension.

## SIGN LANGUAGE PROFICIENCY AND READING COMPREHENSION

Moores and Sweet's study (1990) was one of the first to include explicit measures of signed language skills in an investigation of reading comprehension. They conducted the Language Proficiency Interview (LPI) in American Sign Language (ASL), English-based signing, and spoken English with two groups of students ranging in age from 16 to 18 years. Both groups had the same average hearing loss (above 100 dB), but the first group had deaf parents (n = 65) and the second group had hearing parents (n = 65). The LPI is an interview format usually conducted by native language users; it has a 5-point rating of student proficiency. They used the Stanford Achievement Test to assess reading comprehension grade levels and found that the children of deaf parents had about 6th-grade reading comprehension (i.e., ages 11–12), but the children of hearing parents had about 5th-grade reading comprehension (i.e., ages 10–11). Correlational analyses showed there was a strong correlation between reading and other measures of English-language knowledge. There were moderate correlations between English-based signing and oral LPI scores with reading scores, whereas ASL measures did not show significant correlation with reading skills in either group. One of the explanations offered for the lack of correlation between ASL skills and reading comprehension was the ceiling effect of the LPI in ASL, which creates a lack of variation in student scores.

Mayberry and colleagues (Mayberry 1994; see Chamberlain & Mayberry, 2000) assessed 48 children in three age groups (7–9, 10–12, and 13–15 years). Half of the children came from hearing families in which there was little or no sign language use and half came from deaf families and had been exposed to sign language from birth. ASL comprehension was measured at the sentence and narrative levels using a set of comprehension questions. In contrast to Moores and Sweet's (1990) study, Mayberry found strong positive correlations between ASL comprehension and reading measures (r = .63 to .69). However, those cross-sectional correlations cannot be interpreted as causal effects. Unfortunately, essential variables such as English skills (e.g., spoken English, manually coded English) and the speech perception skills related to them were not taken into account.

Strong and Prinz (1997, 2000) used both expressive and receptive ASL tasks to investigate the correlation of ASL with English literacy skills (including the Woodcock-Johnson Achievement Test battery). They assessed reading at the levels of single vocabulary items, sentences, and paragraphs in a sample of 155 students (8–15 years of age) at a residential school for the deaf. After controlling for nonverbal IQ and age effects, the relationship between ASL and English literacy remained significant. Among the students who attained the higher two (of three) levels of ASL ability there was no significant difference in English literacy between the children of deaf parents and those of hearing parents. This finding was interpreted as evidence that the level of ASL skills and not parental hearing status supported children's English literacy proficiency. Again we must refrain from interpreting the correlations between ASL skills and reading comprehension as causal. It is important to note that neither English language skills nor residual hearing were taken into account in this study.

Hoffmeister (2000) tested English reading comprehension using the Stanford Achievement Test (using norms for deaf and hard-of-hearing students) and complex sentence comprehension in manually coded English in students aged 8 to 15 years. Fifty students were divided into two subsamples based on the amount of their exposure to ASL. The high exposure ASL group not only scored higher on ASL knowledge as assessed by use of a recognition format, but also on the manually coded English task and on reading comprehension. Deaf children exposed more often to ASL performed well on measures of manually coded English. Conversely, those with more exposure to manually coded English demonstrated good ASL grammatical skills. This finding was interpreted as possible evidence for the transfer of skills from one language system to another. Hoffmeister concluded that the correlations between ASL, manually coded English, and reading may have been the result of enhanced language functioning among children with early extensive exposure to language. However, the actual levels of English ability and reading comprehension levels were not reported in the study.

Padden and Ramsey (2000) found significant correlations between reading comprehension scores and ASL grammatical measures in 4th and 5th grade children. ASL and reading achievement were also correlated with the ability to reproduce a fingerspelled word in writing and the ability to write initialized signs presented in a sentence, pointing to a possible role of fingerspelling in the instruction of English as a mediator of the literacy learning process.

Hermans and colleagues (2008) studied the language and literacy skills of deaf children in a bilingual education program in the Netherlands. They found that sign vocabulary predicted reading vocabulary when age, nonverbal intelligence, and short-term memory were controlled. Children with large vocabularies in Sign Language of the Netherlands usually had larger vocabularies in written Dutch, which in turn facilitated reading acquisition. In addition to the possible role of the lexical level as a mediator between sign language skills and reading comprehension, they noted that children who scored in the upper 10 percentiles of written vocabulary tests also tended to have the highest spoken Dutch skills, demonstrated by their comprehension of stories in spoken Dutch and by teacher ratings. Again, this finding accentuates the importance of including spoken language skills in the investigation of the relationships between sign language skills and reading comprehension.

As noted earlier, Moores and Sweet (1990) found significant correlations between proficiency in English-based signing (not ASL) and reading comprehension. This result demonstrates the importance of visually accessible English. Similarly, Convertino and colleagues (2009) did not find a significant correlation between deaf college students' ASL skills and their learning from print (i.e., real-time text). However, learning from sign and print was predicted by the students' reported skills in simultaneous communication.

Mayberry (2007) investigated the effects of age of L1 (ASL) acquisition on reading development in L2 (English). Thirty adults born deaf and first exposed to sign language between birth and 13 years of age were grouped according to their performance on ASL grammatical judgment tasks. Earlier exposure to sign language was not only indicative of better ASL syntactic knowledge, it also exerted a small effect on the outcome of L2, that is, on English reading comprehension. It is worth mentioning that the subgroup of 10 with early access to sign language all had deaf parents; this suggests that it might not only be the age of first exposure, but the quality of signed interaction, as well as other variables associated with growing up in a deaf family, that have an effect on reading comprehension.

Chamberlain and Mayberry (2008) found (again in a group of adults with ASL as their primary language) that a combination of ASL syntactic proficiency and print exposure predicted a very high proportion of the variance in reading comprehension, as measured by the reading comprehension subtest of the Stanford Achievement Test. Grouped by levels of reading comprehension, the mean achievement of the less-skilled readers was between the third and fourth grades, whereas the skilled readers read at an 11th grade level. Interestingly, the age of ASL exposure was not significantly different in the two groups (6.5 vs. 4.2 years).

In conclusion, the majority of previous studies have found positive correlations between high levels of sign language skills and high levels of reading comprehension. This is particularly notable for individuals with early access to sign language, most often growing up with parents who are deaf. However, many of these studies do not report the actual levels of reading comprehension, and others report grade equivalents for deaf students that are far below those of their age peers. Furthermore, it remains unclear whether sign language skills as a first language are naturally transferred via generalized improved conceptual and linguistic proficiency to a spoken language (L2) in written modality, as predicted in Cummins's interdependence hypothesis. Alternatively, it may be that reading comprehension is mainly supported by a teaching methodology that takes advantage of sign language in the instruction of spoken language (written and/or spoken).

Another general weakness of the current state of research is the still restricted knowledge of the mediators between sign language skills and reading comprehension. The studies discussed thus far indicate that it might not be sign language per se, but visual access to the L2 morphosyntactic and sublexical structure via the use of English-based signing (or simultaneous speech/mouthing and sign), as well as fingerspelling, that mediates the literacy learning process. One possible mediator between signed language and literacy is sign vocabulary. Evidently, the preexisting sign language lexicon can be used to understand the meaning of written words. Singleton and colleagues (2004) showed that in a group of 72 deaf elementary school students, those with moderate to high skills in American Sign Language used more diverse and novel/original vocabulary in a written retelling task than those with low ASL skills. They presumably were able to draw upon their semantic knowledge in ASL. In contrast, sign language skills seem to be of no or very limited syntactic benefit with respect to the written form of a spoken language. Even among the group of high-ASL students, functional word use and grammatical accuracy remained pervasive problems. Other possible advantages of sign language skills for reading comprehension are a broader knowledge base (Jackson, Paul, & Smith, 1997) and the use of metacognitive strategies and flexibility (Kelly & Mousley, 2001).

The explanatory power of most of the studies discussed thus far remains limited due to a number of methodological limitations. Important confounding factors not taken into account by many of the studies investigating the relationships between reading and signing skills are residual hearing and spoken language skills. These skills are not only related to the unaided hearing threshold, but more specifically to auditory speech perception with hearing aids or cochlear implants. Better auditory speech discrimination permits more direct access to spoken language and thus more natural learning opportunities and opportunities to use language in everyday conversation. Comprehension of spoken language is known to be a main predictor of reading comprehension (Hoover & Gough, 1990) among hearing students. In addition, many previous studies have not controlled for other variables possibly influencing both reading comprehension and sign language skills, such as age, nonverbal intelligence, working memory, or parental socioeconomic status.

Time of first access to sign language and the quality of sign language input in family and school settings are other possibly confounding factors. In families with parents with normal hearing (about 95% of the parents of children who are deaf or hard of hearing) sign language is often introduced late, when spoken language acquisition remains strongly delayed or hardly possible. Therefore, signing children of hearing parents might be a special group with difficulties in spoken language acquisition that could be related to deficits of intelligence, verbal working memory, executive function, speech motor production, or auditory perception and processing (see the Upper Austrian data discussed later). These variables need to be controlled for in comparisons of the reading skills of children who sign and those who do not.

In a sign-bilingual classroom, we expect that teachers' sign fluencies and their adherence to the bilingual emphasis in their programs will influence reading outcomes. Even an established sign language might not influence reading comprehension if it is not used systematically for the acquisition of the vocabulary, grammar, and text structure of the spoken language and in the development of reading strategies (see Tang, Lam, & Yiu, Chapter 13 of this volume).

Research on this issue is not only complicated by the complexity of the variables that influence the relationship between sign language use and skills and reading comprehension, but also by the small available samples of signing deaf children (or adults). To advance knowledge in the field, two representative studies that included a wide variety of children, families, and specific education-related variables were conducted in Austria (Fellinger, Holzinger, Sattel, Laucht, & Goldberg, 2009).

## AUSTRIAN STUDIES OF BILINGUAL PROGRAMS AND ACADEMIC OUTCOMES

In two samples of deaf school children from different Austrian federal states, the relationship between sign language use and skills and

German reading comprehension was investigated. The research was guided by the following questions.

1. Does sign language *use* as a means of everyday communication in a group of deaf children with profound hearing loss support their acquisition of German (reading comprehension, vocabulary knowledge, grammatical knowledge) when confounding variables are taken into account?
2. Do sign language *skills* contribute directly or indirectly to higher levels of reading comprehension when confounding variables are taken into account?
3. What are the mediating factors between sign language skills and reading comprehension? What is the role of educational variables, specifically the strategic use of sign language in German reading instruction and as a medium of instruction for (all) other subjects?

**Research Methodologies**

The children in our first sample were drawn from a population of 145,000 pupils who were enrolled in grades 1 to 9 during the 2003–2005 school years in Upper Austria (henceforth sample UA). One hundred and eighty-six children with significant permanent hearing loss of at least 40 dB in the better ear, who were registered at the Center for Special Education for the Deaf and Hard of Hearing, were invited to participate in the study. One hundred and sixteen parents agreed to participate and gave their written consent (response rate 62.4%). Seventeen children with performance IQ below 70 and 54 with moderate to severe hearing loss were excluded, as the purpose of this study was to analyze the correlates between sign language and reading comprehension; hence children with better auditory access to spoken language also were excluded. Thus, the final sample consisted of 45 children with profound hearing loss, defined as an unaided hearing threshold of at least 80 dB in the better ear.

The second sample was selected from of a group of 109 children registered at the Centre for Special Education of the Deaf and Hard of Hearing in the federal state of Carinthia (henceforth sample CA) in the 2010 to 2011 school years. Almost all of the caregivers (98.4%) gave written consent for their child to participate in the study. After excluding 16 children with a performance IQ below 70 and all of the students with hearing thresholds below 80 dB, a subsample of 39 children with bilateral profound hearing loss remained. Table 5.1 describes the two samples of profoundly deaf students in Upper Austria and Carinthia.

The average age of the children in both samples was about 11 years, with an age range of 6 to 16 years and an equal distribution of male and female participants. There were no significant differences in

Table 5.1 Comparison of Background Information for Profoundly Deaf Students in Upper Austria and Carinthia

|  | Upper Austria (n = 45) | Carinthia (n = 39) | p value |
|---|---|---|---|
| Age m (sd) | 11.1 (2.9) | 11.0 (2.2) | .944 |
| Male % | 46.7 | 53.8 | .512 |
| Unaided hearing threshold in dB m (sd) | 97.9 (11.1) | 93.9 (16.1) | .183 |
| Age (in months) at fitting of hearing aids m (sd) | 35.8 (28.9) | 23.2 (24.3) | **.037** |
| Cochlear implant users % | 40.0 | 41.0 | .924 |
| Age (in years) at 1st cochlear implantation m (sd) | 4.7 (3.3) | 3.9 (1.8) | .376 |
| Aided hearing threshold M (sd) | 42.9 (11.5) | 41.5 (6.6) | .507 |
| Speech discrimination % m (sd) | 32.6 (30.8) | 48.7 (23.0) | **.009** |
| Parental level of education at least high school % | 20.0 | 31.6 | .227 |
| Parental hearing loss (%) | 4.4 | 20.5 | **.023** |
| Performance IQ m (sd) | 96.8 (14.2) | 98.4 (12.9) | .589 |
| Spoken family language other than German (%) | 22.2 | 12.8 | .262 |

Significant differences (p ≤ 0.05) printed in bold.

residual hearing (unaided hearing threshold) or in the percentage of cochlear-implanted children (about 40%). The age at first fitting of hearing aids was significantly lower for the Carinthian sample, possibly as a consequence of the more recent data collection. They were also doing significantly better in speech discrimination with hearing aids and cochlear implants. As children with learning disabilities had been excluded from the original sample, there was an average performance IQ in both samples. There was a significantly higher proportion of deaf children of parents with hearing loss in the Carinthian sample compared to the Upper Austrian sample (20.5% vs. 4.5%).

It is important to mention the considerable differences between the two federal states with regard to the system of education of children with hearing loss. In Upper Austria the percentage of profoundly deaf children with preferred sign language use is significantly higher than in Carinthia (46.7% vs. 18%). In Carinthia, sign language is used mainly with children of deaf parents (71.4%), whereas in Upper Austria none of the signing deaf children had a parent with hearing loss. The higher percentage of sign language users in Upper Austria might be related to the fact that there is a well-attended special school for the deaf. In contrast, the school for the deaf in Carinthia was closed more than two decades ago. As a consequence, all of the deaf children (except the signing children) in Carinthia are fully mainstreamed in regular classes without peers who are deaf or hard of hearing. As there is no longer a school for the deaf, special teacher resources are allocated to mainstreamed children to a much higher degree than in Upper Austria.

It also is important to recognize the considerable differences in the model of instruction offered to signing deaf students in both provinces. In Carinthia all of the signing deaf students attend a special class for the deaf for children of all ages within a regular school. There is a bilingual model of instruction with native signers present at all times. Reading comprehension is a primary focus of instruction, and sign language is used at a high level as the permanent language of instruction. Written vocabulary and German grammar are taught using sign language. Included in the program is direct teaching of the linguistic aspects of Austrian sign language; this program of instruction makes use of an explicit contrastive approach of language instruction, which is a comparison of sign language structure and meaning with written German. As part of their school day the children attend classes with hearing students, allowing for the use of spoken and/or written language in meaningful interactions. They are accompanied by a signing teacher who interprets for the students if necessary.

In Upper Austria, almost all signing students attend the special school for the deaf; 76% are in small classes exclusively for children with (mostly profound) hearing loss, and a high percentage of the children have learning difficulties and minority backgrounds (Holzinger, 2010, p. 73). At the time of data collection there was only one untrained deaf sign language assistant available for the whole school; this assistant spent a few hours per week assisting in different classes. In addition, there is no structured bilingual program in Upper Austria. Although no formal assessment has been performed, observation suggests that the sign language proficiency of the teachers in Carinthia is considerably higher than that of the teachers in Upper Austria.

**Measures of Achievement**

*Reading Measures*

Reading comprehension was assessed using standardized instruments for assessing reading comprehension in German. At the time of data collection for the Upper Austrian sample, no single measurement suitable for grades 1 to 9 was available. Therefore, a reading comprehension total score was extrapolated from the results of three different tests designed for different grades (Holzinger, 2010). The measures consisted of short authentic texts followed by multiple choice questions that assessed comprehension. For the Carinthian sample, the comprehension of written texts was assessed with a modern standardized measure that makes use of multiple choice questions (Lenhard & Schneider, 2006); this measure was not available at the time of the Upper Austrian study. The ELFE reading test measures the number of correct answers within a limited period of time. Word reading was assessed with the standardized Salzburger Lesetest (Landerl, Wimmer, & Moser, 1997). The assessment required the students to sound out common German words; reading fluency and correctness were rated. In the Austrian system of deaf education, even profoundly deaf children are used to reading words aloud. Correctness was rated by experts familiar with the characteristics of speech productions of deaf and hard-of-hearing children.

*German Language Measures*

The children's German vocabulary knowledge was assessed using a word list (a subtest of the Hamburg Wechsler Intelligence Scales, HAWIK-III), presented in both written and spoken modalities. The children were asked to paraphrase the meaning of each word in their preferred communication system. An additional modern vocabulary test (WWT 6-10, Glück, 2007) was used for the Carinthian sample to assess expressive German vocabulary. Due to the lack of standardized measurements of morphosyntactic knowledge and skills for German-speaking school children, and to exclude any bias related to the modality of the assessment (spoken, written), a variety of methods were used. Holzinger (2010, p. 46) developed a procedure for the written reproduction of sentences presented in print. Furthermore, teachers were asked to assess the student's German morphology and grammar by use of a questionnaire (Holzinger, 2010, p. 244).

In the Upper Austrian sample, comprehension of spoken language (words and utterances) in a face-to-face situation was assessed using the comprehension scales of the German version of the Reynell Developmental Language Scales-III (Sarimski & Süss-Burghart, 2001). In Carinthia, the new German version of the TROG (Test of Reception of Grammar, Bishop, 2003), edited by Fox (2009), was used.

Intelligibility of spoken language was assessed by asking children to sound out German numerals. The speech productions were videotaped and rated for intelligibility through the transcriptions of naïve listeners (Holzinger, 2010, p. 45). Due to time restrictions on the data collection in Carinthia, this procedure could only be performed on the Upper Austrian sample.

*Sign Language Measures*

As is the case for many other sign languages, there are no standardized measures available for Austrian sign language. Furthermore, there are distinct regional varieties, so the use of one standard measure for different regions (e.g., Upper Austria, Carinthia) is not possible. Therefore, to assess the level of signed language skills (as well as spoken language skills) the Profile of Multiple Language Proficiencies (Goldstein & Bebko, 2003) was used. Authentic conversations between the child and an adult native signer (and for spoken language with a non-signing hearing conversation partner) were videotaped and rated by deaf and hearing experts with knowledge of linguistics (Holzinger, 2010). This procedure uses a single scale (levels 1 to 8) that represents different stages of language development in sign language and spoken language. The ratings are largely derived from the morphosyntactic structure of the children's expressive language, which is associated with increases in vocabulary and narrative and conversational skills. The proficiencies range from a pre-linguistic level, through first word combinations, beginning sentences, full simple sentences, compound and complex sentences, to early and full fluency in spoken and signed language. For children with at least basic sign language skills (level 3), receptive sign language grammar was assessed using a procedure adapted from a standardized well-recognized test of German grammar for 4- to 6-year-old children (Wettstein, 1995). Short clips of about 15 videotaped sign utterances of increasing complexity were presented to the children, who were then asked to act them out using play materials. The sample of Austrian sign language structures included simple SOV sentences with non-inflecting verbs, inflecting verbs, grammatical referencing (location of signs), grammatical use of facial mimicry and posture, simple and complex classifiers, and complex causal utterances such as rhetorical questions. For the Upper Austrian sample, a sequence of 14 utterances was used; for the Carinthian sample, the measure adapted by the Centre for Sign Language and Deaf Communication (University of Klagenfurt), which is composed of 17 utterances, was used. There are no norms available for sign language proficiencies in Austrian Sign Language; therefore raw scores of the percentage of correct utterances were calculated. In addition, teachers were asked to rate each student's sign language proficiency using a short questionnaire (Holzinger, 2010, p. 243).

To assess receptive sign language vocabulary, the University of Klagenfurt developed an Austrian Sign Language version of a standardized German vocabulary test (WWT 6-10, Glück, 2007). Due to a lack of norms in Austrian Sign Language, raw scores were calculated to compare the results for individual children. Sign language vocabulary was only assessed for the Carinthian group of deaf students.

*Hearing Measures*

The most recent pure tone thresholds at 500, 1,000, and 2,000 Hz were used to calculate hearing thresholds on the better ear with and without hearing aids or cochlear implants. Speech discrimination was assessed using real word speech audiometry that measured the percentage of words that could be discriminated by hearing alone.

*Cognitive Measures*

To assess performance IQ, the nonverbal scales of the HAWIK-III (the German version of the Wechsler Intelligence Scales) were used. In addition, a series of cognitive skills that might be related to reading comprehension were assessed. Phonological recoding was rated according to the fluency and correctness of sounding out written pseudo-words (Landerl, Wimmer, & Moser, 1997: Salzburger Lesetest). Verbal short-term memory was assessed using the digit span subtest of the HAWIK-III (Wechsler Intelligence Test) for the Upper Austria sample and a different digit span test for the Carinthian sample, which used more recent norms (Nicolay, Rupp, & Rosenkötter, 2003). The digits were presented in spoken language face-to-face situations and simultaneously in signed language, as required.

Further information about the children, their families, and their education was collected by means of parent and teacher questionnaires (Holzinger, 2010, p. 237).

## Sign Language Use and Reading Comprehension Outcomes

*Characteristics of Sign Language Users and Spoken Language Users*

To study the effect of sign language use on reading comprehension, the two regional samples of school children with profound bilateral deafness (unaided hearing threshold >80 dB on the better ear) were each divided into two subgroups based on their respective preferred mode of communication (i.e., spoken or signed language), as reported by their parents.

Table 5.2 presents a description of the two samples and subsamples.

As can be seen from Table 5.2, in the Upper Austrian sample there were no significant differences in the age, sex, performance IQ, unaided hearing threshold, or parental level of education between the two subsamples. There was a higher percentage of cochlear-implanted children among the speaking subsample, but the difference was not statistically significant. As a possible consequence, those who preferred to use spoken language had a significantly better hearing threshold with technical aids (cochlear implants or hearing aids) and slightly better auditory speech discrimination. A significantly higher proportion of the signing children attended the school for the deaf, rather than a mainstream school.

The Carinthian subsamples of speaking and signing children were very similar to each other with respect to age, hearing threshold without technical devices, and performance IQ. However, there was a much

Table 5.2 Comparison of Background Information: Profoundly Deaf Children with Preferred Use of Signed Language versus Spoken Language in Upper Austria and Carinthia

| | Upper Austria | | | Carinthia | | | | |
|---|---|---|---|---|---|---|---|---|
| | Spoken language users (n = 24) | Sign language users (n = 21) | p | Spoken language users (n = 32) | Sign language users (n = 7) | p | p Sign language users UA vs. CA |
| Age m (sd) | 11.4 (3.21) | 10.7 (2.71) | .416 | 10.9 (1.9) | 11.6 (3.3) | .468 | .468 |
| Male % | 37.5 | 57.1 | .188 | 62.5 | 14.3 | **.020** | **.049** |
| Unaided hearing threshold in dB, m (sd) | 96.1 (12.4) | 100.1 (9.2) | .235 | 95.0 (17.4) | 89.3 (6.7) | .401 | **.008** |
| Age (in months) at fitting of hearing aids, m (sd) | 37.5 (24.4) | 33.8 (34.0) | .675 | 26.6 (25.5) | 7.9 (7.8) | .065 | .059 |
| Cochlear implant users % | 50.0 | 28.6 | .143 | 50.0 | 0.0 | **.015** | .111 |
| Age (in years) at 1st cochlear implant, m (sd) | 3.5 (2.5) | 2.8 (2.9) | .344 | 3.9 (1.8) | – | – | – |
| Aided hearing threshold, m (sd) | 35.9 (7.3) | 50.6 (10.4) | **<.001** | 39.8 (5.3) | 49.3 (6.7) | **<.001** | .762 |
| Speech discrimination %, m (sd) | 39.58 (33.2) | 24.5 (26.3) | .102 | 54.2 (20.) | 23.6 (18.9) | **.001** | .930 |
| Parental level of education at least high school level, % | 25.0 | 14.3 | .370 | 38.7 | 0.0 | **.047** | .290 |
| Parental hearing status; deaf parents, % | 8.3 | 0.0 | .176 | 9.4 | 71.4 | **<.001** | **<.001** |
| Performance IQ, m (sd) | 99.9 (14.7) | 93.3 (12.9) | .121 | 99.0 (13.8) | 95.6 (7.6) | .527 | .664 |
| Spoken family language other than German (%) | 16.7 | 28.6 | .338 | 15.6 | 0.0 | .263 | .111 |

Significant differences (p ≤.05) printed in bold.

higher proportion of girls in the small signing sample. In addition, there were no cochlear-implanted children in this group. Therefore, the aided hearing threshold and the speech discrimination results were significantly below the results of the subsample that primarily used spoken language. The most important observation for the interpretation of reading comprehension results and sign language skills are the differences (and similarities) between sign language users in Upper Austria and Carinthia (see rightmost column in Table 5.2). The signing deaf children in both groups were about the same age (10.7 vs. 11.6). There was a significantly higher proportion of girls in the signing subsample in Carinthia. A significantly lower percentage of children in Upper Austria had a parent with hearing loss, whereas there was no significant difference in the level of parental education. The unaided hearing threshold was significantly lower among the Carinthian students. However, probably as a consequence of a significantly lower percentage of cochlear-implanted children, mean speech discrimination results with the use of technical aids were almost identical in the two samples. There were also no significant differences in performance IQ. In Upper Austria 29.6% of children had a minority background, and therefore a spoken family language other than German, whereas there were no children with minority backgrounds among the signing deaf students in Carinthia.

*Language Skills and Reading Comprehension*

Table 5.3 presents the results for reading comprehension and German and signed language skills for both subsamples of children with and without preferred sign language use in Upper Austria and Carinthia.

Due to the use of different reading tests in the two samples, a direct comparison of reading comprehension results is impossible. For the deaf students in Upper Austria, the average level of reading comprehension was about two standard deviations below the hearing norm. The signing deaf children did significantly worse than their peers who relied on spoken language (with a difference of one standard deviation). In Carinthia, the reading comprehension results for the entire sample were within one standard deviation of the hearing norm. These very satisfying results might partly be a consequence of the measurement tool used. To check the validity of ELFE 1-6 for assessing the reading comprehension of the deaf children in Carinthia, it was tested in eight classes of children with normal hearing. According to the available scoring system, which counted the number of correct answers, the instrument proved to be valid for hearing children. However, we found a slightly higher rate of trials and a significantly higher rate of errors in the sample of children with hearing loss compared to the hearing control group (about 30% versus 18%), although these differences were not fully included in the existing scoring system. Therefore, the

Table 5.3 Reading Comprehension, German and Signed Language Skills in Profoundly Deaf Children with Primary Use of Spoken and Signed Language in Upper Austria and Carinthia

| | Upper Austria | | | Carinthia | | | p |
|---|---|---|---|---|---|---|---|
| | Spoken language users (n = 24) | Sign language users (n = 21) | p | Spoken language Users (n = 32) | Sign language users (n = 7) | p | SL users UA vs. CA |
| Reading comprehension composite score, T-value, m (sd) | 34.9 (14.1) | 25.9 (8.8) | .028 | — | — | — | — |
| Reading comprehension ELFE, percentile, m (sd) | — | — | — | 29.2 (27.6) | 45.5 (31.7) | .175 | — |
| Pseudoword reading time, percentile, m (sd) | 65.9 (28.2) | 44.0 (35.2) | .033 | 56.2 (24.1) | 41.3 (33.7) | .202 | .869 |
| Word reading time, percentile, m (sd) | 69.6 (27.7) | 22.8 (22.2) | <.001 | 58.4 (30.7) | 44.0 (26.8) | .291 | .065 |
| Expr. vocabulary German, quotient., m (sd) | 85.2 (27.8) | 65.9 (14.0) | .006 | 86.6 (25.9) | 84.8 (17.2) | .857 | **.007** |
| Expr. grammar German teacher rating, m (sd) | 2.4 (.59) | 1.6 (.48) | <.001 | 2.3 (.78) | 1.5 (.40) | **.012** | .772 |
| Re-writing sentences: morphosyntactic errors %, m (sd) | 7.9 (10.5) | 34.7 (20.6) | <.001 | — | — | — | — |
| Language compreh. German (Reynell), m (sd) | 28.7 (30.6) | 1.0 (0.0) | <.001 | — | — | — | — |
| German language level, m (sd) | 5.2 (1.3) | 2.9 (1.5) | <.001 | — | — | — | — |
| Sign language level (PMLP), m (sd) | — | 4.6 (1.4) | — | — | 6.0 (1.4) | — | **.028** |
| Sign language receptive grammar (percentage correct) | — | 56 (28) | <.001 | — | 85 (15) | — | **.016** |

Significant differences (p ≤.05) printed in bold.

results in the Carinthian sample might include a slight overestimation associated with the test instrument. It is also noteworthy that the subsample of speaking deaf children in CA had somewhat worse auditory speech discrimination results than those in Upper Austria (40% versus 54%). Furthermore, there was a higher degree of mainstreaming of profoundly deaf children and a higher allocation of teacher resources to the mainstreamed students in Carinthia. Remarkably, signing deaf children in Carinthia—in contrast to Upper Austria—were doing better in reading comprehension (though not at a significant level) than the rest of the sample with profound deafness.

With regard to vocabulary knowledge, profoundly deaf students who communicated primarily in spoken language achieved almost identical results in both provinces (about one standard deviation below the norms). However, although the signing students in Carinthia were doing as well as the speaking subsample, the signing deaf sample in Upper Austria demonstrated significantly lower vocabulary knowledge than the students who preferred spoken language (more than one standard deviation less).

For expressive grammar skills, which were assessed by teacher ratings, the situation was different. Both groups of signing students demonstrated significantly worse results than the children who relied mainly on spoken language for their everyday communication.

Although for deaf and hard-of-hearing children in Austria, word reading is no particular challenge (Holzinger, 2010), again the Upper Austrian signing students were doing significantly worse than those who used spoken German, whereas there were no differences between the subsamples in Carinthia.

Due to time restrictions during the data collection, the level of spoken German could only be assessed for the students in Upper Austria using the profile of multiple language proficiencies. As expected, the level of spoken language (lexical and morphosyntactic levels) used in natural conversation was significantly higher for the subsample that used spoken German. Unsurprisingly, signing children achieved a significantly higher signed language level than the subsample who preferred spoken language. However, it is noteworthy that, despite severe limitations of auditory perception in the group of students using spoken German, their average German language level (5.2) was slightly higher than the level of sign language of the children who communicated primarily in the visual mode (4.6). This observation can be interpreted as evidence for the insufficient use of children's potential in the visual-manual modality in the Upper Austrian system of education for the deaf.

Verbal memory (data not included in Table 5.3) in all modes of communication was significantly more delayed in children who use the signed modality.

The level of sign language (PMLP scores) was significantly higher for the signing children in Carinthia than for the signing children in Upper Austria (levels 4.6 versus 6.0, respectively). The Carinthian children had significantly better comprehension of sign language grammar.

In summary, under certain circumstances, proficient sign language use by children with profound hearing loss can be associated with reading comprehension and knowledge of German identical to (or slightly better than) that of profoundly deaf children who communicate primarily via spoken language and have significantly better aided hearing thresholds and auditory speech discrimination (through the use of cochlear implants or hearing aids). However, in the larger Upper Austrian sample, the group of children who preferred sign language for everyday communication were doing significantly worse in reading comprehension, German language knowledge (vocabulary and grammar), and spoken language skills, as measured by their comprehension of spoken German utterances. Evidently, for profoundly deaf children there is no automatic advantage of sign language for reading comprehension achievements. Differences between the two samples that could affect reading outcomes are time of first access to (sign) language and the quality of sign language input, advantages of growing up with deaf parents, the provision of specific models of bilingual instruction, and the level of sign language proficiency. These factors are investigated in the following sections.

## Sign Language Skills and Reading Comprehension

To study the relationship between the level of sign language skills and reading comprehension (research question 2), the data from both study samples were analyzed using bivariate correlations between reading comprehension, sign language level, German language skills, and other possibly confounding variables. Due to very different outcomes for the Upper Austrian and Carinthian samples, the results are presented separately.

*Upper Austrian Sample*

Importantly, in the Upper Austrian sample of pupils with profound deafness, the level of sign language proficiency (PMLP) was significantly negatively correlated with reading comprehension. Sign language level was not correlated, however, with performance IQ. Children with a higher sign language level demonstrated significant deficits in German vocabulary and grammar, comprehension of spoken German, and verbal memory. For sign language receptive grammar, the correlations with reading comprehension were very similar to those with sign language level. The negative correlation with reading comprehension was not significant. However, there were significant correlations (all negative) with German vocabulary and grammar, comprehension of spoken German utterances, intelligibility of spoken German, and the level of German language used in conversation (PMLP). Once these negative correlations between sign language and reading comprehension as well as other German skills were established, other possible correlates with reading comprehension were examined.

For the Upper Austrian sample, reading comprehension was significantly negatively associated with age, which means that the gap between the reading level of the deaf and that of the hearing norm widened each year. There was no significant correlation with the degree of hearing loss, as all of the children in the sample were profoundly deaf. The aided hearing threshold (with hearing aids or cochlear implants) also had no significant influence on reading comprehension. However, aided speech discrimination was highly correlated with reading comprehension. This might be related to the clinical observation that hearing thresholds for non-speech signals can be quite satisfying with the help of cochlear implants. However, a satisfying aided hearing threshold is not necessarily an indication of good speech perception, particularly in those who received their implant rather late. In this sample, the average age at cochlear implantation was 3.4 years.

Another central finding was the highly significant correlation between grammatical and especially vocabulary knowledge of German and reading. Interestingly, phonological recoding was not significantly correlated with reading comprehension. Possibly due to the rather transparent orthography of German and a strong emphasis on phonology in reading instruction at the preschool and school level, phonological recoding was not a major barrier to word recognition for most deaf children. Moreover, deaf children might use other or additional word decoding strategies (e.g., sign and/or finger alphabet decoding).

To summarize the results for the entire Upper Austrian sample, reading comprehension was negatively correlated with sign language skills. However, there were moderate to strong positive correlations with knowledge of German vocabulary and grammar and with spoken German skills, which was demonstrated by auditory perception of words and particularly by the comprehension of spoken utterances in German (Reynell Scales).

To confirm the existence of *specific* correlations between sign language skills (and spoken language skills) and reading comprehension, fixed-ordered multiple regression analyses were conducted controlling the effects of performance IQ, aided speech discrimination, and age.

In step 1 of these regressions, nonverbal intelligence, speech discrimination, and age were entered into the model. The linguistic variables (signed language and German) were entered separately in step 2. As can be seen in Table 5.4, the variables of age, speech perception, and performance IQ explain 44.1% of the variance in reading comprehension. Highly significant additional variables were German grammar

Table 5.4 Predictors of Reading Comprehension in Deaf Students in Upper Austria (threshold dB >= 80; n = 45) by Use of Fixed-Ordered Multiple Regression Analysis

| Step | Independent variable | Standardized Beta-Coefficient | R2 (adjusted) | R2 change |
|---|---|---|---|---|
| 1 | Age | −.504** | 44.1** | 44.1** |
|   | Nonverbal intelligence | .090 | | |
|   | Speech perception (aided) | .461** | | |
| 2 | Verbal memory | .308* | 50.0** | 5.9* |
| 2 | Grammar—composite score | .477** | 61.1** | 17.0** |
| 2 | Expressive vocabulary | .487** | 60.8** | 16.7** |
| 2 | Sign language level (PMLP) | −.277* | 49.7** | 5.6* |
| 2 | Sign language receptive grammar | −.160 | 44.8** | .7 |

and German vocabulary, which explained about 17% of the additional variance. Even after controlling for age, speech perception, and nonverbal IQ, sign language level remained a significant but negative predictor of reading comprehension. Evidently, sign language skills did not advance reading comprehension in Upper Austria.

Among the subsample of sign language users in Upper Austria, the correlations between reading comprehension and sign language level or sign language receptive grammar were not significant, even after controlling for age effects. Consistent with this finding, a comparison of two subsamples of the signing children divided by their relative level of sign language (PMLP: levels 1–4 vs. level 5–9) found that the reading comprehension in the two equal-sized groups was almost identical. There were no significant differences between the subgroups in terms of nonverbal intelligence, parental education, degree of hearing loss, or non-German family language that might affect reading comprehension.

For the sign language users subsample, we particularly investigated the effect of the age of sign language acquisition on sign language, reading comprehension, and German language outcomes. According to parental reports, the age of first regular exposure to sign language varied from the 1st to the 12th year of life. The age of sign language acquisition was within the first 4 years of life for about 50% of the children. The mean age of sign language acquisition was very late (5 years and 2 months). Due to the moderate to strong correlation with age, we controlled for age effects and found significant influences on sign language grammar ($r = -.51$), but not on sign language used in natural conversation (PMLP). Evidently, age of sign language acquisition affects receptive sign language grammar. However, as expected from the results reported in preceding text, there were no age-of-acquisition effects on reading comprehension or German language skills (vocabulary, grammar, or spoken language comprehension). The signing children were further divided into two groups according to their respective level of sign language (10 children each); those with little sign language (up to level 4: full simple sentences) did not have earlier access to sign language compared to those with higher sign language proficiencies (age of sign language acquisition 4 years and 5 months and 5 years and 9 months, respectively. The somewhat later exposure to sign language of those with a higher sign language level can be partly explained by their older age at sign language assessment.

In sum, in the Upper Austrian sample there is no indication whatsoever of an automatic transfer of better sign language skills to better outcomes in reading comprehension, even after controlling for confounding variables such as performance IQ, age, and even speech discrimination with technical aids. The age of sign language acquisition significantly influences sign language syntactic knowledge, as assessed by comprehension of utterances (video clips) with increasing grammatical complexity, but does not affect reading comprehension.

*Carinthian Sample*

As described earlier, and contrary to the results for the Upper Austria sample, the signing deaf students in Carinthia did better in reading comprehension (although the difference was not statistically significant) than the rest of the children with profound hearing loss, despite more pronounced speech perception deficits.

As reported in preceding text, the sign language level of this group, as assessed by the PMLP, was significantly higher than in the Upper Austrian sample (mean scores 6 vs. 4.7). We need to be somewhat cautious when comparing the results for receptive sign language grammar of Carinthian and Upper Austrian students, as a slightly longer assessment was used for the Carinthian variety of Austrian Sign Language, although it assessed a similar level of complexity. Nevertheless, signing deaf children in Upper Austria had a much lower comprehension rate; they comprehended about 56% of the utterances compared to about 85% in the Carinthian sample.

A correlation analysis of the signing deaf children in Carinthia found a positive correlation between the level of sign language and reading comprehension, but it was not significant. Sign language vocabulary was also positively correlated with reading comprehension. Again, the correlation did not attain significance level in the very small sample of Carinthian children. German vocabulary knowledge turned out to be the variable most strongly associated with reading comprehension ($r = .816$, $p = .025$). A regression analysis was used to predict reading outcomes controlling for the effects of performance IQ, age, and speech perception in step 1. After introducing German vocabulary and German grammar separately as step 2, German vocabulary knowledge explained almost 42% of additional variance of reading compared to 17.6% explained by German grammar. A moderate positive correlation was found between spoken language vocabulary and sign language vocabulary (r = .582); however, it remained below significance level. These findings indicate positive relationships between sign language and spoken language vocabulary and confirm the strong impact of spoken language vocabulary knowledge on reading comprehension.

## SUMMARY AND DISCUSSION

In this chapter we investigated the effects of sign language use and sign language skills on reading comprehension. Many previous studies have found correlations between sign language skills and literacy. These positive correlations were interpreted as evidence for Cummins's interdependence hypothesis. According to this theory, sign language proficiencies are assumed to support general cognitive/academic language and problem-solving skills, and these will quasi-automatically facilitate literacy-related skills in another language. The implication is that with the support of sign language as L1, children will learn to read through sufficient, meaningful, and motivating exposure and interaction in L2 print. During this process they will also learn the vocabulary, morphosyntax, and discourse structure of the language itself (Livingston, 1997). Others have recommended explicitly using sign language to systematically teach L2 literacy using contrastive approaches (Neuroth-Gimbrone & Logiodice, 1992; Paul, 1998; Svartholm, 1993, 1994). Different systems of manually coded spoken language and simultaneous communication, including mouthing and fingerspelling, were identified as possible mediators between sign language skills and the written form of L2. Furthermore, as a consequence of universal newborn hearing screening and early provision with hearing aids and cochlear implants, the role of auditory access to spoken language has been increasingly emphasized as a component of language acquisition and reading comprehension.

The results of our analysis of an Upper Austrian sample of profoundly deaf children refute the idea of an automatic transfer of sign language skills as L1 to literacy in L2. However, the small Carinthian sample demonstrates that under certain circumstances sign language as a primary language can be associated with very satisfying reading comprehension outcomes. Moderate correlations between sign language vocabulary and German vocabulary were found. However, they did not attain significance level in the very small group of Carinthian students. German vocabulary and reading comprehension were strongly correlated. These results indicate a possible role of sign language vocabulary as an influence on spoken language vocabulary and reading comprehension (Hermans et al., 2008; Hermans,

Wauters, de Klerk, & Knoors, Chapter 11 of this volume). Sign language grammar was not related to reading comprehension in either sample. However, we need to be aware that for profoundly deaf children much vocabulary learning occurs through print. Deaf learners not only transfer conceptual lexical knowledge from sign to print, but also vice versa.

The Upper Austrian outcomes demonstrate that for profoundly deaf children the introduction and use of sign language as a preferred means of communication does not automatically result in an increase in German vocabulary or grammatical knowledge, nor in an advancement of reading comprehension. Even where there is considerable superiority in the level of sign language compared to the level of spoken language, sign language concepts and linguistic functions are not automatically transferred to reading comprehension in German. Even after controlling for the effects of nonverbal intelligence, speech discrimination with hearing aids or cochlear implants, and age effects, sign language skills explained a small additional variance of reading comprehension outcomes, with a negative correlation. Within the subsample of children who preferred sign language for everyday communication, reading comprehension of those with higher sign language skills was not significantly better than for the rest of the sample. On the other hand, speech discrimination, that is, auditory access to German and comprehension of spoken utterances, was found to be highly correlated with reading comprehension. German vocabulary knowledge and to a smaller degree grammatical knowledge were also shown to be strongly associated with reading outcomes. One cognitive factor significantly positively associated with reading at the text level is verbal short-term memory, which might be interpreted as a marker or correlate of language aptitude. Interestingly, no specific effects of phonological decoding on reading comprehension were found. The rather high transparency of German orthography and a focus on phonologically based reading and spelling instruction in Austria might explain why phonological decoding does not seem to be a specific barrier to reading comprehension for Austrian deaf children.

Comparing the Upper Austrian results with the Carinthian results, we cannot conclude that sign language proficiencies in L1 either hinder or support literacy in German. The differences between the two samples and their environmental conditions allow us to make the following assumptions about the reasons for the better reading comprehension in the Carinthian sample:

A. earlier access to high quality sign language;
B. higher level of students' sign language proficiency;
C. implementation of a high quality sign-bilingual program, including a high amount of print exposure.

As demonstrated in our earlier discussion, among the Upper Austrian sample of signing deaf students, the time of acquisition of sign language proved to be significantly related to the acquisition of sign language grammar; however, it did not correlate with reading comprehension. As expected, and in accordance with Boudreault and Mayberry (2006), the onset of sign language acquisition affects the outcome of sign syntactic knowledge. However, contrary to Mayberry (2007), better sign language skills do not automatically bestow the ability to learn linguistic structure and vocabulary and thus reading comprehension in the L2. Evidently, time of acquisition is not a sufficient condition if other conditions, such as the systematic use of sign language to teach L2 literacy (see point C in preceding text) or a high level of the students' sign language proficiencies (point B) are not met. As can be seen by our Upper Austrian data, early access to sign language, which effects the acquisition of sign language structure, is not necessarily linked to the presence of deaf parents.

According to Cummins's extension of the linguistic interdependence hypothesis, a certain threshold level of one language (cognitive academic language proficiency) might be necessary to support linguistic processes in another language. As reported earlier, the sign language skills of the small Carinthian sample were significantly better than in the Upper Austria sample. However, this high level of sign language skills alone did not show any correlations with reading comprehension. Even the subgroup comparison of Upper Austrian children with low and high levels of signing proficiencies showed no differences in reading comprehension. If not systematically used in deaf education, high proficiency in sign language as L1 does not automatically lead to higher achievements in reading comprehension in L2. From these results we cannot determine whether some sort of natural transfer of L1 sign language skills to L2 literacy is possible just by providing the students with high sign language skills with motivating exposure and opportunities to use L2 print for functional communication. Comparing the environmental conditions of the two Austrian samples and taking into consideration the results of previous studies, we can predict that all three of the conditions mentioned earlier are needed for sign language to support reading acquisition in a second language.

Deaf children need early access to sign language to develop a high level of sign linguistic structure. In the Upper Austrian sample, the students who preferred to use sign language were all children with hearing parents. When these parents were asked about their own sign language competence, one-third reported that it was rather bad, another third reported moderate ability, and another third reported high proficiency. Only 3 out of 25 parents said that they always used signed language when communicating with their deaf child. Fifty percent used signed language with their deaf child always or often; this means that 50% of the families used signing only sometimes, rarely, or never (Holzinger, Fellinger, Hunger, & Beitel, 2007). These data demonstrate that families with deaf children need special support from very early on, and probably ongoing facilitation to advance the level of signed family communication. Well-trained deaf teachers in preschools, kindergartens, and schools are necessary to promote sign language skills and awareness of sign language structure and semantics. However, even within the Upper Austrian subsample of signing children, those with good sign language skills did not automatically demonstrate significantly better reading results.

Explicit and consistent use and enhancement of the students' sign language skills in reading instruction, as well as a permanent focus on reading instruction and opportunities to meaningfully interact in print—as practiced in the Carinthian bilingual program—are necessary for a transfer of signing skills to reading skills. It is a central message of this chapter that specific teaching strategies and approaches are necessary to transfer sign language skills to written German (presumably from very early on). What is of primary importance for the education of Austrian deaf children is not the development of phonological skills, but the use of sign language at a high level of functioning and as a metalanguage to teach German word meaning and sentence and discourse structure.

This study also suggests that speech discrimination with assistive listening devices could explain a significant amount of the variance in reading outcomes. Hearing technology and auditory language input, as well as simultaneous communication, should be used to provide direct auditory access to spoken language. As the prediction of the effect of hearing aid/cochlear implant use on spoken language remains difficult for an individual child, particularly at a very young age, "preventive" use of natural and conventional signing in the early communication needs to be considered. The choice of communication modalities should remain a dynamic and flexible process for families, in accordance with spoken language development and the preferences of the family. By delaying access to sign language for several years, the advantage of a metalanguage and knowledge base for acquisition of spoken and written language might be diminished or be lost.

Opportunities to communicate with hearing peers in mainstreamed school settings, such as those offered as part of the bilingual program in Carinthia, seem to support L2 acquisition, whether in print or in the spoken/heard modality. These results demonstrate that sign language, if introduced late and used insufficiently in families and in the system of education, is of no automatic advantage for the acquisition of reading comprehension, which is a central predictor of academic outcomes, job opportunities, and autonomy in adult life.

# REFERENCES

Akamatsu, C. T., Musselman, C., & Zwiebel, A. (2000). Nature versus nurture in the development of cognition in deaf people. In P. Spencer, C. Erting, & M. Marschark (Eds.), *Development in context: The deaf children in the family and at school* (pp. 255–273). Mahwah, NJ: Lawrence Erlbaum Associates.

Bishop, D. V. M. (2003). *Test for reception of grammar (TROG-2)*. London: Pearson.

Boudreault, P., & Mayberry, R. I. (2006). Grammatical processing in American Sign Language: Age of first-language acquisition effects in relation to syntactic structure. *Language and Cognitive Processes, 21*, 608–635.

Brasel, K. E., & Quigley, S. P. (1977). Influence of certain language and communication environments in early childhood on the development of language in deaf individuals. *Journal of Speech and Hearing Research, 20*, 95–107.

Canale, M., Frenette, N., & Belanger, M. (1987). Evaluation of minority students writing in first and second languages. In J. Fine (Ed.), *Second language discourse: A textbook of current research* (pp. 147–165). Norwood, NJ: Ablex.

Castilla, A. P., Pérez-Leroux, & Restrepo, M. A. (2009). Individual differences and the developmental interdependence hypothesis. *International Journal of Bilingual Education and Bilingualism 12*(1), 1–16.

Chamberlain, C., & Mayberry, R. I. (2008). American Sign Language syntactic and narrative comprehension in skilled and less skilled readers: Bilingual and bimodal evidence for the linguistic basis of reading. *Applied Psycholinguistics 29*, 367–388.

Chamberlain, C., & Mayberry, R. I. (2000). Theorizing about the relation between American Sign Language and reading. In C. Chamberlain, J. P. Morford, & R. I. Mayberry (Eds.), *Language acquisition by eye* (pp. 221–260). Mahwah, NJ: Earlbaum.

Connor, C. M., Hieber, S., Arts, H. A., & Zwolan, T. A. (2000). Speech, vocabulary, and the education of children using cochlear implants: Oral or total communication? *Journal of Speech, Language and Hearing Research, 43*, 1185–1204.

Connor, C. M. & Zwolan, T. A. (2004). Examining multiple sources of influence on the reading comprehension skills of children who use cochlear implants. *Journal of Speech, Language and Hearing Research, 47*, 509–526.

Convertino, C. M., Marschark, M., Sapere, P., Sarchet, T., & Zupan, M. (2009). Predicting academic success among deaf college students. *Journal of Deaf Studies and Deaf Education, 14*, 324–342.

Cumming, A. (1989). Writing expertise and second language proficiency. *Language Learning, 39*, 81–141.

Cummins, J. (1989). A theoretical framework of bilingual special education. *Exceptional Children, 56*, 111–119.

Cummins, J. (1978). Education implications of mother tongue maintenance in minority language groups. *The Canadian Modern Language Review, 34*, 395–416.

Cummins, J. (1986). Empowering minority students: A framework for intervention. *Harvard Education Review, 56*, 18–36.

Cummins, J. (1991). Interdependence of first- and second-language proficiency in bilingual children. In E. Bialystok (Ed.), *Language processing in bilingual children* (pp. 70–89). Cambridge, UK: Cambridge University Press.

Cummins, J. (2000). *Language, power and pedagogy: Bilingual children in the crossfire*. Clevedon, UK: Multilingual Matters.

Cummins, J. (1979). Linguistic interdependence and the educational development of bilingual children. *Review of Educational Research, 49*, 221–251.

Cummins, J. (1981). The role of primary language development in promoting educational success for language minority students. In California State Department of Education (Ed.), *Schooling and language minority students: A theoretical framework*. Los Angeles: Evaluation, Dissemination and Assessment Center, California State University.

Fellinger, J., Holzinger, D., Sattel, H., Laucht, M., & Goldberg, D. (2009). Correlates of mental health disorders among children with hearing impairments. *Developmental Medicine & Child Neurology, 51*(8), 635–641.

Fox, A. (2009). TROG-D, Test zur Überprüfung des Grammatikverständnises. [German version of TROG-2 Test for reception of Grammar-2, Bishop, D.V.M.]. Idstein, Germany: Schulz-Kirchner Verlag.

Gathercole, S. (2006). Non-word repetition and word learning: The nature of the relationship. *Applied Psycholinguistics, 27*, 513–543.

Geers, A. (2003). Predictors of reading skill development in children with early cochlear implantation. *Ear and Hearing, 24*, 59–68.

Geers, A., Brenner, C., Nicholas, J., Uchanski, R., Tye-Murray, N., & Tobey. E. (2002). Rehabilitation factors contributing to implant benefit in children. *Annals of Otology, Rhinology & Laryngology, 111*(5), 127–130.

Geers, A. & Moog, J. (1989). Factors predictive of development of literacy in profoundly hearing-impaired adolescents. *Volta Review, 91*, 69–86.

Glück, C. W. (2007). *Wortschatz- und Wortfindungstest für 6-10-Jährige*. München, Germany: Urban & Fischer.

Goberis, D., Beams, D., Dalpes, M., Abrisch, A., Baca, R., & Yoshinaga-Itano C. (2012). The missing link in language development of deaf and hard of hearing children: Pragmatic language development. *Seminars in Speech and Language, 33*(4), 297–309.

Goldstein, G., & Bebko, J. M. (2003). The profile of multiple language proficiencies: Measure for evaluating language samples of deaf children. *Journal of Deaf Studies and Deaf Education, 8*(4), 452–463.

Haznedar, B. (2006). Persistent problems with case morphology in L2 acquisition. In C. Lléo. (Ed.), *Interfaces in Multilingualism: Acquisition and representation* (pp. 179–206). Hamburg Studies on Multilingualism, Volume 4. Amsterdam; Philadelphia: John Benjamins.

Hermans, D., Knoors, H., Ormel, E., & Verhoeven, L. (2008). The relationship between the reading and signing skills of deaf children in bilingual education programs. *Journal of Deaf Studies and Education of the Deaf, 13*(4), 518–530.

Hoffmeister, R. (2000). A piece of puzzle: ASL and reading comprehension in deaf children. In C. Chamberlain, J. Morford, & R. Mayberry (Eds.), *Language Acquisition by Eye* (pp. 143–163). Hillsdale, NJ: Lawrence Erlbaum Associates.

Holzinger, D. (2010). *Komponenten des Lesens: Determinanten von Leseverständnis bei Kindern mit sensorineuraler Hörstörung*. Habilitation Thesis, Karl Franzens University, Graz.

Holzinger, D., Fellinger, J., Hunger, B., & Beitel, C. (2007). Gebärden in Familie und Schule: Ergebnisse der Cheers Studie in Oberösterreich. *Das Zeichen, 77*, 444–453.

Hoover, W. A., & Gough, P. G. (1990). The simple view of reading. *Reading and Writing: An Interdisciplinary Journal*, 2, 127–160.
Hopf, D. (2005). Zweisprachigkeit und Schulleistung bei Migrantenkindern. *Zeitschrift der Pädagogik*, 51(2), 236–251.
Hornberger, N. (1989). Continua of biliteracy. *Review of Educational Research*, 59, 271–296.
Israelite, N., Ewoldt, C., & Hoffmeister, R. (1992) *Bilingual-bicultural education for deaf and hard-of-hearing students.* Toronto, Canada: MGS Publication Services.
Jackson, D., Paul, P., & Smith, J. (1997). Prior knowledge and reading comprehension ability of deaf and hard-of-hearing adolescents. *Journal of Deaf Studies and Deaf Education* 2(3),172–184.
Kampfe, C. M., & Turecheck, A. G. (1987). Reading achievement of prelingually deaf students and its relationship to parental method of communication: A review of the literature. *American Annals of the Deaf*, 132(1), 11–15.
Kelly, L. (1996). The interaction of syntactic competence and vocabulary during reading by deaf students. *Journal of Deaf Studies and Deaf Education* 1(1), 75–90.
Kelly, R. R., & Mousley, K. (2001). Solving word problems: More than reading issues for deaf students. *American Annals of the Deaf*, 146, 251–262.
King, C., & Quigley, S. (1985). *Reading and deafness.* San Diego, CA: College-Hill Press.
Kovelman, I., Baker, S., & Petitto, L. A. (2008). Age of bilingual language exposure as a new window into bilingual reading development. *Bilingualism: Language and Cognition*, 11(2), 203–223.
Kusché, C. A., Greenberg, M. T., & Garfield, T. S. (1983). The understanding and role-taking ability: A comparison of deaf and hearing children. *Child Development*, 54, 141–147.
Kyle, F. E., & Harris, M. (2006). Concurrent correlates and predictors of reading and spelling achievement in deaf and hearing school children. *Journal of Deaf Studies and Deaf Education*, 11(3), 273–288.
Landerl, K., Wimmer, H., & Moser, E. (1997). *Salzburger Lese- und Rechtschreibtest; Verfahren zur Differentialdiagnose von Störungen des Lesens und Schreibens für die erste bis vierte Schulstufe.* Göttingen, Germany: Verlag Hans Huber.
Lenhard, W., & Schneider, W. (2006). *ELFE 1-6. Ein Leseverständnistest für Erst- bis Sechstklässler.* Göttingen, Germany: Hogrefe.
Livingston, S. (1997). *Rethinking the education of deaf students: Theory and practice from a teacher's perspective.* Portsmouth, NH: Heinemann.
López, L. M., & Greenfield, D. B. (2004). The identification of pre-literacy skills in Hispanic Head Start children. *NHSA Dialog*, 7(1), 61–83.
Marschark, M., Lang, H. G., & Albertini, J. A. (2002). *Educating deaf students: From research to practice.* New York, NY: Oxford University Press.
Mayberry, R. I. (1994). The importance of childhood to language acquisition: Insights from American Sign Language. In J. C. Goodman & H. C. Nusbaum (Eds.), *The development of speech perception: The transition from speech sounds to words* (pp. 57–90). Cambridge, MA: MIT Press.
Mayberry, R. I. (2007). When timing is everything: Age of first-language acquisition effects on second-language learning. *Applied Psycholinguistics* 28, 537–549.
Mayer, C., & Akamatsu C. T. (2011). Bilingualism and Literacy. In M. Marschark & P. E. Spencer (Eds.), *The Oxford handbook of deaf studies, language, and education* (vol. 1, 2nd ed.). New York, NY: Oxford University Press.

Mayer, C., & Wells, G. (1996). Can the linguistic interdependence theory support a bilingual-bicultural model of literacy education for deaf students? *Journal of Deaf Studies and Deaf Education, 1,* 93–107.

Meadow, K. (1968). Early manual communication in relation to the deaf child's intellectual, social, and communicative functioning. *American Annals of the Deaf, 113,* 29–41.

Möhring, A. (2001). The acquisition of French by German pre-school children. An empirical investigation of gender assignment and gender agreement. In S. Foster, Cohen & A. Nizegorodcew (Eds.), *EUROSLA Yearbook* (pp. 171–193). Amsterdam, Netherlands: John Benjamins Publishing.

Moores, D., & Sweet, C. (1990). Relationships of English grammar and communicative fluency to reading in deaf adolescents. *Exceptionality, 1,* 97–106.

Neuroth-Gimbrone, C., & Logiodice, C. (1992). A co-operative bilingual language program for deaf adolescents. *Sign Language Studies, 74,* 79–91.

Nicolay, K., Rupp, A., & Rosenkötter, H. (2003). *Test-CD für die auditiven Funktionen.* Kandern, Germany: Audiva.

Oller, D. K., & Eilers, R. E. (2002). *Language and literacy in bilingual children.* Clevedon Hall, UK: Multilingual Matters.

Padden, C., & Ramsey, C. (2000). American Sign Language and reading ability in deaf children. In C. Chamberlain, J. Morford & R. Mayberry (Eds.), *Language Acquisition by Eye* (pp. 165–189). Hillsdale, NJ: Lawrence Erlbaum Associates.

Paul, P. (1998). *Literacy and deafness: The development of reading, writing, and literate thought.* Boston: Allyn & Bacon.

Pisoni, D. B., Conway, C. M., Kronenberger, W., Horn, D. L., Karpicke, J., & Henning, S. (2008). Efficacy and effectiveness of cochlear implants in deaf children. In M. Marschark & P. Hauser (Eds.), *Deaf cognition: Foundations and outcomes* (pp. 52–101). New York, NY: Oxford University Press.

Reese, L., Garnier, H., Gallimore, R., & Goldenberg, C. (2000). Longitudinal analysis of the antecedents of emergent Spanish literacy and middle school reading achievement of Spanish speaking students. *American Educational Research Journal, 37,* 633–662.

Riches, A., & Genesee, F. (2006). Literacy: Crosslinguistic and crossmodal issues. In F. Genesee, K. Lindholm-Leary, W. Saunders, & D. Christian (Eds.), *Educating English Language learners: A synthesis of research evidence* (pp. 64–108). New York, NY: Cambridge University Press.

Robbins, A. M., Bollard, P. M., & Green, J. (1999). Language development in children implanted with the CLARION cochlear implant. *Annals of Otology, Rhinology, and Laryngology, 177* (Suppl.), 113–118.

Rodda, M., Cumming, C., & Fewer, D. (1993). Memory, learning and language: Implications for deaf education. In M. Marschark & M. D. Clark (Eds.), *Psychological perspectives on deafness* (pp. 339–352). Hillsdale, NJ: Lawrence Erlbaum Associates.

Rothweiler, M. (2006). The acquisition of V2 and subordinate clauses in early successive acquisition of German. In C. Lléo (Ed.), *Interfaces in multilingualism* (pp. 91–113). Amsterdam: John Benjamins Publishing.

Sarimski, K., & Süss-Burghart, H. (2001). *Reynell Developmental Language Scales III: The University of Reading Edition RDLS Manual.* German Version. Unpublished manuscript. Munich, Germany: Kinderzentrum.

Singleton, J., Morgan, D., DiGello, E., Wiles, J., & Rivers, R. (2004). Vocabulary use by low, moderate, and high ASL-Proficient writers compared to hearing ESL and monolingual speakers. *Journal of Deaf Studies and Deaf Education*, 9(1), 86–103.

Singleton, J. L., Supalla, S. J., Litchfield, S., & Schley, S. (1998). From sign to word: Considering modality constraints in ASL/English bilingual education. *Topics in Language Disorders*, 18, 16–29.

Strong, M., & Prinz, P. M. (1997). A study of the relationship between American Sign Language and English literacy. *Journal of Deaf Studies and Deaf Education*, 2, 37–46.

Strong, M., & Prinz, P. M. (2000). Is American Sign Language related to English literacy? In C. Chamberlain, J. Morford, & R. Mayberry (Eds.), *Language acquisition by eye* (pp. 131–163). Hillsdale, NJ: Lawrence Erlbaum Associates.

Stuckless, E. R., & Birch, J. W. (1966). The influence of early manual communication on the linguistic development of deaf children. *American Annals of the Deaf*, 111, 452–460, 499–504.

Svartholm, K. (1993). Bilingual education for the deaf in Sweden. *Sign Language Studies*, 81, 291–332.

Svartholm, K. (1994). Second language learning in the deaf. In I. Ahlgren & K. Hyltenstam (Eds.), *Bilingualism in deaf education* (pp. 61–70). Hamburg, Germany: Signum.

Verhoeven, L. T. (2007). Early bilingualism, language transfer, and phonological awareness. *Applied Psycholinguistics*, 28(3), 426–439.

Verhoeven, L. T. (2001). Transfer in bilingual development: The linguistic interdependence hypothesis revisited. *Language Learning*, 44(3), 381–415.

Vermeulen, A. M. (2007). *Reading skills after cochlear implantation*. Enschede: PrintPartners Ipskamp.

Vernon, M., & Koh, S. (1970). Early manual communication and deaf children´s achievement. *American Annals of the Deaf*, 115, 527–536.

Weber-Fox, C., & Neville, H. J. (1999). Functional neural subsystems are differentially affected by delays in second language immersion: ERP and behavioral evidence in bilinguals. In D. Birdsong (Ed.), *Second language acquisition and the critical period hypothesis* (pp. 23–389). Mahwah, NJ: Lawrence Erlbaum Associates.

Weber-Fox, C., & Neville, H. J. (1996). Maturational constraints on functional specializations for language processing: ERP and behavioral evidence in bilingual speakers. *Journal of Cognitive Neuroscience*, 8, 231–256.

Wettstein, P. (1995). *Psycholinguistischer Sprachentwicklungs- und Sprachverständnistest*. Uster: BSSI.

# 6

# The Influence of Communication Mode on Language Development in Children with Cochlear Implants

Elizabeth A. Walker and J. Bruce Tomblin

Cochlear implants (CIs) are now a common habilitation option for children with profound hearing loss who receive limited benefit from hearing aids. This technology provides children with profound hearing loss access to environmental sounds and has a positive influence on speech perception, speech production, and spoken language skills (Svirsky, Robbins, Kirk, Pisoni, & Miyamoto, 2000). Children with CIs typically reach levels of performance in these areas that surpass those of their non-implanted peers who use hearing aids (L. J. Spencer, Tye-Murray, & Tomblin, 1998; Yoshinaga-Itano, Baca, & Sedey, 2010), but there is wide variation in the degree of benefit that individuals receive from cochlear implants (Sarant, Blamey, Dowell, Clark, & Gibson, 2001). CIs, in combination with early identification and intervention for hearing loss, enable many children with congenital deafness to be educated in regular-education school settings alongside their hearing peers by kindergarten (Geers, Moog, Biedenstein, Brenner, & Hayes, 2009). The advent of CI technology also has resulted in significant changes in approaches to communication and education for children who are deaf.

Much of the research literature on the influence of educational settings for children with CIs focuses on the comparison of different intervention approaches (e.g., auditory-oral communication versus sign language). This chapter will focus on a frequently debated topic among researchers and professionals who work with this population: the choice of communication modality and educational settings for children with CIs. By the 1980s, there were three influential models in deaf education: the bilingual-bicultural model, in which a sign language such as American Sign Language (ASL) or British Sign Language (BSL) is the primary mode of instruction and written/spoken language (e.g., English) is taught as a second language for literacy; total communication, which combines all visual, manual, and auditory components of communication; and the auditory-oral approach, in which children are encouraged to rely on their residual hearing and communicate through spoken language.

## BILINGUAL-BICULTURAL APPROACHES

Among the three main instructional methods, the bilingual-bicultural model is the one most often selected by deaf parents who use sign language. Programs that implement this model base their orientation on the assumption that a strong foundation in one primary language will have positive effects on cognitive, language, and literacy (Carney & Moeller, 1998). This assumption is supported by research demonstrating that deaf children of deaf parents have stronger reading and math skills than deaf children of hearing parents (Meadow, 2005; but see Marschark & Lee, Chapter 9 of this volume). Furthermore, advocates of sign bilingual education propose that bilingual-bicultural approaches facilitate identification with Deaf culture and the Deaf community, which in turn will have a positive long-term impact on social development.

To date, there is little empirical research to support this latter suggestion (Knoors & Marschark, 2012). There also are few studies investigating the spoken language and auditory development of children with cochlear implants who are utilizing a sign bilingual approach. Hyde and Punch (2011) conducted surveys with 247 parents and 151 teachers of children with CIs in Australia. They reported that a small minority of children (6.9%) used Australian Sign Language (Auslan) at home and 9.3% used a bilingual-bicultural approach in school. As Swanwick and Tsverik (2007) acknowledged, evidence-based research on the topic of bilingual-bicultural education and CIs is severely limited by the fact that successful cochlear implant users are rarely placed in sign bilingual programs. Therefore, it can be challenging to determine how sign bilingual approaches complement the goal of cochlear implantation, which is to promote the acquisition of spoken language skills.

Unlike the United States, United Kingdom, and Australia, some countries adopt a sign bilingual approach for educating all children who are deaf, including children with CIs. For example, the Netherlands provides a bilingual program (spoken Dutch and Sign Language of the Netherlands [SLN]) for students who are deaf (see Hermans, De Klerk, Wauters, & Knoors, Chapter 16 of this volume). Parents are encouraged to communicate via sign language, as well as spoken Dutch, and participate in SLN classes (Wiefferink, Spaai, Uilenburg, Vermeij, & De Raeve, 2008). A similar approach is employed in Norway, where Norwegian Sign Language (NSL) is learned as a first language and written/spoken Norwegian is learned as a second language (but see Swanwick, Hendar, Dammeyer, Kristoffersen, Salter, & Simonsen, Chapter 12 of this volume). Wie, Falkenberg, Tvete, and Tomblin (2007) reported that 71% of children implanted in Norway between 1992 and 2001 were educated in a sign bilingual program. As a result, it is feasible to investigate the efficacy of sign bilingual education in children with CIs in these countries without some of the limitations that are inherent in American, Australian, or British research on the relationship between educational setting and language development with a CI. For example, children who use different forms of manual communication such as Cued Speech, Signed English, and ASL can be combined into one group, providing successful CI users access to bilingual education programs.

Wiefferink and colleagues (2008) took advantage of differing educational systems in the Netherlands and the Dutch-speaking part of Belgium (Flanders) to study the effects of sign bilingual language environments on language development in children with CIs. Six Dutch children and 12 Flemish children with CIs participated (age range at implantation: 9 to 27 months of age). The Dutch children used spoken Dutch and SLN in preschool, and all of the parents had learned SLN. The Flemish children relied on spoken Dutch in preschool, supported by signs. Their parents had not learned SLN, although 5 of the 12 parents had taken a course in Simultaneous Communication. Children were assessed at one pre-implant visit, and at 6, 12, 24, and 36 months post-implantation. The Flemish children demonstrated significantly higher scores for receptive and expressive spoken language compared to the Dutch children. Furthermore, the Flemish children (n = 7) who were implanted prior to 18 months of age displayed language skills commensurate with their same-age hearing peers, while the Flemish children (n = 5) implanted after 18 months of age and the Dutch children (all implanted at 20 months of age or older) showed delays relative to their hearing peers. The Dutch children also were assessed for syntactic complexity in spoken language and sign language via two spontaneous language samples conducted with a hearing adult in spoken Dutch and a deaf adult in SLN, respectively. The results showed that the spoken language skills of the Dutch children improved over time, while the syntactic complexity of SLN did not improve.

Wiefferink and colleagues concluded that, overall, the Flemish children, who were educated in spoken Dutch with some sign support, outperformed Dutch children who were educated in a sign bilingual program. The authors did not address the confound of age at implantation, however. The higher scores among the Flemish children may have been influenced by an earlier age at implantation. Researchers have demonstrated a positive impact of earlier implantation on spoken language skills over time (Kirk et al., 2002; Niparko et al., 2010; Tomblin, Barker, Spencer, Zhang, & Gantz, 2005). In addition, the Flemish children had an earlier average age at diagnosis of hearing loss, hearing aid fitting, and enrollment in early intervention, as well as more pre-implant residual hearing—all factors known to influence spoken language outcomes in children with hearing loss (Moeller, 2000; Sininger, Grimes, & Christensen, 2010; Szagun, 2001). The authors also indicated that the Flemish children received better equipment support than the Dutch children, suggesting that the Dutch children may have been without their CIs for extended periods of time due to device malfunctions. There was no report of amount of daily CI use for the participants, but if the Flemish children wore their devices more consistently than the Dutch children, daily use time could also influence language outcomes (Wie et al., 2007). Given the limitations of the study, it is not possible to conclusively state whether children with CIs would benefit more from sign bilingual or spoken language environments. Wiefferink and colleagues recommended that parents initially learn sign language and communicate with their deaf child using spoken language with sign support. This would allow parents to communicate effectively with their young child, while postponing the decision to pursue a sign language or oral educational setting until it becomes clear how adept their child is at perceiving and understanding auditory information from the CI.

Wie and colleagues (2007) conducted the only other study to include a large percentage of children with CIs educated in sign bilingual programs, with the goal of investigating what factors influenced speech recognition scores and speech-recognition growth rate. They evaluated 79 children with prelingual deafness with an average age at implantation of 50 months; 71% of the children were enrolled in a sign bilingual education setting, using NSL and spoken Norwegian. The remaining 29% were enrolled in oral communication educational settings. Results showed that daily CI use time, nonverbal intelligence, and communication mode were the three most important variables for predicting speech recognition. Children enrolled in the oral educational settings had the highest speech recognition scores. Results for the speech-recognition growth rate analysis supported cross-sectional findings; children educated in mainstream settings that relied on spoken language had the fastest growth rate. Based on their findings, Wie and colleagues concluded that there should be an increased focus on speech recognition and production skills in intervention for Scandinavian children with CIs, and recommended a transition in educational approaches from sign language toward spoken language.

In summary, there is limited research on the efficacy of sign bilingual programs for children with CIs. The few published studies were conducted in countries that used sign bilingual programs for all or most students who were deaf (Wie et al., 2007; Wiefferink et al., 2008). Results of both studies suggested that for the children with CIs, those who had more exposure to spoken language with sign support outperformed their peers enrolled in sign bilingual programs in speech-related domains.

Given the limited amount of literature on sign bilingual education and CIs, the remainder of this review will focus on total communication and auditory-oral approaches. These two broad approaches are the ones used most often with deaf children of hearing parents, who have some type of sensory aid (cochlear implants and/or hearing aids). The review will also focus on children with bilateral, severe-to-profound hearing loss who utilize cochlear implants.

There is a small body of literature on the impact of mild-to-moderate hearing loss or otitis media on speech and language development in children (Davis, Elfenbein, Schum, & Bentler, 1986; Elfenbein, Hardin-Jones, & Davis, 1994; Rvachew, Slawinski, & Williams, 1996; Rvachew, Slawinski, Williams, & Green, 1999). Most of these children use spoken language and are in mainstream educational settings (Davis, Shepard, Stelmachowicz, & Gorga, 1981). Although they often demonstrate speech and language deficits, parents and professionals usually do not have to deal with the decision of which intervention approach to select for these children.

## AUDITORY-ORAL APPROACHES

There are several different approaches to implementing an auditory-oral communication modality (OC). All of the approaches share several fundamental assumptions. One is that all children with hearing loss should have the opportunity to learn how to communicate through speech. This is seen as a possibility because very few children are born completely deaf and therefore most can benefit from amplification (Ling, 1984). The primary goal is to see the deaf child mainstreamed in a regular education classroom and integrated into the hearing community as an independent adult. The approaches also share a common dependence on the use of speechreading and audition for communication, to the exclusion of signs or gestures. It is assumed that the acoustic channel must be the primary source of input for the child. The visual channel will develop naturally as a supplement to audition. It is assumed that if the visual channel is emphasized first, the child will learn to rely on visual cues to the detriment of auditory information.

One of the main oralist approaches is called pure oralism or oral/aural (Northern & Downs, 2002). In this approach, children with hearing loss use some form of amplification. They are exposed to spoken language and environmental sounds throughout the day. Training begins with directing the child's visual attention to speechreading. Systematic therapy progresses from teaching the child to perceive and produce isolate sounds, sound combinations, words, and finally, connected speech. Another approach is known as auditory-verbal therapy. It is descended from earlier approaches referred to as acoupedics or unisensory approach (Marschark & Spencer, 2006). This approach is heavily dependent on early identification and amplification, as well as intensive parental involvement in intervention. Training goals are tied to the child's developmental level and are incorporated into daily routines at home. Unlike pure oralism, there is no specific speechreading training. Emphasis is entirely on the auditory mechanism, in the expectation that children will learn to rely on their residual hearing. Auditory-verbal and oral-aural approaches have received sharp criticism in the past, due to their reliance on using only auditory input as the primary linguistic channel. They have experienced a resurgence in recent years due to the success of cochlear implants (Northern & Downs, 2002).

## TOTAL COMMUNICATION APPROACHES

Total communication (TC) is a philosophy that combines auditory, manual, and vocal modes, with the goal of ensuring effective communication by the child. It grew out of research that seemed to indicate that no one method was effective for all children with hearing loss (Ling & Atchley, 1984). It is based on the theory that the simultaneous use of oral and manual communication is mutually reinforcing. It is often emphasized that TC is an educational philosophy, not a communication method. The educator or parent is trying to use whatever communication modality that works to help the child express and comprehend language (Northern & Downs, 2002). It is recommended that the child be exposed to many social communication opportunities with deaf and hearing people, because the implications for TC "go beyond the classroom and involve social and cultural as well as instructional interchange" (Ling & Atchley, 1984; p. 1).

TC is usually implemented in the schools as simultaneous communication (SC), in which the teacher simultaneously combines spoken English with manually coded English (ASL in English word order). This was not the original intent of TC proponents, and frequently the result is that teachers end up stressing one modality over another, depending on their own philosophical bent. SC is also less flexible than the TC philosophy (Marschark & Spencer, 2006). The primary criticism is that TC is a "shotgun approach" to intervention, and the child never becomes adept at one particular system (Northern & Downs, 2002). In addition, research has shown that it is difficult to combine signs and speech effectively at the same time (Marmor & Pettito, 1979; cf., Marschark & Lee, Chapter 9 of this volume). Finally, researchers have expressed concerns about the ability of children to simultaneously process two different modes of language input because of limited memory capacities (Marschark & Spencer, 2006).

It is evident from a review of the history of deaf education that there have been many claims made about the relative advantages of one intervention approach over another. These claims have often been made by professionals with strong philosophical beliefs, and they are not necessarily based on evidence-based, empirical research (Northern & Downs, 2002). Carney and Moeller (1998) advise caution even when interpreting the empirical research on communication modalities. Most of this research is descriptive rather than experimental, and studies tend to focus on characterizing aspects of communication within a certain modality (e.g., Geers & Moog, 1992). These studies will be reviewed in the following section.

## COMPARISONS OF OC AND TC APPROACHES IN CHILDREN WITH HEARING AIDS

The early studies comparing the relative effectiveness of TC versus OC only included children with hearing aids, because cochlear implants for children as young as 2 years of age did not receive approval from the Food and Drug Administration (FDA) until 1990 (P. Spencer, Marschark, & Spencer, 2011). Greenberg and Calderon (1984) described the existing literature comparing OC and TC early intervention programs at that time. The studies they reviewed must be interpreted with some caution because they were all conducted prior to the passage of IDEA, which mandated family-centered early intervention (Part C birth–3 services), as well as universal newborn hearing screening (Joint Committee on Infant Hearing; JCIH, 2007). Nevertheless, Greenberg and Calderon reported that the findings on OC early intervention programs were mostly negative. Most of the children showed significant delays in receptive and expressive language compared to their peers. They also appeared to make little progress in language skills over time. Results did seem to show an advantage for children who were enrolled in intervention earlier or received hearing aids at younger ages. For TC programs, there were very little published data due to its relatively recent emergence (at that time) as an educational option. In general, the literature indicated that children in TC programs demonstrated more positive short-term effects for language outcomes, compared to children in OC programs.

Greenberg, Calderon, and Kusché (1984) investigated the effectiveness of TC programs. They looked at children who were enrolled in a TC program by age 2 years. The program consisted of regular home visits by professionals and home and group sign language classes for parents. These children were compared to another group of children who did not receive consistent intervention services. Both groups started intervention around the same time, but the TC group was exposed to sign language approximately a year earlier than the control group. The limited services that the control group received were mostly focused on auditory-oral communication. During a free play situation with their mothers, the children in the TC group demonstrated more advanced communication than the control group. However, the authors did not mention if the children were using amplification on a regular basis. One limitation of the study was the fact that the experimental group was from an urban area and the control group was from a rural area. This limitation could result in differences (e.g., socioeconomic status) that would present a confound in the results.

Geers, Moog, and Schick (1984) reported on findings that supported an OC approach over TC. They tested children in OC and TC programs on the production of English grammatical structures. All of the children had profound, congenital hearing loss and had been enrolled in intervention since 3 years of age. The study had a cross-sectional design, testing children between the ages of 5 to 9 years. To limit the possibility of selection bias, they excluded any children who had moved from an OC to a TC program. Geers and colleagues found that the TC group achieved significantly better scores when they communicated through sign than spoken language. The OC group outperformed the TC group when all of the children were using oral communication. Based on these findings, the authors concluded that the children exposed to sign language were not developing spoken English at the same pace as manually coded English.

Although they tried to control for selection bias, Geers, Moog, and Schick (1984) acknowledged that the children in the OC program might have shown a propensity for communicating through spoken language at young ages, which was why they were enrolled in an OC program in the first place. If this were the case, it would bias the results because it is not the difference in programs that is the causal factor in group variation, but a difference in the children themselves. Furthermore, the decision to only include children who stayed in OC or TC programs would have resulted in the exclusion of children who struggled with the OC approach and were eventually moved to TC. By eliminating these so-called "oral failures," the authors may have created a biased sample of high-performing children in the OC group. There were additional differences between the two groups that could have influenced the results. The OC children were all in private schools and the children in TC programs were all in public schools. There may have been significant differences in the amount of direct instruction the children were receiving, as well as differences in socioeconomic status (SES). As a final note, the authors reported that both groups of children were significantly delayed compared to their peers, scoring well below 4-year-old normal-hearing children. Regardless of how the two groups performed in comparison to each other, neither group was at language levels expected for their chronological age.

Geers and Schick (1988) went on to compare two groups of children in TC programs, those with deaf parents and those with hearing parents. They hypothesized that the deaf children of deaf parents (D/D group) would perform better on standardized language measures than the deaf children of hearing parents (D/H group) because of the former group's early exposure to (sign) language. Results appeared to support this hypothesis. The two groups showed no differences on expressive language measures at ages 5 and 6. At age 7, the D/D group began to make significant language production gains and the D/H group showed no progress. These results held across three different communication modalities: sign only, sign plus speech, and speech only. Geers and Schick concluded that there was little evidence that knowledge of ASL limits the acquisition of spoken English, because the D/D group showed growth in their oral language skills. Consistent with the results of Geers et al. (1984), both groups were still significantly delayed in their language abilities compared to their normal-hearing peers.

Most studies comparing children in OC versus TC programs have examined outcomes in the preschool and early elementary years, during the early stages of communication development. In contrast, Geers and Moog (1992) investigated oral communication skills in later adolescence. The sample included 227 children tested at 16 and 17 years of age. The primary goal was to investigate the extent to which older children in TC and OC programs developed speech perception and production skills. The two groups were matched on cognitive ability, auditory thresholds, and age. The groups differed on several important variables. Most of the children in the OC group were enrolled in mainstream educational settings, while most of the TC students attended residential schools for the deaf. The TC children also came from families with a lower median income than the OC group. Notably, this study was also one of the first to report on amplification status. Most of the OC children reported that they wore hearing aids most of the time. Less than half of the TC students with hearing parents reported wearing their hearing aids. Most of the TC students with deaf parents reported that they did not wear hearing aids.

The participants were tested on a battery of speech perception, production, and oral language proficiency measures (Geers & Moog, 1992). None of the measures were norm-referenced to an age-matched, normal-hearing comparison group; therefore, the authors did not describe either group's performance in relation to their same-age hearing peers. The OC group performed better than the TC group on all of the tests, except for OC students with thresholds greater than 110 dB HL. The same limitations that were seen in earlier studies still applied, however. Early in the intervention process, clinicians and teachers may have encouraged parents to utilize an OC approach for young children who appeared likely to be successful spoken language users, and may have discouraged an OC approach for children who showed signs of struggling with spoken language development. This initial selection bias would have influenced outcomes at later ages. It is also not surprising that the OC children would perform better on oral language measures, because their education was entirely directed toward improving their proficiency in that mode of communication. Based on the findings, we may conclude that consistent use of amplification promotes oral language proficiency (among those for whom amplification is effective). We can also conclude that the amount of residual hearing influences the acquisition of spoken language, because the children in the OC group with the highest thresholds (greater than 110 dB HL) showed poorer performance on speech perception and production measures than OC students with thresholds between 80 to 110 dB HL.

In conclusion, there were a number of studies investigating speech perception, production, and language outcomes of children in TC versus OC programs during the 1980s and early 1990s (Geers et al., 1984; Geers & Moog, 1992; Geers & Schick, 1988; Greenberg & Calderon, 1984; Greenberg et al., 1984). Much of the work by Geers and her colleagues suggested an OC advantage with respect to spoken language development. The results of these studies should be interpreted with some caution, however, because of possible selection biases in favor of OC approaches. The advent of cochlear implant technology has led to a rather dramatic change in attitudes toward OC and TC educational programs, as the following section describes.

## COMPARISONS OF OC VERSUS TC APPROACHES IN CHILDREN WITH COCHLEAR IMPLANTS

Regardless of the evidence for or against specific intervention approaches, from the 1970s to the 1990s TC was the most frequently used approach in educational settings for deaf children (Northern & Downs, 2002). Approaches to intervention underwent a major shift with the advent of cochlear implants, however. This technology has provided children (and adults) who have profound hearing loss with access to environmental sounds and spoken language, although there is wide variation in the degree of benefit that individuals receive from cochlear implants (Sarant et al., 2001). The technology also has renewed interest in auditory-oral approaches to intervention (Marschark & Spencer, 2006). Some of the research looking at outcomes for children with cochlear implants in relation to intervention approach was equivocal (Dawson, Blarney, Dettman, Barker, & Clark, 1995; Svirsky et al., 2000). Other reports showed positive evidence for auditory-oral approaches (Geers, Nicholas, & Sedey, 2003; Geers, Strube, Tobey, & Moog, 2011; Kirk, Miyamoto, Ying, Perdew, & Zuganelis, 2000; Miyamoto, Kirk, Svirsky, & Sehgal, 1999), although the benefits of OC may be found only in specific areas of communication (e.g., speech perception). Another group of researchers reported that progress in language skills for cochlear-implant users in TC and OC programs depends on the age at which the child receives the implant (Connor, Hieber, Arts, & Zwolan, 2000).

Dawson and colleagues (1995) evaluated receptive vocabulary skills in a group of children who were implanted between 2 and 20 years of age. They found that communication mode did not predict rate of progress in vocabulary, but they acknowledged that their sample included very few children using TC. Robbins, Svirsky, and Kirk (1997) compared 23 children with CIs in OC and TC settings and found equivalent outcomes on global receptive and expressive language measures. Svirsky and colleagues (2000) did not find any differences in global language skills for CI users in TC and OC programs, although the children in OC programs did significantly better when only spoken language was measured. Kirk and her colleagues (2000) found an effect for speech perception abilities in favor of children in OC programs. There were no significant differences between TC and OC groups in terms of rates of vocabulary growth and receptive and expressive language skills.

As cochlear implant technology improves and age at implantation decreases, advantages for auditory-oral intervention approaches have become more apparent. Miyamoto and his colleagues reported that children in auditory-oral programs displayed higher scores on measures of speech perception, speech intelligibility, and expressive language compared to children in TC programs (1999). These findings for speech perception abilities have been replicated in pediatric cochlear implant users from Australia (Sarant et al., 2001) and other centers in the United States (Dunn et al., 2013).

Moog and Geers (2003) summarized the findings of a major study conducted at the Central Institute for the Deaf in St. Louis. The study included 181 children who were 8 to 9 years of age at the time of testing. They were all prelingually deaf with no additional disabilities and were implanted before 5 years of age. The sample was evaluated on a battery of tests, including speech perception, speech production, spoken language, total language (sign plus speech), and reading measures. Use of an auditory-oral approach accounted for a significant proportion of the variance in all areas except literacy. More specifically, Geers, Nicholas, and Sedey (2003) reported that children with CIs educated in OC environments performed significantly better than children in TC settings in terms of narrative production, vocabulary size, and length and complexity of morphosyntax. Moog and Geers concluded that the "ultimate result of this study was to establish the importance of an auditory-oral communication mode to the speech and language development of children after cochlear implantation" (Moog & Geers, 2003, p. 122S).

Seven years later, Geers, Strube, Tobey, and Moog (2011) published a follow-up report on long-term outcomes of children with CIs, including

112 of the original 181 children. Geers and Sedey (2011) reported on the language skills of the cohort. All language measures were administered in SC by examiners experienced in manual communication, regardless of whether or not the children were in OC or TC programs. Children responded in their preferred communication mode. Thus, children's scores were a reflection of their knowledge of the English language, but not exclusively spoken English. Results indicated that a majority of the children performed within one standard deviation of same-age hearing peers on receptive and expressive language and vocabulary measures. Furthermore, Geers and colleagues concluded that early communication mode influenced early language skills, and that the relationship persisted into later adolescence. Almost half of the participants used SC during the first five years of CI use, but by high school, most of the participants reported using an OC approach. There was no evidence that using sign in early childhood had a negative impact on later language development. However, teenagers with CIs who used oral communication demonstrated better overall language skills compared to their peers who relied more heavily on sign language (Geers & Sedey, 2011).

A strength of the study by Geers and colleagues (2011), compared to previous research, was that the investigators examined the children's English language skills in their preferred mode of communication, rather than only emphasizing spoken language performance. The same limitations that existed in earlier literature (Geers & Moog, 1992; Geers & Schick, 1988) remain, however. The children in the OC group may have shown a propensity for communicating via oral language early in childhood, while the children who did not demonstrate this predisposition were moved to TC programs. Geers and colleagues did not report on the amount of daily use, but it is likely that children in the OC group wore their CIs more consistently than children in the TC group and had access to better device maintenance, based on the findings of previous studies (Geers & Moog, 1992; Wiefferink et al., 2008). As a result, the OC children may have outperformed the TC group in later adolescence due to selection bias and consistency of use, not because of the intervention itself. The results by Geers and colleagues (Geers & Sedey, 2011; Geers et al., 2011) provide strong support for the positive influence of OC approaches on communication outcomes of children with CIs, but limitations related to the study should also be taken into account when interpreting the findings. The evidence for a causal connection between communication mode and language outcomes is still not fully evident.

While this research (Geers & Sedey, 2011; Geers et al., 2011) does present positive evidence for the long-term advantages of OC approaches over TC approaches in children with cochlear implants, it overlooks the individual differences that may exist within each group. It also underestimates the possibility that children who use sign prior to implantation and in the early years after CI receipt can still develop age-appropriate communication skills (Hyde & Punch, 2011). Tomblin and colleagues (1999) compared children with cochlear implants to children with hearing aids who were all enrolled in TC educational settings. The children were evaluated on their sentence comprehension skills through sign and speech and their expressive English grammatical abilities. The cochlear implant users performed significantly better than the hearing aid users, suggesting that children with cochlear implants in TC programs can make significant gains in their language abilities.

Another study by Geers, Spehar, and Sedey (2002) specifically examined children with cochlear implants in TC settings. Twenty-seven children participated; 25 had only been enrolled in TC settings, while the other two children started in OC and moved to TC within one year of CI receipt. Geers and colleagues found that there was a wide range of reliance on speech among the participants. Although all of the children were being educated in TC environments, some of them relied primarily on spoken language to communicate, others relied mostly on sign, and still others used a combination of speech and sign. The use of speech was positively correlated with all of the outcome measures (i.e., speech perception, speech production, receptive and expressive language), while the use of sign was negatively correlated with these measures. Consistent with the findings of Tomblin and colleagues (1999), the results indicated that initial placement in a TC environment during early childhood does not preclude later development of auditory and spoken language skills, although the relative emphasis on speech versus sign may affect outcomes. The authors recommended further investigation of the role of speech and sign input at the initial stages of language development (Geers et al., 2002) to further delineate the influence of early sign exposure on later speech and language development.

Other researchers have provided convincing evidence that language outcomes for children who are deaf cannot be ascribed to whether OC is better than TC or vice versa. Connor and colleagues (2000) argued that there is a complex relationship between a child's communication modality, age at implantation, and performance with a cochlear implant. They evaluated articulation skills and receptive and expressive vocabulary in a group of pediatric CI users. All of the participants demonstrated progress on the outcome measures over time, regardless of communication modality. For the articulation measures, the children in OC programs demonstrated significantly greater rates of improvement compared to the children in TC programs. When the OC and TC groups were broken down by age at implantation, there were no significant differences in articulation accuracy for children implanted before age 5. There were also no significant differences between the two groups as a whole on receptive vocabulary measures. Differences emerged again when the groups were separated by age at implantation, with the children in the TC group outperforming children in the OC group on receptive vocabulary measures if they received their implants before age 5. Finally, the TC group showed an advantage over the OC group on expressive vocabulary for children who received implants before age 7. There were no significant differences in expressive vocabulary for children who received their implants between 7 and 10 years of age.

The findings in the studies described thus far (Connor et al., 2000; Geers et al., 2002; Tomblin et al., 1999) have important implications for researchers, clinicians, and families. First, the data indicate that children can benefit from cochlear implants regardless of their communication modality. Second, it is critical that parents and service providers take several factors into consideration before deciding if one intervention approach is preferable to another. Variables such as age at implantation and communication modality interact with one another. While one intervention approach may be appropriate for one child, it might be entirely inappropriate for another child, depending on the parents' goals and the child's intervention history.

One final point that should be considered is that most children's chosen communication modes are not static over time. In the long run, children with CIs will gravitate toward the mode that is more preferable to them as they learn to adjust to the electric signal that the CI provides, as well as to their social and school settings. Watson, Archbold, and Nikolopoulos (2006) followed 176 children for up to 5 years post-implant, dividing them into three groups based on age at implantation (before 3 years of age; 3 to 5 years of age; after 5 years of age). They examined how patterns of communication mode changed during these 5 initial years of CI use. Among all of the children, 61% used OC after 5 years of CI use. Age at implantation had a significant influence on the eventual communication mode; children implanted at younger ages were more likely to change from TC/BSL to OC. Watson, Hardie, Archbold, and Wheeler (2008) replicated those findings in 142 children with CIs, with 114 families reporting that their child had moved from TC/BSL to OC. Six children moved toward greater use of sign language over time. The researchers queried parents on why children changed communication mode, and most parents reported that they were responding to their child's preference for communicating in a certain manner. Parents also stated that they frequently recognized the benefits of using sign language with their child in certain situations, such as swimming pools. These results have important clinical value. Families with a newly diagnosed child may be counseled that early decisions about communication approaches are not fixed for life. Instead, it may be more appropriate to introduce signed communication in combination with spoken language, in order to lay a foundation for later communication development.

## CONCLUSION: A NEED FOR MORE EVIDENCE-BASED RESEARCH ON INTERVENTION APPROACHES FOR CHILDREN WITH CIs

The advantages of different intervention approaches with children who are deaf still require more evidence-based research. Currently, most studies point toward advantages for children in auditory-oral education settings on spoken language outcomes, at least for children with cochlear implants. It should be noted, however, that there are still confounds in this line of research, in that a more advantaged population of children tend to enter OC educational programs (i.e., children in a higher SES who show an early propensity toward success with spoken language). Positive speech and language outcomes for children with CIs are also highly dependent on a number of factors, including amount of residual hearing, age at implantation, amount of daily CI use, and the parents' goals for communication and overall development.

Despite many strong opinions to the contrary, no one has yet produced evidence that sign language prevents children from developing oral language skills, especially when it is utilized early in development. Future research should address the issue of using sign or speech during the initial stages of language learning, and its effects on later language, reading, and psychosocial development. Because of the substantial lowering of the age of identification and intervention over the past 10 years, this line of research is now feasible.

## ACKNOWLEDGMENTS

This work was supported in part by research grants 2P50DC000242-26A1 and R01 DC009560-01 from the National Institutes on Deafness and Other Communication Disorders, National Institutes of Health; grant RR00059 from the General Clinical Research Centers Program, Division of Research Resources, National Institutes of Health; the Lions Clubs International Foundation; and the Iowa Lions Foundation.

## REFERENCES

Carney, A. E., & Moeller, M. P. (1998). Treatment efficacy: hearing loss in children. *Journal of Speech, Language and Hearing Research, 41*(1), S61–S84.

Connor, C. M., Hieber, S., Arts, H. A., & Zwolan, T. A. (2000). Speech, vocabulary, and the education of children using cochlear implants: Oral or total communication? *Journal of Speech, Language and Hearing Research, 43*(5), 1185–1204.

Davis, J., Elfenbein, J. L., Schum, R. L., & Bentler, R. A. (1986). Effects of mild and moderate hearing impairments on language, educational, and psychosocial behavior of children. *Journal of Speech and Hearing Disorders, 51*, 53–62.

Davis, J., Shepard, N., Stelmachowicz, P., & Gorga, M. (1981). Characteristics of hearing-impaired children in the public schools: Part II—psychoeducational data. *Journal of Speech and Hearing Disorders, 46*(2), 130–137.

Dawson, P., Blarney, P., Dettman, S., Barker, E., & Clark, G. (1995). A clinical report on receptive vocabulary skills in cochlear implant users. *Ear and Hearing, 16*(3), 287–294.

Dunn, C. C., Walker, E. A., Oleson, J., Kenworthy, M., Van Voorst, T., Tomblin, J. B.,...Gantz, B. J. (2013). Longitudinal speech perception and language performance in pediatric cochlear implant users: the effect of age at implantation. *Ear and Hearing, 35*, 148–160.

Elfenbein, J. L., Hardin-Jones, M. A., & Davis, J. (1994). Oral communication skills of children who are hard of hearing. *Journal of Speech, Language and Hearing Research, 37*(1), 216–226.

Geers, A., Moog, J., & Schick, B. (1984). Acquisition of spoken and signed English by profoundly deaf children. *Journal of Speech and Hearing Disorders, 49*(4), 378–388.

Geers, A., & Moog, J. S. (1992). Speech perception and production skills of students with impaired hearing from oral and total communication education settings. *Journal of Speech, Language and Hearing Research, 35*(6), 1384–1393.

Geers, A., Moog, J. S., Biedenstein, J., Brenner, C., & Hayes, H. (2009). Spoken language scores of children using cochlear implants compared to hearing age-mates at school entry. *Journal of Deaf Studies and Deaf Education, 14*(3), 371–385.

Geers, A., Nicholas, J. G., & Sedey, A. L. (2003). Language skills of children with early cochlear implantation. *Ear and Hearing, 24*(1 Suppl), 46S–58S.

Geers, A., & Schick, B. (1988). Acquisition of spoken and signed English by hearing-impaired children of hearing-impaired or hearing parents. *Journal of Speech and Hearing Disorders, 53*(2), 136–143.

Geers, A., & Sedey, A. L. (2011). Language and verbal reasoning skills in adolescents with 10 or more years of cochlear implant experience. *Ear and Hearing, 32*(1 Suppl), 39S–48S.

Geers, A., Spehar, B., & Sedey, A. (2002). Use of speech by children from total communication programs who wear cochlear implants. *American Journal of Speech-Language Pathology, 11*(1), 50–58.

Geers, A., Strube, M. J., Tobey, E. A., & Moog, J. S. (2011). Epilogue: Factors contributing to long-term outcomes of cochlear implantation in early childhood. *Ear and Hearing, 32*(1 Suppl), 84S–92S.

Greenberg, M. T., & Calderon, R. (1984). Early intervention outcomes and issues. *Topics in Early Childhood Special Education, 3*(4), 1–9.

Greenberg, M. T., Calderon, R., & Kusché, C. (1984). Early intervention using simultaneous communication with deaf infants: The effect on communication development. *Child Development, 55*, 607–616.

Hearing, Joint Committee on Infant Hearing (2007). Year 2007 position statement: principles and guidelines for early hearing detection and intervention programs. *Pediatrics, 120*(4), 898–921.

Hyde, M., & Punch, R. (2011). The modes of communication used by children with cochlear implants and role of sign in their lives. *American Annals of the Deaf, 155*(5), 535–549.

Kirk, K. I., Miyamoto, R. T., Lento, C. L., Ying, E., O'Neill, T., & Fears, B. (2002). Effects of age at implantation in young children. *Annals of Otology, Rhinology & Laryngology, 111*(189 Suppl), 69–73.

Kirk, K. I., Miyamoto, R. T., Ying, E. A., Perdew, A. E., & Zuganelis, H. (2000). Cochlear implantation in young children: Effects of age at implantation and communication mode. *Volta Review, 102*(4), 127–144.

Knoors, H., & Marschark, M. (2012). Language planning for the 21st century: Revisiting bilingual language policy for deaf children. *Journal of Deaf Studies and Deaf Education, 17*(3), 291–305.

Ling, D. (1984). *Early intervention for hearing impaired children: Oral options.* Boston: College-Hill Press.

Ling, D., & Atchley, T. (1984). *Early intervention for hearing impaired children: Total communication options.* Boston: College-Hill Press.

Marmor, G. S., & Petitto, L. (1979). Simultaneous communication in the classroom: How well is english grammar represented? *Sign Language Studies, 23*, 99–136.

Marschark, M., & Spencer, P. E. (2006). Spoken language development of deaf and hard-of-hearing children: historical and theoretical perspectives. In P. E. Spencer & M. Marschark (Eds.), *Advances in the spoken language development of deaf and hard-of-hearing children* (pp. 3–21). New York, NY: Oxford University Press.

Meadow, K. P. (2005). Early manual communication in relation to the deaf child's intellectual, social, and communicative functioning. *Journal of Deaf Studies and Deaf Education, 10*(4), 321–329.

Miyamoto, R. T., Kirk, K. I., Svirsky, M. A., & Sehgal, S. T. (1999). Communication skills in pediatric cochlear implant recipients. *Acta Oto-laryngologica, 119*(2), 219–224.

Moeller, M. P. (2000). Early intervention and language development in children who are deaf and hard of hearing. *Pediatrics, 106*(3), e43–e52.

Moog, J. S., & Geers, A. (2003). Epilogue: Major findings, conclusions and implications for deaf education. *Ear and Hearing, 24*(1), 121S–125S.

Niparko, J. K., Tobey, E. A., Thal, D. J., Eisenberg, L. S., Wang, N.-Y., Quittner, A. L., & Fink, N. E. (2010). Spoken language development in children following cochlear implantation. *JAMA: The Journal of the American Medical Association, 303*(15), 1498–1506.

Northern, J. L., & Downs, M. P. (2002). *Hearing in children* (5th ed.). Baltimore, MD: Lippincott, Williams, & Wilkins.

Robbins, A. M., Svirsky, M., & Kirk, K. I. (1997). Children with implants can speak, but can they communicate? *Otolaryngology—Head and Neck Surgery, 117*(3), 155–160.

Rvachew, S., Slawinski, E. B., & Williams, M. (1996). Formant frequencies of vowels produced by infants with and without early onset otitis media. *Canadian Acoustics, 24*(2), 19–28.

Rvachew, S., Slawinski, E. B., Williams, M., & Green, C. L. (1999). The impact of early onset otitis media on babbling and early language development. *The Journal of the Acoustical Society of America, 105*, 467–475.

Sarant, J., Blamey, P., Dowell, R., Clark, G., & Gibson, W. (2001). Variation in speech perception scores among children with cochlear implants. *Ear and Hearing, 22*(1), 18–28.

Sininger, Y. S., Grimes, A., & Christensen, E. (2010). Auditory development in early amplified children: factors influencing auditory-based communication outcomes in children with hearing loss. *Ear and Hearing, 31*(2), 166–185.

Spencer, L. J., Tye-Murray, N., & Tomblin, J. B. (1998). The production of English inflectional morphology, speech production and listening performance in children with cochlear implants. *Ear and Hearing, 19*(4), 310–318.

Spencer, P., Marschark, M., & Spencer, L. (2011). Cochlear implants: Advances, issues, and implications. In M. Marschark, P. E. Spencer & P. E. Nathan (Eds.), *The Oxford handbook of deaf studies, language, and education* (vol. 1, pp. 452–471): New York, NY: Oxford University Press.

Svirsky, M. A., Robbins, A. M., Kirk, K. I., Pisoni, D. B., & Miyamoto, R. T. (2000). Language development in profoundly deaf children with cochlear implants. *Psychological Science, 11*(2), 153–158.

Swanwick, R., & Tsverik, I. (2007). The role of sign language for deaf children with cochlear implants: Good practice in sign bilingual settings. *Deafness & Education International, 9*(4), 214–231.

Szagun, G. (2001). Language acquisition in young German-speaking children with cochlear implants: Individual differences and implications for conceptions of a "sensitive phase." *Audiology and Neurotology, 6*(5), 288–297.

Tomblin, J. B., Barker, B. A., Spencer, L. J., Zhang, X., & Gantz, B. J. (2005). The effect of age at cochlear implant initial stimulation on expressive language growth in infants and toddlers. *Journal of Speech, Language and Hearing Research, 48*(4), 853–867.

Tomblin, J. B., Spencer, L., Flock, S., Tyler, R., & Gantz, B. (1999). A comparison of language achievement in children with cochlear implants and children using hearing aids. *Journal of Speech, Language and Hearing Research, 42*(2), 497–511.

Watson, L. M., Archbold, S. M., & Nikolopoulos, T. P. (2006). Children's communication mode five years after cochlear implantation: Changes over time according to age at implant. *Cochlear Implants International, 7*(2), 77–91.

Watson, L. M., Hardie, T., Archbold, S. M., & Wheeler, A. (2008). Parents' views on changing communication after cochlear implantation. *Journal of Deaf Studies and Deaf Education, 13*(1), 104–116.

Wie, O. B., Falkenberg, E.-S., Tvete, O., & Tomblin, J. B. (2007). Children with a cochlear implant: Characteristics and determinants of speech recognition, speech-recognition growth rate, and speech production. *International Journal of Audiology, 46*(5), 232–243.

Wiefferink, C., Spaai, G., Uilenburg, N., Vermeij, B., & De Raeve, L. (2008). Influence of linguistic environment on children's language development: Flemish versus Dutch children. *Deafness & Education International, 10*(4), 226–243.

Yoshinaga-Itano, C., Baca, R. L., & Sedey, A. L. (2010). describing the trajectory of language development in the presence of severe-to-profound hearing loss: A closer look at children with cochlear implants versus hearing aids. *Otology & Neurotology, 31*(8), 1268–1274.

# 7

# Psychosocial Development in Deaf and Hard-of-Hearing Children in the Twenty-first Century

## Opportunities and Challenges

Manfred Hintermair

Numerous studies have shown that deaf and hard-of-hearing (DHH) children face specific challenges in their development. Empirical findings regarding various domains of development reveal that reduced auditory perception and/or its correlates influence a great many processes that are significant for effective and interactive world disclosure, and that special allowances must be made for this when raising and educating these children (Calderon & Greenberg, 2011; Marschark & Wauters, 2011; Trezek, Wang, & Paul, 2011).

With regard to the psychosocial dimension of development, Calderon and Greenberg (2011) stated that good social-emotional development is a crucial prerequisite for a happy and successful life. They described a set of skills that would be required. Among other things, these include good communication skills; the ability to control one's behavior; to understand one's own motivation, feelings, and needs, as well as those of others; the capacity to view any situation from multiple perspectives; and the social competencies needed to build relationships with other people.

The key factor for the successful acquisition of skills in all these domains is "to coordinate affect, cognition, communication, and behavior" (p. 189). Many DHH students unfortunately encounter experiences in their development that are far from optimal and that may make it difficult for them to integrate language, cognition, and affect (Greenberg & Kusché, 1998). At the same time, the development of many other DHH children proceeds successfully, and we now know much about the factors that may influence development positively (see Spencer & Marschark, 2010).

This chapter focuses on the psychosocial development of DHH children. It provides findings that are important for understanding the special needs of DHH children that must be fulfilled in order for them to live a happy life. The role of language and successful communication is given special attention here, and the opportunities that a bilingual approach may provide for good development will be highlighted.

## CHANGING PERSPECTIVES IN PSYCHOLOGY AND EDUCATION

There have been important changes in perspectives on education and psychology that have influenced developments in deaf education over the past decades. Conceptual reorientations such as the salutogenetic model of health, empowerment philosophy, or the results of resilience research no longer focus on deficits (i.e., what does not work), but rather on the developmental strengthening of individual and social variables (i.e., what is available in DHH children and their families that we can use for successful interventions).

In the field of deaf education, this strength-based perspective has influenced both science and practice (Hintermair & Wälder, 2012; Jankowski, 1997; Zand & Pierce, 2011). It has replaced the not very helpful and mostly discriminatory statements of the "psychology of deafness" (Lane, 1992). This change in perspective helps to put the differences in the development of hearing and DHH children in the spotlight. A look at possible differences (note: not deficits!) changes the map of thought and action options: The main focus is not on problems, but on the phenomena of development in the context of deafness. Accordingly, assessment is not used primarily for classification of disorders, but predominantly to understand the developmental phenomena of DHH children and to understand what they mean to the children in their various environments (Rinaldi, Caselli, Onofrio, and Volterra, Chapter 3 of this volume). Furthermore, we are looking for ways to integrate the specific characteristics of being deaf or hard of hearing constructively into education, support, and therapy concepts, and we are using in particular the resources that are available to the children for this endeavor.

Nevertheless, it is important to emphasize that formulating positive goals may not stop us from designating difficulties—on the contrary: from a salutogenic and empowerment perspective of development and health, it is important to keep an eye on the potential developmental challenges of DHH children growing up in a hearing world. Therefore, focusing on the positive developmental goals does not mean that "thinking positively" alone would solve all problems. We need to recognize differences in the development of DHH children and bring them to light in order to adequately address these differences in the design of education and intervention programs. Marschark and Hauser (2008) highlight the special link between adopting a resource-based perspective and its significance for the development of DHH children in saying that hearing loss might "deprive the organism of some of the material resources from which the mind develops, but our inherent resilience ensures that we take advantage of other resources. Thus, the result is not a state of deficiency, but of difference—a difference that has so far failed to receive much attention in educational research and practice" (p. 454). This chapter therefore focuses on psychosocial characteristics of deaf children and adolescents, not from a perspective of "deficiency", but rather from a perspective of "difference." First, however, we should basically consider just what role in particular language plays in children's cognitive and psychosocial development.

## THE ROLE OF LANGUAGE, COGNITION, AND EMOTION FOR CHILD DEVELOPMENT

The linguistic experiences of DHH children are closely linked with aspects of their cognitive and emotional development, so that the interplay of these three domains is essential for a comprehensive understanding of the developmental situation of DHH children.

To understand the significance of language[1] for the development of DHH children, it is important to remember that building up a lexicon and acquiring the grammar of a language are not the only results of language development. One essential characteristic of effective language acquisition is that it plays a decisive role in helping young children to interact with and open up the world. In doing so, they come to recognize and understand both the world and themselves (Prillwitz, 1995). Language thus becomes the place where one's inner mental life is constituted, and people shape themselves and the world with it and in it. This shaping always happens by drawing on other people, so that we are only able to tell our own story and make it comprehensible against the background of our social relationships with others.

Thus, the decisive engine that drives development forward is early access to language. It allows children to open up the world and intrinsically interact with it, so that they obtain a differentiated knowledge of the world. Hart and Risley (1995) showed, in a longitudinal study involving 42 hearing children, the important role of early access to language. The quality of parent-child interactions was a crucial indicator for the later development of the children. What the parents talked about with their children in the first three years of life and how they did it were significant for the language development of children and were predictive of the size of the children's vocabulary and their reading skills when they were in the third grade in primary school.

This clearly shows the important role of early language experiences for the development of children. At the same time, it shows the risk that the development of DHH children runs unless intense linguistic experiences in interactive relationships can be established from very early on. VanDam, Ambrose, and Moeller (2012), in a study involving 22 hard-of-hearing children at the age of 2 years, showed that the language comprehension of children was associated with the number of conversational exchanges, but not with the number of words spoken by adults. This emphasizes the importance of the quality of linguistic interactions for DHH children.

Also related to early access to language and thus relevant for development is access to social interaction and the opportunity to experience a great many things at an early stage in life. Children acquire the social rules, norms, and values that apply in society primarily through exchanging ideas with other people and by talking about experiences, mainly with their parents in their early years, but also, when they grow older, through contact with their peer group and other significant people in their social space. In this respect, the more extensive their social experience, the more differentiated their own canon of values and knowledge of the world become. Through access to language and through as many social contacts as possible, the chance to discover the world in all its diversity also increases accordingly. DHH children can experience hazards in this regard. For example, in the history of deaf education DHH children often were blamed for being egocentric and adhering rigidly to their own opinions (Lane, 1992), and little attention was paid to the social factors that caused this behavior. These factors are closely connected to the lack of social and linguistic-communicative exchanges: " . . . in the absence of diversity, there are no problems to solve, no need for flexibility" (Marschark, 2000, p. 284).

Because of problems with access to language, limitations in incidental learning (Greenberg & Calderon, 2011), and difficulties in dividing attention (Spencer, Swisher, & Waxman, 2004), DHH children are also at risk for developing a fragmented perception of the world. What is particularly important for understanding the psychosocial development of DHH children is the fact that limited linguistic input, in association with a fragmented perception of the world, not only affects children's cognitive development, it affects them emotionally as well; that is, DHH children store everyday experiences affectively as well as linguistically. Accordingly, restricted experiences not only have a clear impact on the acquisition of knowledge and on understanding, but also leave distinct traces in the area of emotional mental states (e.g., self-esteem, self-efficacy, self-confidence). In his model of affect logic, Ciompi (2003) demonstrateed the inseparable unity of the affective and cognitive components involved in any mental performance. Accordingly, all human actions and experiences are not only represented cognitively in the brain, they always have an affective component as well. This determines to what extent the experience in question results in feelings of like or dislike (i.e., is experienced positively or negatively). Ciompi suggested that all cognitive schemata receive a specific affective stamp or "imprint" that is acquired through actions in everyday life, and that people derive the power for their individual development from the affective-emotional side of those schemata. Accordingly, affects are the "energy providers" for cognitive performance: They determine the focus of attention, they regulate access to our different "memory banks," they are the "glue" that binds the various cognitive states together into one meaningful whole, and they determine the hierarchy of a person's thought content (Roth, 2000).

The daily experiences of DHH children are therefore always also events of (less or more intensive) emotional significance closely linked to their linguistic-communicative experiences and to the performance that is expected and required of them in their daily routine, at school or at home. When we look at the development of affect-logic schemata in DHH children from this perspective, it quickly becomes clear that achieving an optimal like-dislike balance while developing these schemata is endangered when communicative conditions are poor, and that this must be taken into account when we are designing support programs.

## PSYCHOSOCIAL DIMENSIONS IN DHH CHILDREN

The following provides a concise overview of results of research addressing the most important domains of psychosocial development of DHH children.

### Self-esteem

In the psychological literature, self-esteem is the emotional and judgmental view of one's own self. It describes the feeling that comes from the experience of being accepted and the experience of competence, participation, and recognition (Brice & Adams, 2011). The sources that self-esteem feeds on are experiences in different areas of life, in which experiences in the family and at school, as well as experiences in extracurricular activities and in contexts outside the family, play a central role. The experiences with peers are particularly important in this respect (Brice & Adams, 2011).

In her meta-analysis of older studies up to the early 1990s, Bat-Chava (1993) stated that it is important to take into account contextual factors in order to understand the development of self-esteem in DHH students properly, for example, the degree of hearing loss, parental hearing status, communication mode used, and the levels of group identification. The studies reviewed by Bat-Chava primarily showed that DHH people with DHH parents, DHH people using sign language, and DHH students who identify strongly with the Deaf community had higher self-esteem.

More recent studies essentially confirm the relevant factors for the development of a good sense of self-esteem. In some of these studies, cultural affiliation plays an important role. Overall, deaf acculturation and bicultural acculturation in particular have proven to be particularly advantageous for the level of self-esteem (Hintermair, 2008; Maxwell-McCaw, 2001). Hintermair (2008), in his study of German DHH adults, further showed that, compared to cultural affiliation, the psychological resources of individuals (life optimism, self-efficacy) were also crucial for the development of self-esteem.

Other studies confirmed the importance of parental hearing status and the use of sign language communication, showing that DHH children with at least one deaf parent, as well as children whose parents were more competent in using sign language, had higher self-esteem values. In a recent study on self-concept and ego development with a representative sample of 68 Dutch DHH adolescents, Van Gent, Goedhart, Knoors, Westenberg, Philip, and Treffers (2012) were able to show that the group of DHH students experienced less pronounced social acceptance and had fewer close friendships than the normal hearing standardization group. Further analysis showed that a higher degree of global self-worth was associated with support for signing during childhood and the quality of parent-child communication.

With respect to educational setting, a study by Yetman and Brice (2002) seems of particular importance because it addresses the social-emotional consequences of inclusive education. They examined self-concept/self-esteem in inclusion or mainstream educational programs in the United States, looking in particular at the number of DHH children in the programs and to what extent this affected their self-esteem. It was found that the DHH children who were together with hearing children for the majority of the time had lower global self-esteem and lower levels in various domains (academic, social, and behavioral self-esteem) than the DHH children who spent rather less time with hearing children. In addition, peer surveys showed that the DHH students were neither preferred nor rejected, but were mostly overlooked or ignored. These results might indicate that contact and exchange with other DHH children is an important aspect of good psychosocial development (see the section on the opportunities and challenges of inclusion later in this chapter).

In recent years, more and more DHH children are provided with a cochlear implant at an early age. There is a growing number of studies available on self-esteem of this group. Most of these studies involve comparisons with groups of hearing children and come to comparable results regarding the level of self-esteem. As an example, in a Danish study using a parental survey on self-esteem and emotional well-being, the data of 164 children with cochlear implants aged from 2 to 17 years were compared with data from a national survey of normal hearing children of the same age. The children with cochlear implants achieved comparable or sometimes higher values in all tested domains of self-esteem and social well-being (Percy-Smith, Caye-Tomasen, Gudman, Jensen, & Thomsen, 2008).

An important study regarding the potential role of bilingual education concepts was conducted by Leigh, Maxwell-McCaw, Bat-Chava, and Christansen (2009). They studied a group of 57 DHH young people, 29 of whom had a cochlear implant and 28 who did not. They collected data using validated measures and gathered information from parents, teachers, and the young people themselves on their cultural affiliation, self-esteem, life satisfaction, and loneliness.

It was found that the cochlear implant users were more hearing-acculturated, while the adolescents without a cochlear implant were Deaf acculturated. Regarding the psychosocial variables (self-esteem, life satisfaction, loneliness), there were no differences between the two groups. The authors therefore noted that the cochlear implant per se does not determine psychosocial well-being, and that bicultural orientation was found in both groups of young people, regardless of whether they had a cochlear implant. Even more important are the conclusions by Leigh and Maxwell-McCaw (2011) in their study on the psychosocial functioning and identity development of children with cochlear implants. They stated that children with cochlear implants can have a clear identity as well as the ability to shift between identity categorizations as the situation demands, and they see this ability as being conducive to mental health.

Given that the findings on the development of children with cochlear implants are very heterogeneous, this may be a strong argument in favor of also having bilingual and bicultural programs available in the rehabilitation process of children with cochlear implants and their families in order to address the diversity of children with cochlear implants and their developmental needs adequately (see Hyde & Punch, 2011). Taken as a whole, this means that different educational options need to be retained, offering a wide palette of educational programs for DHH children (see the later section on opportunities and challenges in deaf education during the early years).

**Quality of Life**

Regarding Health Related Quality of Life (HRQoL), the World Health Organization (WHO) defines quality of life "as individuals' perceptions of their position in life in the context of the culture and value systems in which they live and in relation to their goals, expectations, standards and concerns" (The World Health Organization Quality of Life Assessment Instrument [WHOQOL], 1995, p. 1403).

HRQoL and subjective health are seen as multidimensional constructs that include physical, emotional, mental, social, and behavioral components of well-being and the ability to function from the perspective of the affected. The view is mainly focused on how to integrate socially and participate in all aspects of life appropriate to one's age.

The last few years have also seen more studies on HRQoL in DHH children as well as in children with cochlear implants, rather like the studies on self-esteem. These studies do not lead to unequivocal conclusions, however, as they are difficult to compare due to various factors. There are inconsistencies in the use of the term "quality of life," in the methods accessing HRQL, in the persons acting as informants (parents, teachers, DHH children) and in the educational settings of the students (for a detailed discussion see Hintermair, 2011).

A critical examination of the available studies on quality of life highlights a few patterns. Comparable to the studies on self-esteem, studies focusing exclusively on children with cochlear implants seem to show an overall improvement in their quality of life. For example, Loy, Warner-Czyz, Tong, Tobey, and Roland (2010) conducted a recent study with 88 children with cochlear implants and their families, using the KINDL® questionnaire for measuring HRQoL in children and adolescents. When comparing their findings to data from normal hearing children, the group of implanted children as a whole showed scores comparable to those of the normal hearing peers and their parents. There was an interesting difference between the 8–11-year-old and the 12–16-year-old groups of implanted children. The younger cochlear implant users had lower scores in the family domain than their normal hearing peers, whereas the older cochlear implant users showed lower scores in the school domain than in the evaluations of their parents. Earlier implantation and longer cochlear implant use resulted in higher HRQoL scores.

Studies on DHH students who had varying degrees of hearing loss and used hearing aids instead of cochlear implants showed a tendency for the DHH group to score lower on some scales relating to quality of life than hearing students. This was the case, for example, in a study by Gilman, Easterbrooks, and Frey (2004) that focused on life satisfaction as a key aspect of quality of life. They used the Multidimensional Students' Life Satisfaction Scale to compare both global satisfaction and satisfaction ratings across a number of life domains (family, friends, school, living environment, self) for DHH young people aged between 8 and 18 years and living either in residential settings or attending day school programs. Comparing the results of the DHH students as a collective group with the data from a hearing control group revealed that the scores for global satisfaction and the family, friends, and living environment domains were significantly higher in the hearing group, whereas no differences were observed for the school and self-satisfaction domains.

Again, given the emphasis on inclusion, it is relevant to keep an eye on the quality of life of DHH groups in different educational settings. In this regard, a study by Schick, Skalicky, Edwards, Kushalnagar, Topolski, and Patrick (2013) is of importance. They carried out a study involving 221 DHH adolescents 11–18 years old who had bilateral hearing losses, and used two instruments to measure quality of life. One instrument was the Youth Quality of Life Instrument–Research Version (YQOL-R), a generic measure developed and validated for hearing students; the other was the Youth Quality of Life–Deaf and Hard of Hearing (YQOL-DHH), a new instrument developed for the group of DHH students that takes deaf cultural issues into account. Results with the YQOL-R show that the group of DHH students had significantly lower scores on the Sense of Self domain and the Relationships domain than the normative hearing group, but they achieved comparable scores in the Environment domain and in the total quality of life score. Looking at the different school settings of the DHH students, those attending general schools with DHH programs showed lower scores in all domains than the DHH students attending a school without such programs. Comparison of the group of younger students (11–14 years) with the older group (15–19 years) revealed differences in the Participation domain: The younger students had more positive scores. The authors discussed this result from different perspectives. One point they made is that social interaction issues may have been more important for the older students. Schick and colleagues stressed that the transition into adolescence is a period of rapid change, and functional peer relationships are essential for developing a strong identity. So the challenges for the DHH students going through this phase may well be bigger than for the younger students. Looking at the results obtained with the DHH-specific instrument (YQOL-DHH), there were no differences on any of the domains inspected (Participation, Self Acceptance & Advocacy, and Perceived Stigma), and the students in all school settings reported a positive quality of life. Schick and colleagues interpreted their data as indicating that different educational options may be necessary in the education of deaf students. They also observed that many of the students they asked about quality of life were placed in a school setting appropriate for their needs. They concluded from their results that no one type of school placement seems to be obviously better than others.

Kushalnagar, Topolski, Schick, Edwards, Skalicky, and Patrick (2011) used the same sample as Schick et al. (2013) to explore the role of parent-youth communication for adolescent quality of life. In daily communication, 24% of the students used signs only, 40% speech only, and 36% used sign and speech. Once again, a generic measure (YQOL-R) and a DHH-specific measure for quality of life (YQOL-DHH) were used. The results regarding quality of life showed that the ability of young people to understand their parents' communication correlated positively with their perceived quality of life, regardless of the language modality (sign, speech, or sign/speech). Additionally, those with higher quality of life scores had lower depressive symptoms and lower perceived stigma. The results confirmed the significance of functional parent-child communication for quality of life in DHH students.

To summarize, the data available on HRQL at present indicate some sensitive aspects as important for planning the education of DHH children. Good parent-child communication right from the start seems to be particularly significant for DHH children's quality of life, and the modality used to realize this communication seems to play no significant role. The important thing is that it works! The findings may also explain why the conditions for a good quality of life seem to be much more favorable for DHH children with a cochlear implant. Furthermore, it is essential to keep an eye on changes of the quality of life of DHH children over time, specifically in adolescence. For DHH students, adolescence can be a stage of life with particular challenges regarding communication and participation.

**Emotional and Behavioral Problems**

Despite the fact that the majority of DHH people are mentally healthy and are able to live self-fulfilling lives (Leigh & Pollard, 2011), DHH children and adolescents are at increased risk of mental health problems. Summarizing the research into the socio-emotional problems of DHH students is difficult due to the different methodological approaches, as well as the different additional variables assessed in the current studies. Nevertheless, some trends are clearly visible.

In the majority of the more recent studies, the data consistently show on average a two- to threefold increase in the prevalence rate for socio-emotional problems in DHH students. Van Eldik, Treffers, Veerman, and Verhulst (2004) conclude that, despite some exceptions, "deaf children ... show ... in most studies a higher level of such problems, regardless of who is acting as the informant" (p. 391).

Studies that show low or normal prevalence rates of social and emotional problems in DHH students typically share specific characteristics: First, these are studies in which the DHH children were exclusively or to a large extent attending regular schools. For example, Van Gent, Goedhart, Hindley, Treffers, and Philip (2007) presented data on the mental health of 70 DHH youth aged between 13 and 21 years, using the Child Behavior Checklist (CBCL) and the Teachers' Report Form (TRF) as well as psychiatric examination. Twenty-five percent of the students attended a regular school; the other students attended a school for the deaf. The prevalence rates reported show somewhat lower scores than in other studies that only explored DHH students at schools for the deaf (CBCL: 1.7 times higher; TRF: 1.9 times higher). Regarding emotional and behavioral problems, there were no significant differences for the behavior problems scores when the data were compared with a Dutch norm group, but this was not the case for the emotional problems scores. Here the DHH students had significantly higher problem scores.

Van Gent and colleagues also show that DHH students using spoken language have lower problem scores than students who use sign language. They assume that children with more socio-emotional problems are more often assigned to schools for the deaf, where sign language is used. This concurs with Stinson and Kluwin (2011), who pointed out that the considerable differences currently existing between students at various types of school are not due to the school type itself, but to the individual differences between the students in terms of intelligence and language skills, for example, or even social background or additional disabilities.

Second, in some studies that show lower prevalence rates, this seems to be associated with the educational system for the DHH. DHH students from countries that practice a consistent bilingual education concept show no higher socio-emotional problems when compared with hearing students. In a recent survey, Mejstad, Heiling, and Svedin (2008/2009) studied 111 DHH students in Sweden and used the Strengths and Difficulties Questionnaire (SDQ); 28 students attended a school for the deaf, 23 a school for the hard-of-hearing, and 60 students attended a general school. Parents and teachers of the DHH students, as well as the students themselves, acted as informants. Results revealed almost no differences between the parents', teachers', and students' ratings. Moreover, comparing the findings with data from hearing normative groups in Scandinavian countries also showed no significant differences. The authors attribute this in part to the Swedish educational system, which provides early bilingual intervention for DHH children, along with sign language training for the families. This may well ensure that communication is established early on between the DHH child and its family. In this study there were no gender differences regarding socio-emotional problems, but this was not the case for the type of school that the children attended: Students from schools for the deaf had higher problem scores than students from the other two types of schools.

These results suggest that a secure communication situation seems to be a guarantee for emotional well-being, and therefore it is worthwhile to repeat at this point what has been said earlier: It seems that bilingual concepts can provide a secure access to language for DHH students more reliably than auditory-oral programs that provide access to spoken language only for a part of the population of DHH children. This conclusion is supported by studies that include the quality of communicative competence in any form. Wherever this variable is assessed, it seems to be an important factor in explaining the mental health problems of DHH students: The children who have better competencies always show lower problem scores (Barker, Quittner, Fink, Eisenberg, Tobey, Niparko, and the CDaCI Investigative Team, 2009; Hintermair, 2007). It is important to note that this works regardless of the language modality used by the DHH children (Barker et al., 2009; Dammeyer, 2010; Wallis,

Musselman, & MacKay, 2004). This may be a strong argument for different educational options in deaf education, providing each DHH child with the kind of instruction that works the best for him or her.

## PROSPECTS FOR ENHANCING PSYCHOSOCIAL DEVELOPMENT: EARLY INTERVENTION

In some ways, the opportunities for development in DHH children have never been as good as they are today. Universal newborn hearing screening (UNHS) in particular has opened up new horizons (National Center for Hearing Assessment and Management, 2013). However, in order to maximize the positive effects of UNHS, we must take into account what is known about the parents' situation after diagnosis, we must be familiar with early child development processes, and we must also be aware of the fact that DHH children belong to what is, in many respects, a heterogeneous group (Rinaldi, Caselli, Onofrio, and Volterra, Chapter 3 of this volume). This requires a counseling and intervention concept that is differentiated and open to different methods and approaches. At the moment, however, it seems that counseling after UNHS is dominated by a medical view of hearing loss (Matthijs, Loots, Mouvet, Van Herreweghe, Hardonk, Van Hove, Van Puyvelde, & Leigh, 2012). In many countries, UNHS apparently does not lead to assessing the children's competencies in broad and differentiated ways, so that intervention that is adapted to the needs of the child and the family becomes possible. Instead, most DHH children are placed in auditory-verbal programs, and provision of bilingual early intervention programs is seen as a last resort. This policy may compromise the educational prospects of many DHH children by delaying early access to language. Many DHH children cannot develop their full potential with auditory access to language alone.

A differentiated view on the chances and challenges that the early years pose to DHH children requires a clear understanding of the following aspects: (1) how to assess the parental situation in the light of the UNHS, (2) what the development needs of the children are and what is needed to adequately satisfy these, and (3) what types of intervention are required to ensure good, sustainable child development and to enable families to lead a happy life with their DHH child. The number one guideline for early intervention and education should be to focus firmly on all options that may enable the child to open up the world through communication and interaction and to align one's educational recommendations accordingly.

### The Parents' Situation

For hearing parents of DHH children, the diagnosis of a hearing loss associated with the challenges for communicative interaction with their child may lead to enhanced stress experiences (e.g. Kurtzer-White & Luterman, 2003; Lederberg & Golbach, 2002; Pipp-Siegel, Sedey, & Yoshinaga-Itano, 2002). Some studies indeed showed an enhanced stress level for parents of DHH children compared to parents of hearing children, whereas other studies did not reveal any differences. It is of vital importance to know which factors influence parental stress and, in particular, to emphasize those factors that contribute to low stress levels or to a reduction in stress levels.

Above all, it is the availability of social and personal resources that influence the coping process the most. Other factors are important as well, for example, additional disabilities in the child, communicative competence, and the parents' hearing status (e.g., Asberg, Vogel, & Bowers, 2008; Hintermair, 2006; Luckner & Velaski, 2004; Pipp-Siegel et al., 2002).

Social resources refer to the support that parents of DHH children receive after the diagnosis of their child's hearing loss. It is essential for the parents to get support from their existing social networks (partners, friends, their own parents, neighbors, etc.), as well as from emerging new networks that integrate the support of professionals and the support of DHH adults as well as other parents with DHH children. Personal resources are the psychological characteristics and strengths that help people to cope with difficult situations in life (e.g., life optimism, sense of coherence, self-efficacy, self-esteem), and the specific competence in dealing with the child's hearing loss acquired in the interval after diagnosis (Hintermair, 2006). Luterman (1999) underscored that the most powerful intervention for the DHH child is to have strong, self-confident parents.

So enhancing parents' strengths in their social and personal situation from the very beginning through a family-centered early intervention concept may contribute to low stress levels. This seems to be a good pre-condition for age-appropriate child development (Pipp-Siegel et al., 2002; Pressman, Pipp-Siegel, Yoshinaga-Itano, & Deas, 1999; Pipp-Siegel, Yoshinaga-Itano, Kubicek, & Emde, 2000).

What are the consequences for the design of counseling and intervention services? In answering this question, we need to keep the following points in mind, since they are equally important for the parents of early detected children and for the professionals who work with them and their families (e.g., Young, 2010; Young & Tattersall, 2007):

1. The topic of "coming to grips with the hearing loss" remains at the heart of the matter, even under the conditions set by UNHS! The diagnosis of a hearing loss is a critical life event, and at which time it first enters the lives of parents is of little importance: Dealing with the unexpected and adjusting one's life to accommodate the change is what matters. Precisely

because it is now possible to diagnose children so early in life, thus awakening hopes inspired by the credo of prevention currently circulating in society (namely, "the earlier, the better"), it becomes even more urgent to raise the subjective aspects of early encounters with issues like "handicap," "being different," and so on. This should prevent any mourning of the hoped-for hearing child from being "covered up" by being offered the earliest possible intervention for the child. Young and Tattersall (2007) report in their study on parental experiences after UNHS that the majority of parents were obviously left on their own to cope with the precarious situation of experiencing shock and hope at the same time and having to come to terms with both. It is therefore absolutely essential that we make room for the parental viewpoint very early in the UNHS process (in other words, both in the hospital and later, during the early intervention process) because parents perceive and come to terms with new experiences very differently.
2. The consequences of "covering up" can be brought to light in many different ways: Putting the focus on activity (being able to do something for the DHH child and its development) may well prevent—or at the very least, deflect or bypass—the internal processes of coping with the situation. We must therefore not lose sight of what an early diagnosis means to each different family, and how well they are able to deal with it.
3. In the end, what does the "normality" hope package that the UNHS presents to parents actually mean? The package mainly covers subjects such as "early identification," "early technical care," "aids to quick speech," and so on. Can this convey a differentiated understanding of normality? What exactly is "normal"? Does "normal" mean "as if hearing" (Young & Tattersall, 2007, p. 218)? Are DHH children who do not meet the standards of the hearing world "abnormal"? So how do we balance parental expectations of normality with the promises of normality made by the specialists and cope with both? "What parents may want to hear . . . may not ultimately serve them well" (Young & Tattersall, 2007, p. 218). Are there any alternatives for families to live a happy life with their DHH beyond the hearing paradigm that nevertheless allows them a quality of life of equal value (see also the results of the study by Leigh et al., 2009)?

A single message for parents after UNHS will not fit all (Young & Tattersall, 2005). Even if development conditions for DHH children have significantly improved, individualized parental support strategies are still needed; unfortunately, according to existing data (Matthijs et al., 2012), they are not widely implemented.

## The Children's Situation

What does the UNHS mean for DHH children? The present findings are no reason to fear that early detection could lead to adverse outcomes in social-emotional development as well as in other areas of development (Spencer & Marschark, 2010). On the contrary, the results from the Colorado Home Intervention Project (CHIP) suggest significantly better results in early-diagnosed children (< 6 months) than in later-diagnosed children (Yoshinaga-Itano, 2003, 2006).

In the case of child development, it is helpful to be geared to the basic human needs that are important for good development. Grawe (2007) presented an explanatory model of mental experience and behavior, clarifying the value of early relational experiences for the development of satisfaction and quality of life. Based on the work of Epstein (2003), Grawe (2007) assumed four basic human needs that must be met if an individual is to either undergo a positive development process or develop emotional problems: orientation and control, pleasure versus aversion, attachment, and the increase and protection of self-worth.

Grawe (2007) particularly stressed the need to increase and protect self-worth, since this is a specifically human need. He sees language and reflexion as prerequisites for developing self-worth, because self-perception is largely the result of verbal communication and self-reflective processes, which are, in turn, based on internalized speech. This is a very important aspect when discussing the early development of DHH children, since it points to the importance of multidimensional educational options for DHH children.

When applying Grawe's model to the situation of DHH children, we face certain challenges, especially for the group of DHH children with hearing parents, which is the vast majority of DHH children, comprising over 90% of the cases.

For a (young) child to develop self-worth, it is important to ensure that the child's actions are positively reinforced and that the child can reliably perceive this reinforcement. On the other hand, parents must be able (or must be enabled) to reinforce their DHH child in a suitable way. Many studies have shown that this coordination is or may be much more difficult between hearing parents and their DHH child (Spencer, 2003). Although we know from children with cochlear implants that they are more likely to find better conditions for this task, we also know that not all children with cochlear implants do in fact benefit from the implant in similar ways, so this remains a challenge for all DHH children (Spencer, Marschark, & Spencer, 2011).

To achieve orientation and control, the most important persons in a DHH child's life must be able to express what they feel or what they want to show and explain to their DHH child in the easiest, most fluent, and most differentiated way. It is indeed true that "fluent and intelligible communicative interaction is more important than the kind of communication" (Paul & Quigley, 1990, p. 84). For children to interactively open up the world, it is of the highest priority that the psychological parents truly recognize and understand the children's attempts to organize their perception of the world. Children must get the feeling that they can do this and be sure of it if they are to acquire self-efficacy. Communicative security is highly important for developing this competence, and early access to language is an essential condition for this.

To sufficiently satisfy the need to increase pleasure and decrease aversion, important aspects are fun, warmth, affection, and interest in the interactions between parents, educators, and the DHH child. The interaction of parents and child must be fun, and enjoyment must be mutually meaningful and visible. The educational guidelines for parents that have accompanied deaf education for hundreds of years—phrases such as "you must," "you must not," and so on—limit the mutual experience of joy. It is far more important to focus on the strengths available to parents and children from interaction and to positively reinforce these competencies so as to increase the enjoyment of interaction and communication.

To develop secure attachments, it is necessary to increase sensitivity, meaning the parents' ability to perceive their child's communicative signals. It is also important to optimize responsiveness, which is the parents' willingness to respond to these signals in every possible way. Emotional availability is what counts. On the one hand, we know from several studies that these competencies may be jeopardized in parent-child constellations that do not have the same auditory status (Spencer, 2003). On the other hand, we know from other studies that the emotional availability of parents and child, particularly for "deafness" in the first year of life, is crucial for the child's overall development in later years (Pressman et al., 1999, 2000). The emotional availability of parents and children in the first 12 months contributes significantly to the children's verbal development between the ages of 2 and 3 years. It is necessary, therefore, to focus on and strengthen the mutual emotional availability of parents and child. A recent study shows that emotional availability can be positively promoted by parent training sessions. Reichmuth, Embacher, Matulat, am Zehnhoff-Dinnesen, and Glanemann (2013) have developed a group training program for parents, whose results indicate that parents showed more responsiveness and less inappropriate behavior after training compared to the parents of a control group.

In summary, the message is that securing attachment in the first 12 months as part of communicative interaction is a guarantee for positive development later. In addition, it is most important to recognize the competencies of DHH children early, in order to decide on the best communicative approaches for each child's development. This requires a great deal of basic diagnostic research. In this regard, Geers (2006) urged better methods of assessing the language skills of DHH children at very young ages, regardless of the communication mode. She also called for research to determine the very early factors that indicate which DHH children may be at risk when it comes to developing spoken language. This could be used for more targeted recommendations regarding appropriate early intervention procedures.

### Family-Centered Intervention Services for Families with DHH Children

In recent years, there has been increasing evidence that family-centered intervention for early-diagnosed DHH children and their families seems to be the best guarantee for successful development in general and language development in particular. In a recent Austrian study involving 63 children (mean age 5 years 1 month), Holzinger, Fellinger, and Beitel (2011) have shown that starting family-centered early intervention at an early stage is associated with better linguistic development in early-diagnosed DHH children (Yoshinaga-Itano, 2003, 2006). Thus, it is important to identify what characterizes family-centered intervention. Sass-Lehrer (2012) has recently documented what is necessary when providing effective early intervention for DHH children.

*A Family-Centered Philosophy of Early Intervention*

A family-centered philosophy provides the foundation for effective early intervention programs and practices. Services provided must be culturally sensitive, community-based, collaborative, and developmentally appropriate (Sass-Lehrer, 2012). These principles provide a meaningful, evidence-based framework for practical work with families, which enables the introduction of development, support, and intervention measures that are tailored to the actual life situation of the individual families.

The aim of family-centered work is to strengthen the family's own ability to cope in the context of a differentiated support system. Family-centered early intervention is a process that encourages the parents of the DHH child to take their affairs into their own hands, to discover their own strengths and competencies, and to take these seriously, as well as learning to appreciate the value of solutions they have worked out on their own. Family-centered intervention focuses on the well-being of the families because this is the source of the essential strengths needed for the child's development. So a family-centered approach indicates a definite departure from the traditional understanding of help and of those providing that help. A professional-as-expert model is replaced by a reciprocal family-professional partnership, founded on real trust and understanding (Sass-Lehrer, 2012). Family-centered early intervention does not attempt to persuade parents to "join in" a particular support strategy proposed by the early intervention experts. On the contrary, parents should start by expressing their previous experiences, as well as their wishes, fears, and goals for their child. This is both the starting point for and the driving force behind developments and changes (Sarimski, Hintermair, & Lang, 2013). This approach requires providers of early intervention to see themselves as partners who are interested in and committed to the families and who open themselves up to the world of the family in question and to the experiences and conditions that the family brings to this process (e.g., hearing status of parents, their educational background, and their personal and economic resources).

Furthermore, it is essential for families to be given the opportunity to work together with hearing and DHH experts from different disciplinary backgrounds and perspectives, as well as with other parents of DHH children, so that they learn what it means to be deaf or hard of hearing and what they can do as parents to provide a supportive family environment for their child (Bodner-Johnson, 2003). Most important, families need to become involved. In a study on children whose hearing losses were detected early, Moeller (2000) showed that DHH children from families who were deeply involved had significantly better vocabulary and verbal reasoning skills than children from less involved families.

Finally, it is essential that the programs provide developmentally appropriate counseling and intervention. Program decisions for the DHH child should be made on the basis of what we know about child development and learning, and what we know about the child's social and cultural contexts. This involves facts on general child development as well as differentiated knowledge of DHH child development.

*Counseling in Early Intervention*

Families should be comprehensively informed on the deafness of their child—but not all early intervention centers can (or want to) offer this (Sass-Lehrer, 2012). Making an "informed choice" is necessary for all parents. This implies comprehensive information for selecting and choosing consciously between different pedagogical and educational alternatives that exist. On the one hand, unfiltered, comprehensive, and reliable empirical information has to be given. On the other hand, decision-making must take into account the social and cultural contexts as well as the values and attitudes of families.

Counseling is not simply transmitting information from one person to another. Rather, it is the art of formulating and presenting well-founded, state-of-the-art specialist information as input for discussion and exchange of ideas. Counseling should reflect one's own professional standpoint as well as the viewpoint of the parents and the options available to the children. To do this requires more from the counselor than highly differentiated expert knowledge of the field alone.

Effective counseling and intervention say goodbye to professional fantasies of omnipotence—professionals do not know what the right ways are or what the wrong ones are. This applies especially to the question of which language modality can and should be used, or which should not be used, by parents with a DHH child. Sass-Lehrer (2012) noted that families often report on professional pressure on parents to choose one approach over another. Pressure is ineffective from a family-centered perspective. What is important in this regard is to support parents in regaining control of their situation because this is valuable for strengthening their self-efficacy and competence (Sass-Lehrer, 2012).

Because of the great heterogeneity found in the group of DHH children and their families, we need to have a wide range of offers available as well as the necessary expertise provided by professional teams. This also applies to children with cochlear implants. Nussbaum and Scott (2011) and Gárate (2011) furnished promising theoretical and conceptual considerations on how a bilingual program may help children with cochlear implants and their families to follow a bicultural path in their development (see Hyde & Punch, 2011). Evidence-based data on results from such programs have yet to be provided.

## FUTURE PROSPECTS FOR ENHANCING PSYCHOSOCIAL DEVELOPMENT: CHALLENGES PRESENTED BY INCLUSION

The general trend in recent years has been for more and more DHH children to be educated in integrative settings (OSERS, 2008), and this trend will increase in the future in all Western countries of the world. Whether this will lead to improved developmental results in DHH students is not clear at the moment, but some promising results have been noted in recent research (e.g., Antia, Kreimeyer, & Reed, 2010).

### The Philosophy of Inclusion

An inclusive education claims to be able to give an answer to diversity (UNESCO, 1994; WHO, 2008). Recognition of diversity is a central target of inclusion. Inclusion stands for the right of all children to education and commonality, regardless of their abilities or disabilities, as well as their ethnic, cultural, or social background. Inclusion refers to human rights and requires the school to treat the needs of their student population equally. Inclusion does not want to adjust the terms of the children to the framework of the school, but rather to align the framework to the needs and characteristics of the students.

These basic premises of an inclusion philosophy sound promising, but with respect to DHH children they are linked to crucial questions: How can the requirements of an inclusion philosophy be met adequately? Who ensures that inclusion will be implemented in a way that is valuable for DHH children? Inclusive education has to secure the participation of DHH children in particular. A participatory approach refers to the persons affected and includes them actively in the discourse from the beginning. Their special needs, skills, and abilities have to be considered adequately. This requires considerable professional expertise and negotiating competencies from all stakeholders. Inclusion is a dialogic challenge, and therefore affects DHH children as well as the hearing environment. This means that the DHH child and the persons in its inclusive, thus hearing, environment (teachers, hearing peers) must design experiences by drawing on each other on the basis of mutual empathy and acceptance and must use these experiences fruitfully for common interactions.

**Identity and Inclusion**

The concepts of inclusion and identity are closely intertwined. As inclusion is not a constant state that is eventually reached safely, but requires an ongoing, lifelong balance, identity also has to be negotiated in a lifelong process of identity work. To explain the relationship of inclusion and identity, it is necessary to digress briefly and discuss recent discourses on identity. Working on identity is a process that continuously challenges the individual to handle a range of experiences and requirements in postmodern societies. Establishment of a coherent pattern of experiences and actions is needed (Hintermair, 2008, Leigh, 2009). This new view of identity is closely connected to global social changes in Western societies over the past decades. Living in a "risk society" (Beck, 1992) is associated with a loss of traditions and an increase of fragmentary experiences, and this leads to big challenges for people in devising their identity/identities. Breivik (2005) postulated a need for a new understanding of selves and identities as shifting, flexible, and alert to the necessities of the situation.

We can also see this change of perspective quite clearly in studies on DHH identities. For example, in a recent ethnographic study McIlroy and Storbeck (2011) explored the identity of nine deaf individuals using these people's own narratives. They let the participants tell their life stories, focusing on their experiences either in mainstream settings or at special schools for the deaf. They elaborated a binary conceptualization of identity (deaf identity versus Deaf identity) and proposed a bicultural "dialogue model" that introduces the concept of a "DeaF" identity. The authors state that the capital F in DeaF is meant to highlight the deaf person's fluid postmodern interactions that go beyond the conventional dividing line between Deaf and culturally hearing identities. This supports the position of Ohna (2003), who says that education has to give each DHH child support "to be deaf in his own way" (p. 10).

This viewpoint relates to the perspective of the single individual and reflects the value of cultural diversity, and this is also exactly where the justification and necessity of individual inclusion patterns is to be found. Inclusion education that is well understood, therefore, always has to be an education that bestows identity at the same time. Without a magnifying lens for DHH-specific issues, this endeavor cannot succeed well.

**Psychosocial Risks of Inclusion for DHH Students**

Effective communication, extensive and satisfying participation with other (hearing and DHH) students, and a sense of affiliation or acculturation are important factors that provide good psychosocial development in DHH students. The crux of the matter is to what extent and under which conditions this can be provided for DHH students in inclusive settings; this is important because these are indicators for a strong DHH identity (Stinson & Lang, 1994).

Since the DHH population is a very heterogeneous one and DHH students differ in their learning from hearing students, equal treatment and equal access cannot be applied in the same way with the same structures and support for all DHH students attending general schools (Hintermair & Lukomski, 2010).[2] Every DHH child has unique needs and strengths, and inclusion is meant to fit the needs of DHH students, not the other way around. An inclusive setting for a DHH child is different from an inclusive setting for a blind child or a child with a mental disability. Furthermore, an inclusive setting for one DHH child can look very different from that for another DHH child. Inclusion can become isolation for a DHH child if its implementation is not well thought through.

The issue is complex and multilayered, since for many deaf children being deaf includes being part of a separate culture with a distinct language. But for a hard-of-hearing child or adult who does not use sign language or is not part of the Deaf culture, inclusion is also a challenge (perhaps sometimes more than for Deaf children). The needs of the hard of hearing may easily be ignored because they can "hear" and can "speak," and appear to "pass" for hearing people in some situations. Inclusion, therefore, must take into account how to support a DHH child's full participation in social, political, and economic life by being receptive to the Deaf culture and responsive to the challenges of the child who is hard of hearing. In other words, a deaf or hard-of-hearing child must be granted the right to develop a strong identity as a deaf or hard-of-hearing person and must be provided with barrier-free access to the hearing world. Therefore, it is not enough to follow the legal mandates (in the United States, for example, since 1976 with Public Law 94-142 to the most recent amendments to the IDEA 2004) by including DHH children with hearing individuals and then feeling vindicated and justified. First and foremost, one must consider whether the inclusive setting guarantees that the DHH child will experience access to social and formal information and learning comparable to a hearing child, while also ensuring that the DHH child is not merely a visitor, but a full member of the environment (see Tang, Lam, & Yiu, Chapter 13 of this volume). The intention of inclusion is for DHH students to fully participate in the everyday aspects of society. This intention can, however, backfire when a DHH child is placed with hearing children without addressing the developmental and socialization needs of that DHH child. Physical proximity does not ensure effective social relationships. Hintermair and Lukomski (2010) provided a diagnostic guide regarding the domains that need to be addressed in order to ensure that a DHH child's emotional needs are fulfilled and developmental tasks are achieved. They also addressed the environmental support required to ensure positive development and quality of life.

When considering the most appropriate school environment for DHH students who attend a general school from a psychosocial perspective, attention needs to be paid to particular aspects the their situation (e.g., Cerney, 2007). Frequently, hard-of-hearing children who are able to function orally in quiet one-on-one situations have communication breakdowns in a classroom setting where there are many speakers and the noise level is high. For example, any extraneous noise, such as noisy heating/cooling systems, traffic outside the classroom, or chattering between hearing peers, can also affect the child's concentration. A hearing person learns about human interactions, family dynamics, cultural mores, and world affairs by overhearing conversations at home, school, and the community and by hearing announcements, overhearing phone conversations, and listening to the radio and television or the news. DHH children, in comparison, frequently miss out on these learning opportunities unless these incidental learning situations are made clear to them (Calderon & Greenberg, 2011). Daily interactions in the classroom, such as a rapid rate of discussion, rapid turn-taking, a rapid change of topics, and more than one child talking at a time are also difficult for the DHH child to follow (Cerney, 2004).

The lack of close friendships for DHH children in the mainstream setting (Antia, Kreimeyer, Metz, & Spolsky, 2010; Stinson, Whitmire, & Kluwin, 1996; Van Gent et al., 2012) has critical implications for program planning for their development. Coping with a hearing loss in the mainstream becomes more stressful without the variety of social interaction that can help combat some of the stress. An essential aspect of the social-emotional life of DHH individuals is the communication barrier that leads to social isolation and limited opportunities to practice social skills (Calderon & Greenberg, 2011). One underlying theme is that, for a DHH child, many of the social-emotional issues are not inherent to deafness per se, but are linked directly to the environmental accommodations and the understanding of the deaf experience by others (Lukomski, 2008). Social interaction is not solely about having friends, socializing at school, minimizing one's isolation, or even belonging to a group. Social settings provide rich learning opportunities for language development and also for incidental learning that illuminates the aspects of daily life.

## Co-enrollment Programs in Inclusion

From a psychosocial perspective on deafness and inclusion, in addition to the important role of the DHH child's parents, the highest priority for the DHH child is the role of other DHH persons in his or her life. Many autobiographical reports show the meaning of knowing other DHH people in order to live a happy life as a DHH person. Drolsbaugh (1997), for example, describes how intensely he experienced his first meeting with other DHH children: "I have no idea of how I can adequately describe what it felt like the first time I was surrounded by a whole school of deaf children. It was an awakening, a rebirth of sorts, and all sorts of shackles broke free" (p. 46).

Without such experiences of a common sense of solidarity and relatedness, the development of a secure identity may be at risk. A member of a Deaf Ex-Mainstreamer's Group in the United Kingdom reports on a DHH person's statement when she was confronted with a deaf man's challenge to "be yourself." She replied with the question, "How can you be yourself when you do not know who you are?" (Jones, 2003, p. 26).

In searching for answers on questions like "Who am I?," "Who do I want to be?," or "Where do I belong?," the relationships with other DHH persons may be important in providing impulses, orientation, and a sense of belonging. Although current studies on inclusive experiences of DHH students show many more academic and social benefits than older studies (e.g., Antia, et al., 2010; Stinson & Antia, 1999; Wauters & Knoors, 2008; Wolters, Knoors, Cillessen, & Verhoeven, 2011, 2012), DHH students in inclusive settings may be at risk when it comes to their social-emotional development. This applies especially for those students who are mainstreamed as the only DHH child in a class with normal hearing children, which is the form of inclusion most often practiced, and this holds true for students with all degrees of hearing (Borders, Barnett, & Bauer, 2010).

For those children, out-of-school programs should be held (in the afternoon, on weekends, or during the holidays), where single included DHH students have the chance to meet with other students who are in a similar situation. For example, such a program was provided and evaluated by Gugel, Blochius, and Hintermair (2011). "Hörnix"[3] is a youth club in a German federal state that provides leisure events that are held on weekends, every 2 to 4 weeks, for hard-of-hearing children from 8 to 16 years of age. The leaders of "Hörnix" are young hard-of-hearing adults. They offer play dates, courses on self-defense, theater workshops, workshops on nonverbal communication and sign language, and they enable the children to reflect on what it means to be hard of hearing. Qualitative interviews with 11 children who attended "Hörnix" for over two years showed that the contact with other hard-of-hearing peers was extremely important for their social and emotional well-being, and especially for their sense of identity. Most of the children said that the contact made them aware of the fact that being hard of hearing was a central part of their identity, and that they no longer tried to hide their hearing loss. Also, most of these young people said that their life before "Hörnix" was boring and that the exchange with other hard-of-hearing students helped them to live a happier life than before.

A promising approach regarding academic development and in particular the psychosocial development of included DHH students may be co-enrollment programs, which involve multiple DHH children in a classroom with hearing children. Although, as some authors note, the documentation of the effectiveness of co-enrollment programs is limited and more research is therefore necessary (Wolters et al., 2011), the available results are definitely positive (see Antia & Metz, Chapter 17 of this volume; Tang, Lam, & Yiu, Chapter 13 of this volume; Yiu & Tang, Chapter 14 of this volume; Pérez Martin, Valmaseda, & Morgan, Chapter 15 of this volume; Hermans, De Klerk, Wauters, & Knoors, Chapter 16 of this volume). For example, in a study with 40 hearing and 5 DHH students in two separated classrooms (general education classroom and co-enrollment), Bowen (2008) assessed friendship patterns and other social competencies and attitudes using sociograms, interviews, and videotape analysis. The results show that, first, there were no differences in social acceptance between the DHH and hearing students, and second, that the hearing students in the co-enrollment program had better sign language skills and more positive attitudes toward deafness.

In their study with a co-enrollment group with 4 DHH children and 21 normal hearing peers in a second grade classroom, Wauters and Knoors (2008) also confirmed the data from other studies that DHH students in co-enrollment programs do not differ from their hearing peers with regard to peer acceptance. Good communicative competencies (in spoken and/or sign language) of the DHH and their hearing peers seem to be an important prerequisite for this.

This was confirmed in a recent study by Kramreiter (2011). She presented data from Austria on 17 students, 11 of whom were normal hearing, and 6 who were DHH. The co-enrollment program started in 2005, when all students began their school career in the first class of the primary school. The instruction was conducted by a hearing general education teacher and a hearing teacher for the DHH with sign language competencies, and the teachers team-taught the lessons for the DHH students. Additionally, there was a deaf teacher who worked together with the hearing general education teacher for a couple of hours. The evaluation of this co-enrollment program shows academic benefits for the DHH students comparable with those of the hearing peers. The results for the psychosocial dimension of development were also very satisfactory. All the DHH students liked going to this class, and they felt comfortable there. The majority of the children self-assessed their social relationships as happy and successful. This was confirmed by external ratings from the teachers and the children's parents. All DHH students showed high self-esteem, and had a high motivation to learn. Good coordination and cooperation by the teachers in the program were essential prerequisites for its success.

Marschark and Knoors (2012) argued that co-enrollment programs seem to bridge the gap between the potential educational benefits of mainstream settings and the communicative and social challenges they pose for DHH students better than other mainstream settings. They saw the advantages for this type of program in combining the best practices in regular and special education and potentially protecting DHH students from isolation by offering to them DHH peers in the classroom. As the results of the available studies show, co-enrollment programs not only have the potential to contribute to social acceptance and social learning, but also to academic achievement.

In order to make this happen, the programs need to have a curriculum that infuses content about deafness into the classroom (Gaustad, 1997) as well as metacommunication learning strategies (Kelman & Branco, 2009). Provision of assertiveness training for the DHH students on how to learn to initiate interactions with teachers and peers might be helpful as well (Antia, Stinson, & Gaustad, 2002).

## BILINGUAL DEAF EDUCATION FOR THE PSYCHOSOCIAL WELL-BEING OF DHH CHILDREN: SOME CONCLUSIONS

Research on psychosocial development in DHH children has provided the field of deaf education with a growing body of knowledge about the variables that play an important role in mental health. A number of studies on various relevant psychosocial domains indicate what matters substantially.

All starts with an early, secure parent-child relationship associated with fluent and mutually intelligible communicative interaction. Most studies, whether they investigate self-esteem, quality of life, or socio-emotional problems of DHH children, show that it is important that parent-child communication works, independent of the modality in which the language used for this interaction is realized (spoken language, signing, or both) (Barker et al., 2009; Dammeyer, 2010; Hintermair, 2007; Kushalnagar et al., 2011; Van Gent et al., 2011).

Regarding the considerable diversity of DHH children (Marschark & Knoors, 2012), this is a strong demand, especially for early intervention providers but also for educators working with DHH children at school, to address the needs of all DHH children for effective communication in a way that meets the specific situation of each DHH child. The available results show that it is not particularly useful to put all one's eggs into one basket and thus to favor only a single approach to education: A "one size fits all" concept for deaf education is not beneficial (Marschark & Spencer, 2010).

This still holds, even given the increased opportunities for optimal development of DHH children due to the UNHS and cochlear implantation, since the group of cochlear-implants children is a very heterogeneous one as well (Hyde & Punch, 2011; Szagun, 2001). Deaf education therefore needs a range of programs in order to optimize the chances for all DHH children in the future, no matter how individually different they are. Bilingual educational programs are a necessary ingredient in this array of programs. A considerable number of DHH children may only develop themselves in psychosocially sound ways within the context of a bilingual education program.

Some studies on socio-emotional problems of DHH children show that using sign language in deaf education may be associated with lower prevalence rates of problematic socio-emotional behavior (Mejstad et al., 2008/2009, Sinkonnen, 1994). Although we envisage that in the future more DHH children will use spoken language as their first language as a result of an early diagnosis of hearing loss by UNHS and early provision with a cochlear implant, this should not be taken as an argument against the use of sign language. Knoors and Marschark (2012), for example, suggested that it is valuable to encourage parents of DHH children to learn and use sign language because this could support the children for a better perception of auditory speech, better language comprehension, and improved spoken language vocabulary. We know for quite some time now that the use of sign language need not interfere with the development of spoken language in DHH children (Marschark & Spencer, 2011). On the contrary, to provide parents with DHH children the opportunity to learn to sign in addition to communication in spoken language may enhance the developmental chances for the children and their parents.

We need thorough, differentiated assessment to find out very early which DHH child will most benefit from which educational program(s) for its development (Geers, 2006). For families with DHH children, the providers of early intervention must ensure that parents have been enabled to see that there are many different ways for their child to be deaf or hard of hearing, and that any of these ways may be a viable option in order to become a DHH person with a high overall sense of well-being.

Another important factor for the development of mental health in DHH children, especially related to self-esteem, is early and varying contact with other DHH children and adults, and thus the opportunity to develop a sense of cultural affiliation(s) (Bat-Chava, 1993; Hintermair, 2008; Maxwell-McCaw, 2001). Again, this can be realized in various educational settings adapted to the special needs of each individual DHH child.

Some studies indicate that a bicultural or a Deaf affiliation may be particularly helpful in this respect, but there are also data available that a more hearing-oriented affiliation can contribute to satisfactory self-esteem (Hintermair, 2008). More recent studies, carried out within the context of modern theories on identity construction, indicate that it may be more productive for young people to develop fluid identities (McIlroy & Storbeck, 2011). This is in line with research carried out by Leigh and Maxwell-McCaw (2011) with respect to children with a cochlear implant. They conclude that shifting between identities as the situation demands would be conducive to mental health. To get this on the right track, taking into account the considerable diversity of DHH children, we need various options to meet their needs. This includes the incorporation of bilingual educational experiences (Gárate, 2011; Nussbaum & Scott, 2011).

Allowing DHH children in inclusive settings to experience various linguistic and cultural options seems to be a specific challenge because most of them are the only DHH child in the class or even at the school they are attending. Research indicates that co-enrollment programs where several DHH children share a class with a group of hearing children stimulate DHH children to develop satisfying social relationships and sound emotional well-being (Bowen, 2008; Kramreiter, 2011; Wauters & Knoors, 2008). Apparently, DHH peer contacts are important for well-being. Therefore individually mainstreamed DHH children should be encouraged to meet other DHH children in after-school programs (in the afternoon, on weekends, or in the holidays). Research shows that such programs can contribute to develop a strong identity (Gugel et al., 2012).

To conclude, Leigh (2009) in her seminal work on deaf identities makes clear what is required. She suggests defining characteristics that are important for well-being from the individual's perspective: "How I live my life as a d/Deaf or hard-of-hearing person, how I intermingle with d/Deaf, hard-of-hearing, or hearing others, how I communicate, and with whom I prefer to socialize" (p. 177). She refers to the many unique stories of DHH people that confirm her view that there are many ways to be deaf, Deaf, or hard of hearing. Inclusion will continue to increase in the coming years in deaf education. Its success seems to depend decisively on how the diversity of deaf identities is considered in educational program planning.

For the educators working and living with DHH children, this entails observing the children's development of their identity carefully and going along with them, thereby providing rich experiences that help each single child to be deaf in his or her own way (Ohna, 2003). For this endeavor to be successful, Erting (2003) suggests that educators and teachers should leave aside their own biases and attempt "to see the world through the children's eyes" (p. 376).

No doubt the next few years will be exciting ones for deaf research and deaf education! Because of the diversity in the deaf population, bilingual educational options will continue to occupy an important place in deaf education. Otherwise, individual needs will be insufficiently addressed.

## NOTES

[1] When the term "language" is used throughout this chapter, it always refers to spoken language and sign language unless otherwise explicitly stated.
[2] Portions of this paragraph are based on Hintermair and Lukomski (2010).
[3] "Hörnix" is a combination of two German words: "hear" and "nothing."

## REFERENCES

Antia, S. D., Kreimeyer, K. H., Metz, K. K., & Spolsky, S. (2010). Peer interactions of deaf and hard-of-hearing children. In M. Marschark & P. E. Spencer (Eds.), *Oxford handbook of deaf studies, language, and education* (vol. 1, 2nd ed., pp. 173–187). Oxford; New York: Oxford University Press.

Antia, S. D., Kreimeyer, K. H., & Reed, S. (2010). Supporting students in general classrooms. In M. Marschark & P. E. Spencer (Eds.), *Oxford handbook of deaf studies, language, and education* (vol. 2, pp. 72–92). Oxford; New York: Oxford University Press.

Antia, S. D., Stinson, M. S., & Gaustad, M. G. (2002). Developing membership in the education of deaf and hard-of-hearing students in inclusive settings. *Journal of Deaf Studies and Deaf Education, 7*, 214–229.

Asberg, K. K., Vogel, J. J., & Bowers, C. A. (2008). Exploring correlates and predictors of stress in parents of children who are deaf: Implications of perceived social support and mode of communication. *Journal of Child and Family Studies, 17*, 486–499.

Barker, D. H., Quittner, A., Fink, N. E., Eisenberg, L. S., Tobey, W. A., Niparko, M. D., and The CDaCi Investigative Team (2009). Predicting behavior problems in deaf and hearing children: The influence of language, attention and parent-child communication. *Development and Psychopathology, 21*, 373–392.

Bat-Chava, Y. (1993). Antecedents of self-esteem in Deaf people: A meta-analytic Review. *Rehabilitation Psychology, 38*, 221–233.

Beck, U. (1992). *Risk society. Towards a new modernity.* London: Sage Publications.

Bodner-Johnson, B. (2003). The deaf child in the family. In B. Bodner-Johnson & M. Sass-Lehrer (Eds.), *The young deaf or hard of hearing child: A family-centered approach to early intervention* (pp. 3–33). Baltimore, MD: Paul H. Brooks Publishing.

Borders, C. M., Barnett, D., & Bauer, A. M. (2010). How are they really doing? Observation on inclusionary classroom participation for children with mild-to-moderate deafness. *Journal of Deaf Studies and Deaf Education, 15*, 348–357.

Bowen, S. K. (2008). Coenrollment for students who are deaf or hard of hearing: Friendship patterns and social interactions. *American Annals of the Deaf, 153*, 285–293.

Breivik, J.-K. (2005). *Deaf identities in the making: Local lives, transnational connections*. Washington, DC: Gallaudet University Press.

Brice, P. J., & Adams, E. B. (2011). Developing a concept of self and other: Risk and protective factors. In D. H. Zand & K. J. Pierce (Eds.), *Resilience in deaf children: Adaption through emerging adulthood* (pp. 115–137). New York; Dordrecht; Heidelberg; London: Springer.

Calderon, R., & Greenberg, M. (2011). Social and emotional development of deaf children: Family, school, and program effects. In M. Marschark & P. E. Spencer (Eds.), *The Oxford handbook of deaf studies, language, and education* (vol. 1, 2nd ed., pp. 188–199). New York, NY: Oxford University Press.

Cerney, J. (2007). *Deaf education in America: Voices of children from inclusion settings*. Washington, DC: Gallaudet University Press.

Ciompi, L. (2003). Reflections on the role of emotions in consciousness and subjectivity, from the perspective of affect logic. *Consciousness and Emotion, 4*, 181–196.

Dammeyer, J. (2010). Psychosocial development in a Danish population of children with cochlear implants and deaf and hard-of-hearing children. *Journal of Deaf Studies and Deaf Education, 15*, 50–58.

Drolsbaugh, M. (1997). *Deaf again*. Springhouse, PA: Handwave Publications.

Epstein, S. (2003). Cognitive-experiential self-theory of personality. In T. Millon & M. J. Lerner (Eds.), *Comprehensive handbook of psychology, Vol. 5: Personality and Social Psychology* (pp. 159–184). Hoboken, NJ: Wiley & Sons.

Erting, C. J. (2003). Language and literacy development in deaf children: Implications of a sociocultural perspective. In B. Bodner-Johnson & M. Sass-Lehrer (Eds.), *The young deaf or hard of hearing child: A family-centered approach to early education* (pp. 373–398). Baltimore, MD: Paul H. Brookes Publishing.

Gárate, M. (2011). Educating children with cochlear implants in an ASL/English bilingual classroom. In R. Paludneviciene & I. W. Leigh (Eds.), *Cochlear implants: Evolving perspectives* (pp. 206–228). Washington, DC: Gallaudet University Press.

Gaustad, M. G. (1997). *Deafness intervention with mainstreamed students and teachers: A report of two projects*. Paper presented at the Council for Exceptional Children, Salt Lake City, UT.

Geers, A. (2006). Spoken language in children with cochlear implants. In P. E. Spencer & M. Marschark (Eds.), *Advances in the spoken language development of deaf and hard-of-hearing children* (pp. 244–270). New York, NY: Oxford University Press.

Gilman, R., Easterbrooks, S. R., & Frey, M. (2004). A preliminary study of multidimensional life satisfaction among Deaf/Hard of Hearing youth across environmental settings. *Social Indicators Research, 66*, 143–164.

Grawe, K. (2007). *Neuropsychotherapy. How the neurosciences inform effective psychotherapy.* Mahwah, NJ: Lawrence Erlbaum Associates.

Greenberg, M. T., & Kusché, C. (1998). Preventive intervention for school-age deaf children: The PATHS curriculum. *Journal of Deaf Studies and Deaf Education, 3,* 49–63.

Gugel, J., Blochius, P., & Hintermair, M. (2012). Erfahrungen einzelintegriert beschulter hörgeschädigter Kinder aus Begegnungen mit anderen hörgeschädigten Kindern—Evaluation des Jugendtreffs Hörnix [Experiences of single included deaf and hard of hearing children when meeting other deaf and hard of hearing children—Evaluation of the youth club "Hörnix"]. *Zeitschrift für Heilpädagogik, 63,* 381–388.

Hart, T. R., & Risley, B. (1995). *Meaningful differences in the everyday experience of young American children.* Baltimore, MD: Paul H. Brookes.

Hintermair, M. (2006). Parental resources, parental stress and socioemotional development of deaf and hard of hearing children. *Journal of Deaf Studies and Deaf Education, 11,* 493–513.

Hintermair, M. (2007). Prevalence of socio-emotional problems of deaf and hard of hearing children in Germany. *American Annals of the Deaf, 152,* 320–330.

Hintermair, M. (2008). Self-esteem and satisfaction with life of deaf and hard of hearing people: A resource-oriented approach to identity work. *Journal of Deaf Studies and Deaf Education, 13,* 124–146.

Hintermair, M. (2011). Health-related quality of life and classroom participation of deaf and hard-of-hearing students in general schools. *Journal of Deaf Studies and Deaf Education, 16,* 254–271.

Hintermair, M., & Lukomski, J. (2010). Wie viel Inklusion verträgt der (gehörlose/schwerhörige) Mensch? Eine entwicklungs- und sozialisationspsychologische Skizze [How much inclusion can a (deaf or hard of hearing) person tolerate? A developmental and social psychological framework]. *Das Zeichen, 81,* 88–97.

Hintermair, M., & Wälder, K. (2012). Sense of coherence, emotional stress and coping strategies of hard of hearing people. In C.-H. Mayer & Krause, C. (Eds.), *Exploring mental health: Theoretical and empirical discourses on salutogenesis* (pp. 85–100). Lengerich: Pabst Publishers.

Holzinger, D., Fellinger, J., & Beitel, C. (2011). Early onset of family centered intervention predicts language outcomes in children with hearing loss. *International Journal of Pediatric Otorhinolaryngology, 75,* 256–260.

Hyde, M., & Punch, R. (2011). The modes of communication used by children with cochlear implants and the role of sign in their lives. *American Annals of the Deaf, 155,* 535–549.

Jankowski, K. A. (1997). *Deaf empowerment: Emergence, struggle, rhetoric.* Washington, DC: Gallaudet University Press.

Jones, J. (2003). Lost deaf people and their needs. Part II. In Deaf Ex-mainstreamers Group (Eds.) (2003). *Between a rock and a hard place* (pp. 26–32). Wakefield, UK: DEX.

Kelman, C. A., & Branco, A. U. (2009). (Meta)cognitive strategies in inclusive classes for deaf students. *American Annals of the Deaf, 154,* 371–381.

Kramreiter, S. (2011). Integration von gehörlosen Kindern in der Grundschule mit Gebärdensprache und Lautsprache in Österreich [Integration of deaf children in the primary school with sign language and spoken language in Austria]. Unpublished doctoral dissertation. Vienna: University of Vienna.

Kurtzer-White, E., & Luterman, D. (2003). Families and children with hearing loss: Grief and coping. *Mental Retardation and Developmental Disabilities Research Reviews, 9,* 232–235.

Kushalnagar, P., Topolski, T. D., Schick, B., Edwards, T. C., Skalicky, A. M., & Patrick, D. L. (2011). Mode of communication, perceived level of understanding and perceived quality of life in youth who are deaf or hard of hearing. *Journal of Deaf Studies and Deaf Education, 18,* 47–61.

Lane, H. (1992). *The mask of benevolence: Disabling the Deaf community.* New York, NY: Knopf.

Lederberg, A. R., & Golbach, T. (2002). Parenting stress and social support in hearing mothers of deaf and hearing children: A longitudinal study. *Journal of Deaf Studies and Deaf Education, 7,* 330–345.

Leigh, I. W. (2009). *A lens on deaf identities.* New York, NY: Oxford University Press.

Leigh, I. W., & Maxwell-McCaw, D. (2011). Cochlear implants: Implications for deaf identities. In R. Paludneviciene & I. W. Leigh (Eds.), *Cochlear implants: Evolving perspectives* (pp. 95–110). Washington, DC: Gallaudet University Press.

Leigh, I. W., Maxwell-McCaw, D., Bat-Chava, Y., & Christiansen, J. B. (2009). Correlates of psychosocial adjustment in deaf adolescents with and without cochlear implants: A preliminary investigation. *Journal of Deaf Studies and Deaf Education, 14,* 244–259.

Leigh, I. W., Pollard Jr., R. Q. (2011). Mental health and deaf adults. In M. Marschark & P. E. Spencer (Eds.), *Oxford handbook of deaf studies, language, and education,* (vol. 1, 2nd ed., pp. 214–240). New York, NY: Oxford University Press.

Loy B., Warner-Czyz, A., Tong, L., Tobey, E., & Roland, P. (2010). The children speak: An examination of the quality of life of pediatric cochlear implant users. *Otolaryngology—Head and Neck Surgery, 142,* 247–253.

Luckner, J. L., & Velaski, A. (2004). Healthy families of children who are deaf. *American Annals of the Deaf, 149,* 324–335.

Lukomski, J. (2008). Best practices in planning effective instruction for students who are deaf and hard of hearing. In A. Thomas & J. Grimes (Eds.), *Best practices in school psychology V* (pp. 1819–1822). Washington, DC: NASP Publications.

Luterman, D. (1999). Counselling families with a hearing-impaired child. *Otolaryngologic Clinics of North America, 32,* 1037–1050.

Marschark, M. (2000). Education and development of deaf children—or is it development and education? In P. E. Spencer, C. J. Erting, & M. Marschark (Eds.), *The deaf child in the family and at school* (pp. 275–291). Mahwah, NJ: Lawrence Erlbaum.

Marschark, M., & Hauser, P. C. (2008). What we know and what we don't know about cognition and deaf learners. In M. Marschark & P. C. Hauser (Eds.), *Deaf cognition: Foundations and outcomes* (pp. 439–457). New York, NY: Oxford University Press.

Marschark, M., & Knoors, H. (2012). Sprache, Kognition und Lernen—Herausforderungen an die Inklusion gehörloser und schwerhöriger Kinder

[Language, cognition, and learning: Challenges for inclusion of deaf and hard of hearing children]. In M. Hintermair (Ed.), *Inklusion und Hörschädigung* (pp. 129–176). Heidelberg, Germany: Median.

Marschark, M., & Wauters, L. (2011). Cognitive functioning in deaf adults and children. In M. Marschark & P. E. Spencer (Eds.), *The Oxford handbook of deaf studies, language, and education* (vol. 1, 2nd ed., pp. 486–499). New York, NY: Oxford University Press.

Matthijs, L., Loots, G., Mouvet, K., Van Herreweghe, M., Hardonk, S., Van Hove, G., Van Puyvelde, M., & Leigh, G. (2012). First information parents receive after UNHS detection of their baby's hearing loss. *Journal of Deaf Studies and Deaf Education, 17*, 387–401.

Maxwell-McCaw, D. (2001). *Acculturation and psychological well-being in Deaf and hard of hearing people.* Unpublished doctoral dissertation. Washington, DC: The George Washington University.

McIlroy, G., & Storbeck, C. (2011). Development of deaf identities: An ethnographic study. *Journal of Deaf Studies and Deaf Education, 16*, 494–511.

Mejstad, L., Heiling, K., & Svedin, C. G. (2008/2009). Mental health and self-image among deaf and hard of hearing children. *American Annals of the Deaf, 153*, 504–515.

National Center for Hearing Assessment and Management (2013). The "state" of early hearing detection & intervention in the United States. Retrieved February 27, 2013, from http://www.infanthearing.org/states/index.html.

Nussbaum, D. B., & Scott, S. M. (2011). The cochlear implant education center: Perspectices on effective educational practices. In R. Paludneviciene & I. W. Leigh (Eds.), *Cochlear implants: Evolving perspectives* (pp. 175–205). Washington, DC: Gallaudet University Press.

Ohna, E. S. (2003). Education of deaf children and the politics of recognition. *Journal of Deaf Studies and Deaf Education, 8*, 5–10.

Office of Special Education Programs (OSERS), United States Department of Education, Data Accountability Center (2008). IDEA Part B Educational Environment [Table 2-2]. Retrieved February 28, 2013, from http://www.ideadata.org/arc_toc10.asp#partbLRE.html.

Paul, P. V., & Quigley, S. P. (1990). *Education and deafness.* New York, NY: Longman.

Percy-Smith, L., Cayé-Thomasen, P., Gudman, M., Jensen, J., & Thomsen, J. (2008). Self-esteem and social well-being of children with cochlear implant compared to normal-hearing children. *International Journal of Pediatric Otorhinolaryngology, 72*, 1113–1120.

Pipp-Siegel, S., Sedey, A. L., & Yoshinaga-Itano, C. (2002). Predictors of parental stress in mothers of young children with hearing loss. *Journal of Deaf Studies and Deaf Education, 7*, 1–17.

Pressman, L. J., Pipp-Siegel, S., Yoshinaga-Itano, C., & Deas, A. (1999). Maternal sensitivity predicts language gain in preschool children who are deaf and hard-of-hearing. *Journal of Deaf Studies and Deaf Education, 4*, 294–304.

Pressman, L. J., Pipp-Siegel, S., Yoshinaga-Itano, C., Kubicek, L., & Emde R. N. (2000). A comparison of the links between emotional availability and language gain in young children with and without hearing loss. *The Volta Review, 100*(5) (monograph), 251–277.

Prillwitz, S. (1995). Gebärdensprache in Erziehung und Bildung Gehörloser—Versuch einer Standortbestimmung [Sign language in the education of the deaf—An attempt to look for positions]. *Das Zeichen, 32*, 166–169.

Reichmuth, K., Embacher, A. J., Matulat, P., am Zehnhoff-Dinnesen, A., & Glanemann, R. (2013). Responsive parenting intervention after early diagnosis of hearing-impairment byUniversal Newborn Hearing Screening: The concept of the Muenster Parental Programme. *International Journal of Pediatric and Otorhinolaryngology, 77*, 2030–2039.

Roth, G. (2000). The evolution of consciousness. In G. Roth & M. F. Wullimann (Eds.), *Brain evolution and cognition* (pp. 555–582). New York, NY: Wiley.

Sarimski, K., Hintermair, M., & Lang, M. (2013). *Familienorientierte Frühförderung behinderter Kinder: Theorie und Praxis lebensweltbezogener früher Interventionen* [Family-centered early intervention for children with disabilities: Theory and practice of life-world-related early intervention]. München, Germany: Reinhardt.

Sass-Lehrer M. (2012). Early intervention for children birth to 3: Families, communities, and communication. In L. A. Schmeltz (Ed.), *A resource guide for early hearing detection and intervention* (pp. 10–1–10–16). Retrieved February 07, 2013, from http://www.infanthearing.org/ehdi-ebook/2012_ebook/Chapter10.pdf

Schick, B., Skalicky, A., Edwards, T., Kushalnagar, P., Topolski, T., & Patrick, D. (2013). School placement and perceived quality of life in youth who are deaf or hard of hearing. *Journal of Deaf Studies and Deaf Education, 16*, 512–523.

Spencer, P. E. (2003). Parent-child interaction: Implications for intervention and development. In B. Bodner-Johnson, & M. Sass-Lehrer (Eds.), *The young deaf or hard of hearing child: A family-centered approach to early education* (pp. 333–368). Baltimore, MD: Paul H. Brookes Publishing.

Spencer, P. E., & Marschark, M. (2010). *Evidence-based practice in education deaf and hard-of-hearing students*. New York, NY: Oxford University Press.

Spencer, P. E., Marschark, M., & Spencer, L. (2011). Cochlear implants: Advances, issues, and implications. In M. Marschark & P. E. Spencer (Eds.), *The Oxford handbook of deaf studies, language, and education* (vol. 1, 2nd ed., pp. 452–470). Oxford; New York: Oxford University Press.

Spencer, P. E., Swisher, M. V., & Waxman, R. P. (2004). Visual attention: Maturation and specialization. In K. P. Meadow-Orlans, P. E. Spencer, & L. S. Koester, *The world of deaf infants: A longitudinal study* (pp. 168–188). New York, NY: Oxford University Press.

Stinson, M. S., & Antia, S. D. (1999). Considerations in educating deaf and hard-of-hearing students in inclusive settings. *Journal of Deaf Studies and Deaf Education, 4*, 163–175.

Stinson, M., & Kluwin, T. (2011). Educational consequences of alternative school placements. In M. Marschark & P. E. Spencer (Eds.), *The Oxford handbook of deaf studies, language, and education* (vol. 1, 2nd ed., pp. 47–62). New York, NY: Oxford University Press.

Stinson, M., & Lang, H. (1994). Full inclusion: A path for integration or isolation? *American Annals of the Deaf, 139*, 156–159.

Stinson, M., Whitmire, K., & Kluwin, T. (1996). Self-perceptions of social relationships in hearing-impaired adolescents. *Journal of Educational Psychology, 88*, 132–143.

Szagun, G. (2001). Language acquisition in young German-speaking children with cochlear implants: Individual differences and implications for conceptions of a "sensitive phase." *Audiology & Neuro-Otology, 6,* 288–297.

Trezek, B. J., Wang, Y., & Paul, P. V. (2011). Processes and components of reading. In M. Marschark & P. E. Spencer (Eds.), *The Oxford handbook of deaf studies, language, and education* (vol. 1, 2nd ed., pp. 99–114). New York, NY: Oxford University Press.

UNESCO (1994). The Salamanca statement and framework for action on special needs education. Retrieved June 27, 2013, from http://www.unesco.de/fileadmin/medien/Dokumente/Bildung/Salamanca_Declaration.pdf.

VanDam, M., Ambrose, S. E., & Moeller, M. P. (2012). Quantity of parental language in the home environments of hard-of-hearing 2-year-olds. *Journal of Deaf Studies and Deaf Education, 17,* 402–420.

Van Eldik, T., Treffers, P., Veerman, J., & Verhulst, C. (2004). Mental health problems of Dutch children as indicated by parents' responses to the child behavior checklist. *American Annals of the Deaf, 148,* 390–395.

Van Gent, T., Goedhart, A., Hindley, P., Treffers, A., & Philip, D. A. (2007). Prevalence and correlates of psychopathology in a sample of deaf adolescents. *Journal of Child Psychology and Psychiatry, 48,* 950–958.

Van Gent, T., Goedhart, A. W., Knoors, H. E. T., Westenberg, P. M., Philip D. A., & Treffers, P. D. A. (2012). Self-concept and ego development in deaf adolescents: A comparative study. *Journal of Deaf Studies and Deaf Education, 17,* 333–351.

Wallis, D., Musselman, C., & MacKay, S. (2004). Hearing mothers and their deaf children: The relationship between early ongoing, mode mach and subsequent mental health functioning in adolescence. *Journal of Deaf Studies and Deaf Education, 9,* 2–14.

Wauters, L. N., & Knoors, H. (2008). Social integration of deaf children in inclusive settings. *Journal of Deaf Studies and Deaf Education, 13,* 21–36.

The World Health Organization Quality of Life Assessment Instrument (WHOQOL). (1995). Position paper from the World Health Organization. *Social Science and Medicine, 41,* 1403–1409.

WHO (World Health Organization). (2008). Convention on the Rights of Persons with Disabilities. Retrieved February 07, 2012, from http://www.un.org/disabilities/convention/ conventionfull.shtml.

Wolters, N., Knoors, H. E. T., Cillessen, A. H. N., & Verhoeven, L. (2011). Predicting acceptance and popularity in early adolescence as a function of hearing status, gender, and educational setting. *Research in Developmental Disabilities, 32,* 2553–2565.

Wolters, N., Knoors, H. E. T., Cillessen, A. H. N., & Verhoeven, L. (2012). Impact of peer and teacher relations on deaf early adolescents' well-being: Comparisons before and after a major school transition. *Journal of Deaf Studies and Deaf Education, 17,* 464–482.

Yetman, M., & Brice, P. J. (2002). *Peer relations and self-esteem among deaf children in a mainstream school environment.* Unpublished manuscript, Gallaudet University.

Yoshinaga-Itano, C. (2003). From screening to early identification and intervention: Discovering predictors to successful outcomes for children with significant hearing loss. *Journal of Deaf Studies and Deaf Education, 8,* 11–30.

Yoshinaga-Itano, C. (2006). Early-identification, communication modality, and the development of speech and spoken language skills: Patterns and considerations. In P. E. Spencer & M. Marschark (Eds.), *Advances in the spoken language development of deaf and hard-of-hearing children* (pp. 298–327). New York, NY: Oxford University Press.

Young, A. (2010). The impact of early identification of deafness on hearing parents. In M. Marschark & P. E. Spencer (Eds.), *The Oxford handbook of deaf studies, language, and education* (vol. 2, pp. 241–250). New York, NY: Oxford University Press.

Young, A., & Tattersall, H. (2005). Parents' evaluative accounts of the process and practice of universal newborn hearing screening. *Journal of Deaf Studies and Deaf Education, 10,* 134–145.

Young, A., & Tattersall, H. (2007). Universal newborn hearing screening and early identification of deafness: Parents' responses to knowing early and their expectations of child communication development. *Journal of Deaf Studies and Deaf Education, 12,* 209–220.

Zand, D. H., & Pierce, K. J. (Eds.) (2011). *Resilience in deaf children: Adaption through emerging adulthood.* New York; Dordrecht; Heidelberg; London: Springer.

# 8

# Bilingualism and Bimodal Bilingualism in Deaf People

## *A Neurolinguistic Approach*

Ana Mineiro, Maria Vânia Silva Nunes, Mara Moita, Sónia Silva, and Alexandre Castro-Caldas

Studies on the neurobiology of bilingualism and bimodal bilingualism suggest that when two languages are learned equally, they become represented in the same brain areas. Does this pattern apply to languages that differ greatly in terms of perception, production, and processing requirements, like sign languages? In order to answer these issues, it is important to consider the neural substrate areas of bilingualism and bimodal bilingualism and to link these findings with the variables associated with the context and conditions of language acquisition that may shape and determine the mapping of language in the brain.

### BRAIN, LANGUAGE, AND LANGUAGE DEVELOPMENT

For the vast majority of humans there is a left hemisphere specialization for linguistic functions. The left hemisphere is specialized in solving symbolic and abstract functions, such as language. One avenue to understanding the neural systems that underlie language has been to investigate the brain by examining the consequences of focal lesions. Research investigating hemispheric specialization for sign language concluded that language areas within the left hemisphere are recruited for sign language processing and comprehension. Evidence from lesion studies in spoken languages revealed that only damage to the left hemisphere leads to language impairments.

An impairment in language production or comprehension as a result of brain damage is called aphasia. If there is an impairment in production skills, it is because Broca's area is involved. If comprehension is damaged, Wernicke's area has a lesion. The same damaged areas are found in deaf aphasic signers who have shown the same language impairment patterns (Bellugi & Klima, 2001; Corina, 1998; Emmorey, 2002; Hickok, Klima, & Bellugi, 1996; Poizner, Klima, & Bellugi, 1987).

These results lead us to claim that these particular brain areas are responsible for linguistic processing, regardless of modality (spoken or signed).

The left hemisphere is clearly dominant for both linguistic modalities and the neural asymmetry, which suggests that it is not the motor system or the perceptual mechanisms (audition versus visuospatial processing) that determine the cerebral organization of language. Lesion studies like the one conducted by Hickok, Kritchevsky, Bellugi, and Klima (1996) and Bellugi and Klima (2001) have taught us that language production involves Broca's area regardless of the modality. Broca's area is well known for playing a fundamental role in speech production; it is located just anterior to the primary motor areas involved in the control of lips and tongue. In Hickok, Kritchevsky, Bellugi, and Klima's study of a deaf native signer with left hemisphere lesions mainly in Broca's area, it was found that the signer showed good comprehension but had deficits (bimanual coordination) in sign production. These deficits were specific to sign language production and were not observed when the signer produced non-linguistic hand movements, reinforcing the interpretation that Broca's area is important to the control of speech production and also production in sign language. Data from further research reinforce this interpretation, suggesting that the neural systems underlying language production are invariable regarding spoken or signed languages (Damasio & Damasio, 2000; Fromkin, 2000). It is possible that the frontal mechanisms that sustain phonological working memory are the same as those for similar functions reported for sign language. In this view, the sensory interface system seems to be the main difference between sign and spoken language processing, and both types of languages seem to rely on the same neural substrates (Bellugi & Klima, 2001).

Despite the considerable differences between articulators (vocal tract versus hands), the functional specialization of the neural system is not dependent on the nature of the motor system involved in its production. Congenitally deaf signers have an absence or minimal input from neural areas surrounding the primary auditory cortex, but these areas are nevertheless engaged in processing the visual input of sign languages and so are useful to language functions due to their considerable neuronal plasticity (Emmorey, 2002). More impressive, however, is the finding that in the deaf brain the same neural structures, Broca's area and Wernicke's area (see Figure 8.1) as well as the supramarginal gyrus, are committed to language functions producing and processing complex syntax (Broca's), comprehension (Wernicke's), and semantic and phonological processing (supramarginal gyrus).

This invariance of neural organization across language modalities shows us that our brain evolved to permit a preference for "function" over "form," as Emmorey (2002) has claimed. The coincidence of neural

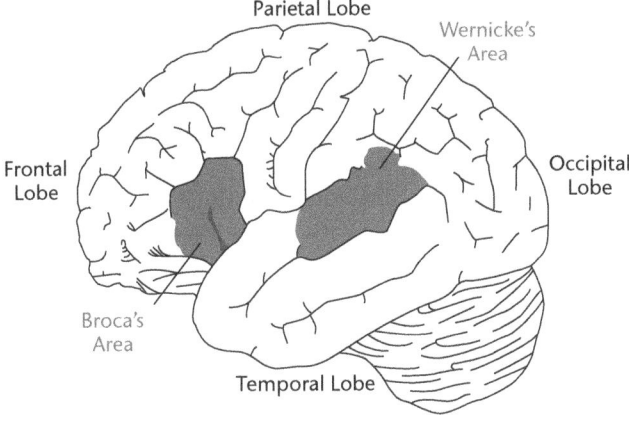

Figure 8.1 Language areas of the human brain.

structures underlying language in both modalities points to a more abstract level of language representation that absorbs the "functional area" for language, regardless of the sensorial and motor systems that are used for language production and transmission.

Nevertheless, and despite a left lateralized hemispheric representation of sign languages, sign languages are more dependent on the right hemisphere for language due to the visual and spatial features of this modality (Bellugi, Klima, & Hickok, 2010; Neville et al., 1997; Neville et al., 1998; Söderfeldt, Rönnberg, & Risberg, 1994). In an event-related potentials (ERP) study, Neville et al. (1997) studied the neural systems that underlie comprehension of open-class words (derivational and constructional "productive" words like nouns, verbs, or adjectives) and closed-class words ("dead words" in terms of lexical productivity, like articles, conjunctions, and auxiliaries). It was found that deaf and hearing native signers showed distinct patterns for open and closed-class in American Sign Language (ASL) signs when compared to English speakers. Regarding English speakers, the ERP response to closed-class words was left lateralized, and for the native ASL signers it was bilateral. This may indicate that there are distinct neural systems—bi-hemispheric activations in the case of sign language and more lateralized activations when it comes to spoken languages—that underlie semantic and grammatical processing in both signed and spoken languages. This also highlights the role of the right hemisphere in sign languages when compared to spoken languages.

A study conducted by Newman, Bavelier, Corina, Jezzard, and Neville (2001) showed that age of acquisition is important for shaping the functional anatomy of the brain in relation to ASL. The authors provided evidence through functional magnetic resonance imaging (fMRI) for a more relevant involvement of right hemisphere structures in ASL processing if the sign language was acquired before puberty. It is difficult to obtain information concerning age of acquisition of spoken languages since late acquisition fortunately is a rarity. From the few cases reported in the literature, the case of Genie (Curtis, 1977) showed that she was able to acquire some language similar to what is found for ASL among late learners. Dichotic listening studies performed with Genie suggested that she was using the right side of the brain more than controls of the same age who had acquired language in the proper time frame. This tendency to process language learning in the right hemisphere, whether in first or second language acquisition, can be found until the learner becomes more proficient in the target language (Xiang, 2012).

However, it seems that there is a difference in modality shaping regarding the role of the right hemisphere in language processing. In the case of deaf individuals, early sign language acquisition implicates more involvement of the right hemisphere than late sign language acquisition. Concerning spoken languages, and bearing in mind that there are not many case studies, acquiring language after puberty promotes a more active role of the right hemisphere in language tasks.

Regarding the involvement of brain shaping in language, the next sections will provide some data and studies reporting the variables involved in language development as well as brain plasticity in deaf and hearing individuals.

## THE BILINGUAL BRAIN

As pointed out by Mechelli and colleagues (2004), humans have a unique ability to learn more than one language. When they do, there is an individual history of acquisition of language that is responsible for shaping the brain from childhood until adulthood, when language is efficiently mastered. When dealing with bilingualism of spoken languages, it is well known that this individual history, in relation to several other aspects such as the degree of proficiency of each language as well as age of acquisition, time of exposure, or even environmental support, is an important issue in understanding the brain mechanisms responsible for processing both languages.

In spite of this individual character, we can still find discussions in the literature on bilingualism regarding the general nature of this adaptation and the factors that have an impact on it. One topic of discussion has been the ways in which bilingualism particularly shapes the language areas. That is, the brain is plastic and adapts to the information that it receives by recruiting the systems that are available.

Language processing is a complex function that involves a number of brain functions related to attention, memory, and cognitive control.

Processing under dual language conditions becomes even more complex. Studies focused on such supplementary cognitive processes have indicated mediation by neural systems during a dual language memory task that are not typically associated with language processing (Hernandez, 2009) and pointed also to distinct specific neural computational demands between first language (L1) and second language (L2) representations (Perani & Abutalebi, 2005). In fact, when people are able to communicate in more than one language, they must control which language they choose to use. Therefore switch control seems to be essential. This additional cognitive processing is trigged by bilingualism (see also Ormel & Giezen, Chapter 4 of this volume).

Based on a review of neuroimaging studies focused on language switching, Abutalebi (2008) and Green (1998) proposed four brain regions that, in addition to their general involvement in cognitive and control functions, are also crucial to bilingual language switching: left dorsolateral prefrontal cortex, anterior cingulate cortex, caudate nucleus, and bilateral supramarginal gyri. Some of these proposed regions were identified by Luk, Green, Abutalebi, and Grady (2012) in a bilingual comparative study using Activation Likelihood Estimation (ALE). Although this study included other brain regions in control switching (such as left middle temporal gyrus and right precentral gyrus), it corroborated the involvement of the caudate nucleus as a critical area for this bilingual language switch control. Crinion and colleagues (2006) also corroborated the use of this critical area, reporting a fundamental role for the left caudate in controlling and selecting the motor sequences that lead to articulation of a selected language, being sensitive to changes in the language and meaning of words. This area seems also to be important for switching in bimodal bilinguals, that is, hearing individuals who use spoken and sign languages (Zou, Ding, Abutalebi, Shu, & Peng, 2012) (see the following section).

These comparative studies suggest that there is no specific brain region that controls bilingual language switching, but that various cortical and subcortical regions employ the left caudate as a critical area for performing this type of switching. The bilingual context is the trigger for these brain switch control regions, which also influence the associated neural areas in bilingual language processing.

Price, Green, and Von Studnitz (1999) have pointed out that the orthography and phonology that are associated with a lexical concept differ from language to language and relate the result to the inhibitory control model of Green (1998). That model suggests that there are language task schemas that link the input from the bilingual lexical semantic system and compete to control outputs from it. Therefore, in order to speak a L2, individuals must inhibit the task schema for word production in the L1. According to this perspective, the process yields a switching cost. The inhibitory mechanism that underlies the control of lexico-semantics is a general cognitive phenomenon (Green, 1998), not a specific mechanism of language processing.

Price, Green, and von Studnitz (1999) pointed to the importance of executive control processes in bilingualism. For instance, it seems that switching between languages in early bilinguals during picture naming involves increased activation in the dorsolateral prefrontal cortex. In an *f*MRI study designed to address separately the question of whether different areas are active for each language in early bilinguals and to investigate the areas that are involved in switching between two languages, Hernandez, Martinez, and Kohnert (2000) found, in accordance with previous studies, that for early bilinguals, processing both languages relies on the same areas. Regarding language switching, they found evidence of dorsolateral prefrontal cortex involvement. The interpretation is that language switching requires executive control and the representation of the two different languages is interpreted as being mediated by systems that usually are not related to language.

Mechelli and colleagues (2004) showed that there is not only functional plasticity, but also structural plasticity in the bilingual brain. With Voxel-based Morphometry (VBM) they showed that learning a second language increases the density of gray matter (GM) in the left inferior parietal cortex and that the degree of structural reorganization in this region is modulated by proficiency and age of acquisition. According to the authors, the relation between GM density and performance may represent a general principle of brain organization. In fact, this effect was greater in the early bilinguals in the left hemisphere and decreased as the age of acquisition increased. The authors suggested that the structure of the human brain is altered by the experience of acquiring an L2 at the same time as the L1. Their results are also important because they verify the importance of the age of acquisition in brain adaptations following bilingualism.

It is commonly held that in early bilinguals who acquire both languages at an early age, similar networks will support both languages, probably due to the availability of similar mechanisms. If a child is exposed to two different spoken languages at the same time, he will recruit similar neural structures for both languages. If the second or subsequent languages are acquired later, however, organization is no longer similar, and the brain will recruit the structures that are the most appropriate for processing new information, undoubtedly making a connection with the previously acquired information. This later acquisition triggers distinct neural associated structures and cognitive processing costs between L1 and L2. The literature on bilingualism of spoken languages supports the idea that the brain areas involved in processing two languages learned simultaneously may be different from those that are involved in processing two different languages learned in distant periods of life or used with different levels of proficiency (e.g., Perani et al., 1998). However, evidence from neuroimaging studies (e.g., Abutalebi, 2008) rejects the claim that early language acquisition of L2 seems to be supported by the same neural foundations responsible for L1 acquisition.

Bilingual speakers may engage different brain paths for processing both languages (Yetkin, Yetkin, Haughton, & Cox, 1996) as a result of the potential role of a number of environmental variables (i.e., proficiency, language exposure, schooling, and age of L2 acquisition), which seem to play an important role in mapping language in the bilingual brain (Abutalebi, Cappa, & Perani, 2005). Neuroimaging studies that have investigated language production and comprehension in bilinguals suggest that if L2 is learned later in life it activates a non-overlapping area of the brain compared to the acquisition of L2 in an early period (Dehaene et al., 1997). Consistent with this idea is the work by Kim, Relkin, Lee, and Hirsch (1997) on early and late bilingual language acquisition, which showed a different physical location for L2 along the periphery of Broca's and Wernicke's regions in the case of late bilinguals, but not in the case of early bilinguals, where the regions are perfectly matched in a overlapping fashion, as the neural substrates for L1 and L2 are shared.

A study of English-French bilingual speakers, all of whom acquired their second language after the age of 7, exhibited shared areas of cerebral activation in the left temporal lobe for all participants when they were using L1, and highly variable areas of activation when they were using L2 (Dehaene et al., 1997). However, a fast growing body of research focusing on both early and late bilinguals with high proficiency showed overlapping activations for L2 in semantic tasks (Chee, Hon, Lee, & Soon, 2001; Illes et al., 1999; Perani et al., 1998). When the proficiency levels were held constant, the age effects decreased. One crucial factor in brain mapping and organization seems to be, therefore, a high proficiency, which increases mental processing of L2 (Perani et al., 2003).

Furthermore, Wartenburger and colleagues (2003) demonstrated, with a neuroimaging paradigm study in which age of language acquisition and proficiency levels were manipulated and both syntactic and semantic tasks were applied, that age of acquisition was only a determinant only for grammar processing. The same does not occur with regard to semantic processing. Age of acquisition only affected cortical representation of the grammar processes, whereas linguistic proficiency mainly influenced the activation of areas related to semantics. Regarding grammatical processing and neural substrates involved in this processing, the perfect overlapping match in neuronal regions only occurred if L2 was acquired at a very early age. Their study was designed with three groups of bilinguals: (1) 11 participants with early acquired L2 during childhood, (2) 12 participants who acquired L2 in adulthood but who attained a high level of proficiency, and (3) 9 participants who acquired L2 later in life and attained limited proficiency. Researchers considered 6 years of age as the critical age for acquiring an L2, and 12 years of age as the limit from which the brain acquires and processes syntax with more difficulty.

In the case of late bilinguals, proficiency is fundamental for brain architecture organization of both grammar and semantics. These findings match the critical period hypothesis (CPH) (Kuhl, 2010; Lenneberg, 1964, 1968; Mayberry, 2010) in language acquisition, which suggests that grammatical processing is dependent on age of acquisition and is based on a neurological competence that needs to be awakened. A high degree of proficiency is indicated as a critical factor for the convergence of L2 representations with those of L1 in language processing such as word production (Chee, Tan, & Thiel, 1999; Klein, Watkins, Zatorre, & Milner, 2006), syntactic processing (Rossi, Gugler, Friederici, & Hahne, 2006), and sentence comprehension (Perani et al., 1998). This reported convergence corroborates Green's (2003) hypothesis, in which the achievement of a proficiency level in L2 promotes a neural convergence of L2 representations with those created for L1.

The importance of proficiency for processing in bilingual brains was revealed in a recent study that analyzed the influence of age of acquisition in terms of the neural correlates of sentence comprehension and word production in two groups with distinct ages of acquisition but with high proficiency in both languages, in this case Italian and Friulian (Consonni et al., 2013). From the reported comparable patterns of neural activations during both cognitive tasks (with focus on the neural representation of nouns and verbs between the two groups), it was found that language proficiency was the main factor in bilingual processing. Bilinguals' grammar proficiency also activates the left thalamus during comprehension of Friulian, as was shown in Wartenburger et al. (2003). Corroborating other studies that have verified language-invariant cortical substrates (e.g., Chan et al., 2008; Willms et al., 2011), the grammatical categories between the two acquired languages seem to remain dissociated, even when acquired at different ages. In this way, the lexicon dependency of L2 on L1 registered by Kroll and Tokowicz (2005), due to the different age of acquisition of L2, is reduced by the proficiency level, in which L2 lexicon representation converges on those created for L1. Consonni and colleagues' (2013) study brings to the fore the fundamental role of language proficiency and language exposure in mapping the neural basis of comprehension and word naming in the bilingual brain.

The functional organization of languages in the bilingual speaker's brain can exhibit substantial differences if we take into account variables such as language use or the context of language use. Perani and colleagues (2003) concluded that a greater portion of brain area is activated in the case of individuals who are exposed less to L2, even if they show great proficiency in that language. Using an *f*MRI paradigm, they studied two groups of early and highly proficient bilinguals (Spanish-born or Catalan-born). Speakers who had Spanish as L1 and lived immersed in Catalan, as assessed by an extensive questionnaire, activated less of the prefrontal cortex for word generation in L2 than speakers who had Catalan as L1 and were less exposed to Spanish (their L2). These exposure-related differences are in line with evidence from previous studies on monolinguals and bilinguals, indicating that experience and practice in language task performance might result in decreased neural activity within the left prefrontal cortex (Abutalebi, 2008; Thompson-Schill, D'Esposito, & Kan, 1999).

In summary, it can be concluded that L2 proficiency and exposure are determinant for lexical semantic processing. In contrast, in the grammatical domain the neural substrate seems to be more dependent on age of acquisition effects (Indefrey, 2006; Perani & Abutalebi, 2005).

The distinction between implicit and explicit language knowledge (Paradis, 2004) could be a good explanation for the lack of differences in brain organization in early and late bilinguals. Early acquisition will lead to implicit knowledge of the language grammar (Ellis, 2008), but late language acquisition will require additional resources of explicit language knowledge and will be based on declarative memory procedures.

This difference between implicit and explicit language knowledge could explain the different activation loci in early and late bilinguals because procedural memory and declarative memory might not be located in co-extensive regions. Evidence from numerous studies has shown us that adult late bilinguals may be faster than early child bilinguals in the initial stages of L2 precisely because they use "shortcuts" to learn explicitly. Children with early L2 acquisition learn broadly and implicitly. They might not use shortcuts, but eventually they attain full native speaker competence through the massive input. This effect is mostly obvious regarding pronunciation of L2 but is no less robust in the domain of grammar (DeKeyser & Larson-Hall, 2005).

In short, there are many factors that influence the bilingual brain, most notably proficiency and age of acquisition, which have an impact on the way in which the brain organizes itself to deal with the difficult task of appropriately representing two languages and voluntarily switching between them. In the case of deaf bilinguals, there are increased challenges in the sense that two modalities and different brain areas are involved. We discuss this issue in the next section.

## THE BIMODAL BILINGUAL BRAIN

Sensory deprivation in one modality, such as deafness, leads to adjustments in the neural development of the existing sensory modalities (Bavelier & Neville, 2002). Research on this neural reorganization has verified a cross-modal reorganization of the auditory cortex to provide the neural substrate with compensatory visual functions that activate single visual functions in parts of the auditory cortex (Lambertz et al., 2005). Thus, when deaf individuals process visual information as linguistic input, their active brain regions correspond to auditory processing (Fine, Finey, Boynton, & Dobkins, 2005; MacSweeney et al., 2004). Existing studies on the localization of neural systems involved in language processing report a significant similarity in the neuroanatomy of signed and spoken languages, suggesting that the neural areas of language are predominantly modality-independent (Hickok, Love-Geffen, & Klima, 2002; Marshall, Atikson, Smulovitch, Thacker, & Woll, 2004).

In addition to the auditory sensory-modality deprivation, the acquisition of two languages in distinct modalities (spoken and signed languages) gives rise to extra neural plasticity in the deaf brain, not only because deaf individuals have to switch between two different languages, but also because their two languages access different sensory-motor systems. In a recent study, Zou, Ding, Abutalebi, Shu, and Peng (2012) found increased gray matter volume in the left caudate brain area in hearing bimodal bilinguals compared to monolinguals. This reinforces the role of the left caudate in language control (see the previous section) for all bilingual populations, regardless of language modality.

Bimodal bilingualism differs from spoken language bilingualism in the production of code-blends instead of code-switches, since the same linguistic information is produced at the same time in both language modalities, rather than selecting just one to communicate. This code-blend phenomenon seems to facilitate the comprehension of two languages with different modalities (Emmorey, Petrich, & Gollan, 2012). This observation stems from production and comprehension tasks in code-blended and single languages performed among early bimodal bilinguals and late bimodal bilinguals of English and ASL. Results show that code-blending production has lower costs for language processing than code-switching, and that dual processing assists the comprehension of both languages by recognition and semantic integration of one language in support of the other. A study by Emmorey, Luk, Pyres, and Bialystok (2008) supported the preference seen in bimodal bilinguals for code-blending rather than code-switching. They reported that in a dual-task with code-blending there were no processing costs for the non-fluent language and that code-blending facilitates lexical access to low-frequency signs. The neural basis and processing of code-blends seem to recruit less activation of the same sensory regions associated with language perception compared with lexico-semantic processing associated regions (Weisberg, McCullough, Petrich, & Emmorey, 2013). This parallel activation has also been verified in hearing. Bimodal bilinguals activate in parallel the phonological and lexical systems of languages with distinct modalities, suggesting that it is possible that linguistic information is transferred across modality as a cross-linguistic processing behavior in bimodal bilingual brains (Shook & Marian, 2012).

Apart from neural plasticity and additional neural associations driven by the absence of auditory sensory modality and bimodal bilingualism processing, the early acquisition of a sign language has been an important issue for addressing the neural regions and mechanisms involved, as well as the benefits of sign language acquisition between birth and early childhood for L1 development and its advantage when acquiring an L2 (sign or spoken language).

Whether sign language acquisition from birth modifies the neural processing of L1 or L2 languages is still being researched. In addition to the typical neural areas associated with processing both (sign and spoken) modality languages without constraint on the chosen modality (Cortina et al., 2003), some neural regions are only active in bimodal bilinguals. Recently, Mayberry, Chen, Witcher, and Klein (2011) tested the effects of age of acquisition by neuroimaging the brains of deaf individuals during grammatical and phonemic-hand judgments, showing that an early age of sign language acquisition provides the classical neural substrates for supporting language processing, in contrast with late sign language acquisition.

The age of acquisition also seems to affect brain lateralization in processing non-manual sign language information (McCullough, Emmorey, & Sereno, 2005), showing left-lateralization in bimodal bilingual deaf signers that has not been detected in bilingual hearing signers. This difference is due to the wide experience of visual non-manual linguistic patterns by deaf signers (Emmorey & McCullough, 2009). Thus, for example, early sign language exposure influences the neural organization for grammatical facial expressions recognition. These studies demonstrate that sign language neural substrates may be close to what is reported for spoken languages, at least in cases of early sign language acquisition and exposure (Neville et al., 1997; Weber-Fox & Neville, 2001).

Nevertheless, as pointed by Penicaud and colleagues (2013), there are no studies exploring how the lack of language input early in life could alter brain development, giving rise to lasting changes in the anatomical organization of the adult brain. Studying a group of congenitally deaf individuals varying in the age of American Sign Language (ASL) acquisition and using voxel-based morphometry (VBM), they explored whether there are local differences in white matter and gray matter concentration across the whole brain related to age of language acquisition. As pointed out by the authors, previous studies using VBM compared white matter (WM) and gray matter (GM) between deaf and hearing individuals, finding that deaf individuals have less white matter than hearing individuals in an area underlying the *planum temporale* and Heschl's gyrus. With VBM they detected two brain areas modulated by age of ASL acquisition, linked to a lower gray matter concentration. Therefore they found that the timing of first language acquisition not only influences the development of the brain functionally but does so neuroanatomically as well, indicating that the effects of early language deprivation and auditory deprivation are not the same. Delayed language acquisition will be associated with changes in the occipital cortex close to the functional area found to be associated with late age of acquisition. The increased gray matter in early learners was interpreted as corresponding to a greater computational power in the visual cortex, leading to a better visual perceptive analysis of the sign language signal.

Early sign language acquisition benefits have been revealed in different fields of language processing. Sign languages seem to provide deaf children with a normal timeline for linguistic development (Wilbur, 2000) and other specific areas of linguistic processing (e.g., Boudreault & Mayberry, 2006; Mayberry & Witcher, 2005). Taking into account the impact of age of sign language acquisition and phonological processing, Mayberry and Witcher (2005) tested sign recognition based on phonological and semantic pairs and non-pairs of ASL signs between native deaf signers and non-native deaf signers. Reaction times increased as the age of ASL acquisition increased, and it was verified that phonological overlapping of prime with target benefited the early signers but inhibited the late signers, revealing that phonological processing is affected by age of language acquisition. Another study concerned with handshape and place of articulation perception (Morford, Grieve-Smith, MacFariane, Staley, & Waters, 2008) observed that phonological and morphological judgments and production of category prototypes of this type also are conditioned by age of acquisition. Taking into account the relation between delayed first language acquisition and exposure with comprehension difficulties, Morford and Carlson (2011) compared deaf native signers and non-native signers in comprehension, processing, and recognition of handshape, location, and signs. The results demonstrated that native deaf signers had better performance in handshape and location parameters and in sign recognition, indicating the significance of a prelingual or early acquisition of sign language in phonological and morphological processing. Another study focusing on spatial relations classifiers (Emmorey et al., 2005) reported activation of the right parietal cortices during a description of object positions while bilingual bimodal hearers are speaking in English, in contrast with monolingual English speakers who only recruit the left parietal cortex (Damásio et al., 2001). With these reports there is congruency about the significant impact of age on phonological and morphological proficiency during sign language acquisition.

Focusing on a higher linguistic level and creating a link between age of acquisition and grammatical judgment, Boudreault and Mayberry (2006) tested whether age of acquisition has different impacts on grammatical judgment. The tasks were performed by three different groups of deaf signers of ASL, according to their ages of ASL acquisition (native, early signers, and late signers). All participants had been exposed to and had used ASL for at least 13 years, making ASL functionally their L1. Age of acquisition appeared to influence response accuracy rather than response latency, with a higher impact on negative structures and on the relation between grammar and age of acquisition, suggesting that delayed L1 acquisition affects the final level of acquisition of morpho-syntax in their L1. To verify these results, Cormier, Schembri, Vinson, and Orfanidou (2012), using the same paradigm tasks, tested whether native, early, and late signers of British Sign Language (BSL) were similar or different in grammatical judgments in BSL. Results confirmed Boudreault and Mayberry's (2006) study, showing that there are significant effects of L1 age of acquisition between birth and 8 years of age on grammatical judgments and underlining that grammatical judgments are affected only by age of acquisition, corroborating Mayberry (1993).

All these studies distinguishing native, early, and late deaf signers emphasize age of sign language acquisition as a major factor in L1 sign language proficiency. However, age of language acquisition not only plays a fundamental role in grammatical judgments in L1, but also influences L2 proficiency with a distinct modality (Mayberry, 2010; Mayberry & Lock, 2003). Nevertheless, deaf individuals do not have the same linguistic experience when they acquire reading skills of a spoken language as hearers do. Reading ability is normally acquired based on associations of letter-sound or whole word-sound, which in deaf individuals is an impracticable methodology. Coding signs, fingerspelling, and internal representations of orthographic letters seems to be the most used methodology for deaf individuals learning to read (Wilbur, 2000).

The absence of spoken language input leads to a different kind of reading decoding by most deaf people compared with hearing individuals (Perfetti & Sandak, 2000). The critical area for reading words is the left visual cortex (the lateral fusiform gyrus in the ventral occipito-temporal cortex), called the visual word form area (VWFA), where segregated activation has been found for phonological and semantic processing (Poldrack et al., 1999). Emmorey, McCullough, Petrich, and Weisberg (2011) found that good skilled deaf readers not only activate the VWFA when reading words, but also activate the left hemisphere for semantic processing. However, activation of this area is limited to semantic segregation, and even though the left hemisphere is activated for reading words, phonological access is incomplete during the word reading task. The deaf individual's ability to understand spoken language also must be taken into account when researching the relation between reading skills and signing competence (Hermans, Knoors, Ormel, & Verhoeven, 2008). This position is consistent with the idea that deaf individuals should have previous knowledge of the language before they try to learn how to write it. This includes not only more face-to-face language contact, which later promotes literacy skills (Mayer & Akamatsu, 2011), but also fits with the view that those deaf individuals who attain better literacy performance skills are those who predominantly use phonological strategies when reading (Brasel & Quigley, 1977; Padden & Ramsey, 2000).

There is a significant relationship between signing and reading skills (Hermans, Knoors, Ormel & Verhoeven, 2008; Hermans, Wauters, De Klerk, & Knoors, Chapter 11 of this volume), evident in the first levels of reading ability. This relationship can constrain the lexical development of L2, resulting in a limited vocabulary and dependence on sign representations rather than words. This point of view is consistent with the idea that a necessary condition for developing literacy in L2 by deaf learners is to have knowledge of the language in its primary, face-to-face form (Mayer & Akamatsu, 2011). Deaf children need to master the alphabetic principle to learn new written words, but being deaf has a severe impact on their phonological awareness (Luetke-Stahlman & Corcoran-Nielson, 2003) and their phonological decoding skills (Adams, 1990; Miller, 2004). As a consequence, most deaf children without cochlear implants will not be able to exploit the natural relations between spoken and written language. Educational programs that include the dimension of learning spoken languages nonetheless possibly can enhance literacy in deaf children. Learning spoken language can develop some sort of articulatory rehearsal that constitutes a procedural phonological memory in the model of working memory (Baddeley, 2003).

It is also reported that some deaf readers access phonology during reading (Perfetti & Sandak, 2000). This observation has been made among deaf readers with linguistic proficiency in sign language and good experience of the spoken language (such as speechreading, good speech intelligibility, and reading proficiency), which allows them to achieve a higher level of reading skill that involves decoding via phonological information from spoken language. Addressing the issue of accessing phonology during reading, an *f*MRI study by MacSweeney, Waters, Brammer, Woll, and Goswami (2008) involved profoundly deaf and hearing individuals making phonological similarity judgments in response to picture pairs. Participants were asked to say whether the spoken English labels rhymed or whether the BSL labels shared the same location (deaf group only). The authors concluded that a very similar network supports phonological similarity judgments made in both English and BSL. Since these languages operate in different modalities, the authors proposed that this phonological processing network is multimodal or possibly supramodal to some extent.

Confirming the effect of L1 proficiency on L2 reading skills, Freel and colleagues (2011) demonstrated that deaf signers with proficiency in ASL have greater competence in reading comprehension compared with deaf signers with low proficiency in ASL, supporting the significance of proficiency in reading skills of L2 as a spoken language (see Holzinger & Fellinger, Chapter 5 of this volume; Marschark & Lee, Chapter 9 of this volume). Findings from that study also emphasized that family education levels influence proficiency in the spoken language and reading skills and thus need to be considered as an additional factor to be included when studying language performance. This feature of family impact is also seen regarding the hearing status of parents. Strong and Prinz (1997) related a greater positive impact on sign language proficiency and reading skills by deaf signers from deaf parents. In a corroborating study, Hoffmeister (2000) studied a group 50 deaf students, ranging from 8 to 18 years old, who had either intensive or limited exposure to ASL. He investigated the relationship between ASL, manually coded English, and English knowledge, finding that regardless of parental status (hearing or deaf) students with greater exposure to ASL were better in all three domains compared to students who had limited exposure to ASL.

In general, concerning L2 acquisition and literacy development, the advantage of being a child of deaf parents is not yet clear (Mayer & Akamatsu, 2011). External factors, such as linguistic and educational variables in reading, were highlighted in one study based on the effects of reading proficiency on lexical processing. Corina, Lawyer, Hauser, and Hirsborn (2013) observed that less-proficient readers activated brain regions normally associated with logographic reading, suggesting the use of different neural areas typically used for orthographic processing by proficient deaf readers and hearing readers. These studies raise questions about the environment of language acquisition and development that must be accounted for when analyzing L2 proficiency and development.

A focus on production rather than reading was the subject of the study by Singleton, Morgan, DiGello, Wile, and Rivers (2004), in which the impact of L1 proficiency on L2 vocabulary was analyzed. Observing the vocabulary frequency of prelingual and postlingual deaf signers, the results indicate that bimodal bilingual prelingual deaf signers have a broader and more varied vocabulary than bimodal bilingual postlingual deaf signers, supporting the critical period hypothesis regarding the impact of first and second language acquisition.

Several studies have focused on the impact of L1 on grammatical judgments in L2, showing that L2 proficiency is constrained by L1 proficiency. Following up on this issue, Mayberry and Lock (2003) conducted a study involving deaf and hearing individuals with different ages of onset in L1 and L2 acquisition. They found that L2 proficiency and grammatical judgments are constrained by the onset age of L1 acquisition independently of L1 or L2 linguistic modality. Later, Boudreault and Mayberry (2006) demonstrated with a timed grammatical judgment task that later acquisition of L1 results in less accuracy in grammatical judgments in L2. These studies suggest that there is a critical age for language acquisition that influences not only L1 proficiency but also proficiency of L2. Also consistent with these results is the neuroimaging study of Wartenburguer and colleagues (2003), which reported that age of acquisition has a greater impact on the neural processing of mechanisms of grammatical judgments than language proficiency, which, in turn, has larger effects on the neural semantic representation processing of L2 than age of acquisition. Therefore, age of acquisition and language proficiency are factors that must be highlighted when studying grammatical judgments and semantic representation.

In contrast with this evidence, recent research (Silva, Mineiro, & Castro-Caldas, 2013; Silva, 2013) has focused on age of acquisition and spoken language effects on Portuguese syntax in deaf individuals, reporting that the age of sign language acquisition has no impact on grammatical tasks. Grammatical performance based on written sentence-picture matching tasks, grammatical judgments of complex sentences, and written tasks revealed only a significant correlation between age of Portuguese acquisition and syntactic performance, revealing no significant impact of L1 on L2.

These studies focusing on the impact of sign language acquisition on the grammatical knowledge of spoken languages thus bring to light contradicting results, revealing the need for further research on this issue. However, it seems that age of acquisition of a sign language influences not only the lexical and semantic representations of language, but also affects the grammatical judgments of the spoken language.

As proficiency of a sign language helps with acquisition of a spoken/written language in deaf signers, the opposite is also found. In grammatical judgment tasks, Cormier and colleagues (2012) reported that late deaf signers, who had first acquired a spoken/written language (English), achieved similar proficiency in sign language as an L2, underlining not only that age of language acquisition is crucial to L2 acquisition but also the importance of bimodal bilingual educational programs for deaf children.

More recently, the impact of L2 on L1 has been addressed by studying bimodal bilinguals, because they were considered to allow for a more precise examination of the effects of L2 experience on the functional brain. In an *f*MRI study comparing deaf and hearing bimodal bilingual speakers of Chinese (L1) and sign language (L2) and monolingual Chinese speakers in a naming picture task in their native language

(L1), Zou and colleagues (2012) were able to examine the effect of L2 on L1 by comparing L1 activation in bilinguals and monolinguals. They found that bimodal bilinguals displayed enhanced functional connectivity across several brain regions. Although previous studies suggested that bilinguals probably apply the neural system of L1 to process L2, the authors were able to show the reverse pattern, in which L2 acquisition induced alteration of the functional brain network. Thus, L2 acquisition seems to influence the neural substrates of language processing in L1.

Bimodal bilingualism is commonly studied based on the language development of L2, considering its performance, context of acquisition, cultural framework, and/or whether the individuals have deaf or hearing parents. It is notable that greater exposure to a sign language stimulates the acquisition of a spoken L2 in deaf learners, and that spoken input assisted by signs during L2 acquisition improves reading (see Hermans, Wauters, De Klerk, & Knoors, Chapter 11 of this volume). Reading involves bimodal phonological knowledge, which has been addressed by reading tasks. But, there are several methods being used to develop and improve the phonological knowledge of a spoken language, and studies report that the use of a phonetic code yields better performance than other strategies. In short, reading, grammatical judgments, morphological processing, and semantic representation in L1 or L2 seem to be affected by age of acquisition, time of exposure to a language, language proficiency, and the language environment. These variables not only affect linguistic performance of both languages in bimodal bilinguals, but also reflect on neural substrates for languages processing and code-blending.

## SUMMARY AND CONCLUSIONS

Distinct linguistic modalities seem to imply the involvement of different cerebral hemispheres during language processing. Apart from the motor programs related to language articulation, sign language requires spatial and movement encoding and decoding that is mainly processed in the right hemisphere. Although studies report left hemisphere dominance for the processing of sign language as well as for spoken languages, bilateral sign language processing with an accentuated involvement of the right hemisphere is driven by early sign language acquisition.

Early bilingualism acquisition involves the same brain areas as early monolingual acquisition. In bilingualism, the left caudate nucleus is responsible for executing code-switching and code-blending. In fact, structural and functional plasticity in bilingual and bimodal bilingual brains seems to be mostly affected by the variables of early acquisition and language proficiency, with the former influencing lexical and semantic representation, and the latter influencing grammatical representation.

However, studies reveal that other factors, such as the context of acquisition, time of exposure, and education, also have an impact on the neural substrates of language and on the propensity for acquiring L1 or an L2 with proficiency. Greater exposure to a sign language seems to improve the acquisition of a spoken/written L2 in deaf learners, and spoken input assisted by signs during L2 acquisition improves reading.

## REFERENCES

Abutalebi, J. (2008). Neural aspects of second language representation and language control. *Acta Psychologica, 128,* 466–478.

Abutalebi, J., Cappa, S. F., & Perani, D. (2005). Functional neuroimaging of the bilingual brain. In J. F. K. Kroll & A. M. De Groot (Eds.), *Handbook of bilingualism: Psycholinguistic approaches* (pp. 497–515). Oxford, UK: Oxford University Press.

Adams, M. J. (1990). *Beginning to read: Thinking and learning about print.* Cambridge, MA: MIT Press.

Baddeley, A. (2003). Working memory: Looking back and looking forward. *Neursocience, 4,* 829–839.

Bavelier, D., & Neville, H. J. (2002). Cross-modal plasticity: Where and how? *Neuroscience, 3,* 443–452.

Bellugi, U., & Klima, E. (2001). Sign Language. In N. Smelser & P. Baltes (Eds.) *International encyclopedia of the social and behavioral sciences* (Vol. 21, pp. 14066–14071). Oxford, UK: Elsevier.

Bellugi, U., Klima, E., & Hickok, G. (2010). Brain organization: Clues from deaf signers with left or right hemisphere lesions. In Luis Clara (Ed.), *Of gesture and word* (pp. 2–17). Lisbon, Spain: Editorial Caminho.

Boudreault, P., & Mayberry, R. I. (2006). Grammatical processing in American Sign Language: Age of first-language acquisition effects in relation to syntactic structure. *Language and Cognitive Processes, 21*(5), 608–635.

Brasel, K., & Quigley, S. (1977). Influence of certain language and communication environments in early childhood on the development of language in deaf individuals. *Journal of Speech and Hearing Research, 20*(1), 95–107.

Chan, A. H. D., Luk, K. K., Li, P., Yip, V., Li, G., Weekes, B., & Tan, L. H. (2008). Neural correlates of nouns and verbs in early bilinguals. *Annals of the New York Academy of Sciences, 1145,* 30–40.

Chee, M. W., Tan, E. W., & Thiel, T. (1999). Mandarin and English single word processing studied with functional magnetic resonance imaging. *The Journal of Neuroscience, 19*(8), 3050–3056.

Chee, M. W., Hon, N., Lee, H. L., & Soon, C. S. (2001). Relative language proficiency modulates bold signal change when bilinguals perform semantic judgments. *NeuroImage 13,* 1155–1163.

Consonni, M., Cafiero, R., Marin, D., Tettamanti, M., Ladanza, A., Fabbro, F., & Perani, D. (2013). Neural convergence for language comprehension and grammatical class production in highly proficient bilingual is independent of age of acquisition. *Cortex, 49*(5), 1252–1258.

Corina, D. P., Poizner, H., & Bellugi, U., Feinberg, T., Dowd, D., & O'Graby-Batch, L. (1992). Dissociation between linguistic and nonlinguistic gestural systems: A case for compositionality. *Brain and Language, 43,* 414–447.

Corina, D. P., Vaid, J., & Bellugi, U. (1992). The linguistic basis of left hemisphere specialization. *Science, 255*(5049), 1258–1260.
Corina, D. P. (1998). Aphasia in users of signed languages. In P. Coppens, Y. Lebrun, & A. Basso (Eds.), *Aphasia in atypical populations* (pp. 261–310). Hillsdale, NJ: Lawrence Erlbaum.
Corina, D. P., San Jose, L., Ackerman, D., Guillemin, A., & Braun, A. (2000). A comparison of neural systems underlying human action and American Sign Language processing. *Journal of Cognitive Neuroscience, supplement,* 414–447.
Corina, D., San Jose-Robertson, L., Guillemin, A., High, J., & Braun, A. R. (2003). Language lateralization in a bimanual language. *Journal of Cognitive Neuroscience, 15*(5), 718–730.
Corina, D., Lawyer, L. A., Hauser, P., & Hirshon, E. (2013). Lexical processing in deaf readers: An fMRI investigation of Reading proficiency. *PLoS ONE, 8*(1), e54696.
Cormier, K., Schembri, A., Vinson, D., & Orfanidou, E. (2012). First language acquisition differs from second language acquisition in prelingually deaf signers: Evidence from sensitivity to grammaticality judgment in British Sign Language. *Cognition, 124*(1), 50–65.
Crinion, J., Turner, R., Grogan, A. Hanakawa, T., Noppeney, U., Devlin, J. T., . . . Price, C. J. (2006). Language control in the bilingual brain. *Science, 312*(5779), 1537–1540.
Curtis, S. (1977). *Genie: A psycholinguistic study of a modern-day "wild child."* New York, NY: Academic Press.
Damasio, A., & Damasio, H. (2000). Aphasia and the neural basis of language. In M.–M. Mesulam (Ed.), *Principles of behavioral and cognitive neurology* (pp. 294–315). Oxford, UK: Oxford University Press.
Damasio, H., Grabowski, T. J., Tranel, D., Ponto, L. L. B., Hichwa, R. D., & Damasio, A. R. (2001). Neural correlates of naming actions and of naming spatial relations. *Neuroimage 13,* 1053–1064.
Dehaene, S., Dupoux, E., Mehler, J., Cohen, L., Paulesu, E., Perani, D., . . . LeBihan, D. (1997). Anatomical variability in the cortical representation of first and second languages. *Neuroreport, 8*(17), 3809–3815.
DeKeyser, R., & Larson-Hall, J. (2005). What does the critical period really mean?. In J. F. Kroll & A. B. de Groot (Eds.), *Handbook of bilingualism: Psycholinguistic approaches* (pp. 88–108). New York, NY: Oxford University Press.
Ellis, N. (2008). Implicit and explicit knowledge about language. In J. Cenoz and N Hornberger (Eds.), *Encyclopedia of language and education* (pp. 119–131). New York, NY: Springer.
Emmorey, K. (2002). *Language, cognition, and the brain: Insights from sign language research.* Mahwah, NJ: Lawrence Erlbaum and Associates.
Emmorey, K., Grabowski, T., McCullough, S., Ponto, L. L. B., Hichwa, R. D., & Damasio, H. (2005). The neural correlates of spatial language in English and American Sign Language: A PET study with hearing bilinguals. *NeuroImage, 24,* 832–840.
Emmorey, K., Luk, G., Pyres, J. E., & Bialystok, E. (2008). The source of enhanced cognitive control in bilinguals: Evidence from bimodal bilinguals. *Psychological Science, 19*(12), 1201–1206.
Emmorey, K., & McCullough, S. (2009). The bimodal bilingual brain: Effects of sign experience. *Brain and Language, 109*(2–3), 124–132.

Emmorey, K., McCullough, S., Petrich, J., & Weisberg, J. (2011, April). *Mapping word reading circuitry for skilled deaf readers*. Poster presented at Cognitive Neuroscience Society meeting. San Francisco, CA.

Emmorey, K., Xu, J., & Braun, A. (2011). Neural responses to meaningless pseudosigns: Evidence for sign-based phonetic processing in superior temporal cortex. *Brain and Language, 117*(1), 34–38.

Emmorey, K., Petrich, J. A. F., & Gollan, T. H. (2012). Bilingual processing of ASL-English code-blends: The consequences of accessing two lexical representations simultaneously. *Journal of Memory and Language, 67*, 199–210.

Fine, I., Finney, E. M., Boynton, G. M., Dobkins, K. (2005). Comparing effects of auditory deprivation and sign language within the auditory and visual cortex. *Journal of Cognitive Neuroscience, 17*(10), 1621–1637.

Freel, B. L., Clark, M. D., Anderson, M. L., Gilbert, G. L., Musyoka, M. M., & Hauser, P. C. (2011). Deaf individuals' bilingual abilities: American Sign Language proficiency, reading skills, and family characteristics. *Psychology, 2*, 18–23.

Fromkin, V. A. (2000). *Linguistics: An introduction to linguistic theory*. Oxford, UK: Blackwell Publishers.

Green, D. W. (1998). Mental control of the bilingual lexico-semantic system. *Bilingualism: Language and Cognition, 1*(2), 67–81.

Hermans, D., Knoors, H., Ormel, E., & Verhoeven, L. (2008). Reading vocabulary learning in deaf children in bilingual education programs. *Journal of Deaf Studies and Deaf Education, 13*(2), 155–174.

Hernandez, A. E., Martinez, A., & Kohnert, K. (2000). In search of the language switch: An fMRI study of picture naming in Spanish-English bilinguals. *Brain and Language, 73*, 421–431.

Hernandez, A. E. (2009). Language switching in the bilingual brain: What's next? *Brain & Language, 109*, 133–140.

Hickok, G., Klima, E. S., & Bellugi, U. (1996). The neurobiology of signed language and its implications for the neural basis of language. *Nature, 381*, 699–702.

Hickok, G., Kritchevsky, M., Bellugi, U., & Klima, E. S. (1996). The role of the left frontal operculum in sign language aphasia. *Neurocase, 2*(5), 373–380.

Hickok, G., Love-Geffen, T., & Klima, E. S. (2002). Role of the left hemisphere in sign language comprehension. *Brain and Language, 82*, 167–178.

Hickok, G., Bellugi, U., & Klima, E. S. (2002). Sign language in the brain. *Scientific American, 284*(6), 58–65.

Hoffmeister, R. J. (2000). A Piece of the puzzle: ASL and reading comprehension in Deaf children. In C. Chamberlain, J. P. Morford, & R. Mayberry (Eds.), *Language acquisition by eye* (pp. 143–163). Mahwah, NJ: Lawrence Erlbaum Publishers.

Illes, J., Francis, W. S., Desmond, J., Gabrielli, J. D. E., Glover, G., Poldrack, R., . . . Wagner, A. D. (1999). Convergent cortical representation of semantic processing in bilinguals. *Brain and Language, 70*, 347–363.

Indefrey, P. (2006). A meta-analysis of hemodynamic studies on first and second language processing: Which suggested differences can we trust and what do they mean?. *Language Learning, 56*(1), 279–304.

Klein, D., Watkins, K. E., Zatorre, R. J., & Milner, B. (2006). Word and nonword repetition in bilingual subjects: a PET study. *Human Brain Mapping, 27*, 153–161.

Kuhl, P. K. (2010). Brain mechanisms in early language acquistion. *Neuron*, 67(5), 713–727.

Kim, K. H., Relkin, N. R., Lee, K. M., & Hirsch, J. (1997). Distinct cortical areas associated with native and second languages. *Nature, 388*, 171–174.

Kroll, J. F., & Tokowicz, N. (2005). Models of bilingual representation and processing: Looking back and to the future. In J. F. Kroll & A. M. B. De Groot (Eds.), *Handbook of bilingualism: Psycholinguistic approaches* (pp. 531–553). New York, NY: Oxford University Press.

Lambertz, N., Gizewsky, E. R., De Greiff, A., & Forsting, M. (2005). Cross-modal plasticity in deaf subjects dependent on the extent of hearing loss. *Cognitive Brain Research, 25*(3), 884–890.

Lenneberg, E. H. (1964). A biological perspective of language. In Eric H. Lenneberg (Ed.), *New directions in the study of language* (pp. 65–88). Cambridge, MA: MIT Press.

Lenneberg, E. H. (1968). The effect of age on the outcome of central nervous system disease in children. In R. L. Isaacson (Ed.), *The neuropsychology of development* (pp. 147–170). New York, NY: Wiley.

Luetke-Stahlman, B., & Corcoran-Nielson, D. (2003). The contribution of phonological awareness and receptive and expressive English to the reading ability of deaf students with varying degrees of exposure to accurate English. *Journal of Deaf Studies and Deaf Education, 8*(4), 464–484.

Luk, G., Green D. W., Abutalebi J., & Grady C. L. (2012). Cognitive control for language switching in bilinguals: A quantitative meta-analysis of functional neuroimaging studies. *Language and Cognitive Processes, 27*(10), 1479–1488.

MacSweeney, M., Grossi, G., & Neville, H. (2004). *Semantic priming in deaf adults: An ERP study.* Poster presented at Proceedings at the Cognitive Neuroscience Society Annual Meeting. San Francisco, CA.

MacSweeney, M., Waters, D., Brammer, M., Woll, B., & Goswami, U. (2008). Phonological processing in deaf signers and the impact of first age language acquistion. *NeuroImage, 40*, 1369–1379.

Marshall, J., Atkinson, J., Thacker, A., Woll, B., & Smulevitch, E. (2004). Aphasia in a user of British Sign Language: Dissociation between sign and gesture. *Cognitive Neuropsychology, 21*(5), 537–554.

Mayberry, R. I. (1993). First-language acquisition after childhood differs from second-language acquisition: The case of American Sign Language. *Journal of Speech and Hearing Research, 36*, 1258–1270.

Mayberry, R. I., & Lock, E. (2003). Age constraints on first versus second language acquisition: Evidence for linguistic plasticity and epigenesis. *Brain and Language, 87*, 369–383.

Mayberry, R. I., & Witcher, P. (2005). What age of acquisition effects reveal about the nature of phonological processing. *CRL Technical Reports, 17*(3), 3–9.

Mayberry, R. I. (2010). Early language acquisition and adult language ability: What sign language reveals about the critical period for language. In M. Marschark & P. Spencer (Eds.), *The Oxford handbook of deaf studies, language, and education* (vol. 2, pp. 281–291). New York, NY: Oxford University Press.

Mayberry, R. I., Chen, J-K., Witcher, P., & Klein, D. (2011). Age of acquisition effects on the functional organization of language in the adult brain. *Brain and Language, 119*, 16–29.

Mayer, C., & Akamatsu, C. T. (2011). Billingualism and literacy. In M. Marschark & P. E. Spencer (Eds.), *The Oxford handbook of deaf studies, language, and education* (vol. 1, pp. 144–155). New York, NY: Oxford University Press.

McCullough, S., Emmorey, K., & Sereno, M. (2005). Neural organization for recognition of grammatical emotional facial expressions in deaf ASL signers and hearing nonsigners. *Cognitive Brain Research, 22*(2), 193–203.

Mechelli, A., Crinion, J. T., Noppeney, U., O'Doherty, J., Ashburner, J., Frackowiak, R. S., & Price, C. J. (2004). Structural plasticity in the bilingual brain. *Nature, 431,* 757.

Miller, P. (2004). Processing of written words by individuals with prelingual deafness. *Journal of Speech, Language, and Hearing Research, 47,* 979–989.

Morford, J. P., Grieve-Smith, A. B., MacFariane, J., Staley, J., & Waters, G. (2008). Effects of language experience on the perception of American Sign Language. *Cognition, 109*(1), 41–53.

Morford, J. P., & Carlson, M. L. (2011). Sign perception and recognition in non-native signers of ASL. *Language Learning and Development, 7*(2), 149–168.

Neville, H. J., Coffey, S. A., Lawson, D. S., Fischer, A., Emmorey, K., & Bellugi, U. (1997). Neural systems mediating American Sign Language: Effects of sensory experience and age of acquisition. *Brain and Language, 57*(3), 285–308.

Neville, H. J., Bavelier, D., Corina, D., Rauschecker, J., Karni, A., Lalwani, A. . . . Turner, R. (1998). Cerebral organization for language in deaf and hearing subjects: Biological constraints and effects of experience. *Proceedings of the National Academy of Sciences, 95,* 922–929.

Newman, A., J., Bavelier, D., Corina, D., Jezzard, P., & Neville, H. J. (2001). A critical period for right hemisphere recruitment in American Sign Language processing. *Nature Neuroscience, 5*(1), 76–80.

Padden, C., & Ramsey, C. (2000). American Sign Language and reading ability in deaf children. In C. Chamberlain, J. Morford, & J. Mayberry (Eds.), *Language acquisition by eye* (pp. 165–189). Mahwah, NJ: Lawrence Erlbaum & Associates.

Paradis, M. (2004). *A neurolinguistic theory of bilingualism.* Amsterdam; Philadelphia: John Benjamins Publishing.

Penicaud, S., Klein, D., Zatorre, R. J., Chen, J. K., & Witcher, P. (2013). Structural brain changes linked to delayed first language acquisition in congenitally deaf individuals. *NeuroImage, 66,* 42–49.

Perani, D., Paulesu, E., Galles, N. S., Dupoux, E., Dehaene, S., Bettinardi V., . . . Mehler J. (1998). The bilingual brain: Proficiency and age acquisition of the second language. *Brain, 121*(10), 1841–1852.

Perani, D., Abutalebi, J., Paulesu, E., Brambati, S., Scifo, P., Cappa, S., & Fazio, F. (2003). The role of age of acquisition and language usage in early, high-proficient bilinguals: A fMRI study during verbal fluency. *Human Brain Mapping, 19*(3), 179–182.

Perani, D., & Abutalebi, J. (2005). The neural basis of first and second language processing. *Current Opinion in Neurobiology, 15*(2), 202–206.

Perfetti, C. A., & Sandak, R. (2000). Reading optimally builds on spoken language: Implications for deaf readers. *Journal of Deaf Studies and Deaf Education, 5*(1), 32–50.

Poizner, H., Klima, E. M., & Bellugi, U. (1987). *What the hands reveal about the brain.* Cambridge, MA: MIT Press.

Poldrack, R. A., Wagner, A. D., Prull, M. W., Desmond, J. E., Glover, G. H., & Gabrieli, J. D. E. (1999). Functional specialization for semantic and phonological processing in the left inferior prefrontal cortex. *NeuroImage*, *10*(1), 15–35.

Price, C. J., Gree, W. D., & von Studnitz, R. (1999). A functional imaging study of translation and language switching. *Brain*, *122*, 2221–2235.

Rossi, S., Gugler, M. F., Friederici, A. D., & Hahne, A. (2006). The impact of proficiency on sytantic second-language processing of German and Italian: Evidence from event-related potentials. *Journal of Cognitive Neuroscience*, *18*(12), 2030–2048.

Shook, A., & Marian, V. (2012). Bimodal bilinguals co-active both languages during spoken comprehension. *Cognition*, *124*, 314–324.

Silva, S., Mineiro, A. & Castro Caldas, A. (2013, January). *How can the early acquisition of sign language and oral language influence the syntactic performance of portuguese?* Paper presented at 3rd International Conference of Sign Linguistics and Deaf Education in Asia. The Chinese University of Hong Kong: Hong Kong.

Silva, S. (2013). *A influência da idade de aquisição da Língua Gestual Portuguesa e da Língua Portuguesa na proficiência gramatical de bilingues surdos*. Master's dissertation, Universidade Católica Portuguesa, 2013.

Singleton, J., Morgan, D., DiGello, E., Wiles, J., & Rivers, R. (2004). Vocabulary use by low, moderate, and high ASL-Proficient writers compared to hearing ESL and monolingual speakers. *Journal of Deaf Studies and Deaf Education*, *9*(1), 86–103.

Söderfeldt, B., Rönnberg, J., & Risberg, J. (1994). Regional cerebral blood flow in sign language users. *Brain and Language*, *46*(1), 59–68.

Strong, M., & Prinz, P. (1997). A study of the relationship between American Sign Language and English literacy. *Journal of Deaf Studies and Deaf Education*, *2*, 37–46.

Thompson-Schill, S. L., D'Esposito, M., & Kan, I. P. (1999). Effects of repetition and competition on activity in left prefrontal cortex during word generation. *Neuron*, *23*(3), 513–522.

Wartenburger, I., Heekeren, H. R., Abutalebi, J., Cappa, S. F., Villringer, A., & Perani, D. (2003). Early setting of grammatical processing in the bilingual brain. *Neuron*, *37*(1), 159–170.

Weisberg, J., McCoullough, S., Petrich, J., & Emmorey, K. (2013, July). *The neural correlates of comprehending ASL-English code-blends*. Poster to be presented at 11th Theoretical Issues in Sign Language Research Conference, University College, London.

Weber-Fox, C., & Neville, H. J. (2001). Sensitive periods differentiate processing of open- and closed-class words: an ERP study of billinguals. *Journal of Speech, Language and Hearing Research*, *44*, 1338–1353.

Wilbur, R. B. (2000). The use of ASL to support the development of English and literacy. *Journal of Deaf Studies and Deaf Education*, *5*(1), 81–104.

Willms, J. L., Shapiro, K. A., Peelen, M. V., Pajtas, P. E., Costa, A., Moo, L. R., & Caramazza, A. (2011). Language-invariant verb processing regions in Spanish-English bilinguals. *NeuroImage*, *57*, 251–261.

Xiang, H. (2012). *The language networks of the brain*. Doctoral dissertation, Radboud Universiteit Nijmegen. ISBN: 9789491027314.

Yetkin, O., Yetkin, F. Z., Haughton, V. M., & Cox, R. W. (1996). Use of functional MR to map language in multilingual volunteers. *American Journal of neuroradiology*, *17*(3), 473–477.

Zou, L., Abutalebi, J., Zinszer, B., Yan, X., Shu, H., Peng, D., & Ding, G. (2012). Second language experience modulates functional brain network for the native language production in bimodal bilinguals. *NeuroImage*, *62*, 1367–1375.

Zou, L., Ding, G., Abutalebi, J., Shu, H., & Peng. D. (2012). Structural plasticity of the left caudate in bimodal bilinguals. *Cortex*, *48*, 1197–1206.

# Part Two
# Education

# 9

# Navigating Two Languages in the Classroom

## *Goals, Evidence, and Outcomes*

Marc Marschark and ChongMin Lee

This chapter concerns bilingualism among deaf students in academic settings. As will become evident in this discussion, this is not meant to be synonymous with or limited to bilingual deaf education insofar as the latter is associated with a more specific meaning. But whatever mode of communication is used in an educational setting with deaf and hard-of-hearing (DHH) learners, its primary goal is the same as it is in a similar setting with hearing students: effective communication between student and teacher as well as among students. In terms of the students, both of those will have specific, long-term effects on cognitive development and social development as well as learning. In terms of the teachers, they also will have implications for classroom management and teacher-student relationships, thus feeding back into their students' cognitive development, social development, and learning (Knoors & Marschark, 2014).

When considering DHH learners, communication in the classroom also has to take into account the fact that most of them come to the classroom not fluent in the language of instruction, whatever it is. Hard-of-hearing students, including those who are hard of hearing by virtue of using cochlear implants, may have better speech and hearing skills than their deaf peers. Nevertheless, the fact that they typically do not have the speech and hearing skills of their hearing age-mates (see Walker & Tomblin, Chapter 6 of this volume) means that they, too, will need special accommodation in the classroom if they are to reach their academic potentials (Marschark, Shaver, Nagle, & Newman, 2014).

Bilingual education is often touted as an effective strategy for addressing the academic, linguistic, and social-emotional needs of DHH students. It frequently is unclear, however, what various educators and investigators mean by bilingual deaf education in practice, and whether it is as effective as is frequently claimed. For DHH youth who primarily use sign language, there clearly are advantages to having fluency in the written/spoken vernacular as well. The importance of the latter for reading and academic attainment is most obvious. Having sufficient spoken language to support interactions with hearing individuals for social, academic, and eventually commercial (e.g., retail interactions, employment) purposes also has advantages, even if it is not a necessity. Nevertheless, many bilingual deaf education programs marginalize spoken language in favor of the written vernacular (see Swanwick, Hendar, Dammeyer, Kristoffersen, Salter, & Simonsen, Chapter 12 of this volume; cf., Lange, Lane-Outlaw, Lange, & Sherwood, 2013).

Knoors and Marschark (2012) pointed out that universal newborn hearing screening, early intervention, digital hearing aids, and cochlear implants have led to an increasing number of deaf children growing up using spoken language. For those who cannot use spoken language or simply do not for whatever reason, sign language provides a fully appropriate—if not exactly equivalent (Marschark & Knoors, 2012)—mode of communication for personal, social, and educational purposes. Sign language also plays an important role in the lives of many deaf individuals who use spoken language but who also desire to be part of the Deaf community and/or interact with deaf individuals who sign. This chapter is not the place to consider either the evidence or the emotions associated with growing up using primarily one language modality or the other. The focus here is limited to the use of sign language and the written/spoken vernacular in the classroom and the extent to which explicit use of both influences achievement among deaf youth. Before considering the evidence with regard to academic outcomes, however, it will be worthwhile to consider several related issues associated with bilingualism, bilingual education, and bilingual deaf education.

## BILINGUALISM AND DEAF LEARNERS: THE BIG VIEW

Bilingualism for DHH children receives support from at least three quarters. One of those emphasizes the importance of a natural sign language (e.g., American Sign Language, ASL) as a potentially important part of deaf children's identity as a member of the linguistic-cultural minority that is the Deaf community (Gregory, 1986; Padden & Humphries, 1988). Beyond recognizing the value of signed languages and the Deaf community, notice that this view represents advocacy for sign language rather than bilingualism per se. Support for DHH children's acquiring two languages generally comes from two more practical perspectives. One is the viewpoint emphasizing the potential for deaf children's acquiring sign language earlier than spoken language. Even if the vernacular (written if not spoken) will be needed at some point for schooling, earlier access to language provides greater opportunities for formal and informal learning as well as language, cognitive, and social development (e.g., see Marschark, 1993, Chapter 5, for a review). The other viewpoint argues that bilingualism per se (e.g., in ASL and English) will support greater academic outcomes for DHH learners with regard to literacy (e.g., Johnson, Liddell, & Erting, 1989) as well as later personal and employment success, what is often referred to as added-value bilingual education.

The sociocultural view of the importance of bilingualism for DHH children, in what typically is referred to as bilingual-bicultural education, seems altogether fitting and proper from both psychological and humanitarian perspectives. Yet we can find no evidence that anyone has investigated the bicultural part of bilingual-bicultural education to evaluate the social-emotional effects of providing DHH children with instruction in either sign language or Deaf culture (but see Hintermair, Chapter 7 of this volume). In a survey of educational programs for DHH students in the United States that describe themselves as bilingual-bicultural programs, LaSasso and Lollis (2003) emphasized both the bicultural and reading components of program curricula. Yet, of the 19 programs they surveyed that described themselves as bilingual-bicultural, only 6 reported that they had a bicultural component in their curriculum.

Although apparently neglected, the social-emotional and social-cultural aspects of bilingual education for deaf students could turn out to be important for language acquisition and academic outcomes as well as for social functioning (see Knoors & Marschark, 2014, Chapter 7). Examinations of bilingualism in hearing children by Lambert (1977) and Cummins (1984), for example, argued that emphasis on acquiring the language of the linguistic majority can place linguistic minority children at a disadvantage in educational environments. Cummins emphasized that attempts to suppress children's use of their first language can lead to feelings of shame and embarrassment that generalize to values and behaviors of their family's linguistic-cultural heritage. Use of the second language (L2) and avoidance of the first language (L1), combined with the associated social-emotional responses, frequently lead to academic difficulties. He therefore argued that it is the school itself, rather than bilingualism, that leads to observed low levels of achievement for children from linguistic minorities, and he emphasized the value of instruction in the child's first language. Of course, there are a variety of issues surrounding a deaf child's "first language" involving both linguistic questions (e.g., whether deaf children's L1 skills theoretically or functionally are equivalent to hearing children's) and minority status (when the majority of deaf children's parents are hearing). However interesting and important they are, these issues, too, are beyond the scope of this chapter (for further discussion of Cummins, see Holzinger & Fellinger, Chapter 5 of this volume; Tang, Lam, & Yiu, Chapter 13 of this volume).

With regard to deaf children, we have identified only a single published study that focused explicitly on *bilingual-bicultural* programming. Andrews, Ferguson, Roberts, and Hodges (1997) reported a study involving seven children attending a bilingual-bicultural program from pre-kindergarten to first grade, all of whom were reported to be functioning at grade level when they reached first grade. The description of the "deaf culture component" of the program (p. 20), however, cited only the availability of classroom technologies (e.g., strobe fire alarms), books and posters containing sign language, and an annual pizza party for deaf children and their hearing families at which deaf adults told stories. The impact of this "deaf culture component" was not evaluated.

We will return to the need for a broader approach to research on bilingual education later. Meanwhile, we will focus on the bilingual aspects rather than the bicultural aspects of educating DHH learners and, in particular, issues associated with having two languages in the classroom. In this regard we consider academic outcomes associated with bilingual education for DHH students as they relate to factors intrinsic and extrinsic to the learner. This will include discussion of research concerning their print literacy, an essential L2 for educational purposes. Questions of whether bilingual programming has demonstrated that deaf children acquire fluency in a signed L1 is a very different matter, and one that we fear has been neglected almost as much as deaf children's acquisition of cultural identities (but see Dammeyer, 2010).

## WHEREFORE ART THOU, BILINGUALISM?

Regardless of whether one is examining specific outcomes of DHH children's bilingualism, for example in cognitive development or print literacy, or bilingual competence per se, it is essential to distinguish bilingualism in educational settings from the use of sign language in the home. Most studies that have reported positive associations between younger DHH students' sign language abilities and academic achievement have focused exclusively on reading, and many of those have involved deaf children of deaf parents (see following discussion). While it seems likely that linguistic and cognitive benefits to deaf children by virtue of having sign language available from birth generally would be facilitative for formal and informal learning, there are two caveats related to the research on reading achievement among those deaf children with deaf parents.

The first caveat concerns deaf parents as academic mentors/models for their deaf children. While the US National Center for Education Statistics (2003) reported that 14% of adults in the United States were functionally illiterate (typically defined as reading and writing at the fourth to fifth grade level), Qi and Mitchell (2012) documented that since 1974 at least 50% of DHH 18-year-olds have continued to score at or below the fourth grade level on the reading comprehension subtest of the Stanford Achievement Test (SAT). Other studies have shown that this situation persists into adulthood (Albertini & Mayer, 2011; Parault & Williams, 2010). This means that many deaf parents will be less than optimal academic models and less able to assist their DHH children with homework or to read with/to them. If deaf children of deaf parents really achieve at higher levels than deaf children of hearing parents, perhaps the use of sign language in the home rather than bilingualism per se might be the key.

That brings us to the second reason for caution in interpreting academic achievement in deaf children of deaf parents as a reflection of bilingualism at home. Simply put, the causal relationship between the two has not been established. Several studies have demonstrated positive associations between early sign language fluency and reading ability (e.g., Padden & Ramsey, 2000; Strong & Prinz, 1997), whereas others have demonstrated a negative association or no relation (e.g., Holzinger & Fellinger, Chapter 5 of this volume; see also Moores & Sweet, 1990). Further, there is also a positive association between early spoken language and reading ability in deaf children (Goldin-Meadow & Mayberry, 2001; Holzinger & Fellinger, Chapter 5 of this volume; Perfetti & Sandak, 2000). It thus appears that when deaf children of deaf parents are observed to read better than expected, early access to language may be a more likely explanation than either sign language or bilingualism per se.

Mayer and Akamatsu (1999) further made the point that while a strong foundation in L1 is necessary for the transfer of skills to an L2, it is not sufficient (Holzinger & Fellinger, Chapter 5 of this volume). In particular, there is no reason to expect skills in a signed L1 to be effective in acquiring print literacy in an L2, any more than oral skills in an L1 benefit acquiring print literacy skills in an L2 (Cummins, 1991). One cannot simply acquire a sign language like ASL, skip the learning of English, and expect to be able to read English. This is not to say that "learning English" means learning to speak English. Mayer and Akamatsu, however, emphasized that whether one likes it or not, spoken language typically provides a bridge to written language that does not have a parallel in sign language. Whether or not *intelligible* speech is essential for that bridge (see Lichtenstein, 1998) and whether or not there are other routes that deaf learners can take to print literacy are matters we will leave to others. For the moment, we also will leave aside the issue that many, if not most, deaf children do not have a particularly "strong foundation" in their L1, whatever it is and however it is acquired. We will return to the issue later in the context of school learning. First, let us consider some of the cognitive and linguistic advantages bestowed by bilingualism and the extent to which they might benefit deaf learners' educational attainment more generally.

## BILINGUALISM AND COGNITION

Because most contemporary treatments of bilingualism among hearing individuals are written in support of its implementation in educational settings, they typically refer to the cognitive benefits resulting from bilingual mastery. Lee (1996) and García and Náñez (2011) noted that studies from the first half of the twentieth century, in contrast, tended either to report negative relationships between bilingualism and cognition or to find no significant relation between them. In their view, those studies generally lacked experimental rigor and were influenced by an anti-immigration sociocultural perspective. More recent studies have indicated that at least among balanced bilinguals, having two languages is associated with greater verbal and nonverbal IQ scores and problem-solving skills (Náñez, Padilla, & Lopez-Máez, 1992), attention (Bialystok, 1999), executive functioning (Carlson & Meltzoff, 2008; see Bialystok & Craik, 2010), and working memory (Bialystok, Craik, Green, & Gollan, 2009).

Peal and Lambert (1962) were among the first investigators to demonstrate the cognitive benefits of bilingualism in children. In the context of French-English bilingualism in Canada, they were interested in the effects of second language learning on verbal and nonverbal intelligence. They found that bilingual fourth graders consistently scored significantly higher than monolingual peers when confounding variables were controlled. In particular, bilingual children's visual-spatial processing and concept formation abilities led Peal and Lambert to conclude that code-switching between languages bestows on children greater mental flexibility and concept formation skills (Bialystok & Craik, 2010). Importantly perhaps, their demonstrations of bilingual advantage rather than disadvantage involved balanced bilinguals, children who were equally fluent in both French and English. Some investigators have argued that the Peal and Lambert sample thus was biased toward children with greater language and cognitive abilities. Nevertheless, studies by Barik and Swain (1975) with children in a French-English bilingual program and Diaz (1985) of children in a Spanish-English bilingual program both showed increasing nonverbal intelligence and metalinguistic awareness over time.

Balanced bilingualism among deaf children likely is harder to come by than it is among children in French-English or Spanish-English immersion programs. And, given the demonstrated cognitive differences between those two populations, as well as between them and hearing individuals (Emmorey, Borinstein, Thompson, & Gollan, 2008; Pisoni, Conway, Kronenberger, Henning, & Anaya, 2010), it is likely that at least some findings from studies involving unimodal (spoken language or sign language) bilinguals will not generalize to bimodal bilinguals (spoken language and sign language).[1] However, bimodal bilingualism—having both a signed language and a written/spoken vernacular—might be expected to carry its own advantages, particularly in the visual-spatial domain. Capirci, Cattani, Rossini, and Volterra (1998), for example, found that teaching Italian Sign Language to hearing children increased their scores on both the Corsi Blocks and the Ravens Progressive Matrices, the latter one of the nonverbal intelligence tests used by Peal and Lambert (1962). The elementary school children in the Capirci et al. study received signed language instruction only 1 hour per week for 7 months during the first year of the program and for 8 months during the second year. Subsequently they showed significantly higher scores on both visual-spatial cognitive tasks than a comparison group of children from the same classes from whom they did not differ at the beginning of the program. Together with findings indicating that some cognitive advantages of being in bilingual homes become apparent as early as 7 months of age, even before a child is producing those languages (Kovács & Mehler, 2009), it would appear that linguistic balance is not a necessary prerequisite for cognitive benefits of bilingualism. Do the languages have to be in the same modality?

Emmorey, Luk, Pyers, and Bialystok (2008) compared (all hearing) bimodal bilinguals, unimodal bilinguals, and monolinguals on a test of attentional control (flanker tasks). The unimodal bilinguals surpassed the other two groups with no apparent benefit to the bimodal bilinguals. Emmorey and colleagues argued that it is experience with the difficult task of dealing with two languages in the same modality that confers the bilingualism advantage (see also Marschark & Hauser, 2012, Chapter 6). Most research into the possible cognitive advantages of bimodal bilingualism, in contrast, has focused particularly on cross-modal language activation (see Ormel & Giezen, Chapter 4 of this volume). Such work suggests the possibility that exposure to signs and their corresponding spoken/written words leads to potential benefits in vocabulary learning. Hermans, Knoors, Ormel, and Verhoeven (2008), for example, conducted a study involving 87 deaf children, 8 to 12 years of age, enrolled in Dutch bilingual education programs where either Sign Language of the Netherlands or Sign-Supported Dutch (see later discussion) was the language of instruction. They reported that the children found it easier to learn written words when they already knew the sign for a concept (see also Andrews, 1988; Wauters, Knoors, Vervloed, & Aarnoutse, 2001). Hermans and colleagues suggested that when a word is encountered repeatedly, the link between it and the sign is strengthened by automatic activation of the latter and, over time, the need for conscious lexical lookup declines. Although the nature of this word-sign activation apparently has not been compared to word-word activation in unimodal bilinguals, it might be that different modalities reduce the possibility of bottlenecks in lexical processing. This, in turn, might help to avoid one of the cognitive disadvantages of unimodal language bilingualism: the slower retrieval of information from long-term memory (Bialystok & Craik, 2010).

With regard to the education of DHH students, we have yet to see studies explicitly examining bilingualism and related cognitive effects in the context of academic learning or achievement (but see discussion of possible implications in Ormel & Giezen, Chapter 4 of this volume). Of particular interest in that regard would be the benefits to executive functioning (Bialystok & Craik, 2010) and metalinguistic skills (Peal & Lambert, 1962), domains in which DHH students' weaknesses have been demonstrated to adversely affect classroom learning (Borgna, Convertino, Marschark, Morrison, & Rizzolo, 2011; Hauser, Lukomski, & Hillman, 2008; Marschark, Sapere, Convertino, Seewagen, & Maltzan, 2004) as well as reading (Banner & Wang, 2011; Kelly, Albertini, & Shannon, 2001). We therefore now turn to bilingualism in deaf education.

## BILINGUALISM, LEARNING, AND SCHOOL

Issues associated with bilingual education for hearing students do not necessarily transfer well to discussions of bilingual deaf education. In part, this is related to unimodal versus bimodal bilingualism differences discussed earlier, but there are other potentially important differences as well. Most notably, delays in language development likely to affect DHH children's learning begin to emerge early in life (Knoors & Marschark, 2014, Chapter 3). Although balanced bilingualism may not be a necessary component for educationally relevant advantages, most DHH children come to school lacking language fluencies (in any modality) comparable to those of hearing peers. We have noted the potential benefits of L1 abilities in the acquisition of an L2, according to Cummins's linguistic interdependence hypothesis, but that transfer requires fluency in L1. It was precisely such issues that led to the move toward bilingual education for DHH children in several countries (Leeson & Sheikh, 2010).

### Bilingualism in Scandinavian Deaf Education

Proponents of bilingual deaf education frequently point to Scandinavia, and Sweden in particular, as potential deaf education models for the rest of the world. Sweden was one of the first countries to offer "universal" bilingual education for deaf students, starting with formal recognition of Swedish Sign Language and the adoption of bilingual programming following the 1980 revision to the Curriculum for Compulsory Education (Heiling, 1998). Bilingual education became the primary approach to educating deaf students in countries such as Norway, the Netherlands, and Denmark, and one option in an array of educational placements in countries like the United States and the United Kingdom.

Swanwick, Hendar, Dammeyer, Kristoffersen, Salter, and Simonsen (Chapter 12 of this volume), however, note the decreasing popularity of bilingual education in Scandinavian countries and the United Kingdom to the point where it now is found primarily in schools for the deaf, which also are experiencing decreasing popularity. In their view, the decline of bilingualism in mainstream deaf education was partly the result of the bilingual deaf education model emphasizing sign language and writing as primary routes to language competency while de-emphasizing spoken language. As many more deaf children gained the potential to acquire spoken language, its marginalization in many deaf education settings clearly sent the wrong message to parents of deaf children, over 95% of whom are hearing. As Swanwick, Hendar, Dammeyer, Kristoffersen, Salter, and Simonsen note, "The emergence of these boundaries around language, policy, and approach seems to work against a concept of bilingual education by constraining choices and provision rather than opening up bilingual and bicultural educational environments for all" (Chapter 12 of this volume).

Swanwick, Hendar, Dammeyer, Kristoffersen, Salter, and Simonsen (Chapter 12 of this volume), Knoors and Marschark (2014), and others have pointed to the positive findings with regard to deaf children's sense of identity and psychosocial well-being in schools and programs designed for deaf children in Scandinavia as well as the United States (e.g., Dammeyer, 2010; Stinson, Whitmire, & Kluwin, 1996). The extent to which those benefits are specifically attributable to sign bilingualism as opposed to deaf children's being accepted in social interactions with similar peers is an empirical question that, as we have seen, remains to be explored (see Antia & Metz, Chapter 17 of this volume). The impact of bilingualism in Sweden with regard to academic performance, however, has been investigated for over 20 years.

Heiling (1998) described a group of deaf eighth graders she had studied in the late 1980s who had started receiving signed communication in preschool. She reported that "[w]hen the children left compulsory school, all were fluent in sign language. Some had been able to develop a relatively good oral language as well, but their interpersonal mode of communication was sign language" (p. 143). Importantly, those students had been exposed primarily to simultaneous communication (speech and sign together, see later discussion) in primary and intermediate school, and it was only in secondary school that "some teachers used sign language exclusively." So, those students would have had only limited access to what is usually considered bilingual deaf education. That limitation notwithstanding, Heiling reported that the students demonstrated higher levels of academic achievement in terms of word knowledge, reading comprehension, and mathematics relative to a 1960s cohort that had been educated exclusively through spoken language. Heiling (1997, cited in Bagga-Gupta, 2004), however, reported that those advantages were not found among students she tested in the early 1990s, students who would have had even more exposure to (true) bilingual education than her earlier sample. Following up on Heiling's studies, Bagga-Gupta (2004) reported that school assessments and evaluations indicated that Swedish deaf students' literacy skills continued to lag behind hearing peers, despite their immersion in bilingual education.

In a more recent investigation, Rydberg, Gellerstedt, and Danermark (2009) examined the educational attainments of more than 2,100 deaf individuals in Sweden, including cohorts educated before and after the initiation of bilingual education. They found that although educational attainments of deaf individuals had increased since deaf education in Sweden became bilingual, the educational attainments of hearing individuals had increased even more, so that the disparity between deaf and hearing achievements remained. Hendar (2009) reached similar conclusions in a government report, concluding that it is difficult for DHH students to achieve high levels of academic achievement, regardless of whether they are enrolled in mainstream or special schools. Overall, Hendar found that students in special schools (those more likely to receive bilingual programming) generally scored lower than their peers in mainstream settings. In a similar study of deaf education in Norway, Hendar (2012, cited in Swanwick, Hendar, Dammeyer, Kristoffersen, Salter, & Simonsen, Chapter 12 of this volume) found that significant numbers of deaf students simply were excluded from the Norwegian student evaluation system apparently in expectation of their low performance.

**Bilingualism and Reading Achievement**

The apparent lack of support in the research literature for bilingual deaf education in any broad sense derives in part from the relative lack of research beyond that focused on the acquisition of literacy skills, with much of the latter focused on vocabulary (e.g., Hermans, Ormel, & Knoors, 2010; Hermans, Wauters, De Klerk, & Knoors, Chapter 11 of this volume; Hermans et al., 2008; Kreimeyer, Crooke, Drye, Egbert, & Klein, 2000). This limitation is somewhat puzzling given the emphasis that commentators have placed on the potential benefits of sign language in domains like science and mathematics (e.g., Harrington, 2000; Lang, 2002; Marschark & Hauser, 2012, Chapter 4). Nevertheless, the focus on literacy is perhaps understandable given its importance for academic attainment and eventual employment, as well as the overarching concern alluded to earlier about bilingual deaf education essentially requiring deaf children to learn to read in their second language.

In their review of the literature, Mayer and Leigh (2010, p. 177) argued that "there is no data to suggest that, as a group, students in bilingual programs are achieving at the age-appropriate language and literacy levels that were predicted when bilingual models were first implemented." In their view, there are two primary issues that have impeded the promise of bilingual deaf education with respect to print literacy. First is the fact that acquiring print literacy as a second language requires proficiency in a first language, something we have noted that most deaf children do not have. Johnston, Leigh, and Foreman (2002) made the same point, arguing that most deaf children and their families begin acquiring sign language too late, and rarely do families and schools have the resources to appropriately immerse them in a sign language environment. Leigh and Johnston (2004) found that among children between 3 and 11 years of age enrolled in a bilingual (Auslan-English) program, only the children with deaf parents demonstrated receptive sign language skills within the normal range (cf., Knoors & Marschark, 2012).

The second impediment to deaf children's acquisition of print literacy in their second language, according to Mayer and Leigh (2010), is the relative inadequacy of their exposure to it. Unlike immigrant children who might use their L1 at home but are surrounded by the L2 in school and community, most DHH children—including those with cochlear implants—will have limited access to the vernacular, at least relative to hearing peers. Mayer and Leigh pointed out that efforts to make the vernacular more accessible to DHH learners through speechreading, fingerspelling, cued speech, and visual phonics have had some success, but none of them has been sufficient to provide DHH students with adequate linguistic information to support age-appropriate literacy (perhaps because they are functional only at the levels of phonemes or words). For proponents of bilingual deaf education, in contrast, the demonstration of significant relations between sign language skills and various measures of reading ability frequently are taken as equivalent to demonstrations of the benefits of bilingual education.

DeLana, Gentry, and Andrews (2007, p. 74) noted that "[i]n the past decade the profession's three national [US] journals . . . have published only one article . . . providing any empirical data specifically on the issue of dual language methodology." They reviewed 16 studies, only four of which were published in peer-reviewed journals, reporting relations of varying strength between ASL skill and English literacy measures. Whether or not the locus of any of those relations can be placed in bilingual programming per se is unclear, but in all but one of those studies (some including the same children), various comparisons indicated positive associations of ASL and literacy-related measures. Possible relations of English language skills and literacy-related measures were not considered.

So how important is it that the L1 of children's bimodal bilingualism be sign language rather than the other way around? First, it is important to re-emphasize the difference between studies purporting to demonstrate better literacy skills among deaf children of deaf parents and those purporting to demonstrate better literacy skills among deaf children who receive bilingual education. As we already have suggested, early sign language skills may be related to reading achievement for the same reason that early spoken language skills are related to reading achievement: Children who have stronger language foundations and linguistic abilities are likely to have better reading skills. The extent to which such abilities derive from early access to effective language versus bilingual education really has not been considered. Demonstrations of simple associations between sign language skills and reading fluency among deaf children of deaf parents, however, likely are confounded.

An early study by Jensema and Trybus (1978) is frequently cited as indicating that having deaf parents leads to stronger reading comprehension. Table 21 of that report indeed showed increases in SAT reading comprehension scores from having no deaf parents, to having one deaf parent, to having two deaf parents. Interestingly, that is the only table in the entire document for which the authors did not indicate whether the differences were statistically significant. In fact, the students with two deaf parents were reported to rely primarily on sign language, while those with one deaf parent relied primarily on spoken language, and both groups scored somewhat higher in reading comprehension than the students with no deaf parents. The authors therefore concluded that "variables other than communication method are operating to give both of these groups a performance advantage over children with hearing parents" (p. 19). Further, Jensema and Trybus's Table 19 shows a significant *positive* relationship between reading comprehension scores and the amount of spoken language used between parents and students and a significant *negative* relationship to the use of sign language from student to parent (that from parent to student was not significant). This finding supports the notion that whatever the reason that deaf children of deaf parents might show reading achievement beyond that of deaf children of hearing parents, it is not a simple consequence of the use of sign language or sign language/written language bilingualism.

Other early studies reported finding deaf students of deaf parents to be reading at higher levels than deaf students of hearing parents, but still well below grade level. Stuckless and Birch (1966) examined reading comprehension as well as other literacy- and school-related abilities in more than 100 deaf students with deaf parents as compared to more than 300 with hearing parents. The deaf students with deaf parents were found to be reading above the level of the students with hearing parents. Yet their average reading level was 4–5 years below grade level. Vernon and Koh (1970) also tested a large group of deaf students and matched smaller groups with deaf versus hearing parents on a variety of relevant factors. Again, the deaf students with deaf parents were reading at levels beyond those with hearing parents but well below the levels of the hearing students.

Brasel and Quigley (1977) explicitly examined the influence of parental hearing status and early linguistic experience in deaf students 10 to 18 years of age with severe to profound hearing losses and minimum IQ scores of 90. The students comprised four groups, a Manual English group of students with deaf parents who had good command of English and who used English-based signing with them from infancy, an Average Manual group with deaf parents who used ASL but were not fluent in written English, and Average Oral and Intensive Oral groups, all of whom had hearing parents and used only spoken language. On both the Test of Syntactic Ability (TSA) and the reading comprehension and language subtests from the SAT, the students who signed outperformed those who used spoken language. In addition, the Intensive Oral group outperformed the Average Oral group, but the Manual English group outscored all three of the other groups.

More recently, links between sign language skill and literacy have been described in conference presentations, published proceedings, and chapters, and have been cited as manuscripts in preparation in works like Chamberlain, Morford, and Mayberry (2000). As noted by DeLana et al. (2007), however, papers in refereed publications remain rare. Strong and Prinz (1997) examined the relationship of ASL skills and English literacy (with IQ controlled) in a group of 160 deaf children with either deaf or hearing mothers, all of whom attended the same school. They found that among 8- to 11-year-old children, ASL skills were not significantly related to English literacy skills for the ones with deaf mothers, although they were for those with hearing mothers. Among 12- to 15-year-olds, skills in the two domains were significantly related for both groups. Information was not provided concerning the relationship of spoken language to literacy scores or the age at which the children with hearing mothers acquired sign language.

Padden and Ramsey (2000) reported a similar study involving 31 deaf children at two grade levels and split between a special school and a mainstream school. Overall, ASL skills were found to be significantly correlated with reading comprehension subtest scores on the SAT, a finding that held for deaf students with hearing parents as well as those with deaf parents (see Rinaldi, Caselli, Onofrio, & Volterra, Chapter 3 of this volume). Results were not reported separately for the two groups or for the two groups in the two settings. Nevertheless, together with the earlier studies, all of these findings support the conclusion that DHH children with better foundational language abilities are likely to be better readers, whether or not they have deaf parents and whether or not they are truly bilingual. The extent to which reading ability might be differentially related to one language mode or another in bilingual children or whether bilingualism per se is the key remains to be examined.

Finally, we are aware of only two studies that explicitly reported educational outcomes of formal bilingual programming for deaf children education in the United States (but see Hermans, De Klerk, Wauters, & Knoors, Chapter 16 of this volume; Holzinger & Fellinger, Chapter 5 of this volume; Tang, Lam, & Yiu, Chapter 13 of this volume). An unpublished report by Nover, Andrews, Baker, Everhart, and Bradford (2002) summarized findings from a 5-year program emphasizing bilingual language planning in one school for the deaf. SAT reading comprehension scores were reported for 168 students aged 8–18 years, 35% of whom had deaf parents. Nover and colleagues found that students between the ages of 8 and 12 years scored significantly higher than the national norms for deaf and hard-of-hearing children. Those scores differed by only 5–25 points (1%) from the norms, and older students scored below the SAT norms (attributed to lesser staff development). Knoors and Marschark (2012) reported that scores on the same test for students of the same age and the same birth years enrolled in another US school for the deaf that applied total communication philosophy scored even higher, exceeding scores of children in the bilingual program in all but one of the five age groups.

Lange and colleagues (2013) reported on the reading and mathematics achievement of DHH students who had been enrolled in a bilingual program incorporating ASL and both spoken and written English. Their achievement growth was compared to a group of predominantly hearing students with the same starting points in achievement and grade levels in reading and mathematics (DHH students with lower levels of achievement were excluded from the study). Although the DHH students' initial progress in the program was behind that of the comparison group, their academic growth in reading exceeded that of their peers after 8.2 years in the program and in mathematics after 2.5 years in the program. Initially, 28% of 61 of the DHH students in the reading study group were at or above average and 19% of 64 students in the math study group were at or above average, according to national norms (overlap between the two groups is unclear). After at least 4 years in the program, 41% of the reading study group was at or above average, and 55% of the students in the mathematics study group were at or above average. The authors concluded that "[w]hereas some groups are lobbying for a one-size-fits-all model to deaf education, research demonstrates a variety of paths for D/HH students to develop academically. Students and parents need educational choices to be available to them and researchers and policy makers need to continue collecting data and monitoring these educational options" (p. 543).

## SIMULTANEOUS COMMUNICATION, BIMODALITY, AND BILINGUAL EDUCATION

Any discussion of navigating the variety of language paths available to DHH students must include simultaneous communication, or sign-supported speech, as it is referred to outside the United States, if only because of its frequent use in DHH classrooms as well as other situations. Signed and spoken languages do not share the same phonological code, thus making simultaneous, equivalent output impossible, but simultaneous communication, in which signs are produced with the grammatical order of the vernacular with accompanying speech (i.e., code-blending), is not uncommon among bimodal bilinguals. Philosophies aside, today's reality is that the majority of both "oral" deaf individuals (often with cochlear implants) and signing deaf individuals (with or without cochlear implants) are likely to function as bimodal bilinguals—using both sign language and written/spoken language—to some extent, at least as young adults if not as children. For example, of the 249 deaf students at Rochester Institute of Technology who were using cochlear implants in the spring of 2013, 74% of them rated their sign language skills as fair to excellent; only 12% said they did not know sign language.

Marschark and Hauser (2012) suggested that simultaneous communication and other vernacular-based sign systems often are used by individuals who are not fluent in a natural sign language, but that fluent teachers might use such sign systems to teach new vocabulary or to support reading. There is no doubt that many individuals who use simultaneous communication do so poorly (Johnson & Erting, 1989) and that teachers who are good users of simultaneous communication usually are good signers as well (see Caccamise, Blaisdell, & Meath-Lang, 1977; Cokely, 1990; Newell, 1978). The interest here is on this educational use of simultaneous communication and its potential for deaf education.

All of the published studies we are aware of that have examined the impact of using simultaneous communication in the classroom have shown that students from 10 years of age to university age learned just as much as they did with other forms of communication (including ASL and Auslan) when teachers were highly skilled in simultaneous communication (e.g., Caccamise et al., 1977; Cokely, 1990; Hyde & Power, 1992; Marschark et al., 2005; Marschark, Sapere, Convertino, & Pelz, 2008; Mollink, Hermans, & Knoors, 2008; Newell, 1978). Mollink, Hermans, and Knoors (2008), for example, found that hard-of-hearing 4- to 8-year-olds remembered more word meanings when words were presented in both spoken Dutch and SLN as compared to signs when they were trained using only spoken Dutch.

In an investigation involving almost 800 DHH college students, Convertino and colleagues (2009) reanalyzed data from several previous studies of learning in mainstream classrooms. Various communication skills, including ASL, spoken English, and speechreading, were assessed using a self-report instrument that had been shown to be valid and reliable for that population. The investigators found that the only language variable to significantly predict learning in mainstream classrooms when other communication, family, audiological, and academic factors were controlled was receptive simultaneous communication skill. Importantly, none of the previous experiments evaluated in that study involved simultaneous communication; all included mainstream instructors with skilled interpreters providing the deaf students with either ASL or English transliteration. The investigators therefore concluded that receptive simultaneous communication abilities reflect language flexibility, an important factor in the profile of persons who are considered bilinguals.

Mayer and Leigh (2010) also raised the possibility of using simultaneous communication to provide access for deaf students to English as a second language, suggesting that such an approach "has the potential to play a significant role not only in bilingual education, but in the education of children who have cochlear implants" (p. 182). Knoors and Marschark (2012) made a similar argument. They pointed out that gestures accompanying spoken language frequently facilitate comprehension (Habets, Kita, Shao, Özyürek, & Hagoort, 2011; Kelly, Özyürek, & Maris, 2010) and suggested that simultaneous communication could be an effective "backup code" for children with cochlear implants. Humphries and colleagues (2012) also provided arguments in favor of signing for children with cochlear implants based largely on the large individual differences and the continuing difficulty in predicting linguistic outcomes following implantation. In essence, this suggests that in the United States, for example, ASL and simultaneous communication might provide a better approach to English literacy than ASL alone. Which DHH students might benefit from such programming in which contexts remains an issue to be explored, but let us consider one possibility a bit further.

### Signing for Children with Cochlear Implants?

The suggestion of using any kind of signing with children who use cochlear implants will seem anathema to many. Spencer, Marschark, and Spencer (2011) reviewed evidence relating to language development in deaf children and found a consistent if small advantage for children using cochlear implants in spoken language programs compared to those in sign language programs. At the same time, however, there is also evidence that early signing can support the development of spoken language by children with cochlear implants (e.g., Connor,

Hieber, Arts, & Zwolan, 2000; Spencer & Tomblin, 2006; Tomblin, Spencer, Flock, Tyler, & Gantz, 1999; Yoshinaga-Itano, 2006). What about its impact on academic achievement?

Spencer, Barker, and Tomblin (2003) examined the reading, writing, and language abilities of 16 deaf students with an average age of 9.8 years. The students had received cochlear implants at an average age of 3.9 years, quite late by current standards, and had an average of 5.9 years experience with them. All were enrolled in mainstream schools where they were supported by sign language interpreters, and all were reported to use simultaneous communication to some extent. The deaf students' reading comprehension scores were only about 10% below those of the comparison group of 16 hearing age-mates (90.1 and 99.5, respectively); they were reading at an average grade level of 3.3 years compared to 3.8 years by the hearing group. The deaf students also lagged behind their hearing peers in writing, which was reliably correlated with language scores for the deaf students but not their hearing peers. Spencer and colleagues emphasized that access to English through cochlear implants provides DHH learners with opportunities for enhancing their language and literacy skills, but the role of sign language and simultaneous communication in supporting those skills was not discussed. Spencer, Gantz, and Knutson (2004) conducted a study with 27 deaf high school students from the same program. They had received cochlear implants between 2 and 13 years of age and had used them for an average of just under 10 years. Despite the relatively late age at implantation, students who used their cochlear implants consistently were found to be reading on par with hearing age-mates, and the group as a whole scored within the normal range. This is a remarkably high level of performance for late-implanted users (cf., Geers, Tobey, Moog, & Brenner, 2008).

Finally, Blom and Marschark (2014) conducted a study involving 40 deaf college students who used cochlear implants. Each student saw two classroom lectures (presented by video), one in which the instructor only spoke and the other in which she used simultaneous communication. There was no difference in scores on a subsequent multiple-choice test for the easier of the two passages (8$^{th}$ to 9$^{th}$ grade level), but the students scored significantly higher with simultaneous communication than with spoken language on the more difficult of the two passages (9$^{th}$ to 10$^{th}$ grade level). The authors concluded that the redundancy offered by simultaneous communication might be helpful for cochlear implant users not only when material is more difficult but also in the classroom and other less than optimal listening environments.

Taken together, the above results suggest that having access to two languages can benefit the language and academic achievement of at least some deaf students with cochlear implants. A similar argument might be made with regard to students with mild hearing losses who hear about as well as those with cochlear implants. Marschark, Shaver, and colleagues (2014) found that such students scored significantly lower than those with moderate hearing losses on the Passage Comprehension, Mathematics, and Social Science subtests of the Woodcock-Johnson III Achievement Tests, while not differing significantly from the students with profound hearing losses. Blackorby and Knokey (2006) obtained similar results with elementary school students.

## NAVIGATING TWO LANGUAGES IN THE CLASSROOM: BILINGUAL EDUCATION AS SAFE HARBOR?

Over the past 30 years, bilingualism and bilingual education for DHH children have gained international attention as means of providing them with the linguistic skills necessary for academic, personal, and eventual employment success. As we have seen, however, the limited research available about such programming is devoted almost exclusively to literacy outcomes, with relatively little attention to how they might influence and be influenced by cognition, learning, or social-emotional functioning (but see Antia & Metz, Chapter 17 of this volume). Understanding the connections and interactions among these domains in bilingual deaf individuals will lead to better understanding of their language abilities, as described by both formal theories (e.g., relating to structural linguistics) and functional theories (e.g., relating to social communication), as well as the impact of such abilities on learning.

With regard to the functional aspects of language, the bilingual experience is quite varied, a situation magnified by the large individual differences among deaf learners. That is, for both hearing and DHH people, the bilingual circumstance of each individual is associated with a different set of social, cognitive, and personal factors that mediate bilingual balance as well as the effects of bilingualism. It therefore is important to recognize that generalizations concerning the outcomes of bilingualism for any population will always be tentative. And, yet, the consequences of bilingualism for educational policy, teaching, cognitive science, and social processes (Bialystok et al., 2009) are just now coming to be explored with regard to DHH individuals.

Meanwhile, a central assumption underlying the placement of DHH students in regular classrooms is that we are able to educate them in that environment as well as or better than we can in separate settings. Success for DHH students in mainstream classrooms, however, requires that information communicated by a hearing teacher for a hearing class is both linguistically accessible and consistent with the knowledge and learning styles of deaf students, that is, that the material is readily learnable. Until recently, there has been little question about the viability of mainstream educational placements, but growing recognition of the generally poor quality of educational interpreting (Napier & Barker, 2004; Sapere, LaRock, Convertino, Gallimore, & Lessard, 2005) and cognitive differences between hearing students and deaf students (Marschark & Knoors, 2012; Pisoni et al., 2010) have forced a re-examination of educational placement for deaf students. The issue has become even more complex with recent demonstrations of unexpected lags in reading achievement by both younger (Nitrouer, Caldwell, Lowenstein, Tarr, & Holloman, 2012) and older (Geers et al., 2008) deaf students with cochlear implants and greater achievement among older students with access to sign language in the classroom (Blom & Marschark, 2014; Spencer et al., 2004). Indeed, studies over the past several years have demonstrated a variety of cognitive differences between hearing students and deaf students that may put the latter, with and without cochlear implants, at an academic disadvantage in the mainstream classroom compared to settings designed for them (Marschark & Knoors, 2012). Unfortunately, even in separate settings—bilingual or not—instructors may be unaware of such differences and thus may be unable to appropriately adjust their interventions and instructional methods.

Bilingualism and bilingual deaf education are based on the assumption that once communication barriers in the classroom have been removed, teaching and learning processes for deaf and hearing students will be much the same (Seal, 2004; Stinson, Elliot, Kelly, & Liu, 2009). Similar assumptions are made with regard to the education of students learning English as a second language. In the case of deaf students, (high-quality) sign language interpreting and real-time text have been assumed to provide them with access to classroom communication comparable to that of hearing peers (see Sapere et al., 2005). Yet recent studies examining deaf students' learning have found that from middle school through college they do not learn any more through sign language than they do from reading, an area in which their difficulties are well-documented (e.g., Borgna, Convertino, Marschark, Morrison, & Rizzolo, 2011; Marschark, Leigh, et al., 2006; Marschark, Sapere, et al., 2009; Stinson et al., 2009). Given the frequent claims about the benefits of sign language in the face of reading challenges (e.g., Johnson et al., 1989; Nover et al., 2002), we expected to find explicit support for bilingualism and bilingual deaf education. The fact that the evidence base is so weak does not mean that they do not have considerable potential (see, for example, the co-enrollment results reported by Antia & Metz, Chapter 17 of this volume; Hermans, De Klerk, Wauters, & Knoors, Chapter 16 of this volume; Kreimeyer, Crooke, Drye, Egbert, & Klein, 2000). One has to be concerned, however, about whether the relevant research simply has not been done or has been done but has not yielded positive results and thus has not been published. If parents, schools, and school systems are going to be asked to embrace bilingual education for DHH students, they need to be provided with evidence of its effectiveness.

## WHERE DO WE GO FROM HERE?

It has been somewhat disconcerting to find that the literature relating to bilingualism, bilingual deaf education, and bilingual-bicultural deaf education is not to be as comprehensive or conclusive as we had expected—and others claim. A number of studies cited earlier compared deaf students who have deaf parents to those who have hearing parents but not to hearing students or hearing norms. On the basis of studies from Sweden (e.g., Rydberg et al., 2009), we need to know whether observed benefits in these domains are incremental or demonstrate the closing of the achievement gap between DHH students and their hearing peers. Older studies frequently found academic advantages for deaf children of deaf parents over their peers with hearing parents, but the differences were small, and the achievement of those students rarely matched that of hearing age-mates.

More recent studies have demonstrated positive relations between sign language skills and literacy (although not other areas of academic achievement), but have failed to distinguish the benefits of early sign language from the benefits of early language. Nevertheless, sign language is easier/earlier acquired than spoken language by at least some deaf children, and thus is available earlier to facilitate the acquisition of further linguistic and cognitive skills necessary for learning. Sign language also may be facilitative for those DHH students who do not have receptive and expressive spoken language skills, or sufficient skills, to fully support their learning in formal and informal settings. Findings suggesting that sign language can benefit both language development (Connor et al., 2000; Tomblin et al., 1999) and academic outcomes (Convertino et al., 2009; Spencer et al., 2004), even for deaf students with cochlear implants, would suggest that the potential academic benefits of sign language or at least signed communication for specific subgroups of DHH students are in need of further investigation. Similarly, it is important to discover what elements of co-enrollment programming are leading to the observed positive outcomes (e.g., Tang, Lam, & Yiu, Chapter 13 of this volume; Hermans, De Klerk, Wauters, & Knoors, Chapter 16 of this volume).

Even if bilingual education is not the best approach to educating all DHH students, it remains an alternative among the broader array of academic approaches to deaf education (Knoors & Marschark, 2012; Lange et al., 2013). Yet the lack of empirical support for bilingual deaf education (let alone bilingual-bicultural deaf education) makes it difficult to argue for the expansion of explicit bilingual education programming for DHH students in any particular form. One likely reason for the lack of strong support for bilingual deaf education—or any other aspect or method of deaf education—is simply the complexity of the issue. DHH students vary more widely than hearing age-mates for a variety of reasons that both contribute to and reflect qualitative and quantitative differences in learning (see Knoors & Marschark, 2014, Chapter 2). Differences between DHH and hearing students as well as among DHH students, particularly with regard to language and cognitive development, make studies of their academic achievement more difficult than they might appear. Earlier we noted the importance of factors such as parental involvement and language ability, but cognitive functioning, early intervention, teacher/instruction variables, and social-emotional functioning also are important for learning and achievement. These differ to some extent between DHH and hearing students and vary more widely among DHH students than hearing students. Not only does this make empirical research difficult, but it means that there is not going to be a single educational method or approach that is optimal for all DHH students. If there is one thing that we have learned from the one-size-fits-all spoken language approach to deaf education it is, as Knoors and Marschark (2014) suggested, "one-size-fits-none."

If the *who, what, when, where,* and *why* of bilingual deaf education remain to be fully elaborated, the necessary directions for future research are fairly clear. Most obvious perhaps are the *who* (which DHH students?) and *when* (at what age?) questions. Both of these, however, will very much depend on the *what* question that concerns which elements of bilingual education (or co-enrollment) beyond bilingualism per se will be most important for DHH students' academic growth. As we indicated earlier, this requires a distinction between bilingualism and bilingual deaf education. There is no doubt that virtually all DHH students will benefit from and need fluency in the written vernacular. The accumulated research evidence also suggests that signed communication will benefit some of those students in some respects (e.g., academic, linguistic, social), but the relative value of natural sign languages versus simultaneous communication (or sign-supported speech) has not been explored.

The relationship between bilingualism at home and bilingualism in school also is in need of investigation. Research into cued speech has shown that its facilitation of print literacy skills among deaf children learning languages such as French and Spanish depend on its use both in school and at home (Leybaert & Charlier, 1996). The difficulties for hearing parents in supporting the sign language needs of DHH students have been broadly discussed, but the likely challenges for many deaf parents to support the written (if not spoken) language needs of their DHH children remains to be investigated. Not unrelated to this issue are the potential benefits of educational programming that is explicitly bicultural. As far as we have been able to determine, the impact of the bicultural part of bilingual-bicultural deaf education on academic, social-emotional, and personal effects have not been explored. The reasons for this are unclear, but they may lie in the not unreasonable assumption that DHH children will benefit from an awareness of their culture and community. Many DHH children, however, will grow up outside that culture and community, and it seems important to determine the extent to which earlier versus later (or no) discovery of a Deaf identity influences individual functioning in various domains. It therefore would be worthwhile to examine ways in which hearing as well as deaf parents support deaf children's acquisition of a Deaf identity and affiliation with the Deaf community and how this is related to the children's educational programming and outcomes.

Another large area of inquiry would involve bidirectional relations of cognitive development/functioning and bilingualism-bilingual education among DHH students. Research has demonstrated that some cognitive differences observed between DHH and hearing individuals that previously were thought to be related to hearing status more recently have been found to have their origins in sign language ability and use (e.g., working memory, face recognition) or in factors totally unrelated to language and hearing status (e.g., sensitivity of peripheral vision; see Marschark & Knoors, 2012, for a review). Differences in memory, problem solving, and other cognitive domains as a function of an individual's preferred language modality have been examined in a number of studies, but their impact on academic achievement has not. To this point, it does not appear that many educators or investigators have explored DHH students' presumed cognitive strengths related to language modality. For example, although some tentative relations between visual-spatial processing and mathematics performance have been documented (e.g., Blatto-Vallee, Kelly, Gaustad, Porter, & Fonzi, 2007; Marschark, Morrison, Lukomski, Borgna, & Convertino, 2013), the potential of that ability as an academic intervention has not been examined. Similarly, DHH students who rely primarily on spoken language have been found to have better sequential memory (e.g., Lichtenstein, 1998), but its potential use in the classroom apparently is unexplored.

While not exhaustive, the preceding examples indicate both the complexity and the potential value of further and broader investigations of bilingual deaf education and of bilingualism among DHH students. Whatever the reasons that such investigations have not been undertaken (or reported) previously, the practical as well as the theoretical implications of such studies are of sufficient importance that they should be driving research agendas both in places where bilingual deaf education is easily available and places where it is less frequent. The extent to which it will be found to benefit particular DHH students with particular backgrounds in particular settings remains to be determined.

Without such research, however, there is no way to know how quickly or slowly bilingual deaf education should move forward, if at all.

## NOTE

1 Whether sign language and written language in the absence of spoken language are truly "bimodal" is an interesting question. Here we will adopt the usage common in the field and will refer to the use of both the signed vernacular and the spoken/written vernacular (with or without spoken language) as bimodal bilingualism.

## REFERENCES

Albertini, J. & Mayer, C. (2011). Using miscue analysis to assess comprehension in deaf college readers. *Journal of Deaf Studies and Deaf Education*, 16, 35–46.

Andrews, J. F. (1988). Deaf children's acquisition of prereading skills using the reciprocal teaching procedure. *Exceptional Children*, 54, 349–355.

Andrews, J. F., Ferguson, C., Hodges, P., & Roberts, S. (1997). What's Up, Billy Jo? Deaf children and bilingual-bicultural instruction in East-Central Texas. *American Annals of the Deaf*, 142, 16–25.

Bagga-Gupta, S. (2004). Literacies and deaf education: A theoretical analysis of the international and Swedish literature. Stockholm: The Swedish National Agency for School Improvement.

Banner, A. & Wang, Y. (2011). An analysis of the reading strategies used by adult and student deaf readers. *Journal of Deaf Studies and Deaf Education*, 16, 2–23

Barik, H. C., & Swain, M. (1975). Three-year evaluation of a language scale early grade French immersion program: The Ottawa study. *Language Learning*, 25, 1–30.

Bialystok, E. (1999). Cognitive complexity and attentional control in the bilingual mind. *Child Development*, 70, 636–644.

Bialystok, E., & Craik, F. I. M. (2010). Cognitive and linguistic processing in the bilingual mind. *Current Directions in Psychological Science*, 19, 19–23.

Bialystok, E., Craik, F. I. M., Green, D. W., & Gollan, T. H. (2009). Bilingual minds. *Psychological Science in the Public Interest*, 10, 89–129.

Blackorby, J., & Knokey, A.-M. (2006, November). A national profile of students with hearing impairments in elementary and middle school: A special topic report from the Special Education Elementary Longitudinal Study. Menlo Park, CA: SRI International.

Blatto-Vallee, G., Kelly, R., Gaustad, M., Porter, J., & Fonzi, J. (2007). Visual-spatial representation in mathematical problem solving by deaf and hearing students. *Journal of Deaf Studies and Deaf Education*, 12, 432–448.

Blom, H. C., & Marschark, M. (2014). Simultaneous communication, cochlear implants, and classroom learning. Manuscript submitted for publication.

Borgna, G., Convertino, C., Marschark, M., Morrison, C., & Rizzolo, K. (2011). Enhancing deaf students' learning from sign language and text: Metacognition, modality, and the effectiveness of content scaffolding. *Journal of Deaf Studies and Deaf Education*, 16, 79–100.

Brasel, K. & Quigley, S. P. (1977). Influence of certain language and communicative environments in early childhood on the development of language in deaf individuals. *Journal of Speech and Hearing Research*, 20, 95–107.

Caccamise, F., Blaisdell, R., & Meath-Lang, B. (1977). Hearing impaired persons' simultaneous reception of information under live and two visual motion media conditions. *American Annals of the Deaf, 122,* 339–343.

Capirci, O., Cattani, A., Rossini, P., & Volterra, V. (1998). Teaching sign language to hearing children as a possible factor in cognitive enhancement. *Journal of Deaf Studies and Deaf Education, 3,* 135–142.

Carlson, S. M., & Meltzoff, A. N. (2008). Bilingual experience and executive functioning in young children. *Developmental Science, 11,* 282–298

Chamberlain, C., Morford, J. P., & Mayberry, R. I. (Eds.) (2000). *Language acquisition by eye.* Mahwah, NJ: Lawrence Erlbaum Associates.

Cokely, D. (1990). The effectiveness of three means of communication in the college classroom. *Sign Language Studies, 69,* 415–439.

Connor, C., Hieber, S., Arts, A., & Zwolan, T. (2000). Speech, vocabulary, and the education of children using cochlear implants: Oral or total communication? *Journal of Speech, Language, and Hearing Research, 43,* 1185–1204.

Convertino, C. M., Marschark, M., Sapere, P., Sarchet, T., & Zupan, M. (2009). Predicting academic success among deaf college students. *Journal of Deaf Studies and Deaf Education, 14,* 324–343.

Cummins, J. (1984). *Bilingualism and special education: Issues in assessment and pedagogy.* Clevedon, UK: Multilingual Matters.

Cummins, J. (1991). Interdependence of first- and second-language proficiency in bilingual children. In E. Bialystok (Ed.), *Language processing in bilingual children* (pp. 70–89). Cambridge, UK: Cambridge University Press.

Dammeyer, J. (2010). Psychosocial development in a Danish population of children with cochlear implants and deaf and hard-of-hearing children. *Journal of Deaf Studies and Deaf Education, 15,* 50–58.

Diaz, R. M. (1985). The intellectual power of bilingualism. *Quarterly Newsletter of the Laboratory of Comparative Human Cognition, 7,* 16–22.

Emmorey, K., Borinstein, H. B., Thompson, R., Gollan, T. H. (2008). Bimodal bilingualism. *Bilingualism: Language and Cognition, 11,* 43–61.

Emmorey, K., Luk, G., Pyers, J. E., & Bialystok, E. (2008). The source of enhanced cognitive control in bilinguals. *Psychological Science, 19,* 1201–1206.

García, E. E., & Náñez, J. E., Sr. (2011). *Bilingualism and cognition: Informing research, pedagogy, and policy.* Washington, DC: American Psychological Association.

Geers, A., Tobey, E., Moog, J., & Brenner, C. (2008). Long-term outcomes of cochlear implantation in the preschool years: From elementary grades to high school. *International Journal of Audiology, 47*(Supplement 2), S21–S30.

Goldin-Meadow, S., & Mayberry, R. I. (2001). How do profoundly deaf children learn to read? *Learning Disabilities Research & Practice, 16,* 222–229.

Gregory, S. (1986). Bilingualism and the education of deaf children. In *Proceedings of the conference on Bilingualism and the Education of Deaf Children: Advances in Practice* (pp. 18–30). Leeds, UK: University of Leeds.

Habets, B., Kita, S., Shao, Z., Özyürek, A. & Hagoort, P. (2011). The role of synchronicity and ambiguity in speech-gesture integration during comprehension. *Journal of Cognitive Neuroscience, 23,* 1845–1854.

Harrington, F. (2000). Sign language interpreters and access for deaf students to university curricula: The ideal and the reality. In R. P. Roberts, S. E. Carr, D.

Abraham, & A. Dufour (Eds.), *The critical link 2: Interpreters in the community*. Amsterdam, Netherlands: John Benjamins Publishing.

Hauser, P. C., Lukomski, J., & Hillman, T. (2008). Development of deaf and hard-of-hearing students' executive function. In M. Marschark & P. C. Hauser (Eds.), *Deaf cognition: Foundations and outcomes* (pp. 286–308). New York, NY: Oxford University Press.

Heiling, K (1997). Döva barns språkliga situation [Deaf children's language situation]. In R. Söderberg (Ed.), *Från joller till läsning och skrivning* (pp. 199–211). Malmö, Sweden: Gleerups.

Heiling, K. (1998). Bilingual vs. oral education. In A. Weisel (Ed.), *Issues unresolved: New perspectives on language and deaf education* (pp. 141–147). Washington, DC: Gallaudet University Press.

Hendar, O. (2009). *Goal fulfillment in school for the deaf and hearing impaired*. Härnösand, Sweden: The National Agency for Special Needs Education and Schools.

Hendar, O. (2012). Elever med hørselshemming i skolen: En kartleggingsundersøkelse om læringsutbytte. [Pupils with hearing impairment in school: A study on learning outcomes]. (Skådalen Publication series No 32). Oslo, Norway: The Research and Development Unit, Skådalen Resource Centre.

Hermans, D., Knoors, H., Ormel, E., & Verhoeven, L. (2008). The relationship between the reading and signing skills of deaf children in bilingual education programs. *Journal of Deaf Studies and Deaf Education, 13*, 518–530.

Hermans, D., Ormel, E., & Knoors, H. (2010). On the relation between the signing and reading skills of deaf bilinguals. *International Journal of Bilingual Education and Bilingualism, 13*, 187–199.

Humphries, T., Kushalnagar, P., Mathur, G., Napoli, D. J., Padden, C., Rathmann, C., & Smith, C. R. (2012). Language acquisition for deaf children: Reducing the harms of zero tolerance to the use of alternative approaches. *Harm Reduction Journal, 9*, 16.

Hyde, M. B., & Power, D. J. (1992). The receptive communication abilities of deaf students under oral, manual and combined methods. *American Annals of the Deaf, 137*, 389–398.

Jensema, C. J., & Trybus, R. J. (1978). *Communication patterns and educational achievement of hearing impaired students*. Washington, DC: Office of Demographic Studies, Gallaudet College.

Johnson, R. E., & Erting, C. (1989). Ethnicity and socialization in a classroom for deaf children. In C. Lucas (Ed.), *The sociolinguistics of the deaf community* (pp. 41–83). New York, NY: Academic Press.

Johnson, R., Liddell, S., & Erting, C. (1989). *Unlocking the curriculum: Principles for achieving access in deaf education*. Gallaudet Research Institute Working Paper 89-3. Washington, DC: Gallaudet University.

Johnston, T., Leigh, G., & Foreman, P. (2002). The implementation of the principles of sign bilingualism in a self-described sign bilingual program: Implications for the evaluation of language outcomes. *Australian Journal of Education of the Deaf, 8*, 38–46.

Kelly, R. R., Albertini, J. A., & Shannon, N. B. (2001). Deaf college students' reading comprehension and strategy use. *American Annals of the Deaf, 146*, 385–400.

Kelly, S. D., Özyürek, A., & Maris, E. (2010). Two sides of the same coin: Speech and gesture mutually interact to enhance comprehension. *Psychological Science, 21,* 260–267.

Knoors, H., & Marschark, M. (2012). Language planning for the 21st century: Revisiting bilingual language policy for deaf children. *Journal of Deaf Studies and Deaf Education, 17,* 291–305.

Knoors, H., & Marschark, M. (2014). *Teaching deaf learners: Psychological and developmental foundations.* New York, NY: Oxford University Press.

Kovács, Á. M., & Mehler, J. (2009). Cognitive gains in 7-month-old bilingual infants. *Proceedings of the National Academy of Sciences of the United States of America, 106,* 6556–6560.

Kreimeyer, K. H., Crooke, P., Drye, C., Egbert, V., & Klein, B. (2000). Academic and social benefits of a co-enrollment model of inclusive education for deaf and hard-of-hearing children. *Journal of Deaf Studies and Deaf Education, 5,* 174–185.

Lambert, W. E. (1977). The effects of bilingualism on the individual: Cognitive and sociocultural consequences. In P. Hornby (Ed.), *Bilingualism: Psychological, social, and educational implications* (pp. 15–27). New York, NY: Academic Press.

Lang, H. G. (2002). Higher education for deaf students: Research priorities in the new millennium. *Journal of Deaf Studies and Deaf Education, 7,* 267–280.

Lange, C. M., Lane-Outlaw, S., Lange, W. E., & Sherwood, D. L. (2013). American Sign Language/English bilingual model: A longitudinal study of academic growth. *Journal of Deaf Studies and Deaf Education, 18,* 532–544.

LaSasso, C., & Lollis, J. (2003). Survey of residential and day schools for deaf students in the United States that identify themselves as bilingual-bicultural programs. *Journal of Deaf Studies and Deaf Education, 8,* 79–91.

Lee, P. (1996). Cognitive development in bilingual children: A case for bilingual instruction in early childhood education. *The Bilingual Research Journal, 20,* 499–522.

Leeson, L., & Sheikh, H. (2010). *Experiencing deafhood: A snapshot of five nations.* Dublin, Ireland: Intersource Group Publishing.

Leigh, G., & Johnston, T. (2004). First language learning in a sign bilingual program: An Australian study. *NTID Research Bulletin, 9,* 1–5.

Leybaert, J., & Charlier, B. (1996). Visual speech in the head: The effect of cued-speech on rhyming, remembering, and spelling. *Journal of Deaf Studies and Deaf Education, 1,* 234–248.

Lichtenstein, E. (1998). The relationships between reading processes and English skills of deaf college students. *Journal of Deaf Studies and Deaf Education, 3,* 80–134.

Marschark, M. (1993). *Psychological development of deaf children.* New York, NY: Oxford University Press.

Marschark, M., & Hauser, P. C. (2012). *How deaf children learn.* New York, NY: Oxford University Press.

Marschark, M., & Knoors, H. (2012). Educating deaf children: Language, cognition, and learning. *Deafness and Education International, 14,* 137–161.

Marschark, M., Leigh, G., Sapere, P., Burnham, D., Convertino, C., Stinson, M., Knoors, H., Vervloed, M. P. J., & Noble, W. (2006). Benefits of sign language interpreting and text alternatives to classroom learning by deaf students. *Journal of Deaf Studies and Deaf Education, 11,* 421–437.

Marschark, M., Morrison, C., Lukomski, J., Borgna, G., & Convertino, C. (2013). Are deaf students visual learners? *Learning and Individual Differences, 25,* 156–162.

Marschark, M., Shaver, D., Nagle, K., & Newman, L. (2014). Predicting the academic achievement of deaf and hard-of-hearing students from individual, household, communication, and educational factors. Manuscript submitted for publication.

Marschark, M., Sapere, P., Convertino, C., Mayer, C., Wauters, L. & Sarchet, T. (2009). Are deaf students' reading challenges really about reading? *American Annals of the Deaf, 154,* 357–370.

Marschark, M., Sapere, P., Convertino, C., & Pelz, J. (2008). Learning via direct and mediated instruction by deaf students. *Journal of Deaf Studies and Deaf Education, 13,* 446–461.

Marschark, M., Sapere, P., Convertino, C., & Seewagen, R. (2005). Access to postsecondary education through sign language interpreting. *Journal of Deaf Studies and Deaf Education, 10,* 38–50.

Marschark, M., Sapere, P., Convertino, C., Seewagen, R. & Maltzan, H. (2004). Comprehension of sign language interpreting: Deciphering a complex task situation. *Sign Language Studies, 4,* 345–368.

Mayer, C., & Akamatsu, C. T. (1999). Bilingual-bicultural models of literacy education for deaf students: Considering the claims. *Journal of Deaf Studies and Deaf Education, 4,* 1–8.

Mayer, C., & Leigh, G. (2010). The changing context for sign bilingual education programs: Issues in language and the development of literacy. *International Journal of Bilingual Education and Bilingualism, 13,* 175–186.

Mollink, H., Hermans, D., & Knoors, H. (2008). Vocabulary training of spoken words in hard-of-hearing children. *Deafness and Education International, 10,* 80–92.

Moores, D., & Sweet, C. (1990). Relationships of English grammar and communicative fluency to reading in deaf adolescents. *Exceptionality, 1,* 97–106

Náñez, J. E., Padilla, R. V., & López-Máez, L. (1992). Bilinguality, intelligence, and cognitive information processing. In R. V. Padilla & A. H. Benavides (Eds.), *Critical perspectives on bilingual education research* (pp. 43–69). Tempe, AZ: Bilingual Press/Editorial Bilingüe.

Napier, J., & Barker, R. (2004). Access to university interpreting: Expectations and preferences of deaf students. *Journal of Deaf Studies and Deaf Education, 9,* 228–238.

National Center for Education Statistics (2003). National assessment of adult literacy. Retrieved March 8, 2013, from http://nces.ed.gov/NAAL.

Newell, W. (1978). A study of the ability of day-class deaf adolescents to compare factual information using four communication modalities. *American Annals of the Deaf, 123,* 558–562.

Nitrouer, S., Caldwell, A., Lowenstein, J., Tarr, E., & Holloman, C. (2012). Emergent literacy in kindergartners with cochlear implants. *Ear and Hearing, 33,* 683–697.

Nover, S., Andrews, J., Baker, S., Everhart, V., & Bradford, M. (2002). ASL/English bilingual instruction for deaf students: Evaluation and impact study. Final report 1997–2002. Retrieved April 2, 2013, from http://www.gallaudet.edu/Documents/year5.pdf.

Padden, C., & Humphries, T. (1988). *Deaf in America*. Cambridge, MA: Harvard University Press.

Padden, C., & Ramsey, C. (2000). American Sign Language and reading ability in deaf children. In C. Chamberlain, J. Morford, & R. Mayberry (Eds.), *Language acquisition by eye* (pp. 165–189). Mahwah, NJ: Lawrence Erlbaum.

Parault, S. J., & Williams, H. M. (2010). Reading motivation, reading amount, and text comprehension in deaf and hearing adults. *Journal of Deaf Studies and Deaf Education, 15*, 120–135.

Peal, E., & Lambert, W. (1962). The relation of bilingualism to intelligence. *Psychological Monographs, 76*, 1–23.

Perfetti, C., & Sandak, R. (2000). Reading optimally builds on spoken language. Implications for deaf readers. *Journal of Deaf Studies and Deaf Education, 5*, 32–50.

Pisoni, D. B., Conway, C. M., Kronenberger, W., Henning, S. & Anaya, E. (2010). Executive function, cognitive control and sequence learning in deaf children with cochlear implants. In M. Marschark & P. E. Spencer, *The Oxford handbook of deaf studies, language, and education* (vol. 2, pp. 439–457). New York, NY: Oxford University Press.

Qi, S., & Mitchell, R. E. (2012). Large-scaled academic achievement testing of deaf and hard-of-hearing students: Past, present, and future. *Journal of Deaf Studies and Deaf Education, 17*, 1–18.

Rydberg, E., Gellerstedt, L. C., & Danermark, B. (2009). Toward an equal level of educational attainment between deaf and hearing people in Sweden? *Journal of Deaf Studies and Deaf Education, 14*, 312–323.

Sapere, P., LaRock, D., Convertino, C., Gallimore, L., & Lessard, P. (2005). Interpreting and interpreter education: Adventures in Wonderland? In M. Marschark, R. Peterson, & E. Winston (Eds.), *Sign language interpreting and interpreter education: Directions for research and practice* (pp. 283–298). New York, NY: Oxford University Press.

Seal, B. C. (2004). *Best practices in educational interpreting* (2nd ed.). Boston: Allyn and Bacon.

Spencer, L. J., Gantz, B. J., & Knutson, J. F. (2004). Outcomes and achievement of students who grew up with access to cochlear implants. *Laryngoscope, 114*, 1576–1581.

Spencer, L. J., Barker, B. A., & Tomblin, J. B. (2003). Exploring the language and literacy outcomes of pediatric cochlear implant users. *Ear and Hearing, 24*, 236–247.

Spencer, L., & Tomblin, J. B. (2006). Speech production and spoken language development of children using "total communication." In P. E. Spencer & M. Marschark (Eds.), *Advances in the spoken language development of deaf and hard-of-hearing children* (pp. 166–192). New York, NY: Oxford University Press.

Spencer, P. E., Marschark, M., & Spencer, L. J. (2011). Cochlear implants: Advances, issues and implications. In M. Marschark & P. E. Spencer (Eds.), *The Oxford handbook of deaf studies, language, and education* (vol. 1, 2nd ed., pp. 452–471). New York, NY: Oxford University Press.

Stinson, M. S., Elliot, L. B., Kelly, R. R., & Liu, Y. (2009). Deaf and hard-of-hearing students' memory of lectures with speech-to-text and interpreting/note taking services. *Special Education, 43*, 45–51.

Stinson, M., Whitmire, K., & Kluwin, T. (1996). Self-perceptions of social relationships in hearing-impaired adolescents. *Journal of Educational Psychology, 88*, 132–143.

Strong, M., & Prinz, P. (1997). A study of the relationship between American Sign Language and English literacy. *Journal of Deaf Studies and Deaf Education, 2*, 37–46.

Stuckless, E. R., & Birch, J. W. (1966). The influence of early manual communication on the linguistic development of deaf children. *American Annals of the Deaf, 111*, 436–480.

Tomblin, J. B., Spencer, L., Flock, S., Tyler, R., & Gantz, B. (1999). A comparison of language achievement in children with cochlear implants and children with hearing aids. *Journal of Speech, Language, and Hearing Research, 42*, 497–511.

Vernon, M., & Koh, S. D. (1970). Effects of early manual communication on achievement of deaf children. *American Annals of the Deaf, 115*, 527–536.

Wauters, L., Knoors, H., Vervloed, M. P. J., & Aarnoutse, C. (2001). Sign facilitation in word recognition. *Journal of Special Education, 35*, 31–40.

Yoshinaga-Itano, C. (2006). Early identification, communication modality, and the development of speech and spoken language skills: Patterns and considerations. In P. Spencer & M. Marschark (Eds.), *Advances in the spoken language development of deaf and hard-of-hearing children* (pp. 298–327). New York, NY: Oxford University Press.

# 10

# Improving Reading Instruction to Deaf and Hard-of-Hearing Students

## Loes Wauters and Annet de Klerk

Reading is probably one of the areas most frequently mentioned as an obstacle for deaf students in their academic achievement. Even though many suggestions have been given from research on the exact sources of reading difficulties, we still do not seem to have found a way to teach all our students to be proficient, confident, and motivated readers.

Reading does not come naturally; it is a skill that one has to learn, or rather that one has to be taught. Most children acquire this skill in school. This means that their teachers need to know how to teach it. What do these teachers need to know about reading and reading instruction in order to effectively teach their students to read? And how can we help teachers incorporate this knowledge in their teaching behavior? These issues will be the focus of this chapter. We will discuss information about reading performance in deaf and hard-of-hearing (DHH) students and factors related to that performance that are relevant to teachers of the deaf. Additionally, an overview of strategies in reading instruction that have been found to be effective in teaching reading to deaf children will be given. Finally, we will provide an example of how we can get teachers to incorporate this knowledge in their teaching behavior in the (reading) classroom.

### THE ISSUE OF READING IN DEAF AND HARD-OF-HEARING STUDENTS IN BILINGUAL EDUCATION

It has often been stated that reading is a challenge for DHH students. The most recent large-scale study on reading achievement in the United States showed that DHH students lag behind their hearing peers, with a median level of reading achievement among DHH 18-year-olds equivalent to that of 9-year-old hearing students (grade 4; Traxler, 2000). This level of achievement had not significantly improved since the first nationwide assessment in 1969 (Qi & Mitchell, 2012). Studies in other countries (United Kingdom, Australia, and the Netherlands) found similar or even lower levels of reading achievement (Conrad, 1979;

Power, 1985, in Power & Leigh, 2000; Wauters, Van Bon, & Tellings, 2006). Even though results on the level of word reading vary, studies on reading comprehension are rather consistent in their findings.

For at least some of the DHH students in bilingual education settings, learning to read coincides with learning the language that they are reading in, and maybe even with learning their first language, sign language (Hermans, Knoors, Ormel, & Verhoeven, 2008a; Hoffmeister, 2000; Marschark & Harris, 1996). Learning to read in a second language is a challenge in itself, but even more so when the learner has little access to the spoken form of that second language that is the basis of the writing system he must learn to tackle. We do not know how deaf readers make the connection between the languages they encounter (Easterbrooks & Beal-Alvarez, 2013). Mayer and Akamatsu (1999) pointed out that there is no evidence that the oral ability in one (first) language facilitates the ability to read and write in another (second) language. If this is the case, Mayer and Akamatsu wondered, why would we expect to see a link between the ability to sign and the ability to read and write English (or any other language)? However, there have been several studies that have shown such a relationship (Chamberlain & Mayberry, 2000, 2008; Hermans, Knoors, Ormel, & Verhoeven, 2008b; Niederberger, 2008; Ormel, Hermans, Knoors, & Verhoeven, 2009; Padden & Ramsey, 1998; Strong & Prinz, 1997). The exact nature of the relation between sign language and written language is unclear, but there seems to be some kind of transfer that can be beneficial for reading development.

The role of spoken language ability should not be underestimated, though. Niederberger (2008), for example, found that children with stronger skills in written language had strong linguistic skills in either sign or spoken language or in both languages (see also Chamberlain & Mayberry, 2000; Harris & Beech, 1998). Furthermore, spoken language and sign language skills have been found to correlate, for example when it comes to receptive vocabulary (Ormel, 2008). Hermans, Ormel, and Knoors (2010) found a significant correlation between sign language and spoken language skills in expressive vocabulary and morphosyntax. This correlation was only found in the older children (5 years and 7 months–8 years and 10 months) and not in the younger children (4 years and 1 month–5 years and 6 months). This led them to introduce the term "cultivated transfer" for the positive effects of practices in bilingual education in which teachers explicitly link the two languages. By explicitly linking signs and words, children's knowledge of sign language is exploited in order for teachers to teach them new vocabulary in the spoken (or written) language. Hermans and colleagues (2008a) suggested that these cultivated associations between the two languages are very valuable in the acquisition of (reading) vocabulary through direct instruction, but that good spoken language skills seem necessary for children to derive word meanings during independent reading. In the end, even though sign language and written language seem to be correlated, deaf children must learn to decode the written representation of the spoken language for which knowledge of that spoken language is beneficial (Mayer, 2007, 2009; Perfetti & Sandak, 2000). Hermans et al. (2008a, 2010) stated that the two languages can work together in reading acquisition. Deaf children are able to rely on their sign language skills to learn the meaning of written words, but eventually they will have to acquire the syntactic and morphological specifications of written words, for which they will need the spoken language.

Universal newborn hearing screening (UNHS) and cochlear implants (CIs) seem to provide the opportunity to better develop spoken language skills, but reading delays have not completely disappeared (Geers, Tobey, Moog, & Brenner, 2008; Harris & Terletski, 2011; Marschark, Rhoten, & Fabich, 2007; Vermeulen et al., 2007). Geers and colleagues (2008) found that the promising reading scores of deaf children with a cochlear implant in elementary schools (Geers & Brenner, 2003) were not completely reflected in the reading scores of the same group in adolescence. As a group, these deaf children did not keep up with their hearing peers, indicating an increase in the reading gap between deaf and hearing students. However, 20% of the children did improve their reading performance relative to their hearing peers.

Harris and Terletski (2011) studied reading in three groups of deaf adolescents (12 to 16 years): 30 early implanted children (< 42 months), 29 late implanted children (> 42 months), and 27 children with hearing aids. Their results showed reading delays in all three groups, again with high variability within the groups. However, differences between the groups were found, with the smallest reading delay (of 2 years) for the group with hearing aids and the largest delay for the early implanted CI group. Of the hearing aid (HA) group, 48% were classified as good readers, compared to 19% of the CI group. The authors concluded that 12- to 16-year-old children with cochlear implants did not read better than their peers with hearing aids. Rather, children with hearing aids read significantly better than early implanted children. However, a significant relation was found with educational setting. Forty-six percent of the children in mainstream settings were good readers, 31% of children in deaf education, and only 6% of children in special units at mainstream schools. Differences between these settings were not statistically tested, but it is interesting to see that children with hearing aids, who were the best readers in this study, were not in mainstream settings (mainstream: 0 HA, 6 late CI, 7 early CI; deaf education: 25 HA, 18 late CI, 12 early CI; special units: 2 HA, 6 late CI, 10 early CI). Also, only a small proportion of the students in special units at mainstream schools were good readers. Harris and Terletski (2011) suggested that schools for the deaf provide specific support for these children to develop their literacy skills.

We can conclude from these studies that even with UNHS and early cochlear implantation the reading gap between deaf and hearing children has not (yet) been closed. Early implanted children seem to make a good start that holds promise for good reading development, but later reading success is not guaranteed. This means that teachers need to monitor the reading development of their students and to continue reading instruction even into adolescence. What do these teachers need to know to support their students' reading development?

## COGNITIVE FACTORS IN DEAF STUDENTS' LEARNING

As noted earlier, reading does not come naturally, especially for DHH children, for whom the language in which they have to read is not fully accessible. However, as Marschark and colleagues (2009) asked: Are deaf students' reading challenges really about reading? What other factors influence deaf students' reading performance? Marschark and colleagues found that deaf students' challenges in reading comprehension are often also reflected in their comprehension of sign language, indicating that there may be more to reading than reading itself. Marschark and Wauters (2008) argued that differences between deaf and hearing students in knowledge, knowledge organization, and cognitive functioning may influence learning. Teachers need to be aware of these differences; deaf children are not simply hearing children who cannot hear. Marschark, Spencer, Adams, and Sapere (2011a, 2011b) discussed differences between deaf and hearing students in the following areas: knowledge and knowledge organization, integration of information and learning, metacognition, memory, and executive function. This section will briefly summarize these differences, as they may be involved in deaf students' learning and thus may influence their reading performance.

### Knowledge and Knowledge Organization

Deaf students are known to have less rich vocabularies and conceptual knowledge than hearing students and, partly because of that, they have a harder time acquiring new word meanings (Easterbrooks & Beal-Alvarez, 2013; Lederberg & Beal-Alvarez, 2011). Differences in semantic knowledge are not only found at the exemplar level, but also at the superordinate level of semantic categorization (Marschark, Convertino, McEvoy, & Masteller, 2004; Ormel, 2008). These differences in knowledge and knowledge organization may influence how deaf readers connect new information to their prior knowledge (Marschark et al., 2011a, 2011b). This means that teachers must provide explicit information and must help students to tie new information to their existing knowledge.

### Integration of Information and Learning

Related to knowledge organization is the integration of information, especially when it comes to reading. Integrating different parts of text or tying new information to prior knowledge is one of the key aspects of reading, also referred to as the ability to make inferences. Skilled readers use their general knowledge to comprehend text and to make inferences. This has been found to be difficult for deaf students, in reading as well as in processing sign language (see Marschark & Wauters, 2008, for an overview). Implications for instruction are that rich contexts have to be provided, prior knowledge has to be activated before reading, and students need to be guided in tying new information to what they already know.

### Metacognition

In order to realize that she does not understand, a reader needs to be able to monitor her own reading processes. Self-monitoring is an important aspect of reading and is found to differ in skilled and less skilled readers. Unskilled readers are less likely to apply monitoring strategies, such as using background information or contextual clues and rereading or looking back in the text, and they often lack the metacognition to realize that they do not understand what they are reading (Mokhtari & Reichard, 2002). The same seems to hold for deaf students (Marschark, Lang, & Albertini, 2002; Strassman, 1997). Strassman suggested that the reading materials used in teaching reading to deaf students are not challenging enough to elicit metacognitive strategies. Teachers should be aware that deaf students are less likely to monitor their own reading process and should explicitly teach them metacognitive strategies and guide them in applying these strategies. We will further discuss this issue in the section on effective reading instruction.

### Memory

Several studies have shown shorter verbal memory spans for deaf than for hearing students (Marschark et al., 2011a, 2011b), indicating that remembering items in a specific order is a challenge for deaf students. More recent studies (Bavelier et al., 2008; Boutla, Supalla, Newport, & Bavelier, 2004; Hall & Bavelier, 2010), however, pointed out that deaf signers have better visuospatial memory. Hall and Bavelier (2010) suggested that these differences in memory are not about deficient performance but about different utilization of the components of (working) memory. Teachers need to know that visuospatial presentation of information may be more effective than sequential presentation, and that it is helpful to practice memory strategies with deaf students (Marschark et al., 2011a, 2011b).

### Executive Function

Executive function (EF) refers to the control system of cognitive processes, such as planning and organizing, working memory, controlling and shifting attention, and inhibition. EF in DHH students is a rather new research topic, and at this point it is not clear how this function develops in DHH children. Much more research is needed in this field, but it is important for teachers to know that EF is a strong predictor of school achievement and that this may have implications for their classroom practice. Difficulties in controlling and shifting attention, for example, would affect the way that teachers need to guide children's attention toward the instruction targets in order to secure full access to instruction (Marschark et al., 2011a, 2011b). DHH students need to get the opportunity to develop these skills, instead of always receiving directions and help in solving tasks (Marschark & Knoors, 2012).

### Implications for Reading Instruction

What should teachers of the deaf take from research on cognitive factors when it comes to reading instruction? Based on research, it seems important to provide explicit information in rich contexts and help students to tie new information to their existing knowledge. Teaching students how to apply metacognitive strategies, such as activating prior knowledge before reading, helps them in tackling reading materials. Teachers should realize that students may have difficulties in planning, organizing, memory, controlling attention, and inhibition (executive functioning), which may influence their (reading) behavior. Also, DHH students often do not apply their knowledge to new tasks (Marschark & Knoors, 2012).

## QUALITY OF INSTRUCTION

So, if teachers provide explicit information in rich contexts, teach metacognitive strategies, and take students' executive functioning into account, would we have proficient deaf readers? No, that would probably not be the case, because there is more to teaching reading than promoting cognitive functioning. Studies on factors predicting academic achievement state that only about 25% of the variance can be explained by student characteristics, parental support, and school placement (Powers, 1999; Stinson & Kluwin, 2011). Stinson and Kluwin suggest that the remaining 75% of the unexplained variance may lie in instructional factors or even the quality of instruction. This factor has received some research attention in the last decade (Hermans, Wauters, De Klerk, & Knoors, Chapter 11 of this volume; Marschark,

Sapere, Convertino, & Pelz, 2008; Marschark, Richardson, Sapere, & Sarchet, 2010). Marschark and colleagues (2008) found that deaf college students can learn as much from a lecture as hearing students when taught by an excellent teacher with experience and skills in teaching deaf students. These teachers seem to adjust their instructional methods to the strengths and needs of deaf students (Marschark et al., 2010). Marschark et al. (2008) pointed out that their findings do not provide any indication on how to educate or support teachers in adjusting their teaching to accommodate deaf students. It is unclear which factors led the teachers in their study to provide effective instruction.

Teachers specialized in deaf education may adjust their instruction in a different way from mainstream teachers (Marschark et al., 2008). In their discussion of the relation between reading and educational setting, Harris and Terletski (2011) also wondered whether "the supportive environment of a school for the deaf provides a better setting for the continuing development of literacy skills" (p. 32). Could the factor of quality of instruction, proposed by Stinson and Kluwin (2011), play a role here? The results of these studies emphasize the need to study how we can provide effective (reading) instruction in the classroom.

## Effective Reading Instruction to Deaf Children

If quality of instruction does indeed play such an important role in academic performance of our students, teachers do not only need to know about reading performance and factors that may influence this performance, but they also need to have knowledge about instructional strategies to teach reading. This section will give an overview of what we know from research about effective reading instruction to DHH students.

Luckner and colleagues (2005) published a review on evidence-based literacy research in deaf education, where they found only 22 studies of literacy and deafness that met the criteria for inclusion in their review, such as inclusion of a control group in the research design. One of the main conclusions of this review was that there is no strong evidence of the effectiveness of reading instruction practices in deaf education. Similar results were found in reviews on specific dimensions of reading, such as vocabulary (Luckner & Cooke, 2010), reading fluency (Luckner & Urbach, 2012), and reading comprehension (Luckner & Handley, 2008). Spencer and Marschark (2010) also stated that "practice in education of deaf and hard-of-hearing students has been based more closely on beliefs and attitudes than on documented evidence from research or the outcomes of interventions" (p. 25). In order to provide evidence-based reading instruction in the classroom, we need to know which practices have been found to be successful. Therefore, we will first discuss what we know about reading instruction to deaf children. We will focus on the five key factors in reading, as discussed by

Easterbrooks and Beal-Alvarez (2013) in their recent book on literacy instruction for DHH students: phonemic awareness, alphabetics (phonics, letter knowledge, and phonological awareness), fluency, vocabulary, and text comprehension. These factors were also incorporated in the work of Schirmer and McGough (2005). We will draw from the work of these authors in our discussion below.

*Phonemic Awareness Instruction and Alphabetics*

Phonemic awareness is the awareness that spoken words are composed of sounds (phonemes) and that these sounds can be manipulated. This awareness supports the alphabetic principle, which is the knowledge that letters (graphemes) correspond to the sounds (phonemes). Even though the research on intervention and instruction of phonemic awareness and alphabetics to deaf readers is too limited to draw any conclusions (Schirmer & McGough, 2005), the importance of explicit instruction in these areas seems rock solid. Also, the potentials of including signs, fingerspellng, and print in this instruction have been studied, and several studies have focused on the promises of Visual Phonics, which will be discussed later.

Miller, Lederberg, and Easterbrooks (2013) studied the viability of explicit instruction in phonological awareness for five deaf children with functional hearing in kindergarten. They examined the effects of phonological awareness instruction, consisting of syllable segmentation, initial phoneme isolation, and rhyme recognition, that was embedded in the emergent literacy intervention Foundations for Literacy (Lederberg, Miller, Easterbrooks, & Connor, 2011), developed for DHH children. Results showed that explicit phonological awareness instruction was effective for these five children with functional hearing.

Apart from this study on phonological awareness instruction, there have been several studies on the use of Visual Phonics (VP), a system of 45 hand and symbol cues that represent the phonemes of spoken English, as a supplement to literacy instruction in deaf education (Beal-Alvarez, Lederberg, & Easterbrooks, 2011; Narr, 2008; Smith & Wang, 2010; Trezek & Malmgren, 2005; Trezek & Wang, 2006; Trezek et al., 2007). These studies have all found significant correlations between the integration of VP into the existing phonics-based reading curriculum and phonological awareness and decoding. Trezek and Wang (2006) studied improvement in word reading and reading comprehension in deaf children in kindergarten and first grade after a year of phonics-based reading instruction supplemented by VP. Both word reading and reading comprehension skills improved. Trezek and colleagues (2007) found similar positive outcomes on phonemic awareness (phoneme segmentation, phoneme deletion, onset and rhyme, and spelling) in a different study where VP was used as a supplement to a different phonics-based reading curriculum.

Narr and Cawthon (2011) studied the experiences of teachers with Visual Phonics. Teachers reported using VP mostly with elementary-age students and mainly for the purpose of phonics instruction and in addition for spelling, phonemic awareness, vocabulary, and articulation. They claimed that VP is easy to use, easy to implement in the existing curriculum, and that it engages students. Teachers felt that the use of VP improved students' phonemic awareness, decoding skills, and to a lesser extent vocabulary and reading comprehension.

In addition to the work on Visual Phonics, Schirmer and McGough (2005) mentioned that previous research showed that deaf readers can learn to recognize words automatically and that young readers may benefit by matching written words with signs or sign print (i.e., graphic representation of the sign, or sign language picture, above each English word), or both. Padden and Ramsey (1998) suggested that the relation between signs, fingerspelling, and print should be embedded in the instruction of word reading by using the techniques of chaining and sandwiching. Andrews (1988; see also Andrews & Mason, 1986) also found that linking print to signs had a positive effect on letter knowledge, vocabulary, and word recognition. Wauters, Knoors, Vervloed, and Aarnoutse (2001) studied the effect of inclusion of signs in training word recognition. They found that 6- to 10-year-old deaf children showed a greater increase in word recognition when words were trained with a combination of spoken words and signs than when they were trained with spoken words only.

*Fluency Instruction*

Fluency is seen as an essential skill in reading development that bridges word reading and text comprehension and can be defined as "the ability to read text quickly, accurately, and with proper expression" (National Reading Panel, 2000, pp. 3–5; Trezek, Wang, & Paul, 2010). Unfortunately, there have been only a few studies on fluency instruction, and even fewer on fluency instruction with deaf readers (Easterbrooks & Beal-Alvarez, 2013; Schirmer & McGough, 2005; Luckner & Urbach, 2012). These studies seem to indicate that independent oral reading and repeated reading are important components of fluency instruction. Schirmer, Therrien, Schaffer, and Schirmer (2009), for example, found a positive effect of rereading instruction on the fluency skills of four DHH children. In a follow-up study (Schirmer, Schaffer, Therrien, & Schirmer, 2012), they added a comprehension monitoring strategy to rereading instruction through the Re-Read-Adapt and Answer-Comprehend (RAAC) intervention. Again, they found a significant improvement in reading fluency. Comprehension improved during the intervention, but it did not generalize to a standardized passage comprehension test.

For deaf children whose primary mode of communication is sign language, reading fluency does not involve oral reading but involves the rendering of printed text through signs. Easterbrooks and Huston (2008) introduced the Signed Reading Fluency Rubric for Deaf Children to assess the fluency when the output of reading is not spoken language but sign language. Signed reading fluency is the ability of the signer to render the printed text into a fluent signed format, containing those signed key elements that demonstrate that the reader has formed a mental visualization of the meaning of the text. Easterbrooks and Huston found a positive relation between students' signed reading fluency and their comprehension of reading passages, suggesting that fluency is important and independent of the modality of the output. The ability to fluently represent what is read in either spoken language or sign has a positive influence on the comprehension of the text. Easterbrooks and Beal-Alvarez (2013) suggest that the Signed Reading Fluency Rubric can also be used as a monitoring tool, because it shows at which points students are struggling and thus where teachers should focus their instruction.

Although no intervention studies have been done, training deaf children to use morphological information in reading seems a viable option to explore as well. Van Hoogmoed, Verhoeven, Schreuder, and Knoors (2011; see also Van Hoogmoed, Knoors, Schreuder, & Verhoeven, 2013) found that deaf children apply morphological information in reading but to a lesser extent than hearing children. Van Hoogmoed et al. (2011, 2013), Gaustad (2000), and Easterbrooks and Stephenson (2006) suggest that morphological processing needs more attention in reading instruction for deaf children. Unfortunately, there is no information yet on the effectiveness of the inclusion of morphological processing in reading instruction on the word reading and fluency skills of deaf children.

*Vocabulary Instruction*

To independently read and understand a text, 98% of the words in that text need to be known to the reader (Hu & Nation, 2000). This shows the importance of vocabulary in the reading process, not only for hearing but also for deaf readers (Kyle & Harris, 2006; 2010). Teachers spend a lot of their time on expanding children's vocabulary through talking with them, reading to them, and through explicit vocabulary instruction. The National Reading Panel (2000) created a taxonomy of vocabulary instruction with five major methods of vocabulary teaching: explicit instruction of word definitions; indirect or implicit instruction through extensive reading; use of multimedia methods; increasing vocabulary learning capacity through reading skills; and use of association methods. Research with deaf students showed positive effects of intensive daily programs, indirect instruction through extensive reading, and the use of computers in vocabulary instruction.

From their review on vocabulary instruction, Schirmer and McGough (2005) suggested that the indirect instruction of vocabulary through extensive reading, as studied by de Villiers and Pomerantz (1992, in Schirmer & McGough, 2005), could be a promising practice. In this instruction, children are supposed to infer word meanings through extensive reading opportunities. However, Schirmer and McGough noted that, given the reading difficulties of deaf children, it would be hard to find texts that are explicit enough for deaf readers to extract word meanings. Another way to provide indirect vocabulary instruction is through storybook reading, especially when storybook reading is an interactive reading process between adult and child, involving questions and dialogue about the story (Fung, Chow, & McBride-Chang, 2005).

In their review on vocabulary research between 1967 and 2008, Luckner and Cooke (2010) found only 10 intervention studies, almost all studying a different intervention. In the intervention studies, positive outcomes were found for the use of computers for vocabulary instruction, and for the integration of words in an intensive daily vocabulary program. All other positive results were descriptive only and should be studied more extensively in order to draw any conclusions about the effectiveness. The same seems true for the recent findings by Aceti and Wang (2010) who found positive results of metacognitively based instruction of multi-meaning words in four deaf, struggling readers (11–13 years old). In this metacognitively based instruction, five metacognitive strategies are incorporated in vocabulary instruction: making predictions, making a picture, relating the information to prior knowledge, self-monitoring through verbalizing confusing points, and self-correction.

Hermans and colleagues (2008a, 2008b, 2010) pointed to the significance of signs in vocabulary learning. Mollink, Hermans, and Knoors (2008) studied the influence of signs in supporting spoken vocabulary development in hard-of-hearing children (kindergarten and first grade). They found that children better remembered word meanings when they were trained using spoken Dutch and signs than when they were trained using spoken Dutch only.

*Text Comprehension Instruction*

Comprehension of what is being read is considered to be the ultimate goal of reading. In the process of achieving this goal, the reader needs to access prior knowledge and to apply reading strategies to monitor comprehension. In their review, Schirmer and McGough (2005) concluded from research on the activation of prior knowledge that building and activating prior knowledge enhances comprehension in deaf readers and that providing extensive information about the topic before reading is more effective than providing only brief information.

Luckner and Handley (2008) examined 27 intervention studies on reading comprehension and found a tentative evidence base for five reading comprehension teaching strategies: explicit comprehension strategy instruction; teaching students story grammar; modified directed-reading thinking activity (DRTA: concept development, sight vocabulary, guided reading, discussion, skill development, and enrichment); activating background knowledge; and using well-written, high-interest text.

Monitoring comprehension facilitates the linking of new information with prior knowledge and supports text-based and knowledge-based inferential processing that is needed for full understanding of the text. Deaf students have been found to use fewer metacognitive strategies than hearing students, and they tend to use less appropriate strategies or to use them for the wrong reasons (Marschark et al., 2002). In addition, they have been found to have difficulty with drawing inferences from text (for reviews, see Marschark & Wauters, 2008; Schirmer & McGough, 2005). Students need to be taught monitoring strategies to achieve text comprehension. Explicit comprehension strategy instruction can be accomplished through steps of direct explanation of the strategy, modeling of the strategy by the teacher, guided practice to assist the students in applying the strategy, and application of the strategy by the students (Luckner & Handley, 2008). The most commonly taught reading strategies are prediction (based on prior knowledge), questioning (to monitor understanding), imagery (creating a mental image), connecting (with prior knowledge), and summarizing.

*Interim Conclusion: Effective Reading Instruction*

There is still a long way to go in establishing evidence-based practices in reading instruction to DHH students, but some conclusions can be drawn from the research discussed thus far. A first conclusion to be drawn is that in order to reach the ultimate goal of understanding what is read, reading instruction should focus on the areas of phonemic awareness, alphabetics, fluency, vocabulary, and comprehension strategies. When children have mastered the decoding process, are able to read fluently, know the words in a text, and can apply monitoring strategies, they will have better chances to understand a text. Promising instruction strategies to help deaf children develop these skills are: the use of Visual Phonics; the use of morphological information; applying techniques to link signs, fingerspelling, and print; providing multiple readings of a text; use of computers; providing an intensive vocabulary program in rich and varied contexts; and explicit strategy instruction.

In their discussion of what deaf students need in the instruction they receive, Marschark and colleagues (2011a, 2011b) suggested the following strategies to help deaf students to reach comprehension: use of concept maps; use of games; explicit instruction, especially when tying new information to existing knowledge; providing practice with strategies; and explaining to students what is expected and why. As Williams

(2012) argued, evidence-based interventions for DHH children can be developed from what has been learned from research with typically hearing children.

But what does this all mean for training our teachers? Marschark and Knoors (2012) stated that the research evidence about effective instructional strategies needs to be translated into actual teaching behavior. Marschark and colleagues (2011b) suggested that the information about effective teaching strategies and about the influence of differences between deaf and hearing students on learning must be incorporated in both pre-service and in-service programs for all educators who work with DHH students. In planning these programs, three criteria should be taken into account (Marzano, 2003): focus on knowledge of the content of instruction, opportunities for active learning, and a coherent and meaningful program of activities. In the remainder of this chapter we will discuss a video coaching project in which at least the first two criteria are met.

## TEACHER TRAINING

Because the quality of instruction and the qualifications of teachers are thought to explain a large part of the variance in students' performance, it seems obvious to invest in teacher training to improve quality, especially in an educational setting as complex as bilingual deaf education. Educators in deaf education agree that reading instruction is one of the priorities in teacher training. Luckner and colleagues (2005) assessed the research and training needs of professionals in deaf education and found that five of the 20 priorities were related to reading, writing, language, and vocabulary. Teaching reading strategies to deaf students was ranked as the third priority, after educating administrators about appropriate services and about how to work within the system to change it. Andrews and Covell (2006) also suggest that teachers of the deaf should be educated in a master's program in which practices in English literacy are part of the curriculum.

Obviously, professionals agree on the need of teacher training in the area of reading instruction. However, creating an effective teacher-training program is not simple (Johnson, 2013; Korthagen, 2010). Teacher training should focus on enhancing teaching behavior. Too often, teachers' theoretical knowledge is not embedded in their classroom behavior, because they are taken up by daily classroom dynamics that directly influence their teaching behavior on the spot (Korthagen, 2010). As Johnson (2013) has pointed out, teachers are constantly challenged to adjust their goals, instruction, materials, activities, and assessments to fit the daily dynamics and changes in teacher requirements, student needs, and organizational issues. Experienced teachers have learned to anticipate and respond to these challenges.

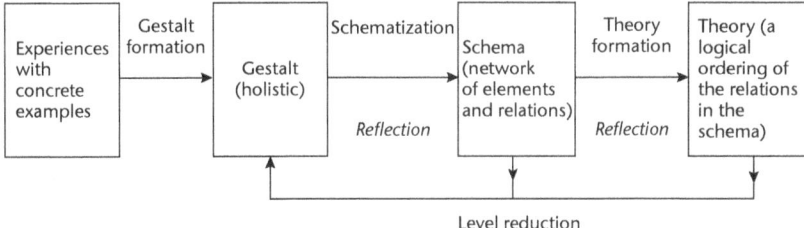

Figure 10.1 The three-level model of learning development by Korthagen (2010).

Korthagen (2010) presented a model of learning development that departs from the assumption that all knowledge is rooted in practical situations (see Figure 10.1). The three-level model suggests that, from the start, theoretical information should be embedded in daily classroom activities. Teacher training should focus on providing opportunities for reflection to help teachers recognize which instruction strategies are effective in certain situations. Through confrontations with comparable situations, teachers are able to develop a network of concepts and relations between situations and their behavior. Teaching behavior can then become self-evident and can be used in a less conscious way, leading to higher quality of instruction.

This three-level model was applied to a small-scale project described in the next section in which video coaching was used to provide teachers with the necessary opportunities for reflection on their reading instruction in the bilingual classroom.

### Effect of Video Coaching on Reading Instruction

Marschark and Knoors (2012) mentioned video coaching as one of the activities to support the training of teachers of the deaf. Coaching teachers may be a way to provide opportunities for teachers to reflect on classroom situations. The International Reading Association (2004) defined literacy coaching as a means of providing professional development to help teachers develop and improve their interventions and instructional skills. Several studies have found a positive effect of teacher coaching on teachers' knowledge and effective reading instruction (Hsieh, Hemmeter, McCollum, & Ostrosky, 2009; Neuman & Cunningham, 2009; Sailors & Price, 2010). Effects were found in primary and secondary education and in both new and experienced teachers.

One way to provide coaching to teachers is through video coaching, a procedure in which teachers are videotaped and receive feedback and guidance to further exploit positive behaviors that are already shown in the video. Again, positive effects of this procedure have been found in teachers, both new and experienced, through reflection on behavior in the videotaped lessons (Fukkink, Trienekens, & Kramer, 2011).

In the study described here, video coaching was used to influence teaching behavior in reading instruction to DHH children. This study was part of a larger project in which we first made an inventory of evidence-based reading practices, resulting in a comprehensive literature review. These evidence-based practices were subsequently illustrated with video clips from actual lessons in deaf education. A DVD with these practices was produced. Following the reasoning of Korthagen's model, just providing the literature review and the DVD to teachers is not enough to improve their reading instruction. They need opportunities to link this theoretical information to their own daily practice. Through discussing their own classroom activities in which they use effective reading instruction strategies, we hoped to help them see the relation between situations, the use of the instruction strategies, and student behavior. From here, they can build their network of relations between situations and actions that helps them to consistently apply the reading instruction strategies in similar situations.

Six K–5 teachers with two to eight years of experience in a school for the deaf in the Netherlands received feedback on their reading instruction through video coaching (experimental group). Three control teachers (kindergarten, first grade, and sixth grade) were videotaped as well, but received overall feedback only after the project was ended. One of them had 25 years of experience in deaf education, and the other two were new teachers with one year of experience in deaf education. Control teachers were told that they were functioning as controls in a project, but they did not know the details of the project and they did not receive any coaching.

The six K–5 teachers in the experimental group were videotaped seven times during reading lessons. They were instructed to teach their lessons as they always did. After videos 2 to 5, they received feedback based on the videos. The first video was used as a baseline for comparison, and the last two were used as follow-up. The three control teachers were videotaped five times, also with a baseline and two follow-up videos, but they did not receive any coaching. Only after the project ended did they receive written feedback based on the videos from their lessons. Table 10.1 shows an overview of the sessions of videotaping and video coaching for the teachers in the experimental group and of videotaping for the control group.

Coaching of the teachers in the experimental group always occurred in the week after the videotaping; 2 to 3 weeks after the coaching session, the next lesson was videotaped. A coaching session lasted between 30 and 45 minutes. The first follow-up (i.e., video session 6) was filmed 2 to 3 weeks after the last coaching session; the second follow-up (i.e., video session 7) was filmed 4 months after the last coaching session.

**Table 10.1 Overview of Videotaping and Video Coaching**

| Experimental group | | Control group | |
|---|---|---|---|
| Videos | Video coaching | Videos | Video coaching |
| 1 | no | 1 | no |
| 2 | yes | 2 | no |
| 3 | yes | - | - |
| 4 | yes | - | - |
| 5 | yes | 3 | no |
| 6 | no | 4 | no |
| 7 | no | 5 | no |

For the control group, the third video was taped at the point where teachers in the experimental group would reach the end of the coaching period. The follow-up videos (video sessions 4 and 5) were filmed, respectively, 2 to 3 weeks and 4 months after video 3. In describing the results of this project, the first five videos for the experimental group will be referred to as the coaching period ("end of coaching" in Figures 10.2 through 10.8). The first three videos for the control group will be referred to as the observation period ("end of observation" in Figures 10.2 through 10.8). The follow-up measurements will just be referred to as first and second follow-up.

Based on the inventory of evidence-based reading practices in the literature review and the DVD, three observation lists were constructed to score teaching behavior: emergent literacy/early literacy (kindergarten), decoding and fluency (grades 1–4), and reading comprehension (grades 5–6). Items on the observation lists referred to practices such as explicit instruction, modeling, and use of signs, print, and fingerspelling. All items on the observation lists were scored on a three-point scale of teacher skills: 1 = inadequate; 2 = adequate; or 3 = good. Inter-rater reliability for scoring of the observation lists was $r = .73$.

Scores on the observation lists were used as input for the feedback that teachers received during the coaching session and for analyses of the results. The coach/researcher selected clips from the video to discuss with the teacher. According to the principles of video coaching and based on the three-level model of learning, feedback would focus on effective instruction strategies that teachers already applied and on providing opportunities for reflection, as well as discussing ways to further incorporate these strategies into their reading lessons.

Items on the observation lists were clustered into 11 aspects of effective reading instruction for analysis (see Table 10.2). Not all aspects were measured (and coached) in all teachers, because the aspects are related to the reading level that is taught in the classroom, and not all aspects apply to all reading levels. For the aspects "fluency instruction"

**Table 10.2 Aspects of Reading Instruction That Were Observed**

| Aspect | Explanation | Phase of reading development |
|---|---|---|
| Efficient use of modalities | The teacher efficiently and consistently utilizes signs, fingerspelling, spoken language, and print. | Emergent/early literacy and decoding and fluency |
| Improving automaticity | The teacher provides opportunities and repetition for improving automaticity of letter knowledge and at word level. | Decoding |
| Variation in reading activities | The teacher varies reading activities through reading of words, sentences, and texts. | Decoding |
| Reading aloud | Where possible, the teacher lets students practice reading aloud without sign support. | Decoding and fluency |
| Fluency instruction (content) | The teacher uses (short) texts and provides opportunities for rereading. | Fluency |
| Fluency instruction (strategy) | The teacher provides cues and practices with morphological structures. | Fluency |
| Reading strategies | The teacher works on reading strategies. | Reading comprehension |
| Reading vocabulary | The teacher works on expanding reading vocabulary. | Reading comprehension |
| Modeling | The teacher applies the principle of modeling (through the "I do, we do, you do" approach).* | All |
| Explain and maintain goal | The teacher explains the goal of the lesson and retains that goal during the lesson. | All |
| Direct instruction | The teacher applies the principles of the direct instruction model. | All |

* In the "I do, we do, you do" approach, the teacher first models the reading strategy or activity (I do), then helps the student in applying the strategy through guided practice (we do), and eventually the student applies the strategy on his own (you do).

(content and strategy), "instruction of reading strategies," and "reading vocabulary," this resulted in too small a group of teachers (one or two) to discuss the results. Therefore, we will only discuss the results of the other seven aspects, namely efficient use of modalities, improving automaticity, reading aloud, modeling, variation in reading activities, direct instruction, and explaining and maintaining the goal of the lesson. The number of teachers also varied for these aspects, as can be seen in Figures 10.2 through 10.8.

The mean score, between 1 and 3, on each of the aspects was derived from a cluster of scores based on a three-point scale of the observation items. Due to the small number of teachers, we are only able to provide descriptive data of the improvement in teaching behavior as explained in Table 10.2. Teaching behavior was considered to have improved when the mean score showed an increase of 0.5 or more. Improvement in teaching behavior in the experimental group was compared to improvement in teaching behavior in the control group, where a difference in improvement between the groups suggests an effect of the video coaching.

*Efficient Use of Modalities*

Research has shown the effectiveness of the combined use of signs, fingerspelling, print, and spoken language in reading instruction. Therefore teachers in the experimental group were coached on the efficient use of these modalities in their reading lessons. These teachers showed an improvement in their skill to effectively and consistently use these modalities after the coaching period, compared to baseline, and were able to retain part of that improvement at follow-up, even 4 months after the coaching stopped. The two control teachers did not improve their skills in efficiently and consistently utilizing the modalities during the observation period or at follow-up. Figure 10.2 shows the changes in teaching behavior after coaching (experimental group) or after the observation period (control group) and at follow-up.

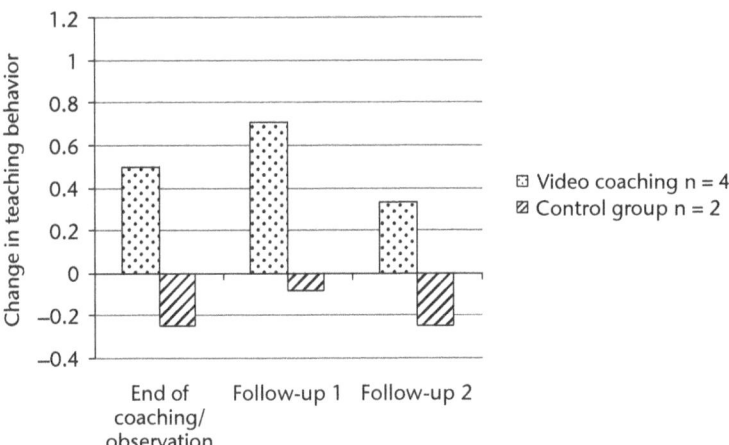

**Figure 10.2** Change in "efficient use of modalities" between baseline and end of coaching, between baseline and follow-up 1, and between baseline and follow-up 2.

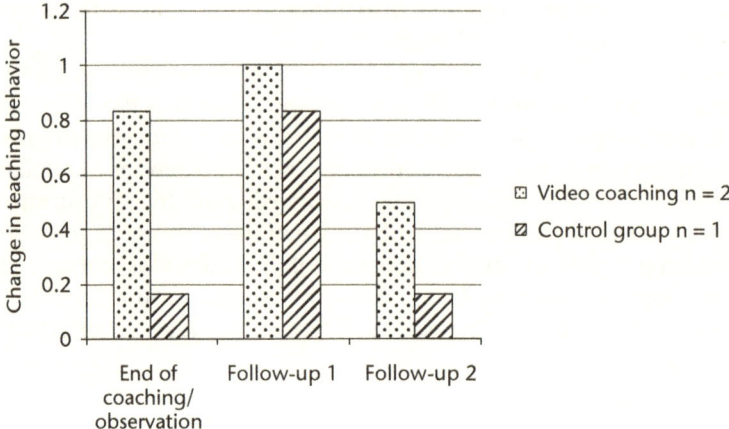

Figure 10.3 Change in "improving automaticity" between baseline and end of coaching, between baseline and follow-up 1, and between baseline and follow-up 2.

*Improving Automaticity*

Two teachers in the experimental group received feedback on their skill in providing opportunities for improving automaticity of letter and word knowledge. Both teachers showed improvement compared to baseline and continued practicing this skill at follow-up (see Figure 10.3). The control teacher did not show improvement during the observation period, but had somehow improved the skill at the first follow-up, and just above the baseline level at the second follow-up.

*Reading Aloud*

Three teachers in the experimental group were coached on providing practice in reading aloud in spoken language to improve fluency skills. Reading aloud was often used in addition to practicing reading in other modalities. As can be seen from Figure 10.4, the control teacher showed an improvement in practicing reading aloud with students during the observation period and at the first follow-up, which was higher than the improvement of the teachers in the experimental group after coaching or at the first follow-up.

*Modeling*

Modeling has often been mentioned as an effective teaching strategy, also in reading instruction for DHH students. The teachers in the experimental group showed an improvement in their modeling skills and managed to retain this improvement even at the second follow-up. The control teachers somewhat decreased their use of modeling skills

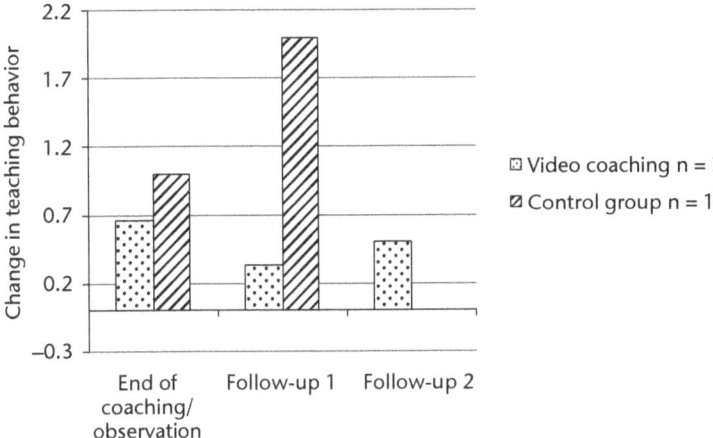

Figure 10.4 Change in "reading aloud" between baseline and end of coaching, between baseline and follow-up 1, and between baseline and follow-up 2.

during the observation period and still showed a decrease at follow-up (see Figure 10.5).

*Variation in Reading Activities*

Using a variety of reading activities in reading lessons is one aspect of using meaningful reading materials. Teachers need to vary their reading activities and reading materials to motivate their students. Both coached teachers in the experimental group showed a small improvement after

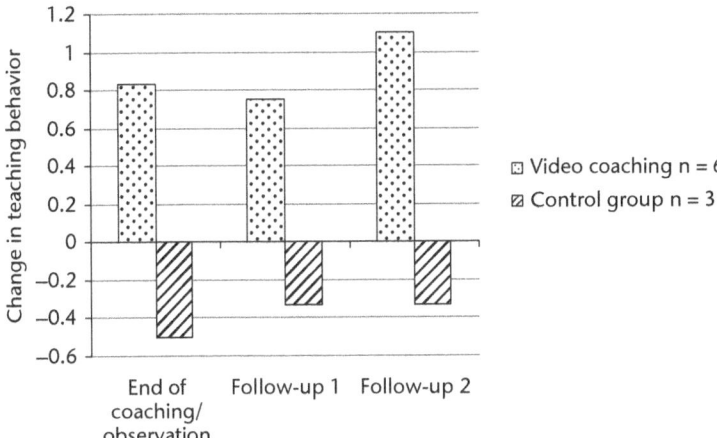

Figure 10.5 Change in "modeling" between baseline and end of coaching, between baseline and follow-up 1, and between baseline and follow-up 2.

262  Bilingualism and Bilingual Deaf Education

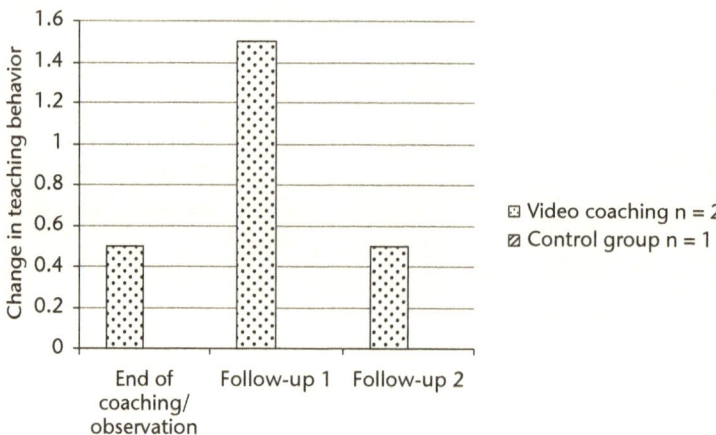

Figure 10.6 Change in variation in reading activities between baseline and end of coaching, between baseline and follow up 1, and between baseline and follow-up 2.

the coaching period, improved even more at the first follow-up, and ended at the same level of improvement at the second follow-up as immediately after coaching (see Figure 10.6). The control teacher did not show any improvement during the observation period and at follow-up.

*Direct Instruction*

The model of direct instruction is a Dutch model of explicit instruction in which teachers go through specific phases during their lessons: daily review of previous content, instruction of new content, guided practice, individual training, reflection, and feedback (Veenman, 1996, 1998). By teaching according to this model of instruction, teachers are applying the skills that are needed for explicit and effective instruction.

The teachers in the experimental group showed a better improvement in applying the principles of the direct instruction model after coaching than the control teachers did after the observation period, but at follow-up the control teachers showed similar or even better improvement than the experimental group (see Figure 10.7).

*Explain and Maintain the Goal of the Reading Lesson*

One aspect of the direct instruction model is that teachers should always start their lesson explaining the goal of the lesson to the students. In addition, they should be able to maintain that goal during their lesson. We found this aspect to be hard for many teachers. The teachers in the experimental group improved their use of this teaching strategy after coaching, but did not retain this improvement at both follow-up measurements. The control teacher showed a higher score at the second follow-up without being coached (see Figure 10.8).

Improving Reading Instruction    263

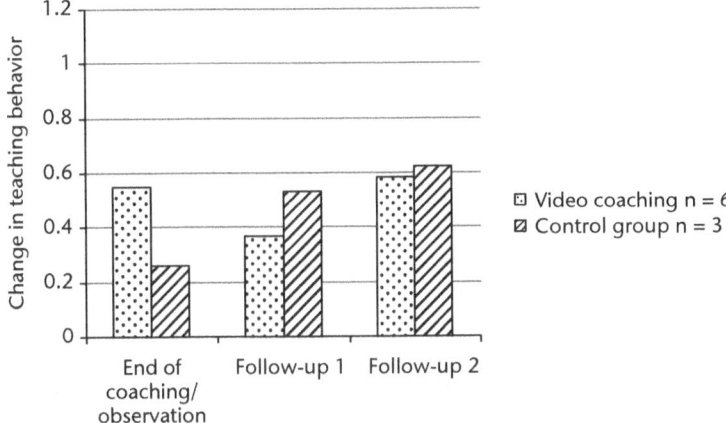

Figure 10.7 Change in "direct instruction" between baseline and end of coaching, between baseline and follow-up 1, and between baseline and follow-up 2.

*Interim Conclusion: Effects of Video Coaching on Reading Instruction*

Through video coaching we aimed at the second level of learning, the development of a network of concepts and relations between situations and teaching behavior. When teachers learn to identify the situations in which certain instruction strategies are effective, they can apply these strategies more consistently to improve reading instruction. Although it concerns a small group of teachers in the experimental group, and the

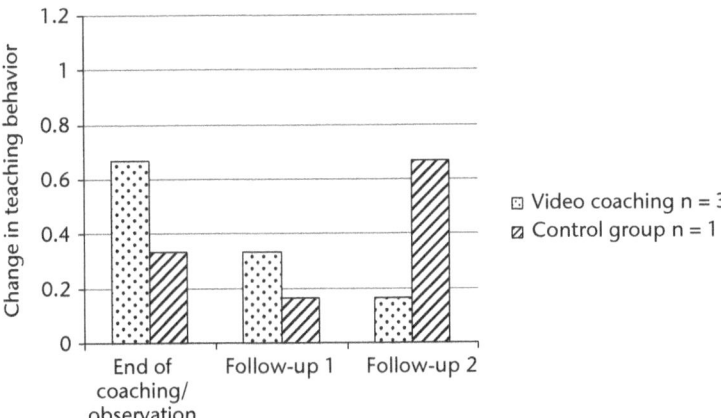

Figure 10.8 Change in "explaining and maintaining goal" between baseline and end of coaching, between baseline and follow-up 1, and between baseline and follow-up 2.

results have to be carefully interpreted, the video coaching technique adopted in the current study led to improvement on six of the seven analyzed aspects, contrary to the performance of teachers in the control group who did not improve over the same period. On four of these aspects—"efficient use of modalities," "modeling," "variation in reading activities," and "improving automaticity"—the difference between the experimental group and the control group continues to exist at follow-up. On the aspect "explaining and maintaining the goal of the lesson," the teachers in the experimental group did not manage to retain the improvement. On "direct instruction" the teachers retained their improvement, but the teachers in the control group also managed to improve their skills in this period, probably caused by efforts from the school management to improve direct instruction at the school level.

These results suggest that it is possible to positively affect teaching behavior in the reading lessons through video coaching. Teachers in the experimental group perceived the feedback as pleasant and meaningful, and commented that it helps to have the opportunity to watch video clips of their own lessons with the coach because it provides a good opportunity for them to reflect on their behavior. This reflection is necessary to build networks in the second level of the three-level model of learning development by Korthagen (2010).

## SUMMARY AND CONCLUSIONS

Learning to read is a challenge for deaf children, and teaching deaf children to read is a challenge for teachers, certainly in an educational concept as complex as bilingual education. This chapter focuses on what teachers should know about teaching reading to DHH children and how we can help them to incorporate this knowledge in their teaching behavior.

Apart from cognitive factors affecting deaf students' learning, quality of instruction is thought to contribute largely to students' academic performance. What is it that teachers need to do to accommodate their instruction to the needs of DHH students? Reviews have shown that reading instruction to DHH students should focus on several areas: phonemic awareness, alphabetics (letter knowledge, phonological awareness, and phonics), fluency, vocabulary, and text comprehension. Easterbrooks and Beal-Alvarez (2013) also mentioned the factor motivation as an important aspect in reading instruction, but immediately state that little is known about how we can teach motivation. However, teachers need to know that students who are internally motivated will probably learn to read more easily than students who are less motivated.

Instruction strategies that have been found to be effective in the above-mentioned reading areas are the following: explicit instruction in phonological awareness, use of Visual Phonics, matching written words with signs and spoken words, independent oral reading, repeated reading, use of morphological information, intensive vocabulary programs, building and activating prior knowledge, and explicit instruction of reading and monitoring strategies.

Apart from knowledge about cognitive factors in deaf students' learning process, teachers need to know about these effective teaching methods. Just having this theoretical knowledge is not enough, though. We have used the three-level model of learning development by Korthagen (2010) to explain that teachers need many experiences with certain teaching situations and need to reflect on these situations in order to incorporate their knowledge in their behavior unconsciously. Through reflection, teachers learn which instruction strategies are more effective in certain situations. By consistently applying these effective strategies in the right situations, they can improve their reading instruction. Video coaching seems to be one way to accomplish this, as is shown in the study described in this chapter. Video coaching was used to incorporate effective reading instruction strategies into the behavior of teachers of the deaf. The teachers in this study showed changes in their behavior in terms of "efficient use of modalities," "modeling strategies," "provision of a variety of reading activities," "explaining and maintaining goals," and "improving automaticity at letter and word level." Although these results were found in a small group of teachers, they are promising for teacher education related to the teaching of reading. When given the opportunity to reflect on their own behavior through video coaching, teachers of DHH students are indeed able to change their behavior in the reading classroom. Through video coaching two of the criteria of effective in-service programs (Marzano, 2003) were realized: focus on knowledge of the content of instruction and opportunities for active learning.

## REFERENCES

Aceti, K. J., & Wang, Y. (2010). The teaching and learning of multimeaning words within a metacognitively based curriculum. *American Annals of the Deaf, 155*(2), 118–123.

Andrews, J. F. (1988). Deaf children's acquisition of prereading skills using the reciprocal teaching procedure. *Exceptional Children, 54,* 349–355.

Andrews, J. F. & Covell, J. A. (2006). Preparing future teachers and doctoral-level readers in deaf education: Meeting the challenge. *American Annals of the Deaf, 151,* 464–475.

Andrews, J. F., & Mason, J. M. (1986). How do deaf children learn about prereading? *American Annals of the Deaf, 131,* 210–217.

Bavelier, D., Newport, E. L., Hall, M. L., Supalla, T., & Boutla, M. (2008). Ordered short-term memory differs in signers and speakers: Implications for models of short-term memory. *Cognition, 107*(2), 433–459.

Beal-Alvarez, J. S., Lederberg, A. R., & Easterbrooks, S. R. (2011). Grapheme-phoneme acquisition of deaf preschoolers. *Journal of Deaf Studies and Deaf Education, 17*(1), 39–60.

Boutla, M., Supalla, T., Newport, E. L., & Bavelier, D. (2004). Short-term memory span: Insights from sign language. *Nature Neuroscience, 7*, 997–1002.

Chamberlain, C., & Mayberry, R. I. (2000). Theorizing about the relation between American Sign Language and reading. In C. Chamberlain, J. P. Morford, & R. I. Mayberry (Eds.), *Language acquisition by eye* (pp. 221–259). Mahwah, NJ: Lawrence Erlbaum Associates.

Chamberlain, C., & Mayberry, R. I. (2008). American Sign Language syntactic and narrative comprehension in skilled and less skilled readers: Bilingual and bimodal evidence for the linguistic basis of reading. *Applied Psycholinguistics, 29*, 367–388.

Conrad, R. (1979). *The deaf schoolchild*. London: Harper and Row.

Easterbrooks, S., & Beal-Alvarez, J. (2013). *Literacy instruction for students who are deaf and hard of hearing*. New York, NY: Oxford University Press.

Easterbrooks, S. R., & Huston, S. G. (2008). The signed reading fluency of students who are deaf/hard of hearing. *Journal of Deaf Studies and Deaf Education, 13*(1), 37–54.

Easterbrooks, S. R., & Stephenson, B. (2006). An examination of twenty literacy, science, and mathematics practices used to educate students who are deaf or hard of hearing. *American Annals of the Deaf, 151*, 385–397.

Fukkink, R. G., Trienekens, N., & Kramer, L. J. C. (2011). Video feedback in education and training: Putting learning in the picture. *Educational Psychology Review, 23*, 45–63.

Fung, P., Chow, B. W., & McBride-Chang, C. (2005). The impact of a dialogic reading program on deaf and hard-of-hearing kindergarten and early primary school-aged children in Hong Kong. *Journal of Deaf Studies and Deaf Education, 10*(1), 82–95.

Gaustad, M. G. (2000). Morphographic analysis as a word identification strategy for deaf readers. *Journal of Deaf Studies and Deaf Education, 5*(1), 60–80.

Geers, A., & Brenner, C. (2003). Background and educational characteristics of prelingually deaf children implanted by five years of age. *Ear and Hearing, 24*, 2S–14S.

Geers, A., Tobey, E., Moog, J., & Brenner, C. (2008). Long-term outcomes of cochlear implantation in the preschool years: From elementary grades to high school. *International Journal of Audiology, 47*, S21–S30.

Hall, M. L., & Bavelier, D. (2010). Working memory, deafness, and sign language. In M. Marschark and P. E. Spencer (Eds.), *Oxford handbook of deaf studies, language, and education* (vol. 2, pp. 458–471). New York, NY: Oxford University Press.

Harris, M., & Beech, J. (1998). Implicit phonological awareness and early reading development in prelingually deaf children. *Journal of Deaf Studies and Deaf Education, 3*, 205–216.

Harris, M., & Terletski, E. (2011). Reading and spelling abilities of deaf adolescents with cochlear implants and hearing aids. *Journal of Deaf Studies and Deaf Education, 16*(1), 24–34.

Hermans, D., Knoors, H., Ormel, E., & Verhoeven, L. (2008a). Modeling reading vocabulary learning in deaf children in bilingual education programs. *Journal of Deaf Studies and Deaf Education, 13*, 155–174.

Hermans, D., Knoors, H., Ormel, E., & Verhoeven, L. (2008b). The relationship between the reading and signing skills of deaf children in bilingual education programs. *Journal of Deaf Studies and Deaf Education, 13,* 518–530.

Hermans, D., Ormel, E., & Knoors, H. (2010). On the relation between the signing and reading skills of deaf bilinguals. *International Journal of Bilingual Education and Bilingualism, 13*(2), 187–199.

Hoffmeister, R. (2000). A piece of the puzzle: ASL and reading comprehension in deaf children. In C. Chamberlain, J. Morford, & R. Mayberry (Eds.), *Language acquisition by eye* (pp. 143–163). Mahwah, NJ: Lawrence Erlbaum Associates.

Hsieh, W., Hemmeter, M. L., McCollum, J. A., & Ostrosky, M. M. (2009). Using coaching to increase preschool teachers' use of emergent literacy practices. *Early Childhood Research Quarterly, 24,* 229–247.

Hu, M., & Nation, P. (2000). Unknown vocabulary density and reading comprehension. *Reading in a Foreign Language, 13*(1), 403–430.

International Reading Association (2004). *The role and qualifications of the reading coach in the United States.* Newark, DE: Author.

Johnson, H. A. (2013). Initial and ongoing teacher preparation and support: Current problems and possible solutions. *American Annals of the Deaf, 157*(5), 439–449.

Korthagen, F. A. J. (2010). Situated learning theory and the pedagogy of teacher education: Towards an integrative view of teacher behavior and teacher learning. *Teaching and Teacher Education, 26,* 98–106.

Kyle, F. E., & Harris, M. (2006). Concurrent correlates and predictors of reading and spelling achievement in deaf and hearing school children. *Journal of Deaf Studies and Deaf Education, 11*(3), 273–288.

Kyle, F. E., & Harris, M. (2010). Predictors of reading development in deaf children: A 3-year longitudinal study. *Journal of Experimental Child Psychology, 107,* 229–243.

Lederberg, A. R., & Beal-Alvarez, J. (2011). Expressing meaning: From communicative intent to building vocabulary. In M. Marschark & P. E. Spencer (Eds.), *Oxford handbook of deaf studies, language, and education* (vol. 1, 2nd ed., pp. 258–275). New York, NY: Oxford University Press.

Lederberg, A. R., Miller, E. M., Easterbrooks, S. R., & Connor, C. M. (2011). *Foundations for literacy.* Unpublished curriculum. Atlanta: Georgia State University.

Luckner, J. L., & Cooke, C. (2010). A summary of the vocabulary research with students who are deaf or hard of hearing. *American Annals of the Deaf, 155*(1), 38–67.

Luckner, J. L., & Handley, C. M. (2008). A summary of the reading comprehension research undertaken with students who are deaf or hard of hearing. *American Annals of the Deaf, 153*(1), 6–36.

Luckner, J. L., Muir, S. G., Howell, J. J., Sebald, A. M., & Young, J. (2005). An examination of the research and training needs in the field of deaf education. *American Annals of the Deaf, 150*(4), 358–368.

Luckner, J. L., Sebald, A. M., Cooney, J., Young, J., & Muir, S. G. (2005/2006). An examination of the evidence-based literacy research in deaf education. *American Annals of the Deaf, 150*(5), 443–456.

Luckner, J. L., & Urbach, J. (2012). Reading fluency and students who are deaf or hard of hearing: Synthesis of the research. *Communication Disorders Quarterly, 33*(4), 230–241.

Marschark, M., Convertino, C., McEvoy, C., & Masteller, A. (2004). Organization and use of the mental lexicon. *American Annals of the Deaf, 149*(1), 51–61.

Marschark, M., & Harris, M. (1996). Success and failure in reading: The special case (?) of deaf children. In C. Cornoldi & J. Oakhill (Eds.), *Reading comprehension difficulties: Processes and intervention* (pp. 279–300). Mahwah, NJ: Lawrence Erlbaum Associates.

Marschark, M., & Knoors, H. (2012). Educating deaf children: Language, cognition, and learning. *Deafness and Education International, 14*(3), 136–160.

Marschark, M., Lang, H. G., & Albertini, J. A. (2002). *Educating deaf students: From research to practice*. New York, NY: Oxford University Press.

Marschark, M., Rhoten, C., & Fabich, M. (2007). Effects of cochlear implants on children's reading and academic achievement. *Journal of Deaf Studies and Deaf Education, 12*(3), 269–282.

Marschark, M., Richardson, J. T. E., Sapere, P., & Sarchet, T. (2010). Approaches to teaching in mainstream and separate postsecondary classrooms. *American Annals of the Deaf, 155*(4), 481–487.

Marschark, M., Sapere, P., Convertino, C. M., Mayer, C., Wauters, L., & Sarchet, T. (2009). Are deaf students' reading challenges really about reading? *American Annals of the Deaf, 154*(4), 357–370.

Marschark, M., Sapere, P., Convertino, C., & Pelz, J. (2008). Learning via direct and mediated instruction. *Journal of Deaf Studies and Deaf Education, 13*(4), 546–561.

Marschark, M., Spencer, P. E., Adams, J., & Sapere, P. (2011a). Evidence-based practice in educating deaf and hard-of-hearing children: Teaching to their cognitive strengths and needs. *European Journal of Special Needs Education, 26*(1), 3–16.

Marschark, M., Spencer, P. E., Adams, J., & Sapere, P. (2011b). Teaching to the strengths and needs of deaf and hard-of-hearing children. *European Journal of Special Needs Education, 26*(1), 17–23.

Marschark, M., & Wauters, L. (2008). Language comprehension and learning by deaf students. In M. Marschark & P. Hauser (Eds.), *Deaf cognition: Foundations and outcomes* (pp. 309–350). New York, NY: Oxford University Press.

Marzano, R. J. (2003). *What works in schools: Translating research into action*. Alexandria, VA: ASCD.

Mayer, C. (2007). What really matters in early literacy development of deaf children. *Journal of Deaf Studies and Deaf Education, 12*(4), 411–431.

Mayer, C. (2009). Issues in second language literacy education with learners who are deaf. *International Journal of Bilingual Education and Bilingualism, 12*(3), 1–11.

Mayer, C., & Akamatsu, C. T. (1999). Bilingual-bicultural models of literacy education of deaf students: Considering the claims. *Journal of Deaf Studies and Deaf Education, 4*(1), 1–8.

Miller, E. M., Lederberg, A. R., & Easterbrooks, S. R. (2013). Phonological awareness: Explicit instruction for young deaf and hard-of-hearing children. *Journal of Deaf Studies and Deaf Education, 18*(2), 206–227.

Mokhtari, K., & Reichard, C. A. (2002). Assessing students' metacognitive awareness of reading strategies. *Journal of Educational Psychology, 94*, 249–259.

Mollink, H., Hermans, D., & Knoors, H. (2008). Vocabulary training of spoken words in hard-of-hearing children. *Deafness and Education International, 10*, 80–92.

Narr, R. F. (2008). Phonological awareness and decoding in deaf/hard-of-hearing students who use Visual Phonics. *Journal of Deaf Studies and Deaf Education, 13*(3), 405–416.

Narr, R. F., & Cawthon, S. W. (2011). The "Wh" questions of *Visual Phonics*: What, who, where, and why. *Journal of Deaf Studies and Deaf Education, 16*(1), 66–78.

National Reading Panel (2000). *Report of the National Reading Panel. Teaching children to read: An evidence-based assessment of the scientific research literature on reading and its implication for reading instruction.* Washington, DC: US Department of Health and Human Services.

Niederberger, N. (2008). Does the knowledge of a natural sign language facilitate deaf children's learning to read and write? Insights from French Sign Language and written French data. In C. Plaza Pust & E. Moralez-Lopez (Eds.), *Sign bilingualism: Language development, interaction, and maintenance in sign language contact situations* (pp. 39–50). Amsterdam; Philadelphia: John Benjamins Publishing.

Neuman, S. B., & Cunningham, L. (2009). The impact of professional development and coaching on early language and literacy instructional practices. *American Educational Research Journal, 46*, 532–566.

Ormel, E. (2008). *Visual word recognition in bilingual deaf children.* Unpublished dissertation, Radboud Universiteit Nijmegen, the Netherlands.

Ormel, E., Hermans, D., Knoors, H., & Verhoeven, L. (2009). The role of sign phonology and iconicity during sign processing: The case of deaf children. *Journal of Deaf Studies and Deaf Education, 14*, 436–448.

Padden, C., & Ramsey, C. (1998). Reading ability in signing deaf children. *Topics in Language Disorders, 18*, 30–46.

Perfetti, C. A., & Sandak, R. (2000). Reading optimally builds on spoken language: implications for deaf readers. *Journal of Deaf Studies and Deaf Education, 5*, 32–50.

Power, D., & Leigh, G. R. (2000). Principles and practices of literacy development for deaf learners: A historical overview. *Journal of Deaf Studies and Deaf Education, 5*, 3–8.

Powers, S. (1999). The educational attainments of deaf students in mainstream programs in England: Examination results and influencing factors. *American Annals of the Deaf, 144*(3), 261–269.

Qi, S., & Mitchell, R. E. (2012). Large-scale academic achievement testing of deaf and hard-of-hearing students: Past, present, and future. *Journal of Deaf Studies and Deaf Education, 17*, 1–18.

Sailors, M., & Price, L. R. (2010). Professional development that supports the teaching of cognitive reading strategy instruction. *The Elementary School Journal, 110*, 301–322.

Schirmer, B. R., & McGough, S. M. (2005). Teaching reading to children who are deaf: Do the conclusions of the National Reading Panel apply? *Review of Educational Research, 75*, 83–117.

Schirmer, B. R., Schaffer, L., Therrien, W. J., & Schirmer, T. N. (2012). Reread-adapt and answer-comprehend intervention with deaf and hard of hearing readers: Effect on fluency and reading achievement. *American Annals of the Deaf, 156*(5), 469–475.

Schirmer, B. R., Therrien, W. J., Schaffer, L., & Schirmer, T. N. (2009). Repeated reading as an instructional intervention with deaf readers: Effect on fluency and reading achievement. *Reading Improvement, 46*, 168–177.

Smith, A., & Wang, Y. (2010). The impact of Visual Phonics on the phonological awareness and speech production of a student who is deaf: A case study. *American Annals of the Deaf, 155*(2), 124–130.

Spencer, P. E., & Marschark, M. (2010). *Evidence-based practice in educating deaf and hard-of-hearing students.* New York, NY: Oxford University Press.

Stinson, M. S, & Kluwin, T. N. (2011). Educational consequences of alternative school placements. In M. Marschark & P. E. Spencer (Eds.), *The Oxford handbook of deaf studies, language, and education* (vol. 1, 2nd ed., pp. 47–62). New York, NY: Oxford University Press.

Strassman, B. K. (1997). Metacognition and reading in children who are deaf: A review of the research. *Journal of Deaf Studies and Deaf Education, 2*(3), 140–149.

Strong, M., & Prinz, P. M. (1997). A study of the relationship between American Sign Language and English literacy. *Journal of Deaf Studies and Deaf Education, 2*, 37–46.

Traxler, C. B. (2000). The Stanford Achievement Test, 9th edition: National norming and performance standards for deaf and hard-of-hearing students. *Journal of Deaf Studies and Deaf Education, 5*, 337–348.

Trezek, B. J., & Malmgren, K. W. (2005). The efficacy of utilizing a phonics treatment package with middle school deaf and hard-of-hearing students. *Journal of Deaf Studies and Deaf Education, 10*(3), 256–271.

Trezek, B. J., & Wang, Y. (2006). Implications of utilizing a phonics-based reading curriculum with children who are deaf or hard of hearing. *Journal of Deaf Studies and Deaf Education, 11*(2), 202–213.

Trezek, B. J., Wang, Y., & Paul, P. V. (2010). Processes and components of reading. In M. Marschark & P. E. Spencer (Eds.), *Oxford handbook of deaf studies, language, and education* (vol. 1, 2nd ed., pp. 99–114). New York, NY: Oxford University Press.

Trezek, B. J., Wang, Y., Woods, D. G., Gammp, T. L., & Paul, P. V. (2007). Using Visual Phonics to supplement beginning reading instruction for students who are deaf or hard of hearing. *Journal of Deaf Studies and Deaf Education, 12*(3), 373–384.

Van Hoogmoed, A. H., Knoors, H., Schreuder, R., &Verhoeven, L. (2013). Complex word reading in Dutch deaf children and adults. *Research in Developmental Disabilities, 34*, 1083–1089.

Van Hoogmoed, A. H., Verhoeven, L., Schreuder, R., & Knoors, H. (2011). Morphological sensitivity in deaf readers of Dutch. *Applied Psycholinguistics, 32*, 619–634.

Veenman, S. (1996). Effectieve instructie in het special onderwijs [Effective instruction in special education]. *Speciaal Onderwijs, 66*, 123–131.

Veenman, S. (1998). Leraargeleid onderwijs: directe instructie [Teacher directed education: direct instruction]. In J. D. Vermunt & L. Verschaffel (Eds.),

*Onderwijzen van kennis en vaardigheden. Onderwijskundig lexicon* [Teaching knowledge and skills. Educational lexicon] (3rd ed., pp. 27–47). Alphen a/d Rijn, Netherlands: Samson.

Vermeulen, A. M., Van Bon, W., Schreuder, R., Knoors, H., & Snik, A. (2007). Reading comprehension of deaf children with cochlear implants. *Journal of Deaf Studies and Deaf Education, 12*(3), 283–302.

Wauters, L. N., Van Bon, W. H. J., & Tellings, A. E. J. M. (2006). Reading comprehension of Dutch deaf children. *Reading and Writing: An Interdisciplinary Journal, 19,* 49–76.

Wauters, L., Knoors, H., Vervloed, M. P. J., & Aarnoutse, C. (2001). Sign facilitation in word recognition. *Journal of Special Education, 35*(1), 31–40.

Williams, C. (2012). Promoting vocabulary learning in young children who are d/Deaf and hard of hearing: Translating research into practice. *American Annals of the Deaf, 156*(5), 501–508.

# 11

# Quality of Instruction in Bilingual Schools for Deaf Children

*Through the Children's Eyes and the Camera's Lens*

Daan Hermans, Loes Wauters, Annet de Klerk, and Harry Knoors

### BILINGUAL DEAF EDUCATION IN THE NETHERLANDS

As in other countries, deaf and hard-of-hearing (DHH) students in the Netherlands are educated in regular schools and in special schools (see Swanwick, Hendar, Dammeyer, Kristoffersen, Salter, & Simonsen, Chapter 12 of this volume). Compared to other countries, however, many more DHH students are educated in schools for the deaf. In 2012, a total of 1,667 DHH students were educated in primary or secondary schools; 604 of these students were profoundly deaf without multiple disabilities (CBS, 2013). Seventy percent of those deaf students were taught in special schools for the deaf; 30% were educated in regular schools. As a result of the introduction of universal newborn hearing screening (UNHS) early in the twenty-first century and the decrease in the age of cochlear implantation, this pattern is changing.

Schools for the deaf in the Netherlands have a bilingual policy. In 1998, schools for the deaf signed an agreement with the government arranging for the introduction of Sign Language of the Netherlands (SLN), together with spoken and written Dutch. In return for the promise to cooperate in curriculum planning, schools received extra funding for teacher training in SLN, for the employment of deaf teachers, and for developing special curricula for SLN, Dutch, and Deaf culture. These curricula have been developed in recent years in web-based formats, under the motto Sprong Vooruit (Leap Forward).

Bilingual education was introduced as a way to increase the access of profoundly deaf children to language by delivering an input of SLN as early as possible, while at the same time using Dutch in both spoken and written format (Knoors, 2007; Knoors & Fortgens, 1995). The idea was that increased access to language, and more specifically to the language of instruction, would help deaf children to learn more at school and to achieve better academically. Furthermore, it was also assumed that hard-of-hearing children with too little access to spoken Dutch could profit from a bilingual input in their development. Bilingual education thus was expected to increase the quality of instruction and education for deaf children. The question is whether and to what extent this really happened (see Holzinger & Fellinger, Chapter 5 of this volume). This question is all the more important because the key characteristics of deaf children have considerably changed since the introduction of bilingual deaf education. In the early years of bilingual education, very few deaf children in the Netherlands had received cochlear implants. This changed in 2002 because beginning in that year, the expenses related to implant surgery and the rehabilitation program were covered by health insurance plans. Today, 90–95% of all young profoundly deaf children without severe additional disabilities are implanted, most of them at the age of 1 year. A considerable proportion of very young deaf children now have bilateral implants. Increasingly, deaf children with multiple disabilities also are being implanted. This change has had consequences for language policy in schools for the deaf, leading to more prominence of spoken Dutch and to flexibility in the actual arrangement of language input in SLN and Dutch (Knoors & Marschark, 2012).

## QUALITY OF EDUCATION AND INSTRUCTION

It is quite normal that children vary in development and in achievement. However, this variation is comparatively large in DHH children. Stinson and Kluwin (2011) reviewed the effects of school placement (general versus special education) on academic achievement of deaf students. They concluded that educational placement explained only a very small proportion of the variance, less than 5%. Student characteristics such as learning potential and parental support explained considerably more variance, up to 25%. But the largest part remained unexplained. Stinson and Kluwin (2011) put forward the hypothesis that quality of instruction and education might be a key factor in this, since in many studies of academic achievement of deaf students, quality of education is not measured. Stinson and Kluwin (2011, p. 54) concluded:

> . . . although it is easy on a theoretical and experiential basis to describe significant process differences among the placement types, seldom have instructional factors (much less quality of instruction) entered into the analysis of between-placement differences. One could easily speculate that much of the 75% of unexplained variance lies there.

Instruction is important for students' learning. Its importance is already evident during preschool (Pianta et al., 2005), but remains so in other levels of education. Effective instruction becomes even more important in bilingual education programs, because these programs are by definition very complex. Students need to achieve proficiency in two languages, not only with respect to basic communication skills, including vocabulary and grammatical knowledge, but also with respect to literacy and higher order thinking (Lindholm-Leary, 2005). Marzano (2003; Marzano, Pickering, & Pollock, 2001) identified various effective instruction techniques for the education of hearing students. Summarizing content, generating and testing hypotheses, reinforcement, cooperative learning, and doing homework are examples of these evidence-based techniques.

Knoors and Hermans (2010) summarized research into the quality of education for deaf students. They started from models of educational effectiveness (Creemers, 1994; Scheerens & Bosker, 1997; Walberg, 1984) that incorporate various factors that influence achievement, typically grouped in three domains: society, school, and classroom. In their review, Knoors and Hermans focused on classroom factors. Specifically, they looked at language of instruction, instructional strategies and adaptations, teacher-student relationships, and classroom management. Knoors and Hermans concluded that "the picture of the quality of instruction for deaf students that emerges from the research literature available is at best fragmented" (p. 68). At that time, they already had begun to study various aspects related to classroom instruction in order to get a better, empirically supported picture of the quality of instruction in deaf education in general and bilingual deaf education in particular. Three studies will be reported in this chapter, focusing, respectively, on language of instruction in relation to learning gain, teacher activities and students' involvement, and students' perceptions of teaching quality and teacher-student relationships, thus at least partly looking at bilingual deaf education through the children's eyes. First, however, we will aim the camera lens at achievement by discussing actual achievement data of deaf students in (bilingual) schools for the deaf in the Netherlands.

## ACHIEVEMENT OF DUTCH DEAF STUDENTS

For the purposes of our first study, we collected achievement data of 174 DHH children, grades 1 to 6, from four special schools for deaf children with bilingual education programs. These children had no additional disabilities. The achievement data consisted of test scores (the national CITO tests) on mathematics, spelling, and reading comprehension. The data reflect the progress that children make in one year: Achievement = DA / DAE * 100, where DA stands for Didactic Age (number of months at school, counted from grade 1) and DAE for Didactic Age Equivalent (level in a particular subject, expressed in months). The norm percentage is 100%.

Compared to this norm, the percentages for bilingually educated DHH children for mathematics, spelling, and reading comprehension were, respectively, 58%, 50% and 45%. This indicates a serious gap between the achievements of DHH children in bilingual schools for the DHH and those of hearing children in regular schools. At the end of primary education, deaf students have acquired only half the knowledge that they should have acquired. These figures are, in a sense, disappointing, given all the attempts that professionals at schools made to improve instruction and education. We are certainly not dealing with unmotivated teachers—quite the contrary. Further, these achievement outcomes are consistent with those reported in the literature in various other countries (Hendar, 2009; Rydberg, Gellerstedt, & Danermark, 2009). It therefore seems important that we look for explanatory factors. One of the areas that might account for the results obtained is quality of instruction. Among the instructional factors that are related to achievement are, by definition, language of instruction, teaching activities and student engagement, and teacher-student relationships. We therefore explored these factors empirically.

## LANGUAGE OF INSTRUCTION AND LEARNING GAINS

Given the fact that many deaf students lack proficiency in spoken language and in sign language and that, partly as a consequence of this, they also experience significant problems in reading and writing, it should come as no surprise that deaf students tend to learn significantly less from instruction than hearing students do. Marschark, Sapere, Convertino, and Seewagen (2005) studied learning gain, the amount of content that students learned from instruction in one lesson, in deaf and hearing college students. Deaf students received instruction, mediated by sign language interpreters with varying amounts of experience. The study showed that deaf students with deaf parents did not learn more than those with hearing parents and that both groups of deaf students learned significantly less than hearing students. Marschark et al. argued that either mediated instruction is the problem, or the deaf students were unable to comprehend the instruction fully. Alternatively, hearing instructors may use instruction techniques that are less effective for deaf students.

In a later study, Marschark, Sapere, Convertino, and Pelz (2008) showed that deaf students are able to learn as much from direct instruction as from interpreter-mediated instruction, provided both (signing) teachers and interpreters have excellent sign language skills. That study also showed that deaf students are able to attain equal amounts of learning gain if differences in prior knowledge are controlled for and if they are taught by skilled teachers of the deaf. This result was obtained irrespective of the hearing status of the teacher and of the use of spoken or sign language by the student. In a re-analysis of 10 previous experiments, Convertino and colleagues (2009) were able to demonstrate that, after controlling for family, audiological, and academic factors, the deaf students' receptive skills in simultaneous communication were the only significant predictor of learning gain, even if the language of instruction had not involved simultaneous communication. Convertino et al. argued that their results likely reflected that flexibility in dealing with spoken or signed language of instruction is crucial, rather than the proficiency level in simultaneous communication. That sign language proficiency does not lead to more learning gain compared to instruction using written language has been found in various other studies (Borgna et al., 2011; Marschark, et al., 2006; Marschark et al., 2009; Stinson, Elliot, Kelly, & Liu, 2009). According to Knoors and Marschark (2014), these and other studies suggest that "if deaf students are taught by a skilled teacher of the deaf who is aware of their cognitive abilities, the location of the classroom in a regular or separate school and the mode of classroom communication is of lesser importance" (p. 225).

In bilingual education in the Netherlands, it was assumed for a long time that deaf students in primary and secondary education would learn best if sign language was the language of instruction. Given the studies carried out in the United States and the observations of Dutch teachers that the variability of children's proficiency in sign and spoken language has grown, teachers no longer seem sure that the instruction of deaf children in SLN is the sole most effective way of delivering the curriculum. As a consequence, in many schools for the deaf, the language policy has changed, grouping children in classrooms according to the language of instruction they are said to prefer. So, children who were judged by the teacher to be more proficient in sign language are grouped together and receive instruction in SLN, whereas children who are judged to be more proficient in spoken Dutch are also grouped together and receive instruction in either Sign Supported Dutch (SSD) or spoken Dutch. Given the small number of deaf children in schools, clustering is not easy. It often results in classes that are made up of children with varying ages or levels of development. The question then is whether clustering on the basis of assumed language of preference really leads to improved learning. Is there any empirical support for the assumption that, for instance, instruction in SSD promotes learning for children who prefer SSD to a larger extent than instruction in sign language or vice versa?

A study was carried out comparing learning gain in SLN versus SSD in DHH children. This study included 40 children, 26 DHH and 14 hearing. The group of 26 DHH children consisted of 11 boys and 15 girls. Five children were moderate-severely deaf and 21 children profoundly deaf. Sixteen DHH children were unilaterally (14) or bilaterally

(2) implanted, but no data were available about the age of implantation. The chronological ages of the children varied between 7;0 and 12;1 years, with an average of 9;6 years. Nonverbal IQ data were available for 25 out of 26 DHH children, varying between 80 and 120, with a mean of 101 (the national average for hearing children is 100). The remaining child was not intellectually disabled. All children were enrolled in special schools for deaf children with a bilingual education program using SLN and written and spoken Dutch.

The group of 14 hearing children consisted of 6 boys and 8 girls. All hearing children were in mainstream education. Their ages varied between 7;3 and 10;0 years, with an average of 8;6 years. The language preference of the DHH children was determined either by extracting information from the children's files at school or through a questionnaire administered to the teachers. Thirteen DHH children were said to prefer Sign Supported Dutch (SSD) and thirteen children SLN.

A match-mismatch paradigm was used, replicating the study by Marschark et al. (2005) with college students. The materials used in this Dutch study were based on four storybooks that are frequently used in regular and special schools. The stories were about the planet earth, the moon, head lice, and the bat (animal). The stories lasted between 5 and 10 minutes. Each of the stories was recorded on video in spoken Dutch (for the hearing children), SSD (for the DHH children), and SLN (for the DHH children). The average length of the stories was 5.8 minutes for spoken Dutch, 7.0 minutes for SSD, and 9.5 minutes for SLN. The Dutch, SSD, and SLN versions of each story were told by a very experienced, fully certified sign language interpreter who had been working with deaf children for more than 20 years.

For each of the stories, 10 multiple-choice questions were developed as test items for the pre- and post-test. To minimize the impact of large differences in the pre-test on the amount of knowledge that hearing and DHH children could actually acquire, information in the stories was constructed in ways that most children would not have this information available as prior knowledge. An example of one of the questions is "Question: What is the smallest continent? Answers: A. Australia, B. The Netherlands, C. Oceania, and D. Africa." In all, 40 multiple-choice questions were developed, 10 for each story. The hearing children received all four stories in spoken Dutch. The DHH children received two stories in SLN and two stories in SSD.

Children were tested individually in two sessions of approximately 45 minutes. In each session, two stories, two pre-tests, and two post-tests were administered. On the first day, half of the DHH children started with a story in SSD, followed by a story in SLN. On the second day, the same group of DHH children started with a story in SLN, followed by a story in SSD. For the other half of the children, the order in which the stories were administered was the other way around.

**Table 11.1 Percentages of Correct Scores of DHH and Hearing Students**

|  | Preferred modality | | | Non-preferred modality | | |
| --- | --- | --- | --- | --- | --- | --- |
|  | Pre-test | Post-test | Learning gain | Pre-test | Post-test | Learning gain |
| Hearing students | 31.79 | 67.68 | 52.34 | x | x | x |
| DHH students | 32.50 | 58.45 | 38.35 | 26.54 | 54.23 | 36.93 |

The actual scores of the children are listed in Table 11.1. Learning gains were defined as the differences between children's scores on the pre-test and post-test (post-test score – pre-test score) as a function of the margin available for learning ((100 – pre-test score) * 100). In other words, a child's learning gain was defined as: "Learning gain = ((post-test score – pre-test score) / (100 – pre-test score)) * 100."

The learning gains of hearing children were significantly higher than the learning gains of DHH children. Hearing children had a mean learning gain of 52% of the test items, whereas DHH children obtained a gain of 38% of the test items in their preferred modality and 37% in their non-preferred modality.

The learning gains of the DHH children in the modality they preferred and the learning gains in the modality they did not prefer did not differ significantly. Furthermore, in line with the findings of Marschark et al. (2005) obtained with DHH college students, the mean learning gains of DHH children in SLN (37.34% of all items) were equally high in comparison to the mean learning gains of DHH children in SSD (37.94% of all items).

The finding that DHH children learned as much in SLN as in SSD does not come as a complete surprise given previous studies in the United States. Those studies, however, involved college students, while we obtained these results for DHH children in primary education. One possible explanation might be that the stories in SLN and SSD were not different enough, because of the overlap in sign vocabulary and, to the extent that sign language grammar can be combined with spoken Dutch, in grammatical structures. An alternative explanation might be that the sign language proficiency of these students is simply not good enough in order to be able to extract sufficient information from complex sign language grammar. This last alternative seems not implausible given the problems of deaf children with hearing parents in acquiring SLN, even if they are placed in bilingual programs (e.g., Hermans, Knoors, & Verhoeven, 2009; Hermans, Ormel, & Knoors, 2010). Ensuring qualitatively good sign language input seems to be a serious problem for hearing parents and hearing teachers (Knoors & Marschark, 2012). For these parents and teachers, SLN is a foreign language that they have to master. Although research is surprisingly limited, there are indications that the actual proficiency that parents and teachers reach in sign language often is rather limited. This may be a consequence of a lack of sign language training, but it should also be acknowledged that many adults simply do not have the language aptitude to learn a foreign language successfully. As a consequence, the input that deaf children receive in sign language is less rich and less well-structured than would normally be the case with first language input.

More remarkable is the present finding that DHH children in this study learned as much in the preferred as in the non-preferred mode of communication. One could argue that their teachers, who are often hearing, simply are not good at identifying the language and modality preference of their students. On the other hand, the groupings were based in part on information taken from assessment files of the children. An alternative explanation could be in line with that of Convertino and colleagues (2009), namely, that the communicative flexibility of deaf students accounts for this result. Clearly, more research is needed, but if this result is found in future replication studies, one would certainly have to question the current policy in Dutch deaf education of grouping students according to their language and modality preference.

## TEACHER ACTIVITIES AND STUDENT ENGAGEMENT

One of the most important activities in the classroom is instruction by the teacher. There are various different approaches to instruction, some more behaviorally oriented (e.g., explicit instruction), others more from a cognitive perspective (constructivist models). Some of these approaches are rather formal sequences of steps and relatively teacher-directed; others emphasize student initiatives and active learning to a greater extent (Orlich, Harder, Trevisan, & Brown, 2012). No one model seems to be ideally suited for all students, all subjects, all phases of knowledge acquisition, and all grades. But central to all approaches is the attempt to enhance students' engagement during the lessons (Marks, 2000). Students' engagement during the learning process is one the major predictors of their social and cognitive outcomes (Finn, 1993), and enhancing students' engagement in the classroom is one of the major challenges for educators (Steinberg, 1996).

Various instructional approaches influence student engagement and learning in students in different manners. Central to behaviorally oriented approaches to instruction is the assumption that direct (explicit) instruction is one of the more effective ways of teaching (Veenman, Denessen, Van Den Oord, & Naafs, 2003). High quality of instruction is associated with establishing high levels of student engagement, resulting in comparatively high levels of achievement. Within this educational approach, the manner in which teachers structure their lessons is, therefore, one of the major research topics (Veenman, 1996, 1998).

Direct instruction is thought to be most effective when teachers go through specific phases during their lessons: daily review of previous content, instruction of new content, guided practice, individual training, reflection, and feedback. In general, instruction time ideally is relatively short, thus not tapping too much into the attention resources of students.

To us, studying teaching activities and student engagement in bilingual programs for deaf students is one way of assessing the quality of instruction in these programs. In our study, five primary school classes with DHH children participated. Four of these classes were located in two special schools for DHH children with bilingual programs. One class was part of the co-enrollment program for DHH and hearing children reported on by Hermans, De Klerk, Wauters, and Knoors (Chapter 16 of this volume). In this program, small groups of DHH children are included in regular classrooms with hearing students. All are co-taught by a teacher of the deaf and a regular teacher. The co-enrollment class was included in the study because we wanted to compare instruction and engagement in both types of educational settings. The number of DHH children in the classes in the special schools varied between four and nine. The children's ages varied between 9;0 and 11;2 years with an average of 10;4 years. The co-enrollment class consisted of 25 hearing students and 3 DHH students, aged 10;9 to 12;0, with an average of 11;0. All three schools involved in this study adhere to the direct instruction approach in their educational philosophy.

To assess the structure of lessons in and DHH children's engagement during the lessons, we administered an observation instrument developed by Roelofs (1993), the COMMIT/GEA. This instrument assesses various aspects of the structuring of lessons. The observation instrument uses a time-sampling method consisting of intervals of 20 seconds. During the first 7 seconds the teacher activity and the engagement of one student are observed. These variables are scored during the next 13 seconds. In the next cycle of 20 seconds, the teacher activity and the engagement of a different student are observed and scored. This cycle is repeated until the lesson is finished.

In general, the COMMIT/GEA instrument identifies two major phases during direct instruction: "instruction to the class" and "individual processing of the instruction." Within each phase, several different teacher activities can be identified. During the phase of "instruction to the class," the teacher activates the children's existing knowledge on a particular subject. She or he subsequently explains the new content to the students and then provides guided practice. During the phase of "individual processing of instruction," the teacher's activities include providing individual help to students, giving feedback to students, exerting control, and preparation of the next lesson. The COMMIT/GEA instrument also contains a category "remaining activities," which consists mainly of procedural activities such as waiting for students to be quiet after a disruption. This category comprised approximately 10% of the time in both the special schools and the co-enrollment program, and was not included in the analyses reported here.

The engagement of students during the lessons was studied by observing their behavior during both phases, following Roelofs, Veenman, and Raemakers (1994). We focused on only one aspect of student engagement: "time-on-task." Roelofs et al. considered this aspect of student engagement as the core component of student engagement and learning in the classroom. The students' behavior was scored as "engaged" when they paid attention to their teacher in the instruction phase (in these instances they were looking at the teacher) or when they were working on their exercises during the individual processing of the instruction. When children were not paying attention, were waiting, or were absent from the classroom (for instance, for speech therapy), their behavior was scored as "not engaged."

In each of the five classes, five lessons on mathematics were observed. The lessons lasted between 15 and 55 minutes, with an average of 34 minutes. Half of the lessons were observed and scored by one observer, while the other half of the lessons were observed and scored by two observers to assess inter-observer reliability. Inter-observer reliability was high (Cohen's kappa = 0.89).

In Table 11.2 the results obtained with the COMMIT/GEA instruments are shown for the four classes in the special schools and for the class in the co-enrollment program. Statistical analyses were restricted

Table 11.2 Setting, Teaching Activity, and Students' Involvement

|  | Special | Co-enrollment |
|---|---|---|
| Teacher activities |  |  |
| Instruction to the class | 23% | 51% |
| 1. Activating existing knowledge | 4% | 2% |
| 2. Instruction new knowledge | 10% | 28% |
| 3. Guided exercises | 9% | 21% |
| Individual processing of instruction | 77% | 49% |
| 1. Individual help | 41% | 30% |
| 2. Feedback | 9% | 8% |
| 3. Control | 11% | 7% |
| 4. Organization | 16% | 4% |
| Students' involvement |  |  |
| Task oriented | 63% | 80% |
| Not task oriented | 11% | 7% |
| Waiting/procedural activities | 9% | 8% |
| Not present in the classroom | 17% | 5% |

to the results obtained in the four classes in special schools and the co-enrollment class.

In general, there was less instruction to the whole class in special schools and more individual help and exerted control during the individual processing of instruction. Furthermore, DHH children were less task-oriented, but mainly because they were out of class more (for instance, for speech therapy).

Although the present results may not be generalized to all bilingual schools for the deaf in the Netherlands, the data indicate that it is fruitful to study teaching activities in relation to students' engagement. As pointed out earlier, all three schools involved in this study adhere to the direct instruction approach in their educational philosophy. The data from this study reveal that teachers in the two special schools spent considerably less time on the first phase of direct instruction (instruction to the class), in comparison to the teachers in the co-enrollment program. Although the classes are much smaller in size in special schools, the students' skills in a particular subject vary widely. Teachers may find it difficult to attune their instruction to the levels of the students in their class. They may have to resort to individualized instruction due to the different skill levels of students. Alternatively, the small class sizes in special schools may tempt teachers into a more individualized approach in order to provide their students with maximum access to the instruction.

## STUDENTS' PERCEPTIONS OF QUALITY OF INSTRUCTION

Finally, we also studied the DHH students' perceptions of the quality of instruction, including their relationships with their teachers. This is an approach that may offer significant insights into quality of instruction. Castelijns (1996) stated the following about students' perceptions:

> If one talks with students and is sincerely interested in their views about what school means to them, one will soon notice that they have outspoken, remarkably well articulated views. When students talk about school they prove to possess sharp observation skills and balanced ways of expression. Even more so, the views that students share provide schools with valuable and applicable information. (p. 5, our translation)

Quality of instruction is a concept that includes many aspects (Hendriks, Doolaard, & Bosker, 2001; Knoors & Hermans, 2010). Obviously, didactic characteristics of instruction are an important aspect, but task adaptation, classroom climate, relationships with peers, and relationships with teachers are also important. We wanted to study the students' perceptions of these various aspects of the instructional context, but were particularly interested in the perceived quality of teacher-student relationships, since the quality of these relationships is important for achievement at various levels of education, starting as early as preschool (Hamre & Pianta, 2001; Pianta & Steinberg, 1992). Greater closeness between teachers and students and better contact positively influence student motivation, irrespective of ethnic background or gender (Den Brok, Van Tartwijk, Wubbels, & Veldman, 2010). When students are more motivated, in turn, they attend more to instruction and as a result learn more. Teacher-student relationships are influenced by factors such as gender and ethnicity (Jerome, Hamre, & Pianta, 2009).

A high quality of teacher-student relationship is even more important for students with disabilities. These students often have experienced negative parent-child interactions, resulting in behavior problems. They are at risk for maladjustment at school and for developing mental health problems later in life. For these students, positive teacher-student relationships could be a protective factor for their emotional and social development. Unfortunately, studies repeatedly show that teacher-student relationships are valued as less positive by students with disabilities compared to non-disabled students (Eisenhower, Baker, & Blacher, 2007; Lapointe, Legault, & Batiste, 2005; Murray & Greenberg, 2001).

There is only limited research into the quality of teacher-student relationships in deaf education (for an overview, see Knoors & Marschark, 2014). There is some evidence that deaf college students prefer being taught by deaf teachers, partly because they think these teachers are more effective in their teaching (Lang, Dowaliby, & Anderson, 1994; Lang, McKee, & Conner, 1993), but those assumptions have not been validated. In one study, the same pattern was found in deaf children in primary and secondary education, but the researchers could not find an association between the hearing status of teachers of the deaf and the academic achievement of deaf students (Roberson & Serwatka, 2000).

Wolters, Knoors, Cillessen, and Verhoeven (2012) studied peer and teacher-student relationships cross-sectionally in 759 grade 6 (672 hearing, 87 deaf) and 840 grade 7 (736 hearing, 104 deaf) students in the Netherlands. In grade 6, 35 deaf students were in mainstream and 52 in special education, whereas in grade 7, 42 deaf students were in mainstream and 62 in special education. Students rated their relationships with their teachers and their well-being on two six-item scales. All items had three response options. The scales were taken from the Dutch School Questionnaire (Smits & Vorst, 1990). Teacher support turned out to be an important predictor of well-being in both grade 6 and 7 in special education, but only in grade 6 (so only in primary education) of mainstream education. Deaf and hearing students in mainstream education in general experienced more teacher support than those in bilingual deaf education.

In our study we included 145 DHH children and 355 hearing children. The group of 145 DHH students consisted of 80 boys and 63 girls. All these students were enrolled in special schools for deaf children with a bilingual education program, using both Sign Language of the Netherlands (SLN) and (spoken and written) Dutch. Their ages varied between 8;2 and 13;3 years, with an average age of 10;9 years. The hard-of-hearing children (32) all had hearing aids, while most of the deaf children (87 out of 113) had cochlear implants. No data were available on the age of implantation. All judgments of the DHH students are about hearing teachers. The group of 353 hearing children consisted of 181 boys and 172 girls. All hearing children were enrolled in a regular school. Their ages varied between 8;0 and 12;1 years, with an average of 10;8 years.

For the purpose of the present study we administered an adapted version of the ZEBO (Zelf Evaluatie Basis Onderwijs: Self Evaluation Primary Education) developed by Hendriks and Bosker (2003) to the DHH and hearing students. The ZEBO consists of several questionnaires that broadly assess the quality of education as perceived by students, teachers, and school directors (Hendriks, Doolaard, & Bosker, 2001). We administered the questionnaire that was developed to assess students' perceptions of the quality of education.

This questionnaire consists of 70 statements divided over seven scales. For each statement (e.g., "I like my teacher"), students had to indicate to what extent they agree with the statement (1 = Disagree; 2 = Neutral; 3 = Agree). The first scale is achievement pressure. We grouped the items of this scale into three subcategories: pressure felt by the child, positive encouragement by the teacher, and negative feedback on the quality of student work. The second scale addresses both teacher-student relationship and perceived teacher support. The third scale focuses on didactics. We grouped the items of this scale into the following categories: the structuring of lessons and the effectiveness of explanations. The fourth scale deals with peer relationships. The items of this scale were categorized under the headings "acceptance by peers" and "quantity of social relations." Task adaptation is the fifth scale. Items were grouped into two categories: the difficulty level of classroom tasks and the amount of redundancy. The sixth scale is time for task, and the seventh scale is labeled classroom climate. The items of this scale are grouped as addressing either level of quietness or management skills of teachers.

As the original ZEBO instrument consisted of grammatically complex sentences judged to be too difficult for DHH children in primary education to comprehend (in both Dutch and in SLN), the ZEBO was adapted. Overall, we made two types of adjustments. First, the grammatical complexity of most of the sentences was reduced, often by splitting up grammatically complex sentences. For instance, the sentence

"When I do not understand what the teachers says, I have to wait for a long time before the teacher helps me" was changed to "I do not understand what the teachers says. Then I have to wait for a long time before he helps me." Second, infrequent words were replaced by more frequent alternatives. The written version of the ZEBO was administered to hearing children, whereas the version administered to DHH students (Sign Supported Dutch, SLN, or written Dutch) was picked in consultation with the students' teachers.

Table 11.3 lists the average scores of the DHH and hearing students on the various scales of the ZEBO and their subcategories. Only differences in scores on the scales themselves, not on the subcategories, were tested statistically. On six of the seven scales, the judgments of DHH students differed significantly from those of their hearing peers. Only the results of these scales are reported here.

DHH students felt significantly more achievement pressure than their hearing peers. More specifically, they felt more pressure in terms of their workload at school, they experienced more negative feedback from the teacher on the quality of their work, and experienced less positive encouragement. Teacher-student relationships were valued

Table 11.3 Students' Perceptions about Quality of Instruction

| Scale/category | DHH students | Hearing students |
|---|---|---|
| 1. Achievement pressure | 2.45 | 2.27** |
| Felt by the child | 2.59 | 2.28 |
| Positive encouragement by teacher | 2.37 | 2.50 |
| Negative feedback on quality of work | 2.37 | 1.89 |
| 2. Teacher-student relationship | 2.50 | 2.64** |
| Relationship | 2.42 | 2.58 |
| Support | 2.54 | 2.68 |
| 3. Didactics | 2.47 | 2.37** |
| Structuring of lessons | 2.41 | 2.21 |
| Effectiveness of explanation | 2.55 | 2.63 |
| 4. Peer relationships | 2.49 | 2.65** |
| Acceptance by peers | 2.50 | 2.61 |
| Quantity of social relations | 2.48 | 2.68 |
| 5. Task adaptation | 1.93 | 1.92 ns |
| The difficulty level of classroom tasks | 1.94 | 1.83 |
| Amount of redundancy | 1.89 | 2.16 |
| 6. Time for task | 2.00 | 2.23** |
| 7. Classroom climate | 2.08 | 2.00* |
| Level of quietness | 2.09 | 2.08 |
| Management skills of teachers | 2.08 | 1.93 |

*$p < .05$, **$p < .01$

significantly lower by DHH students compared to hearing students. The relationship itself and the level of support by teachers were judged less positively.

The didactics of teachers were scored significantly lower by DHH students than by hearing students. Although DHH students perceived their lessons to be more structured in comparison to hearing students, at the same time they rated their teachers' abilities in explaining the content lower than hearing students did. This seems to confirm the less positive evaluation of teacher support on the teacher-student relationship scale.

DHH students rated peer relationships significantly lower than their hearing counterparts. Both peer acceptance and quantity of social relations were scored less positively.

Time for task was perceived to be significantly less by DHH students, meaning that they thought they had less time to complete tasks. At the same time, classroom climate was rated significantly higher by DHH students, due to higher judgments of classroom management of teachers by these students.

In summary, with respect to the classroom as a social entity, DHH students valued their relationships with their deaf peers and with their teachers less than hearing students did. Focusing on the classroom as instruction environment, DHH students experienced less time for tasks, more classroom management but less support and less effective explanations by their teachers, and thus they rated achievement pressure higher than hearing students.

The results therefore seem to reveal two clear and consistent patterns. On the one hand, the less positive relationships that DHH students, compared to hearing students, experience with their (hearing) teachers seem to be reflected in experiencing less positive encouragement and more negative judgments. On the other hand, the higher management skills of DHH students' teachers seem to be reflected in more structured lessons, but at the same time instruction was seen to be characterized by less effective explanations, less time on task, and, maybe as a consequence, more difficult classroom tasks and more achievement pressure. Why is it that DHH students in these Dutch bilingual schools are less satisfied with instruction and social relations than hearing students are? One would expect that bilingual deaf education would be an ideal educational environment, given the fact that the most accessible language for most DHH students, sign language, is used and that there are many DHH peers. All teachers in this study, however, were hearing. It is tempting to conclude that this is all about mismatches in hearing status and lack of sensitivity and responsiveness due to communication difficulties, the implication being that results would be more positive in the case of deaf teachers of the deaf. However, alternative interpretations should not be overlooked. The results we obtained may also be a reflection of differences between DHH and hearing students in metacognitive skills or of differences in characteristics of special versus general education. Some studies have pointed out that DHH students in special education in the Netherlands, thus in bilingual deaf schools, have typically more additional learning or mental health problems than those in regular schools (Coppens, Tellings, Van der Veld, Schreuder, & Verhoeven, 2012; Kouwenberg, Rieffe, Theunissen, & Oosterveld, 2012). Clearly, more research is needed to uncover factors that might be responsible for the relatively negative judgments of DHH students in bilingual education.

## QUALITY OF INSTRUCTION AND DEAF EDUCATION

The studies we reported in this chapter were not designed to generally evaluate bilingual deaf education. We did not compare achievement data of DHH students in bilingual programs with those of students in auditory-oral programs in the past. Nor did we compare programs of deaf education in a controlled study, distributing students to the conditions randomly. Even if we wanted to accomplish this, it would have led to an impossible mission. First, methods of education are strongly intertwined with educational settings, for example, bilingual programs being almost synonymous with special education and monolingual programs with mainstream education. Second, randomized distribution of deaf students to programs would clearly be inappropriate and unethical. This does not mean, however, that the results obtained are of no importance to those involved in bilingual deaf education. Simply put, those who expected bilingual deaf education to close the gap in achievement between deaf and hearing children are clearly proven wrong by Dutch achievement data. Our results concerning academic achievement of DHH students in bilingual programs in the Netherlands presented in this chapter indicate that, on average, they learn approximately half the amount of what hearing students learn in a year. This remaining gap is confirmed by recent research on the effects of bilingual deaf education in other countries (Hendar, 2009; Rydberg et al., 2009; see Swanwick, Hendar, Dammeyer, Kristoffersen, Salter, & Simonsen, Chapter 12 of this volume).

The question, of course, may be raised as to whether it is realistic to expect DHH students to achieve similarly to hearing students. The impact of congenital or early deafness on development in general and language development in particular is profound. And the most accessible language to DHH students, a sign language, is not the language of most (95%) of their parents, thus leading to varying delays in accessible first language input. Furthermore, research in the Netherlands seems to indicate that deaf students in special deaf education, and thus in bilingual programs, have considerably more developmental challenges than deaf and hearing peers in mainstream education. Still, it may be feasible to compare their achievements with those of typically developing hearing students in regular schools, as long as only students without additional disabilities are included and comparisons are characterized by careful and correct control of potential differences between deaf and hearing learners. Given the complexity of all these issues, it seems wise to be cautious with interpretations of differences.

But this is only part of the story. Our research also indicates that the quality of instruction in bilingual schools of the deaf is less than hoped for in a number of aspects. Student engagement is negatively influenced by pull-out activities such as individual speech therapy; teacher support is judged to be less in quality; and teacher-student relationships are valued lower by students than one might wish. All this may negatively influence the academic achievement of deaf students in bilingual programs. The results of our experiments also question the validity of the assumption that because of its accessibility for DHH students, SLN is also the most effective language of instruction. More flexibility with respect to the choice of language of instruction in bilingual deaf education and an increased focus on other factors (e.g., didactic techniques) that might contribute to learning by deaf students might be a wise way to move forward (see Knoors & Marschark, 2012).

At the same time, the relationship of deaf students with their teachers definitely requires more attention, as does the enhancement of teachers' sensitivity and responsiveness in teaching their students. Furthermore, our results also point out that paying specific attention to teacher training and to on-the-job coaching of teachers to the didactic aspects of teaching is not a luxury, but a necessity (see Wauters & De Klerk, Chapter 10 of this volume). If we want education of DHH students in general, and the complex bilingual deaf education in particular, to be successful in bringing about proper academic achievement in DHH students, focusing on the long-lasting question of language choice seems simply not enough. It might even distract us from the rather more important questions, those directly related to quality of instruction.

## REFERENCES

Borgna, G., Convertino, C., Marschark, M., Morrison, C., & Rizzolo, K. (2011). Enhancing deaf students' learning from sign language and text: Metacognition, modality, and the effectiveness of content scaffolding. *Journal of Deaf Studies and Deaf Education, 16,* 79–100.

Castelijns, J. (1996). *Beelden van bekwaamheid: Een onderzoek naar de implementatie en effecten van het programma Responsieve instructie voor leerkrachten in groep 1 en 2 van de basisschool* [Images of competence: A study into the implementation and effects of the program Responsive instruction for teachers in kindergarten]. Doctoral dissertation, University of Utrecht, the Netherlands.

CBS. (2013). Retrieved on April 25, 2013, from www.cbs.nl.
Coppens, K. M., Tellings, A., Van der Veld, W., Schreuder, R., & Verhoeven, L. (2012). Vocabulary development in children with hearing loss: The role of child, family, and educational variables. *Research in Developmental Disabilities*, 33(1), 119–128.
Convertino, C. M., Marschark, M., Sapere, P., Sarchet, T., & Zupan, M. (2009). Predicting academic success among deaf college students. *Journal of Deaf Studies and Deaf Education*, 14, 324–343.
Creemers, B. P. M. (1994). *The effective classroom*. London: Cassell.
Den Brok, P., Tartwijk, J., Wubbels, T., & Veldman, I. (2010). The differential effect of the teacher-student interpersonal relationship on student outcomes for students with different ethnic backgrounds. *British Journal of Educational Psychology*, 80(2), 199–221.
Eisenhower, A. S., Baker, B. L., & Blacher, J. (2007). Early student-teacher relationships of children with and without intellectual disability: Contributions of behavioral, social, and self-regulatory competence. *Journal of School Psychology*, 45, 363–383.
Finn, J. D. (1993). *School engagement and students at risk*. US Department of Education, Office of Educational Research and Improvement, National Center for Education Statistics.
Hamre, B. K., & Pianta, R. C. (2001). Early teacher-child relationships and the trajectory of children's school outcomes through eight grade. *Child Development*, 72(2), 625–638.
Hendar, O. (2009). *Goal fulfillment in school for the deaf and hearing impaired*. Härnösand, Sweden: The National Agency for Special Needs Education and Schools.
Hendriks, M. A., Doolaard, S., & Bosker, R. J. (2001). School self-evaluation in the Netherlands: Development of the ZEBO-instrumentation. *Prospects*, 31(4), 503–518.
Hendriks, M. A., & Bosker, R. (2003). *ZEBO instrument voor zelf-evaluatie in het basisonderwijs* [ZEBO instrument for self-evaluation in primary education]. Enschede, Netherlands: Twente University Press.
Hermans, D., Knoors, H., & Verhoeven, L. (2009). Assessment of sign language development: The case of deaf children in the Netherlands. *Journal of Deaf Studies and Deaf Education*, 15, 107–119.
Hermans, D., Ormel, E., & Knoors, H. (2010). On the relation between the signing and reading skills of deaf bilinguals. *International Journal of Bilingual Education and Bilingualism*, 13(2), 187–199.
Jerome, E., Hamre, B., & Pianta, R. (2009). Teacher-child relationships from kindergarten to sixth grade: Early childhood predictors of teacher-perceived conflict and closeness. *Social Development*, 18, 915–945.
Kouwenberg, M., Rieffe, C., Theunissen, S. C., & Oosterveld, P. (2012). Pathways underlying somatic complaints in children and adolescents who are deaf or hard of hearing. *Journal of Deaf Studies and Deaf Education*, 17(3), 319–332.
Knoors, H. (2007). Educational responses to varying objectives of parents of deaf children: A Dutch perspective. *Journal of Deaf Studies and Deaf Education*, 12(2), 243–253.
Knoors, H., & Fortgens, C. (1995). Het Rotterdamse tweetaligheidsproject: Twee talen voor dove kleuters [The Rotterdam Bilingual Project: Two languages for deaf toddlers]. *Van Horen Zeggen*, 35(1), 4–11.

Knoors, H., & Hermans, D. (2010). Effective instruction for deaf and hard-of-hearing students: Teaching strategies, school settings, and student characteristics. In M. Marschark & P. E. Spencer (Eds.), *The Oxford handbook of deaf studies, language, and education* (vol. 2, pp. 57–71). New York, NY: Oxford University Press.

Knoors, H., & Marschark, M. (2012). Language planning for the 21st Century: Revisiting bilingual language policy for deaf children. *Journal of Deaf Studies and Deaf Education, 17*(3), 291–305.

Knoors, H., & Marschark, M. (2014). *Teaching deaf learners: Psychological and developmental foundations.* New York, NY: Oxford University Press.

Lang, H., McKee, B., & Conner, K. (1993). Characteristics of effective teachers: A descriptive study of perception of faculty and deaf college students. *American Annals of the Deaf, 138,* 252–259.

Lang, H. G., Dowaliby, F. J., & Anderson, H. (1994). Critical teaching incidents: Recollection of deaf students. *American Annals of the Deaf, 132*(2), 119–127.

Lapointe, J. M., Legault, F., & Batiste S. J. (2005). Teacher interpersonal behavior and adolescents' motivation in mathematics: A comparison of learning disabled, average, and talented students. *International Journal of Educational Research, 43*(3), 39–54.

Lindholm-Leary, K. (2005). *Review of research and best practices on effective features of dual language education programs.* Washington, DC: Center for Applied Linguistics.

Marks, H. M. (2000). Student engagement in instructional activity: Patterns in the elementary, middle, and high school years. *American Educational Research Journal, 37*(1), 153–184.

Marschark, M., Sapere, P., Convertino, C., Mayer, C., Wauters, L., & Sarchet, T. (2009). Are deaf students' reading challenges really about reading? *American Annals of the Deaf, 154,* 357–370.

Marschark, M., Sapere, P., Convertino, C., & Pelz, J. (2008). Learning via direct and mediated instruction by deaf students. *Journal of Deaf Studies and Deaf Education, 13,* 446–461.

Marschark, M., Sapere, P., Convertino, C., & Seewagen, R. (2005). Access to postsecondary education through sign language interpreting. *Journal of Deaf Studies and Deaf Education, 10,* 38–50.

Marschark, M., Leigh, G., Sapere, P., Brunham, D., Convertino, C., Stinson, M., Knoors, H., Vervloed, M. P. J., & Noble, W. (2006). Benefits of sign language interpreting and text alternatives for deaf students' classroom learning. *Journal of Deaf Studies and Deaf Education, 11*(4), 421–437

Marzano, R. J. (2003). *What works in schools: Translating research into action.* Alexandria, VA: ASCD.

Marzano, R. J., Pickering, D., & Pollock, J. E. (2001). *Classroom instruction that works.* Alexandria, VA: ASCD.

Murray, C., & Greenberg, M. T. (2001). Relationships with teachers and bonds with school: Social emotional adjustment correlates for children with and without disabilities. *Psychology in the Schools, 38,* 25–41.

Orlich, D. C., Harder, R. J., Callahan, R. C., Trevisan, M. S., & Brown, A. H. (2012). *Teaching strategies: A guide to effective instruction.* Belmont, CA: Wadsworth Publishing.

Pianta, R. C., & Steinberg, M. S. (1992). Teacher-child relationships and the process of adjusting to school. *New Directions for Child Development, 57*, 61–80.
Pianta, R. C., Howes, C., Burchinal, M., Bryant, D., Clifford, R., Early, C., & Barbarin, O. (2005). Features of pre-kindergarten programs, classrooms, and teachers: Do they predict observed classroom quality and child-teacher interactions? *Applied Developmental Science, 9*(3), 144–159.
Rydberg, E., Gellerstedt, L. C., & Danermark, B. (2009). Toward an equal level of educational attainment between deaf and hearing people in Sweden? *Journal of Deaf Studies and Deaf Education, 14*, 312–323.
Roelofs, E. C. (1993). *Teamgerichte nascholing en coaching: Een experimentele studie in scholen met combinatieklassen* [Team directed education: An experimental study of schools with combined classes]. Doctoral dissertation, University of Nijmegen, the Netherlands.
Roelofs, E., Veenman, S., & Raemaekers, J. (1994). Improving instruction and classroom management behaviour in mixed-age classrooms: Results of two improvement studies. *Educational Studies, 20*(1), 105–126.
Roberson, J. L., & Serwatka, T. S. (2000). Student perceptions and instructional effectiveness of deaf and hearing teachers. *American Annals of the Deaf, 153*(3), 328–343.
Scheerens, J., & Bosker, R. (1997). *The foundations of educational effectiveness.* Oxford, UK: Pergamon.
Smits, J. A. E., & Vorst, H. C. M. (1990). *Schoolvragenlijst [School Questionnaire].* Amsterdam, the Netherlands: Harcourt Test Publishers.
Steinberg, L. (1996). *Beyond the classroom: Why school reform has failed and what parents need to do.* New York, NY: Simon and Schuster.
Stinson, M. S., Elliot, L. B., Kelly, R. R., & Liu, Y. (2009). Deaf and hard-of-hearing students' memory of lectures with speech-to-text and interpreting/note taking services. *Special Education, 43*, 45–51.
Stinson, M. S, & Kluwin, T. N. (2011). Educational consequences of alternative school placements. In M. Marschark & P. E. Spencer (Eds.), *The Oxford handbook of deaf studies, language, and education* (vol. 1, 2nd ed., pp. 47–62.). New York, NY: Oxford University Press.
Veenman, S. (1996). Effectieve instructie in het special onderwijs [Effective instruction in special education]. *Speciaal Onderwijs, 66*, 123–131.
Veenman, S. (1998). Leraargeleid onderwijs: Directe instructie [Teacher directed education: Direct instruction]. In J. D. Vermunt & L. Verschaffel (Eds.), *Onderwijzen van kennis en vaardigheden: Onderwijskundig lexicon* [Teaching knowledge and skills: Educational lexicon] (3rd ed., pp. 27–47). Alphen a/d Rijn, the Netherlands: Samson.
Veenman, S., Denessen, E., Van Den Oord, I., & Naafs, F. (2003). Direct and activating instruction: Evaluation of a preservice course. *The Journal of Experimental Education, 71*3), 197–225.
Walberg, H. J. (1984). Improving the productivity of America's schools. *Educational Leadership, 41*(8), 19–27.
Wolters, N., Knoors, H., Cillessen, A., & Verhoeven, L. (2012). Impact of peer and teacher relations on deaf early adolescents' well-being: Comparisons before and after a major school transition. *Journal of Deaf Studies and Deaf Education, 17*(4), 463–482.

# 12

# Shifting Contexts and Practices in Sign Bilingual Education in Northern Europe

## *Implications for Professional Development and Training*

Ruth Swanwick, Ola Hendar, Jesper Dammeyer,
Ann-Elise Kristoffersen, Jackie Salter, and Eva Simonsen

This chapter reviews concepts and approaches in bilingual education for deaf children and proposes changes in thinking and in practice. From a Northern European perspective, we explore how shifts in educational policy and developments in knowledge and technology have changed language learning for deaf children in Norway, Sweden, Denmark, and the United Kingdom. We show how existing language practices necessitate the conceptualization of a new model of learning and deafness that is situated within a global view of language and culture. We also discuss the implications for practice and professional development of a more plural view of language, learning, and deafness that situates deaf children's multimodal and multilingual language development with a contemporary view of bilingualism.

Use of the term "deaf" in this chapter refers to any level of hearing loss significant enough to have an impact on language development and learning. This includes mild, moderate, severe, and profound categories in audiological terms. This term also communicates the cultural and linguistic aspects of deafness. However, as a point of clarification, we note that discussions of bilingual education have hitherto focused largely on severely and profoundly deaf pupils, especially in Nordic contexts.

In discussing a group of countries that have over the last 30 years engaged with the paradigm of bilingual education for deaf children, we present a critical discussion of what has been learned from this shared journey and perspective. Although roundly debated and critiqued, the sign bilingual movement enjoyed a period of creativity and growth during the 1980s and 1990s in each of these countries. The linguistic study of sign languages burgeoned, and the increasing role of sign languages in education spawned the development of innovative teaching practices and materials (Arnesen, Enerstvedt, Høie, & Vonen, 2002; Knight & Swanwick, 2002; Mahshie, 1995; Svartholm, 1993; Vonen, 1997). This cultural view of deafness, language, and learning opened doors and presented new challenges in research and practice and created a buzz in the deaf education community. Scandinavian countries led the way by readily adopting sign languages as an educational entitlement for deaf children, supported by special curricula for bilingual bimodal education (Opplæringslova, 1998; Skolöverstyrelsen, 1983). This inspired other countries, in particular the United Kingdom, which looked to these models for guidance on developing bilingual policy and practice (Swanwick, 2010).

There is no standardized model in Nordic countries that measures this bilingual approach. In each of the settings, however, some general positive effects for deaf children have been reported. The studies concern issues such as identity and psychosocial well-being (Bagga-Gupta, 2000; Dammeyer, 2010), early development of language and communication (Lewis, 1995; Mahshie, 1995; Smith, Gregory, & Wells, 1997), and improved access to the curriculum and to peer interaction in the classroom as well as support for the development of early literacy skills (Dammeyer, 2013; Kristoffersen & Simonsen, 2012, 2014).

However, we identify concerns about the direction and future of bilingual education for deaf children. Even though deaf children are becoming more bilingual, and indeed multilingual, current discourses of language and deafness still create boundaries around language pedagogy that are neither authentic nor helpful for developing practice. In practical terms, deaf children are able to move across language borders and boundaries, but languages policies are not moving with them (and do not seem fluid enough to do so). For example, many deaf children switch between sign and spoken languages in their everyday lives in different contexts for different purposes. They engage in what we can call "translanguaging" by mixing and switching modalities, but language policies do not account for this flexibility of language in use. Further, deaf children's increasingly sophisticated access to the sounds of speech means that more and more deaf children have access to one or two spoken languages outside the school context, even though they may be using sign language at school for access to the curriculum. Language policies that place delineations between sign and spoken language do not properly reflect or enable practitioners to plan for the learning needs of these multilingual and bimodal learners.

We propose a need to look again at bilingual education for deaf children in the light of a growing knowledge base, a global inclusion context, and fast-moving developments in technology. To this end we provide a synthesis of what has been learned from our common and distinct experiences of bilingual education in Denmark, Norway, Sweden, and the United Kingdom. We explore ways of reframing this approach and the implications for research, practice, and professional development.

## THE JOURNEY TO BILINGUAL EDUCATION

During the 1980s, ideas about educating deaf children bilingually began to develop in each of these national contexts. This was against the background of concerns about deaf children's attainments within traditional approaches (Conrad, 1979; Widel, 1993). These concerns coincided with growing worldwide research demonstrating sign languages as naturally evolving rule-governed languages that share similarities with each other and with other spoken languages (Brennan & Colville, 1984; Kyle & Woll, 1985). This prompted the recognition of sign language as the primary language for deaf children with severe and profound deafness in Denmark, Norway, and Sweden, with a particular role for special schools as bilingual educational environments in the 1980s. New knowledge and a growing acceptance of bilingualism as a strength, not a hindrance, in the learning context raised the visibility of sign language in education and research as well as in the media.

In Sweden, Norway, and Denmark, the concept of bilingual education as a legal right and individual entitlement drove legislative changes and curriculum transformation that fully engaged parents of deaf children (Arnesen et al., 2002; Svartholm, 1993; Vonen, 1997). The terminology to describe language provision was used differently in each national context, but the educational goal in each case was to provide a bilingual and bicultural education for deaf children to ensure early language acquisition and equal access to the curriculum (Ministry of Education, 1991; Opplæringslova, 1998; SFS 1980, 64).

In each of these countries, curricula and syllabi were adapted to sign language as the language of education for deaf children. In Norway, the right to bilingual bimodal tuition (Opplæringslova, 1998, Chapter 2, Section 2–6) was accompanied by the introduction of a national separate bilingual curriculum for deaf students (Vonen, 2007). Any deaf child in his or her local school was entitled to a bilingual, bimodal education. In Sweden, special schools for deaf children became officially bilingual in 1981. Similarly in Denmark, changes in the early 1980s resulted in legislative reform in 1991, making access to sign language in schools a legal entitlement (Lewis, 1994; Ministry of Education, 1991; Widel, 1993). To implement these changes, teachers were trained to use sign language and to teach according to the new curricula, and sign language courses for parents were established in Nordic countries. For example, in Norway parents are offered a 40-week sign language training program over a 16-year period, which provides accommodation and travel expenses and compensation for loss of wages. This extensive and expensive program has proved to be very successful, according to an extensive external evaluation report (Rambøll, 2011). Parents state that they have been able to acquire sign language competence sufficient to support their children in their homework and to communicate with them in a way that enables family members to participate on an equal level.

In the United Kingdom, developments were not on the same national scale as in Scandinavia, as they were not supported by language legislation or curricular change. However, bilingual education developed rapidly in some regions, as teachers felt empowered through having a language that they could use to deliver the curriculum. These developments were supported by national practitioner and researcher groups that worked together to create a definition of sign bilingualism and guidelines for practice (Pickersgill & Gregory, 1998). A Teacher of the Deaf Program was established at the University of Leeds to train and support teachers to work with bilingual pupils. This activity provoked a lively period of new research and development work in deaf education in the United Kingdom (Gregory & Swanwick, 2012; Knight & Swanwick, 2002).

Without legislative impetus, bilingual provision developed sporadically rather than systematically in the United Kingdom across all types of mainstream and special school provision. By contrast, in Norway, Sweden, and Denmark, the entitlement to bilingual education functioned as a substantial claim for the maintenance of separate schools for deaf students, as the only way of offering bilingual educational environments for the fulfillment of this legal right. This effectively divided deaf children into two language groups in terms of either language preference or audiological criteria. In the case of Norway, parents were offered bilingual education for their children, in special schools for the deaf as well as in mainstream education. Still, parent guidance agencies, both in the medical and the educational field, tended to present parents with an obligation to make a choice between spoken or signed language for communication with their child (Simonsen, Kristoffersen, & Hjulstad, 2009a).

In Sweden and Denmark, severely and profoundly deaf pupils were entitled to bilingual education in special schools, and those with unilateral, mild, and moderate hearing loss were educated in their local schools through spoken language or in "center schools" (mainstream schools with units resourced for deaf children). With the introduction of sign language as a subject for hearing pupils in primary, secondary, and adult education in 1995 in Sweden, sign language shifted from being a method of communication only for deaf pupils in special schools to being one of many languages used in Sweden at large (SOU 2006:54, p. 63).

## CURRENT ISSUES

The shaping of provision and separate grouping of children in Norway, Denmark, and Sweden seems to have allowed boundaries between languages and language approaches to occur. A parallel issue emerged in the United Kingdom as bilingual education became established within some schools and services. As confidence grew in the use of British Sign Language (BSL) in education, the role of spoken language development became somewhat eclipsed in educational language planning. The conceptualization of the sign bilingual model (at that time) emphasized sign and written modalities as the pathways to language competency (Svartholm, 1995, 2010). This meant that the development of spoken language pathways was given less of a focus in policy and practice (see, for example, Hansen, 1990; Heiling, 1995; Johnson, Liddell, & Erting, 1989; Mahshie, 1995).

The emergence of these boundaries around language, policy, and approach actually works against a concept of bilingual education by constraining language choices in educational provision, rather than opening up bilingual and bicultural educational environments for all. For example, language planning in a sign bilingual language environment might not include enough spoken language exposure for some pupils' developing bilingual skills, and equally, the lack of access to sign language in an auditory/oral environment might inhibit some deaf pupil's curriculum understanding. This separation is inflexible and does not reflect how children develop and use languages in their daily lives, or how they make transitions between languages. It is also "undemocratic," as it removes true language choice from children, placing it in the hands of policymakers.

### The Potential of Technologies

Since the 1990s, cochlear implants have revolutionized the audiological management for children with a profound hearing loss (see Walker & Tomblin, Chapter 6 of this volume). At the same time, the development of digital technologies has transformed hearing aids, and the range of auditory implants (middle ear implants, bone anchored hearing aids, and brainstem implants) has greatly improved access to audition for different levels and types of hearing loss. In addition, the development of screening and diagnostic techniques has resulted in the introduction of newborn hearing screening programs, allowing congenitally deaf babies to be identified very shortly after birth. Further developments in the field have enabled audiologists to successfully fit hearing aids and cochlear implants to very young children, thus enabling their access to audition during the first year of life (Archbold, 2010; Tetzchner, 2012). Although cochlear implants have benefited many profoundly deaf children, including those with complex and additional needs

(Edwards, 2007; Johnson, DesJardin, Barker, Quittner, & Winter, 2008; Meinzen-Derr, Wiley, Grether, & Choo, 2010), there do remain deaf children for whom implants are not affording the expected benefits. Research and educational provision must continue to seek to understand and meet the needs of these pupils (Danielsson & Hendar, 2010; Punch & Hyde, 2011).

Such technologies are now giving profoundly deaf children increased opportunities and potential for the development of spoken language(s) and, of course, are changing their language profiles. Studies in the United Kingdom show that particularly after early implantation, children will reduce their use of sign language, even though they may pick it up again later in life (Watson, Archbold, & Nikolopoulos, 2006). More studies of this nature are needed that address issues related to the language transitions that children make.

A greater understanding of nuances and variability of language use would seem to be essential for language planning in the educational context so that practitioners are able to take full account of the changing roles of sign languages and sign support systems in deaf children's lives. Such an approach would look across deaf children's lifelong language abilities, rather than separately at sign language or spoken language development at a very young age (often the case in CI studies; Kunnskapssenteret, 2011; Percy-Smith et al., 2006; Tortzen, 2008). A continuum of language provision all in one place would alleviate the tension experienced by parents trying to make either/or choices between spoken language and sign language approaches; such choices require that they predict the language needs and development trajectories of their deaf children (Simonsen, Kristoffersen, & Hjulstad, 2009b). We have much to learn from families of deaf children who speak of the "communication journey" that takes place after implantation (Wheeler, Archbold, Hardie, & Watson, 2009), rather than conceptualizing language and language approaches as categorical or bounded systems.

The pragmatic and responsive approach that deaf children and their families adopt toward the use of sign and spoken language informs us of the need to move beyond policy-driven distinctions between spoken and sign language use and to look for a more plural view of language and learning. This plurality is growing apace as assistive technologies provide deaf individuals with equal and personal access to information, global communication, and social networking (Breivik, 2005; Valentine & Skelton, 2008). A plural view of languages throughout deaf education (not framed as unique to a bilingual perspective) would bring about changes to our knowledge base of deaf children's languages and cultures and would provoke the development of tools to capture the language demographics of our populations, as well as diverse individual language profiles. This would change our approach to language planning for schools and services and individuals to include attention to all multilingual and multimodal skills and to provide pathways for children to make short- and long-term transitions between languages for different purposes at different times in their lives. Deaf children and their parents would be met with the opportunities to develop spoken and sign languages in one space, where movement across and between languages, or translanguaging, is seen as the norm and part of a life-long repertoire of language skills.

**The Inclusion Agenda**

The rapid development of technology coincided with a global inclusion agenda articulated in the Salamanca Agreement of 1994 and an impetus to educate more deaf children in mainstream. Societies' aspiration for inclusion has reshaped deaf education, which hitherto was being organized around the choice of language approach (auditory/oral, total communication, or bilingual). The trend in these four countries is now moving toward a reduction in special schools and increased inclusive provision for deaf pupils, either individually or as part of a resourced center within a mainstream school. In Norway, Denmark, and Sweden, bilingual education was located mainly in the special schools, which was probably the only way to implement the reform at that time. A consequence was limited use of sign language in other settings, turning the schools for the deaf into "sign-language islands."

In Denmark, there are today three special schools for the deaf that offer sign language as a part of education. Of the 100 deaf pupils attending these schools, the majority have additional or complex needs. Almost all children with cochlear implants attend ordinary classes in mainstream schools or are part of small groups in "center schools" where support in sign language is restricted. There are no official statistics on how many deaf children there are in the Danish public schools.

In Sweden, there are currently six special schools for the deaf, which offer a bilingual education for approximately 400 pupils, and eight mainstream schools that are technically adapted to deaf pupils. The concept of bilingualism has changed from a sign-written definition to a more pluralistic praxis with sign-written and spoken languages. Sign language for hearing pupils is offered as a subject in these latter schools. This is unique compared to the opportunities that many other countries offer for deaf and hearing pupils. Even though the subject (sign language for hearing children) is not heading toward bilingual competence, it is a very good choice for many pupils. A governmental proposal declares that sign language should be given the same status as any other foreign language in upper secondary education when pupils apply to higher education. If this proposal passes, it will strengthen sign language in Sweden in accordance with the Swedish Language Act (SFS 2009:600) and will give opportunities for cross-language activities for deaf and hearing pupils.

In Norway, the shift has also been away from special schools and classes for the deaf to mainstream education, where the deaf students are placed individually among hearing peers. The number of students in special schools for the deaf has been reduced from about 140 in 2002 to 69 in 2010 (Kunnskapsdepartementet, 2011). The Norwegian parliament has decided to close down the existing state schools for the deaf, except for one school in Trondheim in central Norway.

In the United Kingdom, schools for the deaf have also closed or have become increasingly adapted for deaf children with additional and complex needs. More than 80% of deaf children in the United Kingdom are now educated in mainstream schools, with a small proportion in resourced centres or units within these (Archbold, Nikolopoulos, O'Donoghue, & Lutman, 1998, 2002; Consortium for Research into Deaf Education [CRIDE], 2012). The special schools that do exist offer varied language provision. Some describe themselves as "using an auditory/oral approach" (without the use of sign language), whereas others describe themselves as having a "bilingual philosophy" or offering a broad-based approach (English and BSL) under the umbrella term of "total communication."

The majority of deaf children are now in mainstream education, and it is important that we evaluate the breadth of language support available here. Even though technologies enable more deaf children to access the mainstream curriculum, they may still need some kind of (sign or spoken) language or other visual support for learning. Engaging with the mainstream curriculum language demands, interacting with a number of different teachers every day (in generally poor acoustic conditions), and the increased use of group work represent major learning challenges for these pupils (Archbold & Mayer, 2012; Kristoffersen & Simonsen, 2012).

These changes in patterns of educational placement and developments in technology have not resolved the general issue of underachievement in deaf education. The proportion of deaf pupils who do not reach national goals is still disquieting. There are no differences between the countries in this matter. In the last 6–7 years, attainment data have been collected in the United Kingdom, Norway, and Sweden that confirm international findings showing that even after many educational reforms, a gap in attainment still exists between deaf pupils and their hearing counterparts (Hendar, 2008, 2012; Powers, 1999; Stacey, Fortnum, Barton, & Summerfield, 2006; Thoutenhoofd, 2006; Tymms, Brien, Merrell, Collins, & Jones, 2003).

## CHANGING LANGUAGE APPROACHES

From this shared perspective, we suggest that a review of the concept of bilingual education cannot be done in isolation. It entails a rethink of what we mean by language learning in this field. The lessons that we have learned about language and learning in bilingual education are pertinent to all deaf children: First, the fact that deaf children's language and communication profiles are changing may result in much greater potential for multilingual and multimodal language experience. Second, the educational context has become increasingly focused on inclusive provision, providing a much wider experience of language practices but also presenting language and learning challenges in the classroom. Third, the prevailing issues of underachievement and access to language and learning need to be addressed within a language framework that recognizes the range of language resources that individuals draw on for learning and that is responsive to the transitions that they make between their languages over time and on a daily basis. All three issues require a perspective on language and language support that recognizes the breadth and diversity of language experience. This rethinking will break down boundaries between language policy and practice that have re-emerged and will shift debate around practice to center less on issues of modality and more on diagnosing, understanding, and meeting the changing communication needs of deaf children (Gregory & Swanwick, 2012). New pedagogies are needed that are not lodged with a language approach but which embrace a broader understanding of the linguistic experiences of young deaf people and their families. If we are to develop more differentiated, responsive, flexible, and relevant language approaches that anticipate and respond to deaf children's sign, spoken, and written language(s), we need to develop our knowledge of the wider language practices of deaf children and their families. This information would inform our "language planning" for all deaf children (Knoors & Marschark, 2012).

## A NEW LANGUAGE MODEL?

We suggest looking to a new model of language and deafness that explores the benefits of multilingual and multimodal practices as part of a repertoire of language competences and socially embedded language practices in deaf children's everyday lives (Heller, 2007). This mirrors a shift toward "plurilingualism" in discourses of language learning and pedagogies (Council of Europe, 2007) that recognize the repertoire of communicative resources of individuals as flexible, changing, and transversal repertoires that are bought into play within culturally complex environments (Blackledge & Creese, 2010; Garcia, 2009).

This stepchange in our thinking deconstructs concepts of discrete routes to the mastery of spoken or sign language in isolation and suggests instead a focus on the interrelationship and interactions between sign and spoken languages. This will "democratize" (Little, 2011, p. 392) language education for deaf children by challenging established language constructs and ownership of language approaches that are legitimized in the educational context. We have taken hold of "communication" in our field as the central issue, and perhaps now it is time to think more holistically about language and learning.

**Implications for Research**

This stepchange will require more research about the "language landscape" (Crowe, McLeod, & Ching, 2012) in deaf education. This is important for our developing understanding of deafness and the related language experience and is vital for planning educational support and intervention. Although we know that multilingualism presents very specific issues of identity and language preference for deaf children and their families, there are only a very small number of studies worldwide that have attempted to collect information about these issues (Albertorio, Holden-Pitt, & Rawling, 1999; Arnesen et al., 2008; Crowe et al., 2012; Grimes, Thoutenhoofd, & Byrne, 2007; Türker-Van der Heiden, 2011, 2012).

There are gaps in our knowledge about deaf children's multilingualism, which is increasing because of globalization and technology. Research into deaf children's language experience currently centers on sign language and spoken language development in English-speaking populations, in a mutually exclusive fashion. Missing from this research is attention to the language experience and use of deaf children in less economically developed and non-English speaking counties. Even in English-speaking countries, we lack information about the spoken languages other than English that deaf children and young people increasingly use at home (Cline & Mahon, 2010). In the United Kingdom, for example, we know that 14% of the deaf school population (more that 10,000 children) use more than one spoken language at home, but we do not know what these languages are (CRIDE, 2012). There is similar emerging research in Norway (Türker-Van der Heiden, 2011, 2012). These are significant gaps in our knowledge that need to be explored in order for bilingual deaf education to develop and respond to the multilingual and multimodal potential of deaf children.

We need research that constructs a demographic picture or "language map" of deaf children's cultures and signed and spoken language. Ethnographic work of this nature has begun in some contexts, but our knowledge is very incomplete (Albertorio et al., 1999; Arnesen et al., 2008; Crowe et al., 2012; Grimes et al., 2007). Together with this language demographic research, we also need to develop tools and approaches that accurately describe individual spoken, sign, and bimodal linguistic repertoires. Longitudinal case studies (such as Dammeyer, 2012) or qualitative in-depth studies of deaf children's language development across modalities (such as Cramér-Wolrath, 2013) will contribute to wider understandings of multimodal and multilingual language development and will open up new research agendas for language and learning.

### Implications for Practice

Practically, this new knowledge would provide an internationally relevant framework on which to organize language teaching, learning, and assessment in deaf education. This framework would establish globally shared objectives, standards, pedagogical approaches, and language terminologies. For the classroom, we could expect to see new tools for language assessment and planning, and curricula for teaching all linguistic varieties in deaf education.

In the United Kingdom, practitioners are taking these ideas forward as they review their provision and their approach to "language planning" in response to the issues raised by Knoors and Marschark (2012). A group of bilingual schools and services are looking at the way in which they ensure that language policies and approaches are differentiated and responsive to the increasingly diverse population of deaf children who use sign, spoken, and written languages, and for 15% a spoken language other than English at home. This critical review marks a change in perspective on the roles of sign, spoken, and bimodal language use and a shift in practice toward a new plurilingual view of deaf children's language experience and skills. The outcome of this work thus far suggests that practitioners are already rethinking how deaf children's language experience and use are described and categorized in schools. They express a need to shrug off the straitjacket of language ideologies in deaf education as they conceptualize new approaches to their work. They note the need for flexible and mindful use of a language repertoire that offers spoken, sign, and manually coded forms of English as appropriate for the individual. They describe the tools that they currently have for language assessment and planning as inadequate for the changing and diverse language skills of the population. They are looking instead for ways of profiling all deaf children's multilingual and multimodal skills and the transitions that they make across and between languages.

### Implications for Professional Development

The daily support and long-term management of the complex language issues in deaf education should be addressed by practitioners who are equipped to diagnose and plan individual language and learning programs. This is problematic in contexts where no specific training is required for teaching or supporting deaf children in school. In Norway, for example, some teachers may be trained in special needs education and/or in Norwegian sign language, but this is not mandatory. In Denmark, teachers working with children with hearing impairment often take extra courses in audiology, literacy, general special education, and audio-verbal therapy. There are no formal educational requirements for teachers of the deaf. To support the national and international aims of inclusion, special teacher training in Sweden was replaced in 1990 by special educator training (Mattson & Hansen, 2009). These special educators supervise the teachers in their school, but do not necessarily teach deaf pupils (Bagga-Gupta & Domfors, 2003). These changes have de-skilled practitioners in deaf education to the extent that teacher knowledge of technical aids, sign language, and differentiation strategies cannot be assumed. A qualification study in southern Sweden 2009 predicts that the number of teachers with specific knowledge of deafness and learning will decline in the next 5–10 years (Johnsson, 2009), leaving a depleted resource of specialist and skilled special teachers of the deaf, and the situation is the same in Norway.

In the United Kingdom, the picture is a little more optimistic, as a specialized mandatory teacher of the deaf training is still required. However, not all deaf pupils are supported by qualified teachers of the deaf in the classroom. Teachers of the deaf only account for approximately 47% of the workforce supporting deaf children within education. A further 48% are a variously skilled body of deaf and hearing professionals who teach and support deaf children in preschool and nursery, schools, and colleges, and for whom there is a clear lack of recognized professional training, status, and associated qualifications. They include teaching assistants (TAs), communication support workers (CSWs) and deaf adults (CRIDE, 2012).

The international field of deaf education thus comprises a diverse group of professionals who are variously qualified (or not), working with a heterogeneous population where complex factors impact on learning. Furthermore, there exists a diversely skilled body of professionals who teach and support deaf children in schools and colleges for whom recognized professional status and associated qualifications are lacking.

This variable international picture of professional expectation and a lack of current networks between training institutions are problematic within a field where the development and dissemination of knowledge-based practice is a priority. This could be addressed globally and locally. An internationally established network of researchers and practitioners would provide a forum for the identification of shared professional development priorities. Through collaborative working and sharing of data, this network could develop training techniques and approaches that build on local established expertise but that are globally relevant. Such an initiative may provide avenues for importing knowledge from research into classroom practice in order to improve deaf children's learning and achievement. These are the research and practice outputs that we need in the current educational context, where there is an increasing emphasis on attainment data, accompanied by imposed curriculum initiatives lacking an evidence base, a reduction of professional development opportunities, and a dearth of research into development and training in this field.

At a local level, there are ways of facilitating professional development beyond formal training. For many practitioners, professional development is about questioning, challenging, and developing their own work and engaging with research questions within their working context (Swanwick & Kitchen, 2012, 2013). In the United Kingdom, a number of action research partnerships between practitioners and researchers have been developed to facilitate this. Supported by researchers, practitioners are designing and implementing action research projects to investigate their own questions. This national model of collaborative working has empowered schools and services to take hold of and become part of the research agenda and to recognize their own potential for researching learning issues in a real-world context (Carter & Swanwick, 2012). The unique feature of this work is that it is practitioner-led. The role of the researchers is to sustain the momentum of the activities and lightly "hold the shape" of the projects. Regular Action Research Symposiums provide the forum for dissemination of this work within and beyond the United Kingdom. This way of working with practitioners develops genuine and productive research-practice partnerships and opens up dialogue both nationally and internationally about new ways of envisioning the interface between research and practice.

## SHIFTING CONTEXTS AND PRACTICES: CONCLUSIONS

This chapter has presented perspectives from four Northern European countries that made great strides in developing bilingual education policy and practice in the 1980s and 1990s. This involved a proactive engagement with new ideas and thinking around concepts of deafness, language, and learning. When we first began to describe and teach deaf children as bilingual (or sign bilingual), the focus was on the development of a signed and a spoken language, and the term "bilingual" was new in deaf education. We ask now if that term is adequate to describe the language experience and profiles of deaf children now in our educational systems.

Research and practice in this area has tended to categorize and separate language approaches, rather than take a pluralistic view. We suggest that this has inhibited the development of an integrated research perspective within and across these domains and has led to ideological positions that have polarized policy, practice, and educational discourses across an international stage (Simonsen, 2007; Swanwick, 2010). We argue for a new way of looking that goes beyond discrete questions about the development of one language or the other to connect these questions, looking across deaf children's sign and spoken language (bimodal and bilingual) resources and experiences.

This requires a shift of focus in deaf education away from questions of language policy to questions of language and learning, which ask what language, mix, or mode is appropriate in a specific learning situation. A pluralistic perspective on early language acquisition would ensure that deaf children continue to have opportunities to learn and develop language skills and competencies without restrictions. To take this further, we need to develop our knowledge of deaf children's language practices in the learning context. Practitioners engage with this knowledge on a daily basis as they mediate language policy, practice, and learning issues; professional development and teacher education can therefore focus on these issues. However, alongside this, we need ongoing transaction between research and practice which ensures that the lived language and learning experiences of deaf children are reflected in the policy and research discourses in deaf studies and deaf education.

## REFERENCES

Albertorio, J. R., Holden-Pitt, L., & Rawlings, B. (1999). Preliminary results of the Annual Survey of Deaf and Hard of Hearing Children and Youth in Puerto Rico: The first wave. *American Annals of the Deaf, 144*(5), 386–394.

Archbold, S. (2010). *Deaf education, changed by cochlear implantation?* Nijmegen, Netherlands: Radboud University Nijmegen, University Medical Centre.

Archbold, S. M., Nikolopoulos, T. P., Lutman, M. E., & O'Donoghue, G. M. (2002). The educational settings of profoundly deaf children with cochlear implants compared with age-matched peers with hearing aids: Implications for management. *International Journal of Audiology, 41*(3), 157–161.

Archbold, S., Nikolopoulos, T. P., O'Donoghue, G. M., & Lutman, M. E. (1998). Educational placement of deaf children following cochlear implantation. *British Journal of Audiology, 32*(5), 295–300.

Archbold, S., & Mayer, C. (2012). Deaf education: The impact of cochlear implantation? *Deafness & Education International, 14*(1), 2–15.

Arnesen, K., Enerstvedt, R. T., Engen, E. A., Engen, T., Høie, G., & Vonen, A. M. (2008). The linguistic milieu of Norwegian children with hearing loss. *American Annals of the Deaf, 153*(1), 65–77.

Arnesen, K., Enerstvedt, R. T., Høie, G., & Vonen, A. M. (2002). *Tospråklighet og lesing/skriving hos døve barn: En kartlegging av grunnskoleelever og deres språklige situasjon [Bilingualism and literacy among deaf children in primary school].* Skådalen Publication Series No 16. Oslo, Norway: Skådalen Resource Centre.

Bagga-Gupta, S. (2000). Visual language environments: Exploring everyday life and literacies in Swedish Deaf bilingual schools. *Visual Anthropology Review, 15*, 95–120.

Bagga-Gupta, S., & Domfors, L. (2003). Pedagogical issues in Swedish Deaf education. In L. Monaghan, C. Schmaling, K. Nakamura, & G. Turner (Eds.), *Many ways to be deaf: International and sociocultural variation* (pp. 67–88). Washington, DC: Gallaudet University Press.

Blackledge, A., & Creese, A. (2010). *Multilingualism*. London, UK: Continuum.

Breivik, J. K. (2005). *Deaf identities in the making: Local lives, transnational connections*. Washington, DC: Gallaudet University Press.

Brennan, M., & Colville, M. D. (1984). *Words in hand: A structural analysis of the signs of British Sign Language* (2nd ed.). Edinburgh, UK: Moray House College/Carlisle BDA.

Carter, A., & Swanwick, R. (2012). Action research makes a difference. BATOD Magazine, March edition, 40–44.

Cline, T., & Mahon, M. (2010). Deafness in a multilingual society: A review of research for practice. *Educational and Child Psychology, 27*(2), 41–49.

Conrad, R. (1979). *The deaf school child: Language and cognitive function*. London, UK: Harper & Row.

Council of Europe. (2007). *Common European Framework of Reference for Languages: Learning, teaching, assessment*. Cambridge, UK: Cambridge University Press.

Cramér-Wolrath, E. (2012). Attention interchanges at story-time: A case study from a deaf and hearing twin pair acquiring Swedish sign language in their deaf family. *Journal of Deaf Studies and Deaf Education, 17*(2), 141–162.

Consortium for Research into Deaf Education (CRIDE). (2012). Report on 2012 survey on educational provision for deaf children. Retrieved from The National Deaf Children's Society (NDCS) website: http://www.ndcs.org.uk/professional_support/national_data/uk_education_.html.

Crowe, K., McLeod, S., & Ching, T. Y. C. (2012). The cultural and linguistic diversity of 3-year-old children with hearing loss. *Journal of Deaf Studies and Deaf Education, 17*(4), 421–438.

Dammeyer, J. (2010). Psychosocial development in a Danish population of children with cochlear implants and deaf and hard-of-hearing children. *Journal of Deaf Studies and Deaf Education, 15*, 50–58.

Dammeyer, J. (2012). A longitudinal study of pragmatic language development in three children with cochlear implants. *Deafness and Education International, 14*(4), 217–232.

Dammeyer, J. (2013). Literacy skills among deaf and hard of hearing students and students with cochlear implants in bilingual/bicultural education. *Deafness and Education International*. doi:10.1179/1557069X 13Y.0000000030

Danielsson, B., & Hendar, O. (2010). Cochlear implants—not always enough? BATOD Magazine, September edition, 30–31.

Edwards, L. (2007). Children with cochlear implants and complex needs: A review of outcome research and psychological practice. *Journal of Deaf Studies and Deaf Education, 12*, 258–268.

García, O., & Baetens, B. H. (2009). *Bilingual education in the 21st century: A global perspective*. Malden, MA: Wiley-Blackwell.

Gregory, S., & Swanwick, R. (2012). The sign bilingual movement. BATOD Magazine, March edition, 11–13.

Grimes, M., Thoutenhoofd, E. D., & Byrne, D. (2007). Language approaches used with deaf pupils in Scottish schools: 2001–2004. *Journal of Deaf Studies and Deaf Education, 12*(4), 530–551.

Hansen, B. (1990). Trends in the progress towards bilingual education for deaf children in Denmark In S. Prillwitz, & T. Vollhaber, (Eds.), *Sign language research*

and application: Proceedings of the International Conference on Sign Language Research and Application (pp. 51–62). Hamburg, Germany: Signum Press.
Heiling, K. (1995). *The development of deaf children: Academic achievement levels and social processes*. Hamburg, Germany: Signum.
Heller, M. (2007). *Bilingualism: A social approach*. Basingstoke, UK: Palgrave Macmillan.
Hendar, O. (2008). *Måluppfyllelse för döva och hörselskadade i skolan [Goal fulfillment in school for the deaf and hearing impaired]*. Örebro, Sweden: Specialskole myndigheten.
Hendar, O. (2012). *Elever med hørselshemming i skolen: En kartleggingsundersøkelse om læringsutbytte [Pupils with hearing impairment in school: A study on learning outcomes]. Skådalen Publication series No 32*. Oslo, Norway: Skådalen Resource Centre.
Johnsson, K. (2009). *Kompetensinventering. [Qualification survey]*. Örebro, Sweden: Specialpedagogiska skolmyndigheten.
Johnson, K. C., DesJardin, J. L., Barker, D. H., Quittner, A. L., & Winter, M. E. (2008). Assessing joint attention and symbolic play in children with cochlear implants and multiple disabilities: Two case studies. *Otology & Neurotology, 29*, 246–250.
Johnson, R. E., Liddell, S. K., & Erting, C. J. (1989). *Unlocking the curriculum: Principles for achieving access in deaf education. Gallaudet Research Institute Working Paper 89-3*. Washington, DC: Gallaudet University.
Knight, P. A., & Swanwick. R. A. (2002). *Working with deaf pupils: Sign bilingual policy into practice*. London: David Fulton Publishers.
Knoors, H., & Marschark, M. (2012). Language planning for the 21st century: Revisiting bilingual language policy for deaf children. *Journal of Deaf Studies and Deaf Education, 17*(3), 291–305.
Kristoffersen, A. E., & Simonsen, E. (2012). Teacher-assigned literacy events in a bimodal bilingual preschool with deaf and hearing children. *Journal of Early Childhood Literacy*. August 24, doi:10.1177/1468798412453731
Kristoffersen, A. E., & Simonsen, E. (2014). Exploring letters in a bimodal bilingual nursery school with deaf and hearing children. *European Early Childhood Education Research, 22*(4).
Kunnskapsdepartementet. (2011). *Læring og fellesskap [Learning and community]*. St.meld. 18 (2010–2011). Oslo: Kunnskapsdepartementet.
Kunnskapssenteret. (2011). *Kommunikasjonsformer for barn med cochleaimplantat. Systematisk oversikt* [Cochlear implant and communication modality, a review]. Rapport fra Kunnskapssenteret nr 15–2011. Oslo, Norway: Kunnskapssenteret. http://www.kunnskapssenteret.no/Publikasjoner/Kommunikasjonsformer+for+barn+med+cochleaimplantat.13075.cms.
Kyle, J., & Woll, B. (1985). *Sign language: The study of deaf people and their language*. Cambridge, UK: Cambridge University Press.
Lewis, W. (1995). *Bilingual teaching of deaf children in Denmark (Description of a project 1982–1992)*. Aalborg, Denmark: Døveskolernes Materialelaboratorium.
Lewis, W. (1994). *Tegnsprog som fag: Undervisningsvejledning* [Sign-language subjects and curriculum: Guide for teachers]. Aalborg, Denmark: Døveskolernes materialelaboratorium.
Little, D. (2011). The Common European Framework of Reference for Languages: A research agenda. *Language Teaching, 44*, 381–393.

Mahshie, S. N. (1995). *Educating deaf children bilingually with insights and applications from Sweden and Denmark.* Washington, D.C.: Gallaudet University, Pre College Programs.

Mattson, E. H., & Hansen, A. M., (2009). Inclusive and exclusive education in Sweden: Principals' opinions and experiences. *European Journal of Special Needs Education, 24*(4), 465–472.

Meinzen-Derr, J., Wiley, S., Grether, S., & Choo, D. I. (2010). Language performance in children with cochlear implants and additional disabilities. *The Laryngoscope, 120*, 405–413.

Ministry of Education. (1991). *Bekendtgørelse om faget tegnsprog I folkeskolen.* [Ministerial order on the subject of sign language in school]. Copenhagen, Denmark: Ministry of Education. Retrieved from https://www.retsinformation.dk/forms/R0710.aspx?id=73740&exp=1.

Opplæringslova. (1998). Lov om grunnskolen og den vidaregåande opplæringa [The Education Act]. http://www.lovdata.no/all/nl-19980717-061.html.

Percy-Smith, L., Jensen, J. H., Josvassen, J. L., Jønsson, M. H., Andersen, J., Samar, C. F., Thomsen, J. C., & Pedersen, B. (2006). Forældrevurdering af talesprog og generel trivsel hos børn med cochleaimplantat [Parents' rating of oral language and well-being among children with cochlear implant]. *Ugeskrift for Læger 168*(33), 2659–2664.

Pickersgill, M, & Gregory, S. (1998). *Sign bilingualism: A model.* Wembley, UK: Adept Press.

Powers, S. (1999). The educational attainments of deaf students in mainstream programs in England: Examination results and influencing factors. *American Annals of the Deaf, 144*(3), 261–269.

Punch, R., & Hyde, M. (2011). Communication, psychosocial, and educational outcomes of children with cochlear implants and challenges remaining for professionals and parents. *International Journal of Otolaryngology, 4*, 1–10. doi:10.1155/2011/573280

Rambøll. (2011). *Evaluering av opplæringsprogram for foreldre til døve og hørselshemmede barn* [Evaluation of educational program for parents of deaf and hard of hearing children]. Oslo, Norway: Rambøll Management Consulting.

SFS 1980:64. *Förordning om mål och riktlinjer i 1980 års läroplan för grundskolan* [National curriculum for Compulsory Education]. Stockholm, Sweden: Utbildningsdepartementet.

SFS 2009:600. *Språklagen* [Swedish Language Act]. Stockholm, Sweden: Kulturdepartementet.

Simonsen, E. (2007). Competing perspectives in research and professional work with young deaf children. In M. Hyde & G. Høie (Eds.), *To be or to become: Language and learning in the lives of young deaf children.* Skådalen Publication Series no. 25. Oslo, Norway: Skådalen Resource Centre.

Simonsen, E., Kristoffersen, A. E., & Hjulstad, O. (2009a). Great expectations: Perspectives on cochlear implantation of deaf children in Norway. *American Annals of the Deaf. 154*(3), 263–273.

Simonsen, E., Kristoffersen, A. E., & Hjulstad, O. (2009b). *Hva skjer i klasserommet? Rapport fra prosjektet Inkluderende opplæring for barn med cochleaimplantat* [What's going on in the classroom? Report from the project Inclusive education for children with cochlear implants]. Skådalen Publication Series No 29. Oslo, Norway: Skådalen Resource Centre.

Skolöverstyrelsen. (1983). *Läroplan för specialskolan: Kompletterande föreskrifter till Lgr 80* [National curriculum for special school]. Stockholm, Sweden: Liber utbildningsförlaget.

Smith, S. D., Gregory, S., & Wells, A. (1997). Language and identity in sign bilingual deaf children. *Deafness and Education, 21*(3), 31–38.

SOU 2006:54. *Teckenspråk och Teckenspråkiga: Översyn av teckenspråkets ställning.* [Sign language and sign language users: Review of the status of sign language]. Stockholm, Sweden: Fritzes Offentliga Publikationer.

SOU 2011:33. *Med rätt att välja: Flexibel utbildning för elever som tillhör specialskolans målgrupp* [The right to choose: Flexible education for pupils belonging to the target group of special school]. Stockholm, Sweden: Fritzes Offentliga Publikationer.

Stacey, P. C., Fortnum, H. M., Barton, G. R., & Summerfield, A. Q. (2006). Hearing-impaired children in the United Kingdom, I: Auditory performance, communication skills, educational achievements, quality of life, and cochlear implantation. *Ear and hearing, 27*(2), 161–186.

Svartholm, K. (2010). Bilingual education for deaf children in Sweden. *International Journal of Bilingual Education and Bilingualism, 13*(2), 159–174.

Svartholm, K. (1995). Bilingual education for the deaf: Evaluation of the Swedish model. *Proceedings from The XII World Congress of the World Federation of the Deaf.* (pp. 413–417). Vienna, Austria.

Svartholm, K. (1993). Bilingual education for the deaf in Sweden. *Sign Language Studies, 81,* 291–332.

Swanwick, R. (2010). Policy and practice in sign bilingual education: Development, challenges and directions. *International Journal of Bilingual Education and Bilingualism. 13*(2), 147–158.

Swanwick, R., & Kitchen, R. (2013). Pathway for professionals. BATOD Magazine, May edition, 34–36.

Swanwick, R., Kitchen, R., & Salter, J. (2012). Priorities for professional development. BATOD Magazine: December edition, 6–7.

Tetzchner, S. V. (2012). *Utviklingspsykologi [Developmental psychology].* Oslo, Norway: Gyldendal.

Thoutenhoofd, E. (2006). Cochlear implanted pupils in Scottish schools: 4-year school attainment data (2000–2004). *Journal of Deaf Studies and Deaf Education, 11*(2), 171–188.

Tortzen, A. (2008). *Danske børn med cochlear implant: Undersøgelse af Forældres erfaringer og valg* [Danish children with cochlear implant: An evaluation of parents' experiences and choices]. Virum, Denmark: Videnscenter for Hørehandicap.

Türker-Van der Heiden, E. (2011). *Studies on deaf immigrants.* Paper presented at 8th International Symposium in Bilingualism. Oslo, Norway: University of Oslo.

Türker-Van der Heiden, E. (2012). *Hørselshemmede med minoritetsbakgrunn* [Deaf students with a minority background]. Paper presented at NOA Conference Norsk som andrespråk [Norwegian as a secondary language]. Oslo, Norway: University College.

Tymms, P., Brien, D., Merrell, C., Collins, J., & Jones, P. (2003). Young deaf children and the prediction of reading and mathematics. *Journal of Early Childhood Research, 1*(2), 197–212.

Vonen, A. M. (1997). *1997, Et merkeår i døveundervisningens historie*. Skådalen Publication. Series no. 2. Oslo, Norway: Skådalen Resource Centre.

Valentine, G., & Skelton, T. (2008). Changing spaces: The role of the Internet in shaping Deaf geographies. *Social & Cultural Geography, 9*(5), 469–485.

Widel, J. (1993). *Døves kultur [Deaf culture]*. Alborg, Denmark: Døveskolernes Materialecenter.

Watson, L. M., Archbold, S. M., & Nikolopoulos, T. P. (2006). Children's communication mode fi years after cochlear implantation: Changes over time according to age at implant. *Cochlear Implants International, 7*(2), 77–91.

Wheeler, A., Archbold, S. M., Hardie, T., & Watson, L. M. (2009). Children with cochlear implants: The communication journey. *Cochlear Implants International, 10*(1), 41–62.

# Part Three

# Bilingual Education in Co-enrollment Settings

# 13

# Language Development of Deaf Children in a Sign Bilingual and Co-enrollment Environment

Gladys Tang, Scholastica Lam, and Kun-man Chris Yiu

The impetus for linguistic research on American Sign Language (ASL) and British Sign Language (BSL) between the 1960s and the 1980s (Klima & Bellugi, 1979; Kyle & Woll, 1985; Stokoe, Casterline, & Croneberg, 1965) has led to a continuous growth of linguistic evidence of the properties of many natural signed languages throughout the world. That work has confirmed that the abstract principles of structural organization observed in spoken languages are also shared by signed languages (see Brentari, 2010; Pfau, Steinbach, & Woll, 2012; Sandler & Lillo-Martin, 2006, for updates of the existing literature). Some studies in the 1980s also examined how deaf or hearing children born to deaf parents acquired signed language. The results revealed a developmental profile resembling that reported in the acquisition literature of spoken languages (Lillo-Martin, 1991; Newport & Meier, 1985; Petitto, 1983, 1987, 1990).

Contrary to the burgeoning of positive research findings based on sign linguistics and sign language acquisition, however, there was a lack of consensus on the role of natural signed language in raising and educating deaf children. Generally speaking, research findings revealed that deaf children lagged behind their hearing age norms in oral language, reading comprehension, and literacy development in the spoken language. The controversy regarding the linguistic advantage of deaf children born to deaf parents in literacy development still persists. While some studies documented early sign language advantage among deaf children born to deaf parents (Chamberlain & Mayberry, 2000; Hoffmeister, 2000; Padden & Ramsey, 2000; Singleton, Supalla, Litchfield, & Schley, 1998; Strong & Prinz, 1997; Wilbur, 2000), a recent study by Wauters, Van Bon, and Tellings (2006) reported that deaf children whose home language was spoken language performed better than deaf children born to deaf parents, both in terms of word identification and reading comprehension. Despite such contradictory findings, the increasing interest in natural signed language has triggered the establishment of sign bilingual programming for deaf children primarily in special settings in different parts of Europe, the United Kingdom, the United States, Australia, and Canada (see Swanwick, Hendar, Dammeyer, Kristoffersen, Salter, & Simonsen, Chapter 12 of this volume).

Views regarding sign bilingual programming have been quite polarized (see Marschark & Lee, Chapter 9 of this volume; Pérez Martin, Valmaseda Balanzategui, & Morgan, Chapter 15 of this volume). Also, increasingly, sign bilingual programming has been facing the challenge of a global trend of inclusive deaf education supported by advanced hearing technology such as cochlear implantation, which results in increasing opportunities for severe and profoundly deaf children to study in mainstream settings (Swanwick & Marschark, 2010). In those settings, signed language support is being reduced to a bare minimum, or is nonexistent. This phenomenon sometimes comes with the misconception among educators and parents that learning signed language impedes deaf children's spoken language development. The approach of sign bilingualism and co-enrollment in mainstream deaf education aims to address this issue. In this chapter, we report on some preliminary findings of the grammatical development of 20 severe to profoundly deaf children studying in a mainstream setting that adopted sign bilingualism and co-enrollment as two overarching philosophies for educating and raising deaf children. We focus on examining the development of the deaf children's grammatical knowledge of oral Cantonese, written Chinese, and Hong Kong Sign Language (HKSL) because knowledge of grammar has been argued to be an indispensable component in boosting literacy development in spoken language and educational attainment, among other factors (Spencer & Marschark, 2010).

## SIGN BILINGUAL PROGRAMMING

Typical sign bilingual programs take natural signed languages as deaf learners' first language (L1), which is purported to support their literacy development in spoken language as their second language (L2), despite the fact that almost 95% of these learners are born to hearing parents. Proponents of this approach to educating deaf children render it important to support Deaf identity and culture in deaf children's overall development because they are perceived to be linguistically different, rather than pathologically at risk (Grosjean, 1986, 1994, 2010a, 2010b; Hoffmeister, 2000; Lane, Hoffmeister, & Bahan, 1996; Padden & Humphries, 1988; Wilbur, 2000). Many of these programs draw on Cummins's (1981) interdependence hypothesis, which assumes that there is a common, core proficiency between Language X (L1) and Language Y (L2), allowing unidirectional and subsequently bidirectional transfer of linguistic as well as conceptual knowledge between the two languages. Note that Cummins's arguments usually center on the transfer of lexical and phonological, as well as literacy, academic, and conceptual skills. He does not explicitly reject the transfer of syntactic or morphosyntactic knowledge, but suspects that transfer may not be possible when two languages are structurally dissimilar at the surface level (Cummins, 2005).

The concept of "sign bilingual programming" to date is embraced by different educators with different forms of school practices or even different forms of signing and visual communication systems (Carlson, Morford, Shaffer, & Wilcox, 2010; Swanwick, Hendar, Dammeyer, Kristoffersen, Salter, & Simonsen, Chapter 12 of this volume). As noted earlier, views regarding the use of sign bilingual programming in special settings to support deaf children's language and literacy, as well as educational attainment, are polarized. On the one hand, continual research in different natural signed languages, as well as their acquisition by deaf children, supports the tenet that early exposure to signed language brings decided advantages in literacy skills, reading comprehension, and educational outcomes (Mayberry, 2007), as well as cognitive benefits like theory of mind (Schick, De Villiers, De Villiers, & Hoffmeister, 2007; Tomasuolo, Valeri, Di Renzo, Pasqualetti, & Volterra, 2012). On the other hand, the efficacy of sign bilingual programing has been criticized for not producing sufficient empirical evidence to meet the expectations that it has promised to offer—in particular, filling the gap of literacy development and educational attainment between sign bilingual deaf children and their hearing age norms (Knoors & Marschark, 2012; Mayer & Leigh, 2010; Spencer & Marschark, 2010). Also, Cummins's transfer view has been criticized for being theoretically unsound when applied to deaf education because (1) it fails to capture the fact that many hearing parents of deaf children cannot provide deaf children with a strong signed language foundation as L1, (2) ASL and English demonstrate distinct differences in terms of linguistic organizations at the surface level, (3) lack of a print form for signed language makes the transfer of print knowledge to a spoken language impossible, and (4) it is difficult for deaf children to engage in discourses of academic discussions due to the difficulty in accessing speech as L2 (Holzinger & Fellinger, Chapter 5 of this volume, Mayer, 2009; Mayer & Akamatsu, 2003; Mayer & Leigh, 2010; Mayer & Wells, 1996).

Despite these arguments, in some studies deaf children's early signed language skills were found to be correlated positively with vocabulary knowledge and reading comprehension in spoken language, although a gap existed when compared with the hearing age norms (Chamberlain & Mayberry, 2008; Freel, Clark, Anderson, Gilbert, Musyoka, & Hauser, 2011; Hermans, Knoors, Ormel, & Verhoeven,

2008; Hoffmeister, 2000; Padden & Ramsey, 2000; Singleton, Morgan, DiGello, Wiles, & Rivers, 2004; Strong & Prinz, 1997; Wilbur, 2000). One crucial issue is natural signed language input. Goldin-Meadow and Mayberry (2001) found that deaf children who failed to obtain sufficient natural language input or who received only Manually Coded English as input failed to reach native-like proficiency or a satisfactory level in either language. Mayberry and Lock (2003) also found that first language exposure being delayed until age 6 or older would have a negative impact on deaf children's grammatical development and reading comprehension.

On the oral language front, recent years have seen the introduction of newborn hearing screening and early cochlear implantation. Many studies on children with implants showed improvement in speech perception or language production with potentials for reaching age-appropriate oral language abilities. Nonetheless, children with implants still demonstrated variable outcomes, and some continued to fall short of their chronological age peers in literacy skills, reading comprehension skills, and educational attainment (Archbold & Mayer, 2012; Caselli, Rinaldi, Varuzza, Giuliani, & Burdo 2011; Geers, Moog, Biedenstein, Brenner, & Hayes, 2009; Hammer, 2010; Marschark, Sarchet, Rhoten, & Zupan, 2010). In terms of current educational practices in many countries, children with early implants are mainstreamed and are subject to a mode of education that is either purely auditory-oral or auditory-visual with visual communication systems such as cued speech, contact signs, manually coded spoken language, and the like because these strategies are assumed to bring deaf children in "direct" and "visible" contact with spoken language (Mayer & Leigh, 2010). Under those circumstances, exposure to natural signed language appears to be superfluous and will only be accessible to deaf children when diagnostics show that they fail to demonstrate development in oral language. On some occasions, they will be advised to return to special settings for their education. As such, sign bilingual programming in those settings sometimes becomes the shelter for these so called "underperformed" deaf children, and it is the only time when they begin to acquire signed language, as late learners with not on par language learning outcomes.

The preponderance of cochlear implantation at the expense of early signed language input is being counteracted by the proposal of nurturing bimodal bilingualism with deaf children to safeguard optimal language acquisition during the critical period. Involved researchers argue that the success rate of cochlear implantation is still highly variable, and linguistic deprivation during deaf children's critical period of language acquisition will lead to long-term negative impacts on their language, literacy, cognitive, and social development (Humphries et al., 2012). In fact, what seems to be lacking in the controversy of sign bilingual programming is information about the processes of bilingual acquisition when deaf children are exposed to a signed language and a spoken language in the acquisition environment, enabling them to acquire two languages stemming from different modalities simultaneously.

## RESEARCH ON BIMODAL BILINGUAL ACQUISITION

Recent years have seen a shift of orientation in signed language acquisition research, which is from monolingual to bimodal bilingual acquisition by either deaf children born to deaf or hearing parents, or hearing children born to deaf parents (i.e., CODAs). When language is perceived as innately endowed in humans, deaf children are no different from any ordinary child having the potential for acquiring more than one language, if given appropriate linguistic input. Therefore, the concept of children becoming bimodal bilinguals just develops naturally from theories of linguistics and language acquisition (Grosjean, 2010a; Lillo-Martin, 2008; Van den Bogaerde & Baker, 2005). The capacity of utilizing two grammatical systems simultaneously in language production (i.e., code-blending) has been examined in the context of interactions between deaf caregivers and child CODAs (Baker & Van den Bogaerde, 2008, on Dutch and Sign Language of the Netherlands, SLN), adult CODAs (Emmorey, Bornstein, & Thompson, 2005, on ASL and English), and deaf child acquirers (Donati & Branchini, 2013, on Italian and Lingua dei Segni Italiana, LIS; Fung & Tang, 2013, on Cantonese and HKSL). Taken together, code-blending is evidential of the interactions of two developing linguistic systems in language performance and is subject to principles of natural language organization. From an educational perspective, the recognition of code-blending enables researchers to distinguish it from simultaneous communication (SimCom). Code-blending reflects the linguistic processing of a signed language and a spoken language in language production, while SimCom is basically driven by the syntax of the spoken language where individual signs, primarily lexical in nature, are being incorporated into the spoken language syntax in language production in a serial fashion.

## HOW FEASIBLE IS IT TO INTRODUCE SIGNED LANGUAGE IN MAINSTREAM SETTINGS?

As discussed earlier, sign bilingual programming is implemented primarily in special settings that cater to deaf learners with severe to profound hearing loss. Deaf children with mild or moderate hearing losses usually study in mainstream settings and have little signed language exposure. This practice of early educational placement divides deaf children between these two learning environments with different ideologies (Swanwick, 2010). Nevertheless, the use of signed language through sign interpretation in mainstream settings to support learning is being practiced in some countries. However, there are concerns over its quality (Russell, 2010), as well as the sociocultural consequences of the interpreter and the deaf learner being perceived as out-group in the classroom environment (Schick, Williams, & Kupermintz, 2005).

In the United States and Australia, positive effects are observed when Deaf paraprofessionals are recruited to support deaf students in mainstream settings. Their presence raises the Deaf awareness and metalinguistic awareness among hearing students as well as deaf students of the differences between spoken language and signed language (McKee, 2005). As for deaf students in mainstream settings, there have been studies showing that learning signed language in addition to speech raises grade-level scores (DeLana, Gentry, & Andrews, 2007) and supports social interactions between deaf students and their hearing peers (Bowen, 2008).

## CO-ENROLLMENT PROGRAMMING

Knoors and Marschark (2012) argued that there is no single method of communication to satisfy the wide diversity of strengths and weaknesses of individual deaf learners in their education, and it is only practical to consider a variety of approaches to satisfy their diverse needs. They further suggested that co-enrollment be another option for educating deaf children in mainstream settings. In other words, the breaking of barriers of language and educational settings to accommodate deaf children's diverse needs may open up new venues for exploring ways of enhancing literacy development and educational outcomes.

Co-enrollment has the intrinsic characteristics of having both deaf and hearing students learning together in a regular classroom setting. Unlike conventional mainstream settings with just one or two deaf students, co-enrollment distinguishes itself from other forms of practices by a critical mass of deaf students enrolled in a regular class of hearing students, team-taught by a Deaf teacher and a hearing teacher. Since the creation of the "Tripod Program" in the United States (Kirchner 1994), there has been an increasing number of co-enrollment programs for deaf and hearing students worldwide, in (1) Madrid, Spain (Pérez, Valmaseda Balanzategui, & Morgan, Chapter 15 of this volume) (2) The Netherlands (Hermans, de Klerk, Wauters, & Knoors, Chapter 16 of this volume), (3) Arizona, United States (Antia & Metz, Chapter 17 of this volume), (4) Italy (Ardito, Caselli, Vecchietti, & Volterra, 2008), and (5) Tainan, Taiwan (Hsing & Su, 2013). From a bilingual acquisition perspective, we argue that co-enrollment programming in mainstream settings may offer an acquisition-rich environment in terms of linguistic input, as both signed language and spoken language become the language of instruction as well as the language of daily interactions between the deaf and the hearing participants, students and teachers alike. As in special schools for deaf students, Deaf children of Deaf parents, Deaf adults, or senior students become the sources of linguistic input to the younger ones.

Being a relatively new approach for educating deaf children, research findings to substantiate its efficacy are just emerging (see Antia & Metz, Chapter 17 of this volume; Hermans, De Klerk, Wauters, & Knoors, Chapter 16 of this volume). Most studies focused on initial gains, especially gains in vocabulary knowledge in the spoken language. Based on scores on the Stanford Achievement Test (Harcourt Brace & Company, 1997), Kreimeyer, Crooke, Drye, Egbert, and Klein (2000) examined the language outcomes of 15 deaf students in grades 2 through 4 after 3 years of co-enrollment programming. The deaf students were observed to perform at grade level in reading vocabulary but not in reading comprehension. Four years later and after 7 years of operation, McCain and Antia (2005) studied another 5 co-enrolled deaf students and found that their reading scores were better than the deaf norms but were still below the hearing age norms. Hermans, De Klerk, Wauters, & Knoors (Chapter 16 of this volume) also observed a significant growth rate in receptive vocabulary in Dutch with 12 co-enrolled deaf students, although a gap still existed when compared with the hearing age norms. Taken together, co-enrollment programming yielded some initial gains in terms of vocabulary knowledge, but long-term gains at the higher linguistic levels, as involved in reading comprehension, require further investigation.

## THE HONG KONG CO-ENROLLMENT STUDY

Reviewing a series of research projects, Spencer and Marschark (2010) identified a number of factors that impact the literacy development of deaf children. A noticeable difficulty in grammatical attainment among deaf learners was observed, which hindered both their reading and writing development (King & Quigley, 1985), as well as automaticity and processing time of print materials (Kelly, 2003). To add to the literature on co-enrollment, we examined the development of grammatical knowledge of oral Cantonese, written Chinese, and HKSL of 20 severe and profoundly deaf children studying in a sign bilingual and co-enrollment program in Hong Kong. We addressed the fundamental question of whether there is cross-modal interaction of linguistic knowledge among the languages in question, as suggested by Mayer to be unlikely or by Cummins to be suspect due to highly dissimilar linguistic structures. It is important to verify whether a relationship exists in the development of grammatical knowledge of these languages, as our ultimate goal is to improve the literacy skills of severe and profoundly deaf children.

## Sociolinguistic Context

The language policy of Hong Kong stipulates that students should be proficient in oral Cantonese (which is most children's L1), written Chinese (which is based on Mandarin grammar and is most children's early L2), and English (another L2 introduced at more or less the same time as written Chinese). In other words, when formal schooling begins at age 2 or 3, young children in Hong Kong will be exposed to Mandarin Chinese and English input in a parallel fashion. Note that the social milieu of Hong Kong does not encourage "written Cantonese" (i.e., written Chinese based on Cantonese grammar), with the arguments that certain Cantonese words may not have equivalent written forms, and those that exist are neither standardized nor recognized officially. Therefore, written Chinese in Hong Kong is based on Mandarin grammar but pronounced in Cantonese.

As most parents use Cantonese at home, the prospect of becoming bilingual or trilingual rests upon access to input in the educational context. In the syllabi of kindergarten and primary education, a greater proportion of time is allotted to promoting the acquisition of written Chinese and English. From a deaf perspective, the task of acquiring language in a learning environment like Hong Kong is intriguing because deaf children must mediate with these languages not only in language acquisition terms but also in terms of using them to access education. Seen in this light, there may be many facets of language acquisition by deaf children raised in the Hong Kong environment, depending on whether they have acess to HKSL, types of schools they go to and level of hearing loss. For instance, some deaf children studying in mainstream settings who have no access to HKSL will develop Cantonese in a monolingual fashion in early childhood. They will then acquire English and the written form of Mandarin Chinese as L2s. The rapid expansion in the use of Putonghua in primary and secondary education in Hong Kong also means that students are required to learn Putonghua as a second oral language in addition to Cantonese, over and above written Chinese based on Mandarin grammar. As such, students are taught to read written Chinese using both Cantonese and Putonghua pronunciation.

While a majority of deaf students are being mainstreamed with no support of HKSL, a very small number of deaf students study in special school settings where teachers of the deaf have been encouraged to use either speech or total communication in educating their students. It is against this sociolinguistic milieu that the Jockey Club Sign Bilingualism and Co-enrollment in Deaf Education Programme (i.e., the SLCO Programme) was set up in Hong Kong in 2006. Studying under this program, deaf and hearing children are expected to add HKSL to their linguistic repertoire, becoming "multilingual" in every sense of the word, although in this project we adopted a broader definition of "bilingualism" as having knowledge of more than one language. As the name of the SLCO Programme suggests, sign bilingualism and co-enrollment are the two overarching philosophies for raising and educating deaf children in this setting. Practically, the SLCO Programme hopes to introduce one more option to the existing oralist approach to deaf education in Hong Kong.

### Children in the SLCO Program

Twenty deaf children studying from primary 1 (i.e., K-2 in the US system) to primary 5 (i.e., K-6 in the US system) were identified for the current study based on three criteria: (1) they enrolled in the SLCO Programme at the third and final year of kindergarten education, hence one full year of intensive, initial exposure to HKSL; (2) they had severe to profound hearing loss (i.e., average hearing thresholds higher than 70 dB); (3) they had no other disabilities. Nine deaf students did not participate in the current study, either because they had been diagnosed as having additional disabilities (i.e., 2 students), did not join the SLCO Program at kindergarten (i.e., 4 students), or they had only unilateral, mild, or moderate hearing loss (i.e., 3 students).

For those who had been selected for the study, their ages ranged from 7;7 to 13;5 (average 10;2). Fourteen of them were implanted at an average age of 2;5. For the six deaf children who wore hearing aids, one was diagnosed to be not suitable for implantation due to the lack of a cochlear in either ear, and hearing aids were fitted instead. The average age of fitting of hearing aids with these children was 1;4. Among them, four were born to Deaf parents, and they studied at three different grades. Two of them had Mainland Chinese backgrounds with exposure to Chinese Sign Language through their parents. The rest of the deaf children were born to hearing parents. Table 13.1 summarizes the backgrounds of the 20 deaf children in the analysis, in terms of their chronological age, gender, types of hearing devices, parents' hearing status, hearing level in the better ear (in dB), age of oral Cantonese input, written Chinese input, and HKSL input.

### Assessment Procedures

*Hong Kong Cantonese Oral Language Assessment Scale: Cantonese Grammar (HKCOLAS-CG)*

Few tools on assessing syntactic and morphosyntactic knowledge of Cantonese have been designed, and HKCOLAS was the first standardized tool targeting children from kindergarten 3 (i.e., K-1) to primary 6 (i.e., K-7) (T'sou, Lee, Tung, Chan, Man, & To, 2006). There were 7 subscales in the package. In the current study, the subscale "Cantonese Grammar" (HKCOLAS-CG) was chosen. The tasks of this subscale included picture selection (i.e., verbal comprehension), responses to questions (i.e., verbal

Table 13.1 Background of the Deaf Participants

| Codes | Gender | Hearing level (dB) | Chrono-logical age | Parents' hearing status | Hearing device | Duration of written Chinese input | Duration of Cantonese input | Duration of HKSL input | Age of written Chinese input | Age of Cantonese input | Age of HKSL input |
|---|---|---|---|---|---|---|---|---|---|---|---|
| C1-1-CTY | F | 88 | 10;8 | Hearing | CI | 98 | 118 | 75 | 2;6 | 0;9 | 4;4 |
| C1-2-HST | F | 118 | 12;11 | Hearing | CI | 113 | 131 | 74 | 3;6 | 2;0 | 6;8 |
| C1-3-LKY | M | 105 | 12;8 | Hearing | CI | 110 | 135 | 75 | 3;6 | 1;3 | 6;4 |
| C1-4-SMC | M | 93 | 11;9 | Deaf | HA | 111 | 136 | 129 | 2;6 | 0;4 | 1;0 |
| C1-5-TKH | M | 108 | 13;5 | Hearing | CI | 93 | 136 | 74 | 5;8 | 2;0 | 7;2 |
| C2-1-CYF | M | 108 | 9;9 | Hearing | CI | 87 | 98 | 62 | 2;6 | 1;6 | 4;6 |
| C2-2-SMY | F | 72 | 10;3 | Deaf | HA | 93 | 110 | 123 | 2;6 | 1;0 | 0;0 |
| C2-3-TWK | M | 107 | 11;10 | Hearing | HA | 82 | 103 | 62 | 5;0 | 3;2 | 6;7 |
| C2-5-WCY | M | 87 | 11;6 | Hearing | HA | 96 | 102 | 72 | 3;6 | 2;11 | 5;6 |
| C2-6-WSY | F | 120 | 11;5 | Hearing | HA | 107 | 133 | 62 | 2;6 | 0;3 | 6;2 |
| C3-1-CKY | F | 93 | 9;3 | Hearing | HA | 69 | 83 | 56 | 3;6 | 2;2 | 4;6 |
| C3-2-CKW | F | 97 | 9;7 | Hearing | CI | 85 | 95 | 56 | 2;6 | 1;7 | 4;10 |
| C3-5-OTN | F | 118 | 9;7 | Hearing | CI | 85 | 90 | 56 | 2;6 | 1;11 | 4;10 |
| C3-6-TSM | F | 108 | 8;11 | Hearing | CI | 65 | 98 | 56 | 3;6 | 0;7 | 4;2 |
| C4-1-CNW | F | 88 | 8;2 | Deaf | CI | 62 | 81 | 79 | 3;0 | 1;3 | 1;6 |
| C4-2-CWK | F | 120 | 8;11 | Hearing | CI | 65 | 82 | 43 | 3;6 | 2;0 | 5;3 |
| C4-3-CWL | F | 120 | 8;11 | Hearing | CI | 65 | 82 | 43 | 3;6 | 2;0 | 5;3 |
| C4-4-CHY | F | 80 | 8;7 | Hearing | CI | 49 | 68 | 32 | 4;6 | 2;9 | 5;10 |
| C4-5-GTC | F | 95 | 8;3 | Deaf | CI | 69 | 92 | 87 | 2;6 | 0;6 | 1;0 |
| C5-4-SLY | F | 117 | 7;7 | Hearing | CI | 61 | 72 | 43 | 2;6 | 1;6 | 3;11 |

comprehension), grammaticality judgment (i.e., verbal comprehension), and picture description (i.e., verbal expression). There were 89 test stimuli for assessing knowledge of functional categories, complex sentences, and compound sentences with logical connectives. To accommodate deaf children's verbal comprehension, an audio-visual mode in test condition was developed with permission of the publisher. HKCOLAS was adopted as a formal measurement when the deaf children entered the SLCO Programme at the primary level. The children were tested on an individual basis under the aided condition, and the scoring method strictly observed the procedures specified in the package. Since the current study did not aim at comparing deaf children's performance with age norms, raw scores were used instead of standard scores.

*Assessment of Chinese Grammatical Knowledge (CGA-Primary and KG)*

As tools for assessing deaf children's syntactic and morphosyntactic knowledge of written Chinese were lacking, a new assessment instrument—*Assessment of Chinese Grammatical Knowledge* (i.e., CGA-Primary and KG)—was developed, based on analyses of Chinese linguistics and child language acquisition in Chinese. In the current study, the package CGA-Primary was adopted. It was an online assessment, containing 136 test items distributed over 15 syntactic and morphosyntactic structures. There were four tasks to the assessment: word reordering, picture selection, picture-sentence matching, and fill-in-the-blank. The task instructions were presented in Cantonese or HKSL in a video format. In the current study, the assessment was conducted in a computer room at school.

*Hong Kong Sign Language Elicitation Tool (HKSL-ET)*

This tool was developed to profile the HKSL development of deaf children in terms of their HKSL production and judgments of grammaticality. The grammatical components included wh-questions, yes/no questions, negation and modals, classifier constructions, non-manual adverbials, and verb agreement. These linguistic structures were reported in previous studies either in terms of the linguistics of HKSL or its acquisition (Tang & Sze, 2002, Tang, 2003; Lee 2006; Tang, 2007; Tang, Sze, & Lam, 2007; Tang, Lam, Sze, Lau, & Lee, 2008; Lam, 2009). There were two major components of HKSL-ET: (1) one judgment task, as our goal was to assess deaf children's knowledge of appropriate non-manual adverbials and syntactic word order of wh-questions, negation, and modals; and (2) three production tasks, namely picture description for eliciting classifier predicates, elicited producton for word order of negation, wh-questions, and yes-no questions, as well as story retelling for modals and verb agreement. All production data were transcribed using ELAN and scored with reference to a set of criteria based on reported analyses of HKSL.

## Outcome Assessments

Table 13.2 shows the scores of the three assessments and some of the factors to be adopted in the current analysis. At the outset, our goal was to verify whether any relationship existed between the development of grammatical knowledge of oral Cantonese, written Mandarin, and HKSL. Pearson Product correlational analyses were used to verify if there was any linear progression among the scores based on HKCOLAS-CG, CGA-Primary, and HKSL-ET. The results indicated that there was a significantly positive correlation between HKCOLAS-CG and CGA-Primary, suggesting that the development of grammatical knowledge between the two varieties of Chinese was highly related. The linear relationship between CGA-Primary and HKSL-ET was also significantly correlated, as was the linear relationship between HKCOLAS-CG and HKSL-ET. These findings suggest that the children's developing grammars of the three languages were highly correlated, to the extent that the development of one language may predict a commitment development of the other. One possible interpretation is that these three languages may share some common underlying cross-linguistic properties beyond the surface level. Hence, from a language acquisition

Table 13.2 Deaf Children's Performance on HKCOLAS-CG, CGA, and HKSL-ET

| Codes | HKCOLAS-CG (%) | CGA (%) | HKSL-ET (%) |
| --- | --- | --- | --- |
| C1-1-CTY | 83.13 | 89.71 | 75.13 |
| C1-2-HST | 38.55 | 80.15 | 45.84 |
| C1-3-LKY | 34.94 | 74.26 | 61.33 |
| C1-4-SMC | 83.13 | 88.97 | 78.67 |
| C1-5-TKH | 36.14 | 72.06 | 50.55 |
| C2-1-CYF | 32.53 | 57.35 | 53.26 |
| C2-2-SMY | 75.90 | 92.65 | 63.18 |
| C2-3-TWK | 81.93 | 84.56 | 57.86 |
| C2-5-WCY | 61.45 | 88.97 | 71.92 |
| C2-6-WSY | 45.78 | 84.56 | 47.72 |
| C3-1-CKY | 83.13 | 93.38 | 47.95 |
| C3-2-CKW | 44.58 | 76.47 | 43.58 |
| C3-5-OTN | 31.33 | 52.21 | 25.64 |
| C3-6-TSM | 78.31 | 85.29 | 49.19 |
| C4-1-CNW | 32.53 | 61.76 | 45.21 |
| C4-2-CWK | 50.60 | 59.56 | 44.21 |
| C4-3-CWL | 61.45 | 79.41 | 45.98 |
| C4-4-CHY | 27.71 | 50.00 | 49.36 |
| C4-5-GTC | 49.40 | 84.56 | 63.41 |
| C5-4-SLY | 24.10 | 29.41 | 32.23 |

perspective, the acquisition of a certain property of one language will have a positive effect on the other, as the result suggests.

Hermans, Ormel, and Knoors (2010) reported a lack of significant interaction between signing and vocabulary skills initially with younger learners under age 5;1, when they had just entered primary education. They hypothesized that transfer would only take place when there was some threshold knowledge of SLN in place. To investigate this issue, we asked if duration of exposure (i.e., sustained input) had any effect on the interactions of grammatical knowledge of the three languages. The deaf children were divided into two groups based on the criterion of 60 months of language exposure to each of the three languages (approximately 5 years).

For the eight deaf children with fewer than 60 months of exposure to each of the languages, correlational analyses showed that there was a highly significant interaction between oral Cantonese and written Chinese only. This could be due to the relatively earlier access to oral Cantonese and written Chinese before joining the SLCO Program, or the typological proximity between the two linguistic systems. There was a moderately significant interaction between written Chinese and HKSL, but no significant correlation between oral Cantonese and HKSL was observed. Since these deaf children were only exposed to HKSL when they joined the SLCO Program, a weaker relationship was expected, probably due to their lack of threshold knowledge of HKSL. In this way, the current finding is similar to that reported in Hermans et al. (2010). For the remaining 12 deaf children who had sustained input from the three languages for longer than 60 months, significant interactions were observed between each language pair.

One interpretation of the findings is the crucial role played by the duration of sustained input from each of the three languages, which consistently bolster the relationships among them. In other words, the longer the deaf children were immersed in the co-enrollment environment, the stronger the relationship between the languages. Such a relationship was first observed between oral Cantonese and written Chinese, and eventually extended to HKSL with either variety of Chinese. The closer relationship between oral Cantonese and written Chinese is expected due to linguistic proximity, as well as early access to both languages by deaf children with the support of hearing aids or cochlear implants, in addition to speech and language therapy training.

Since the sample size was quite small and eyeballing the data found interesting individual variation, we decided to run a cluster analysis to group the deaf children statistically based on their performance in the three assessments. Centroid Method (with squared Euclidean distance measure) of hierarchical clustering was applied to categorize the children based on their performance on HKCOLAS-CG, CGA-Primary, and HKSL-ET. Two clusters of deaf children resulted, with two deaf children C3-5-OTN and C5-4-SLY being filtered out as outliers because of their extremely poor performance (hence difficult to measure and qualify in the cluster analysis. Table 13.3 presents the distribution of the deaf children according to their cluster membership. Next, some variables were isolated in order to examine the underlying attributes that formed these two clusters. A non-parametric analysis (Spearman Correlation) was applied, incorporating the variables of hearing level in the better ear, speech perception, and hearing devices, as well as initial age of oral Cantonese, written Chinese, and HKSL input. Note that for speech perception, scores were obtained based on the deaf children's performance in the *Cantonese Lexical Neighborhood Test* (i.e., CLNT, Yuen et al., 2008). Results showed that speech perception, hearing devices, and age of first sign language exposure correlated significantly with the forming of the two clusters, while other factors did not yield any significant relationships (e.g., hearing level, age of written Chinese input, age of Cantonese input). These findings suggest that a complex relationship exists between speech perception abilities, hearing devices, and age of sign language input, which impacts deaf children's development of grammatical knowledge in oral Cantonese, written Chinese, and HKSL. Table 13.3 summarizes the distribution of the deaf children within each cluster. In what follows, we will qualitatively describe the two clusters of deaf children.

A few observations can be made regarding the two clusters of deaf children. First, the mean scores of the three tests were much higher in cluster A than in cluster B, suggesting that the deaf children in cluster A were better at developing grammatical knowledge of the three languages than those in cluster B. Among the three tests, HKCOLAS-CG revealed a more obvious difference between clusters (i.e., mean scores: A = 73.09% vs. B = 38.15%), which is understandable, as the CLNT scores (i.e., speech perception) of the deaf children in cluster A were much higher than those in cluster B (i.e., mean scores: A = 91.56% vs. B = 43.56%). In other words, despite sharing a similar level of hearing loss, those deaf children with better speech perception abilities were able to perform well on the oral language assessment. Hence, speech perception is a crucial determinant for developing Cantonese grammar in the Hong Kong context, in the absence of a formal written mode for this dialect of Chinese.

Second, even though 8 out of 9 deaf children in cluster B had a cochlear implant but 5 out of 9 deaf children in cluster A wore hearing aids, on average, the deaf children in cluster A performed better than those in cluster B. This suggests that hearing devices may not be a factor for predicting language performance as far as this study is concerned.

Third, all deaf children in clusters A and B showed a better command of grammatical knowledge of written Chinese (i.e., CGA-Primary) than oral Cantonese (i.e., HKCOLAS-CG) and HKSL (i.e., HKSL-ET). This

Table 13.3 Clusters of Deaf Children Based on HKCOLAS-CG, CGA and HKSL

| Codes | HKCOLAS-CG (%) | CGA (%) | HKSL-ET (%) | CLNT (%) | Hearing level (dB) | Hearing device | Parents' hearing status | Age/duration of Cantonese input (month) | Age/duration of written Chinese input (month) | Age/duration of HKSL input (month) |
|---|---|---|---|---|---|---|---|---|---|---|
| Cluster A | | | | | | | | | | |
| C1-1-CTY | 83.13 | 89.71 | 75.13 | 100.00 | 88.00 | CI | Hearing | 0;9 (118) | 2;6 (98) | 4;4 (75) |
| C1-4-SMC | 83.13 | 88.97 | 78.67 | 100.00 | 93.00 | HA | Deaf | 0;4 (136) | 2;6 (111) | 1;0 (129) |
| C2-3-TWK | 81.93 | 84.56 | 57.86 | 72.00 | 107.00 | HA | Hearing | 3;2 (103) | 5;0 (82) | 6;7 (62) |
| C3-6-TSM | 78.31 | 85.29 | 49.19 | 100.00 | 108.00 | CI | Hearing | 0;7 (98) | 3;6 (65) | 4;2 (56) |
| C3-1-CKY | 83.13 | 93.38 | 47.95 | 92.00 | 93.00 | HA | Hearing | 2;2 (83) | 3;6 (69) | 4;6 (56) |
| C2-2-SMY | 75.90 | 92.65 | 63.18 | 92.00 | 72.00 | HA | Deaf | 1;0 (110) | 2;6 (93) | 0;0 (123) |
| C4-3-CWL | 61.45 | 79.41 | 45.98 | 84.00 | 120.00 | CI | Hearing | 2;0 (82) | 3;6 (65) | 5;3 (43) |
| C2-5-WCY | 61.45 | 88.97 | 71.92 | 96.00 | 87.00 | HA | Hearing | 2;11 (102) | 3;6 (96) | 5;6 (72) |
| C4-5-GTC | 49.40 | 84.56 | 63.41 | 88.00 | 95.00 | CI | Deaf | 0;6 (92) | 2;6 (69) | 1;0 (87) |
| Average | 73.09 | 87.50 | 61.48 | 91.56 | 95.89 | | | 1;6 (102.67) | 3;3 (83.11) | 3;7 (78.11) |
| Cluster B | | | | | | | | | | |
| C1-2-HST | 38.55 | 80.15 | 45.84 | 8.00 | 118.00 | CI | Hearing | 2;0 (131) | 3;6 (113) | 6;8 (74) |
| C3-2-CKW | 44.58 | 76.47 | 43.58 | 84.00 | 97.00 | CI | Hearing | 1;7 (95) | 2;6 (85) | 4;10 (56) |
| C2-6-WSY | 45.78 | 84.56 | 47.72 | 0.00 | 120.00 | HA | Hearing | 0;3 (133) | 2;6 (107) | 6;2 (62) |
| C1-3-LKY | 34.94 | 74.26 | 61.33 | 0.00 | 105.00 | CI | Hearing | 1;3 (135) | 3;6 (110) | 6;4 (75) |
| C1-5-TKH | 36.14 | 72.06 | 50.55 | 68.00 | 108.00 | CI | Hearing | 2;0 (136) | 5;8 (93) | 7;2 (74) |
| C2-1-CYF | 32.53 | 57.35 | 53.26 | 4.00 | 108.00 | CI | Hearing | 1;6 (98) | 2;6 (87) | 4;6 (62) |
| C4-1-CNW | 32.53 | 61.76 | 45.21 | 64.00 | 88.00 | CI | Deaf | 1;3 (81) | 3;0 (62) | 1;6 (79) |
| C4-4-CHY | 27.71 | 50.00 | 49.36 | 72.00 | 80.00 | CI | Hearing | 2;9 (68) | 4;6 (49) | 5;10 (32) |
| C4-2-CWK | 50.60 | 59.56 | 44.21 | 92.00 | 120.00 | CI | Hearing | 2;0 (82) | 3;6 (65) | 5;3 (43) |
| Average | 38.15 | 68.46 | 49.01 | 43.56 | 104.89 | | | 1;7 (106.56) | 3;6 (85.67) | 5;4 (61.89) |
| Outliers | | | | | | | | | | |
| C3-5-OTN | 31.33 | 52.21 | 25.64 | 32 | 118 | CI | Hearing | 1;11 (90) | 2;6 (85) | 4;10 (56) |
| C5-4-SLY | 24.1 | 29.41 | 32.23 | 12 | 117 | CI | Hearing | 1;6 (72) | 2;6 (61) | 3;11 (43) |

phenomenon was most obvious among the deaf children of cluster B. It seems that with these children, better grammatical knowledge of written Chinese (i.e., CGA-Primary) and HKSL (i.e., HKSL-ET) compensates for their poor speech perception abilities (i.e., CLNT) and poor performance in oral Cantonese (i.e., HKCOLAS-CG). In fact, as most children only learned HKSL when they entered the SLCO Program, it stands to reason that the HKSL scores of some deaf children were lower than those of the other two languages.

Fourth, more children in cluster A displayed a balanced performance with the three language assessments, much more so than the children of cluster B, most of whom scored lower than 50% in either HKSL-ET or HKCOLAS-CG, or both. Fifth, there was little difference in the initial age of exposure to oral Cantonese (cluster A = 1;6 vs. cluster B = 1;7) and written Chinese (cluster A = 3;3 vs. cluster B = 3;5), probably due to the universal hearing screening policy in Hong Kong and the relatively more uniform age of formal schooling among the children. However, the age of exposure to HKSL was much younger with children in cluster A than in cluster B (cluster A = 3;7 vs. cluster B = 5;4). A closer examination found a concentration of deaf children born to deaf parents. There were three in cluster A and only 1 in cluster B. It seems that the combined effects of early sign language exposure, early fitting of hearing aids, and strong speech perception abilities supported the development of the three languages with these children in the study. Deaf children with poor speech perception, on the other hand, would rely more on HKSL and written Chinese in their language performance, due to their relatively poor oral language input and output.

## IMPLICATIONS OF THE FINDINGS

This study of language acquisition by a group of severe and profoundly deaf children in a sign bilingual and co-enrollment program found a significantly positive relationship between their development of syntactic and morphosyntactic knowledge of oral Cantonese, written Chinese, and HKSL. Also, we observed no adverse effects on the development of oral Cantonese or written Chinese when the deaf children were acquiring HKSL; otherwise, statistically, we should be expecting a negative correlation between the scores of HKCOLAS-CG and HKSL or CGA-Primary and HKSL (cf. Spencer & Marschark, 2010). The results do not seem to show a significant difference in the types of hearing technology these children were prescribed with, as most children in cluster A were fitted with hearing aids rather than cochlear implants and they performed better than those in cluster B. However, as there were deaf children born to deaf parents in cluster A, their better performance may skew the results somewhat. What we have learned from the current study is that, for severe and profoundly deaf children, speech perception abilities rather than hearing levels have an effect on the development of oral Cantonese grammar.

In fact, positive interactions in deaf children's assessments based on vocabulary, narratives, and reading comprehension between a signed language and a spoken language have been reported in recent studies (Hermans et al., 2010, on SLN and Dutch; Menéndez, 2010, on Catalan Sign Language and English; Niederberger, 2008, on Langue des Signes Française and French). Some other studies went further by adopting a bilingual processing model, with evidence revealing cross-modal activation of sign language knowledge (e.g., phonological or semantic) during written word recognition by sign bilinguals (Morford, Wilkinson, Villwock, Piñar, & Kroll, 2011, on ASL in English word recognition by deaf adults; Ormel, Hermans, Knoors, & Verhoeven, 2012, on SL in Dutch word recognition by deaf children; see Ormel & Giezen, Chapter 4 of this volume).

The current study adds to the pool of evidence of this positive relationship through examining severe and profoundly deaf children's syntactic and morphosyntactic knowledge of three target languages. It should be pointed out that we made no specific attempts in this study to compare the linguistic structures of the three languages cross-linguistically and by way of which we isolated certain "direct" evidence of cross-linguistic transfer in the data. Instead, we examined deaf children's grammatical knowledge at the broader level by designing stimuli that reflect the syntax or morphosyntax of the three languages, as all natural languages are bound to display such properties through various means.

How do we explain such a phenomenon? One plausible interpretation of the significantly positive correlations between the language pairs could be maturation. As the deaf children were drawn from P1 to P5, and if the linguistic environment was conducive enough, we should be expecting growth of grammatical knowledge of each of the languages over time, hence the positive correlations. A plausible outcome of increasing grammatical knowledge of the three languages may result in cross-linguistic transfer during the course of language development. Indeed, acquisition studies constantly allude to the transfer of linguistic knowledge from L1 to L2 in second language acquisition or from the more dominant to the less dominant language in bilingual acquisition. If this assumption holds, then the findings may suggest that cross-modal, linguistic transfer of grammatical knowledge between a signed language and a spoken language at some higher linguistic levels is likely. This runs counter to some earlier claims that surface structural differences or the lack of a print form in a signed language does not encourage cross-modal transfer of linguistic knowledge (Mayer & Akamatsu, 2000; Mayer & Wells, 1996, p. 105). As noted earlier, although Cummins emphasizes the possibility of transfer of conceptual and linguistic knowledge from one language to the other, he also casts doubt on the possibility of linguistic transfer in some specific domains of linguistic knowledge, especially syntactic and morphosyntactic knowledge of dissimilar languages. The current findings run counter to his assumptions.

The earlier observation by Hermans and colleagues (2010) that initial cross-modal transfer is unlikely when there is insufficient threshold knowledge of language also found some support in the current study. When systematic exposure to the three languages was less than 60 months, the lack of correlation initially between the scores of HKSL and oral Cantonese was observed. This is understandable because most of these children did not develop HKSL until after they had joined the SLCO Programme, and acquiring oral Cantonese solely via the auditory-oral mode was difficult initially, given their speech perception abilities. However, a significant correlation between oral Cantonese and written Chinese, and between HKSL and written Chinese, was observed with this group of children. For oral Cantonese and written Chinese, it may be due to the benefit of the early intervention policy of Hong Kong, where deaf children are fitted with either hearing aids or cochlear implants, enabling early exposure to oral Cantonese and subsequently written Chinese.

If the transfer view holds, unimodal, cross-linguistic transfer at the syntactic and morphosyntactic level is likely with similar languages, and written Chinese may support the long-term development of oral Cantonese. Second, the closer relationship between HKSL and written Chinese also suggests that severe and profoundly deaf children rely heavily on HKSL and written Chinese in their language development. It is especially crucial with those children who have poor speech perception abilities. Still another possibility is that there is no "direct" transfer per se, but the "multilingual" learning environment offers enriched linguistic input from different languages, which supports deaf children's overall language development (Volterra, personal communication).

How do we situate our current findings with reference to Cummins's interdependence hypothesis? Although this hypothesis on L1 transfer is narrowly defined and is hypothesized to be applicable to general conceptual knowledge and certain domains of linguistic knowledge only, one can still align this transfer view with current theories of language acquisition, particularly the concept of cross-linguistic influence in second language acquisition and bilingual acquisition. According to these paradigms of linguistic research, abstract knowledge of principles and parameters of Universal Grammar manifest themselves in natural languages, hence the possibility of linguistic transfer given certain conditions. In accounting for code-blending within the framework of distributed morphology, for instance, Lillo-Martin, Koulidobrova, de Quadros, and Chen (2012) argued that bimodal bilinguals have one computational system but two lexicons at their disposal. In deriving the structure, they may transfer knowledge of syntax from one language to the other. In spelling out the structure, bimodal bilinguals may employ two independent phonetic forms (i.e., speech and sign), hence the code-blending phenomenon.

In the context of the current study, such a facility of transferring linguistic knowledge at the abstract level may be perceived as having a scaffolding effect, supporting deaf children's dynamic processes of bilingual acquisition rather than hindering them, resulting in the positive correlation between HKCOLAS-CG, CGA-Primary and HKSL-ET. We observed that at least deaf children from cluster A demonstrated such effects. In language acquisition terms, language learners are bound to utilize their developing linguistic resources to support the acquisition process at any given point of development, be it second language acquisition or bilingual acquisition.

Adopting the premise that deaf children may undergo bilingual acquisition, a highly dynamic bioprogram across the life span, it is important to analyze the timing of input of the languages involved and the nature of linguistic input in the home and school environment, as they play a pivotal role in supporting bilingual if not multilingual development. In terms of the timing of linguistic input, bimodal bilinguals may acquire two languages in either a simultaneous or sequential fashion. Simultaneous bilingual acquisition refers to the processes whereby children are given early exposure to two languages between ages 0–3. Early exposure to a second language between ages 4–6 (i.e., before formal schooling begins) and after mastering an L1 will be characterized as sequential bilingual acquisition (Meisel, 2004). Therefore, the acquisition of signed language and spoken language by CODAs naturally pertains to simultaneous bilingual acquisition. However, Deaf children born to Deaf parents nowadays also stand a good chance of undergoing simultaneous bilingual acquisition to some extent. They receive early signed language input through their parents; at the same time, universal hearing screening and fitting of hearing devices at an early age enable them also to gain early access to spoken language input, as evidenced by those deaf children born to deaf parents in both clusters A and B.

As for deaf children born to hearing parents, one has to accept the fact that they seldom enjoy the facility of signed language input as L1 in the home environment. That situation underlies the usual arguments against diverting deaf children's attention to acquiring a signed language initially, especially when cochlear implantation suggests chances of success (Mayer & Leigh, 2010). However, it is possible to assume that, given sufficiently early linguistic input, deaf children born to hearing parents may undergo a relatively longer period of simultaneous bilingual acquisition when compared with their "Deaf of Deaf" peers and typically developing bilingual child acquirers. In fact, it is sometimes difficult to draw a clear-cut distinction between simultaneous and sequential bilingual acquisition processes, even in typical acquisition conditions. In monolingual first language acquisition, age 3 marks the mastery of certain fundamental properties of the target language grammar (Guasti, 2004, offers an excellent summary), but not its entirety.

The acquisition literature also reveals that full attainment of some specific domains of syntax, such as long passives, will occur at age 6 (Borer & Wexler, 1992), or development of formal representations of semantic, as well as pragmatic and discourse knowledge, will extend into adolescence (Nippold, 1988). In other words, even under typical conditions, early L2 acquisition may occur in parallel with advanced L1 acquisition. Put in the context of deaf children born to hearing parents, if universal hearing screening and early intervention are in place to ensure early access to spoken language input, these children may also be candidates for simultaneous or sequential bilingual acquisition if they are given early and sustained input in signed language, albeit not in the home context as reported in typical bilingual acquisition studies. For those who do not develop strong speech perception abilities due to various reasons, an early injection of signed language input is only to their advantage. This echoes Goldin-Meadow and Mayberry's (2001, p. 226) observation that "early detection of hearing loss, early entry into an educational system, and early and continuous contact with fluent signers together may go a long way toward ensuring that profoundly deaf children have access and learn a language."

If the assumption holds that deaf children raised in a sign bilingual and co-enrollment environment enjoy an early access to signed language and undergo simultaneous or sequential bilingual acquisition, Cummins's earlier stipulation for a strong, initial L1 foundation and some threshold knowledge of L2 in order for transfer to take place becomes redundant. Also, the promotion of signed language being deaf children's L1 needs to be redefined, on grounds of the timing of L1 input to delineate simultaneous and sequential bilingual acquisition, as discussed previously. Where deaf children have the opportunities for early exposure to more than one language and develop knowledge of these languages accordingly, it is likely that they will have both spoken language and signed language as their L1s in a simultaneous or sequential acquisition fashion. For some sign bilingual deaf children, especially those with poor speech perception abilities, HKSL may become their dominant language in due course; for some others it may become their less dominant language, as opposed to oral Cantonese or written Chinese, given the benefits of cochlear implantation, and some deaf children may choose the oral path (Archbold & Mayer, 2012; Mayer &

Leigh, 2010). It is at least a bottom-up decision from the learners, rather than a top-down one from the educators.

The second factor is the nature of linguistic input. The crux of the matter is whether deaf children are given the opportunity for immersion in an acquisition-rich environment with sustained input in both signed language and spoken language. From a simultaneous bilingual acquisition perspective, dual language input has been generally accepted to be beneficial to bilinguals in the spoken language literature (Genesee, 2009). Thordardottir (2011) also claimed that bilingual children need at least 40% of waking hour exposure to a language if their competence in that language is to be comparable to that of monolingual children. The positive effects of linguistic immersion on the bilingual development of hearing children born to deaf parents were also reported in Kanto, Huttunen, and Laakso (2013).

In other words, when deaf children undergo bilingual development while at the same time using the languages to access education—especially for severe and profoundly deaf children such as those from the SLCO Program—the school environment is crucial, as it is the breeding ground of linguistic input, especially HKSL. In addition to immersion in naturalistic spoken language input through daily interactions with hearing peers and teachers, the critical mass of deaf children and Deaf teachers also sustains the input in HKSL in the co-enrollment environment. The daily presence of Deaf teachers in the classrooms (i.e., 6–8 in the current co-enrollment setting), in particular, alleviates the pressure on the hearing teachers in conveying the curriculum content in two different modalities and thus safeguards adequate linguistic input when the signing skills of the hearing teachers are still improving.

The current study shows that this sustained dual/trio linguistic input creates an acquisition rich environment in a way akin to immersion programs in Canada whereas in the current context for deaf children's bilingual if not multilingual development, and more importantly, their access to a regular curriculum. This is especially true for severe and profoundly deaf children born to hearing parents who do not receive input in signed language at home; the early, sustained input in spoken and signed language as occurred in a co-enrollment environment becomes crucial in supporting their sign bilingual acquisition. In fact, some signed language acquisition studies already indicate that deaf children's linguistic output can potentially surpass their "impoverished" or "inconsistent" input, given a sustained period of signed language exposure (Singleton & Newport, 2004; Senghas & Coppola, 2001).

## CONCLUDING OBSERVATIONS

Swanwick, Hendar, Dammeyer, Kristoffersen, Salter, and Simonsen (Chapter 12 of this volume) argue that instead of adopting a polarized view separating language from educational approaches, it would be more beneficial, if not healthier, if the field of deaf education were injected with a view of linguistic pluralism, accepting the differences in strengths and weakness of the different modes of communication in the educational process for deaf children. The sign bilingual and co-enrollment approach to deaf education as implemented in the Hong Kong context shares this objective, coming from research on sign linguistics and bilingual acquisition. As Grimes, Thoutenhoofd, and Byrne (2007) claim, parents must be well informed about a menu of options before they decide on a monolingual approach to educating their deaf child. This is just as important as when parents opt for a sign bilingual approach; sign bilingual development is to be expected and should be viewed as an enrichment rather than as a disadvantage.

Finally, as the SLCO Program is still at the stage of experimentation, the initial findings are encouraging but highly preliminary for reasons such as the reliability and validity of the new assessment tools for measuring deaf children's linguistic competence in different target languages. Presently, the small number of students in the program was also due to the small size of the deaf student population in Hong Kong (i.e., about 5,000 school-age deaf students from kindergarten to upper secondary and all hearing levels). In addition, the lack of a written form for oral Cantonese also prevents the researchers from developing assessment tools using this mode. Also, HKCOLAS-CG which was conducted primarily via verbal comprehension may be biased against those deaf children with poor speech perception abilities in the testing condition. Information from their verbal production may give an additional dimension of their oral Cantonese abilities. Future research may involve comparative analysis of deaf children studying in a co-enrollment environment as against those in regular mainstream settings, to further evaluate the efficacy of the sign bilingual and co-enrollment approach in the broader context of deaf education in Hong Kong.

### ACKNOWLEDGMENTS

The authors would like to acknowledge the generous funding support of The Hong Kong Jockey Club Charities Trust for the project "Jockey Club Sign Bilingualism and Co-enrollment in Deaf Education Programme" (2006–2014).

### REFERENCES

Archbold, S., & Mayer, C. (2012). Deaf education: The impact of cochlear implantation? *Deafness & Education International*, 14(1), 2–15.

Ardito, B., Caselli, M. C., Vecchietti, A., & Volterra, V. (2008). Deaf and hearing children reading together in school. In C. Plaza-Pust & E. Morales-López

(Eds.), *Sign bilingualism* (pp. 137–164). Amsterdam: John Benjamins Publishing.

Baker, A., & Van den Bogaerde, B. (2008). Codemixing in signs and words in input to and output from children. In C. Plaza-Pust & E. Morales-López (Eds.), *Sign bilingualism: Language development, interaction, and maintenance in sign language contact situations* (pp. 1–27). Amsterdam: John Benjamins Publishing.

Borer, H., & Wexler, K. (1992). Bi-unique relation and the maturation of grammatical principles. *Natural Language and Linguistic Theory, 10*(2), 147–189.

Bowen, S. K. (2008). Co-enrollment for students who are deaf or hard of hearing: Friendship patterns and social interactions. *American Annals of the Deaf, 153*(3), 285–293.

Brentari, D. (2010). *Sign languages*. Cambridge, UK: Cambridge University Press.

Carlson, M. L., Morford, J. P., Shaffer, B., & Wilcox, P. P. (2010). The educational linguistics of bilingual deaf education. In F. M. Hult (Eds.), *Directions and prospects for educational linguistics* (pp. 99–115). Heidelberg, Germany: Springer.

Caselli, M. C., Rinaldi, P., Varuzza, C., Giuliani, A., & Burdo, S. (2012). Cochlear implant in the second year of life: Lexical and grammatical outcomes. *Journal of Speech, Language, and Hearing Research, 55*(2), 382–394.

Chamberlain, C., & Mayberry, R. I. (2000). Theorizing about the relationship between ASL and reading. In C. Chamberlain, J. P. Morford, R. I. Mayberry (Eds.), *Language acquisition by eye* (pp. 221–260). Mahwah, NJ: Lawrence Erlbaum Associates.

Chamberlain, C., & Mayberry, R. I. (2008). American Sign Language syntactic and narrative comprehension in skilled and less skilled readers: Bilingual and bimodal evidence for the linguistic basis of reading. *Applied Psycholinguistics, 29*(03), 367–388.

Cummins, J. (1981). The role of primary language development in promoting educational success for language minority students. In California State Department of Education (Ed.), *Schooling and language minority students: A theoretical framework* (pp. 3–49). Los Angeles: Evaluation, Dissemination and Assessment Center, California State University.

Cummins, J. (1991). Interdependence of first- and second-language proficiency in bilingual children. In E. Bialystok (Ed.), *Language processing in bilingual children* (pp. 70–89). Cambridge, UK: Cambridge University Press.

Cummins, J. (2005). *Teaching for cross-language transfer in dual language education: Possibilities and pitfalls*. Paper presented at TESOL Symposium on Dual Language Education: Teaching and learning two languages in the EFL setting. Bogazici University, Istanbul, Turkey, September 23, 2005.

Cummins, J. (2006). *The relationship between American Sign Language proficiency and English academic development: A review of the research*. Unpublished paper for the Ontario Association of the Deaf, Toronto, Ontario, Canada.

DeLana, M., Gentry, M. A., & Andrews, J. (2007). The efficacy of ASL/English bilingual education: Considering public schools. *American Annals of the Deaf, 152*(1), 73–87.

Donati C., & Branchini, C. (2013). Challenging linearization: Simultaneous mixing in early bimodals. In T. Biberauer & I. Roberts (Eds.), *Challenges to linearization* (pp. 93–128). Berlin: Mouton de Gruyter.

Emmorey, K., Borinstein, H. B., & Thompson, R. (2005). Bimodal bilingualism: Code-blending between spoken English and American Sign Language. In J. Cohen, K. T. McAlister, K. Rolstad, & J. MacSwan (Eds.), *Proceedings of the 4th International Symposium on Bilingualism* (pp. 663–673). Somerville, MA: Cascadilla Press.

Freel, B. L., Clark, M. D., Anderson, M. L., Gilbert, G. L., Musyoka, M. M., & Hauser, P. C. (2011). Deaf individuals' bilingual abilities: American Sign Language proficiency, reading skills, and family characteristics. *Psychology*, 2(1), 18–23.

Fung, C. H.-M., & Tang, G. (2013). *Simultaneous acquisition of Hong Kong Sign Language and Cantonese: Violation of code-blending grammar*. Paper presented at the 1st Symposium on Sign Language Acquisition, Universidade Católica Portuguesa, Lisbon, Portugal.

Geers, A. E., Moog, J. S., Biedenstein, J., Brenner, C., & Hayes, H. (2009). Spoken language scores of children using cochlear implants compared to hearing age-mates at school entry. *Journal of Deaf Studies and Deaf Education*, 14(3), 371–385.

Genesee, F. (2009). Early childhood bilingualism: Perils and possibilities. *Journal of Applied Research on Learning (Special Issue)*, 2, 1–21.

Goldin-Meadow, S., & Mayberry, R. I. (2001). How do profoundly deaf children learn to read?. *Learning Disabilities Research & Practice*, 16(4), 222–229.

Grimes, M., Thoutenhoofd, E. D., & Byrne, D. (2007). Language approaches used with deaf pupils in Scottish Schools: 2001–2004. *Journal of Deaf Studies and Deaf Education*, 12(4), 530–551.

Grosjean, F. (1986). Bilingualism. In J. V. Van Cleve and C. Baker-Shenk (Eds.), *Gallaudet encyclopedia of deaf people and deafness*, (vol. 3, pp. 179–182). New York, NY: McGraw-Hill.

Grosjean, F. (1994). Sign bilingualism: Issues. In K. Brown (Ed.), *The encyclopedia of language and linguistics*. Oxford, UK: Pergamon Press.

Grosjean, F. (2010a). *Bilingual: Life and reality*. Cambridge, MA: Harvard University Press.

Grosjean, F. (2010b). Bilingualism, biculturalism, and deafness. *International Journal of Bilingual Education and Bilingualism*, 13(2), 133–145.

Guasti, M. T. (2004). *Language acquisition: The growth of grammar*. Cambridge, MA: MIT Press.

Hammer, A. (2010). *The acquisition of verbal morphology in coclear-implanted and specific language impaired children Language*. Doctoral dissertation. Leiden University, LOT Dissertation Series 255, Utrecht.

Harcourt Brace & Company (1997). Stanford Achievement Test-9 (9 Ed.) San Antonio, TX: Harcourt Brace & Company.

Hermans, D., Ormel, E., & Knoors, H. (2010). On the relations between signing and reading skills of sign bilinguals. *International Journal of Bilingual Education and Bilingualism*, 13(2), 187–199.

Hermans, D., Knoors, H., Ormel, E., & Verhoeven, L. (2008). The relationship between the reading and signing skills of deaf children in bilingual education programs. *Journal of Deaf Studies and Deaf Education*, 13(4), 518–530.

Hoffmeister, R. J. (2000). A piece of the puzzle: ASL and reading comprehension in Deaf Children. In C. Chamberlain, J. P. Morford & R. Mayberry (Eds.), *Language acquisition by eye* (pp.143–146). Mahwah, NJ: Lawrence Erlbaum Associates.

Hsing, M-H., & Su, S-F. (2013). *A sign bilingual plus partial inclusion experiment for young deaf students in Taiwan: Benefits and challenges*. Paper presented at the 3rd International Conference on Sign Linguistics and Deaf Education in Asia, January 30–February 2, 2013, The Chinese University of Hong Kong.

Humphries, T., Kushalnagar, P., Mathur, G., Napoli, D. J., Padden, C., Rathmann, C., & Smith, S. R. (2012). Language acquisition for deaf children: Reducing the harms of zero tolerance to the use of alternative approaches. *Harm Reduction Journal*, 9(1), 1–9.

Kanto, L., Huttunen, K., & Laakso, M. L. (2013). Relationship between the linguistic environments and early bilingual language development of hearing children in Deaf-parented families. *Journal of Deaf Studies and Deaf Education*, 18(2), 242–260.

Kelly, L. P. (2003). The importance of processing automaticity and temporary storage capacity to the differences in comprehension between skilled and less skilled college-age deaf readers. *Journal of Deaf Studies and Deaf Education*, 8(3), 230–249.

King, C., & Quigley, S. (1985). *Reading and deafness*. San Diego, CA: College-Hill Press.

Kirchner, C. J. (1994). Co-enrollment as an inclusion model. *American Annals of the Deaf*, 139(2), 163–164.

Klima, E. S., & Bellugi, U. (1979). *The signs of language*. Cambridge, MA: Harvard University Press.

Knoors, H., & Hermans, D. (2010). Effective instruction for deaf and hard-of-hearing students: Teaching strategies, school settings and student characteristics. In M. Marschark & P. E. Spencer (Eds.), *The Oxford handbook of deaf, language, and education* (vol. 2, pp. 57–71). New York, NY: Oxford University Press.

Knoors, H., & Marschark, M. (2012). Language planning for the 21st century: revisiting bilingual language policy for deaf children. *Journal of Deaf Studies and Deaf Education*, 17(3), 291–305.

Komesaroff, L. R., & McLean, M. A. (2006). Being there is not enough: Inclusion is both deaf and hearing. *Deafness and Education International*, 8(2), 88–100.

Kreimeyer, K. H., Crooke, P., Drye, C., Egbert, V., & Klein, B. (2000). Academic and social benefits of a co-enrollment model of inclusive education for deaf and hard-of-hearing children. *Journal of Deaf Studies and Deaf Education*, 5(2), 174–185.

Kyle, J., & Woll, B. (1985). *Sign Language: The study of deaf people and their language*. New York, NY: Cambridge University Press.

Lam, S. (2009). *Early phrase structure in Hong Kong Sign Language*. Unpublished PhD thesis, The Chinese University of Hong Kong.

Lane, H. L., Hoffmeister, R., & Bahan, B. J. (1996). *A journey into the Deaf-world*. San Diego, CA: Dawn Sign Press.

Lee, J. (2006). *Negation in Hong Kong Sign Language*, Unpublished MPhil. thesis. The Chinese University of Hong Kong.

Lillo-Martin, D. C. (1991). *Universal grammar and American Sign Language: Setting the null argument parameters*. Dordrecht, Netherlands: Kluwer.

Lillo-Martin, D. (2008). Sign Language acquisition studies: Past, present and future. In Ronice Müller de Quadros (Ed.), *Sign languages: Spinning and unraveling the past, present and future. TISLR9, forty-five papers and three posters from the 9th Theoretical Issues in Sign Language Research Conference* (pp. 244–263). Petrópolis, Brazil: Editora Arara Azul.

Lillo-Martin, D., Koulidobrova, H., de Quadros, R. M., & Chen Pichler, D. (2012). Bilingual language synthesis: Evidence from WH-Questions in bimodal bilinguals. In A. K. Biller, E. Y. Chung, & A. E. Kimball (Eds.), *BUCLD 36 Proceedings*. Somerville, MA: Cascadilla Press.

Marschark, M., Sarchet, T., Rhoten, C., & Zupan, M. (2010). Will cochlear implants close the reading achievement gap for deaf students? In M. Marschark and P. Spencer (Eds.), *The Oxford handbook of deaf studies, language, and education* (vol. 2, pp. 127–143). New York, NY: Oxford University Press.

Marschark, M., & Spencer, P. E. (2010). Promises(?) in deaf education: From research to practice and back again. In M. Marschark and P. E. Spencer (Eds.), *The Oxford handbook of deaf studies, language and education* (vol. 2, pp. 1–14). New York, NY: Oxford University Press.

Mayberry, R. I. (2007). When timing is everything: Age of first-language acquisition effects on second-language learning. *Applied Psycholinguistics, 28*(3), 537.

Mayberry, R. I., & Lock, E. (2003). Age constraints on first versus second language acquisition: Evidence for linguistic plasticity and epigenesis. *Brain and Language, 87*(3), 369–384.

Mayer, C. (2009). Issues in second language literacy education with learners who are deaf. *International Journal of Bilingual Education and Bilingualism, 12*(3), 325–334.

Mayer, C., & Wells, G. (1996). Can the linguistic interdependence theory support a bilingual-bicultural model of literacy education for deaf students? *Journal of Deaf Studies and Deaf Education, 1*(2), 93–107.

Mayer, C., & Akamatsu, C. T. (2003). Bilingualism and literacy. In M. Marschark & P. Spencer (Eds.). *The Oxford handbook of deaf studies, language and education* (pp. 136–147). New York, NY: Oxford University Press.

Mayer, C., & Leigh, G. (2010). The changing context for sign bilingual education programs: Issues in language and the development of literacy. *International Journal of Bilingual Education and Bilingualism, 13*(2), 175–186.

McCain, K. G., & Antia, S. D. (2005). Academic and social status of hearing, deaf, and hard of hearing students participating in a co-enrolled classroom. *Communication Disorders Quarterly, 27*(1), 20–32.

McKee, R. L. (2005). As one deaf person to another: Deaf paraprofessionals in mainstream schools. *Deaf Worlds, 21*(1), 1–48.

Meisel, J. (2004). The bilingual child. In T. K. Bhatia & W. C. Ritchie (Eds.), *The handbook of bilingualism* (pp. 91–113). Oxford, UK: Blackwell.

Menéndez, B. (2010). Cross-modal bilingualism: Language contact as evidence of linguistic transfer in sign bilingual education. *International Journal of Bilingual Education and Bilingualism, 13*(2), 201–223.

Morford, J. P., Wilkinson, E., Villwock, A., Piñar, P., & Kroll, J. F. (2011). When deaf signers read English: Do written words activate their sign translations? *Cognition, 118*, 283–292.

Morgan, G., & Kegl, J. (2006). Nicaraguan Sign Language and theory of mind: The issue of critical periods and abilities. *Journal of Child Psychology and Psychiatry, 47*(8), 811–819.

Newport, E., & Meier, R. (1985). The acquisition of American Sign Language. In D. I. Slobin (Ed.), *The cross-linguistic study of language acquisition* (vol. 1, pp. 881–930). Hillsdale, NJ: Lawrence Erlbaum Associates.

Nippold, M. A. (Ed.). (1988). *Later language development: Ages 9 through 19*. Austin, TX: Pro-Ed.

Niederberger, N. (2008). Does the knowledge of a natural sign language facilitate deaf childrens' learning to read and write? Insights from French Sign Language and written French data. In C. Plaza-Pust & E. Morales-López (Eds.), *Sign bilingualism* (pp. 29–50). Amsterdam: John Benjamins Publishing.

Ormel, E., Hermans, D., Knoors, H., & Verhoeven, L. (2012). Cross-language effects in written word recognition: The case of bilingual deaf children. *Bilingualism: Language and Cognition, 15*(2), 288–303.

Padden, C. A., & Humphries, T. L. (1988). *Deaf in America: Voices from a culture*. Cambridge, MA: Harvard University Press.

Padden, C., & Ramsey, C. (2000). American Sign Language and reading ability in deaf children. In C. Chamberlain, J. Morford, and R. Mayberry (Eds.), *Language acquisition by eye* (vol. 1, pp. 65–89). Mahwah, NJ: Lawrence Erlbaum Associates.

Peterson, N. R., Pisoni, D. B., & Miyamoto, R. T. (2010). Cochlear implants and spoken language processing abilities: Review and assessment of the literature. *Restorative Neurology and Neuroscience, 28*(2), 237–250.

Petitto, L. A. (1983). From gesture to symbol: The relation between form and meaning in the acquisition of personal pronouns in American Sign Language. *Papers and Reports on Child Language Development, Stanford University, 22*: 100–107.

Petitto, L. A. (1987). On the autonomy of language and gesture: Evidence from the acquisition of personal pronouns in American Sign Language. *Cognition, 27*(1), 1–52.

Petitto, L. A. (1990). The transition from gesture to symbol in American Sign Language. In V. Volterra & C. J. Ertin (Eds.), *From gesture to language in hearing and deaf children* (pp. 153–161). Berlin, Germany: Springer Heidelberg.

Pfau, R., Steinbach, M., & Woll, B. (2012). *Sign language: An international handbook. Handbooks of linguistics and communication science*. Berlin. Germany: Mouton de Gruyter.

Pisoni, D. B., Conway, C. M., Kronenberger, W. G., Horn, D. L., Karpicke, J., & Henning, S. C. (2008). Efficacy and effectiveness of cochlear implants in deaf children. In M. Marschark & P. C. Hauser (Eds.), *Deaf cognition: Foundations and outcomes*, (pp. 52–101). New York, NY: Oxford University Press.

Plaza-Pust, C., & López, E. M. (2008). Sign Bilingualism: Language development, interaction and maintenance in sign language contact situation. In C. Plaza-Pust & E. Morales-López (Eds.), *Sign bilingualism* (pp. 333–379). Amsterdam, Netherlands: John Benjamins Publishing.

Russell, D. 2010. *Inclusion or the illusion of inclusion: A study of interpreters working with deaf students in inclusive education settings*. Manuscript. University of Alberta, Canada.

Sandler, W., & Lillo-Martin, D. (2006). *Sign language and linguistic universals*. Cambridge, UK: Cambridge University Press.

Schick, B., Williams, K., & Kupermintz, H. (2005). Look who's being left behind: Educational interpreters and access to education for deaf and hard-of-hearing students. *Journal of Deaf Studies and Deaf Education, 11*(1), 3–20.

Schick, B., de Villiers, P., de Villiers, J., & Hoffmeister, R. (2007) Language and theory of mind: A study of deaf children. *Child Development, 78*(2), 376–396.

Senghas, A., & Coppola, M. (2001). Children creating language: How Nicaraguan Sign Language acquired a spatial grammar. *Psychological Science*, 12(4), 323–328.

Singleton, J. L., Supalla, S., Litchfield, S. I., & Schley, S. (1998). From sign to word: Considering modality constraints in ASL/English bilingual education. *Topics in Language Disorders*, 4, 16–29.

Singleton, J. L., & Newport, E. L. (2004). When learners surpass their models: The acquisition of American Sign Language from inconsistent input. *Cognitive Psychology*, 49(4), 370–407.

Singleton, J. L., Morgan, D., DiGello, E., Wiles, J., & Rivers, R. (2004). Vocabulary use by low, moderate, and high ASL-proficient writers compared to hearing ESL and monolingual speakers. *Journal of Deaf Studies and Deaf Education*, 9(1), 86–103.

Spencer, P. E., & Marschark, M. (2010). *Evidence-based practice in educating deaf and hard-of-hearing students*. New York, NY: Oxford University Press.

Stokoe, W. C., Casterline, D. C., & Croneberg, C. G. (1965). *A dictionary of American Sign Language on linguistic principles*. Washington, DC: Gallaudet University Press.

Strong, M., & Prinz, P. (1997). A study of the relationship between American Sign Language and English literacy. *Journal of Deaf Studies and Deaf Education*, 2, 37–46.

Supalla, S. J., & Cripps, J. H. (2008). Linguistic accessibility and deaf children. In B. Spolsky & F. M. Hult (Eds.), *The handbook of educational linguistics* (pp. 174–191). Oxford, UK: Blackwell.

Swanwick, R. (2010). Policy and practice in sign bilingual education: Development, challenges and directions. *International Journal of Bilingual Education and Bilingualism*, 13(2), 147–158.

Swanwick, R., & Marschark, M. (2010). Enhancing education for deaf children: Research into practice and back again. *Deafness and Education International*, 12(4), 217–235.

T'sou, B., Lee, T., Tung, P., Chan, A., Man, Y., & To, C. (2006). *Hong Kong Cantonese oral language assessment scale*. Hong Kong: City University of Hong Kong Press.

Tang, G. (2003). Verbs of motion and location in Hong Kogn Sign Language: Conflation and lexicalization. In K. Emmorey (Ed.), *Perspectives on classifier constructions in sign languages* (pp. 143–163). Mahwah, NJ: Lawrence Erlbaum Associates.

Tang, G. (2006). *A linguistic dictionary of Hong Kong Sign Language*. Hong Kong: Chinese University Press.

Tang, G. (2007). *Grammaticalizing FINISH into a perfective aspect marker in HKSL*. Paper presented at The Workshop on Acquisition of Functional Categories in Asian Languages, December 26, 2007, The Chinese University of Hong Kong.

Tang, G., & Sze, F. (2002). Nominal expressions in Hong Kong Sign Language: Does modality make a difference? In R. P. Meier, K. Cormier, & D. Quinto-Pozos (Eds.), *Modality and structure in signed and spoken languages* (pp. 296–321). Cambridge, UK: Cambridge University Press.

Tang, G., Sze, F., & Lam, S. (2007). Acquisition of simultaneous constructions by deaf children of Hong Kong Sign Language. In M. Vermeerbergen,

L. Leeson, & O. Crasborn (Eds.), *Simultaneity in signed languages* (pp. 283–316). Amsterdam, Netherlands: John Benjamins Publishing.

Tang, G., Lam, S., Sze, F., Lau, P., & Lee, J. (2008). Acquiring verb agreement in HKSL: Optional or obligatory. In R. M. de Quadros (Eds.), *Proceedings of theoretical issues in sign language research conference 9*. Petrópolis, Brazil: Editora Arara Azul.

Thordardottir, E. (2011). The relationship between bilingual exposure and vocabulary development. *International Journal of Bilingualism, 15*(4), 426–445.

Tomasuolo, E., Valeri, G., Di Renzo, A., Pasqualetti, P., & Volterra, V. (2013). Deaf children attending different school environments: Sign language abilities and theory of mind. *Journal of Deaf Studies and Deaf Education, 18*(1), 12–29.

Van den Bogaerde, B., & Baker, A. (2005). Code mixing in motherchild interaction in deaf families. *Sign Language and Linguistics, 8*(1–2), 1–2.

Wauters, L. N., Van Bon, W. H. J., & Tellings, A. E. J. M. (2006). Reading comprehension of Dutch deaf children. *Reading and Writing, 19*, 49–76.

Watson, L. M., Archbold, S. M., & Nikolopoulos, T. P. (2006). Children's communication mode five years after cochlear implantation: Changes over time according to age at implant. *Cochlear Implants International, 7*(2), 77–91.

Wilbur, R. B. (2000). The use of ASL to support the development of English and literacy. *Journal of Deaf Studies and Deaf Education, 5*(1), 81–104.

Yuen, K. C. P., Ng, I. H. Y., Luk, B. P. K., Chan, S. K. W., Chan, S. C. S., Kwok, I. C. L., & Tong, M. C. F. (2008). The development of Cantonese Lexical Neighborhood Test: A pilot study. *International Journal of Pediatric Otorhinolaryngology, 72*(7), 1121–1129.

# 14

# Social Integration of Deaf and Hard-of-Hearing Students in a Sign Bilingual and Co-enrollment Environment

Kun-man Chris Yiu and Gladys Tang

Recent advancement in research on sign linguistics and sign language acquisition has enabled us to reconsider the possibility that signed language may partner with spoken language in supporting the linguistic, cognitive, and psychosocial development of deaf and hard-of-hearing (DHH) children. As such, sign bilingual programming has been promoted to maximize the educational opportunities of DHH students and their literacy development (Grosjean, 2010; Padden & Ramsey, 2000; Plaza-Pust & López, 2008; Swanwick, Hendar, Dammeyer, Kristoffersen, Salter, & Simonsen, Chapter 12 of this volume). Although this mode of education has been conventionally adopted in special settings, recent developments in deaf education also attempt to incorporate sign bilingualism into mainstream settings supported by co-enrollment practices. Such attempts imply that sign bilingualism transcends the physical boundaries defined by segregation and inclusion in deaf education, and that co-enrollment draws on not only DHH students' but also hearing students' existing linguistic, intellectual, as well as psychosocial resources in the process of mutually supporting each other's bilingual education (see Hintermair, Chapter 7 of this volume).

One crucial question regarding educating DHH students in a mainstream setting is whether social integration between DHH and hearing students can be achieved. This question derives from concerns about DHH students experiencing difficulty in integration or gaining social membership when educated in a majority hearing school community (Keating & Mirus, 2003; McKee, 2008; Stinson & Antia, 1999; Tvingstedt, 1995).

In this chapter, we will add to the literature on social integration by examining this phenomenon among a group of DHH and hearing students being educated using the philosophies and practices of sign bilingualism and co-enrollment in deaf education in the Hong Kong context. Specifically, we ask whether social acceptance assumes a bilateral process in a co-enrollment environment, or whether it interacts with DHH students' attitudes toward their own deafness and hearing students' attitudes toward their DHH peers. We also ask whether oral language proficiency is a precondition for social integration in a co-enrollment setting, a research question that needs further exploration in the face of new approaches to educating DHH students in mainstream settings.

## SOCIAL INTEGRATION

Broadly speaking, social integration refers to the creation of a "society for all," including the disadvantaged or vulnerable groups and persons (United Nations, 2005). Over the past few decades, the prevailing education philosophy for children with hearing loss saw a drastic shift from special (or segregated) education to inclusive education (Spencer & Marschark, 2010), with a goal of social integration of DHH students, in addition to equal learning opportunities in the hearing majority school community.

According to Stinson and Antia (1999), social integration is technically defined as students' abilities to interact with, make friends with, and be accepted by peers. The extent of *social interactions, social relationships*, and *social acceptance* by hearing peers as well as DHH peers reveals how well DHH students are assimilated into the school community. In this chapter, we will focus on factors contributing to the *social acceptance* of DHH students in a co-enrollment program, which we believe underlies the broader perception or attitudes toward integrating DHH students into a hearing majority community.

DHH students who are being accepted into the school/class community gradually develop a feeling of belongingness, or "membership," in contrast to "visitorship." As "members," they are perceived to be an integral part of the school community by their peers, sharing a set of social values and perceptions that defines their membership. This concept of membership or "citizenship" offers a philosophical backdrop against which we examine how a co-enrollment setting infused with an inclusive culture makes DHH students feel that they are being accepted and valued and, most important of all, allows for their unique educational needs to be met (Anita, Stinson, & Gaustad, 2002, p. 214).

## SOCIAL INTEGRATION IN INCLUSIVE DEAF EDUCATION

Although inclusive deaf education has become a global trend, "to access an inclusive, quality and free primary education and secondary education on an equal basis with others" is considered the right of children with disabilities, including DHH students (United Nations Convention on the Rights of Persons with Disabilities, 2006, Article 24 (2b)). However, physical proximity or physical placement alone does not provide sufficient conditions for social inclusion of DHH students in public schools (Antia, 1982; Antia et al., 2002; Bunch, 1994; Keating & Mirus, 2003). Reviewing a number of studies conducted in different European countries, Dammeyer (2010, p. 51) found that the prevalence rates of psychosocial difficulties of DHH students, regardless of their educational settings, ranged from 20% to 50%. In his study of 334 Danish students aged 6–19, the prevalence rate of psychosocial difficulties of DHH students was 3.7 times greater than their hearing counterparts. Where social relationships are concerned, DHH students tend not to be well adjusted in mainstream settings in terms of social interactions with hearing peers (Antia & Kreimeyer, 1996; Arnold & Tremblay, 1979; Keating & Mirus, 2003), social acceptance (Antia & Kreimeyer, 1997; Kluwin, Stinson, & Colarossi, 2002; Saur, Layne, Hurley, & Opton, 1986), and social relationships (Nunes, Pretzlik, & Olsson, 2001; Tvingstedt, 1995). Thus many DHH students in mainstream settings may perceive themselves as "visitors" rather than "members" of their school/class communities. Antia, Jones, Luckner, Kreimeyer, and Reed (2011) found that compared with hearing norms, approximately 25% of the DHH students had a decrease in social skills over a period of five years.

Nevertheless, contradictory findings have been reported, where the social outcomes of DHH students from mainstream settings were found to be comparable to their hearing counterparts (Andersson, Olsson, Rydell, & Larsen, 2000; Leigh, Maxwell-McCaw, Bat-Chava, & Christiansen, 2009). While reporting similar positive social outcomes, Wauters and Knoors (2008, p. 30) also observed that their 14 DHH students (with 4 in co-enrollment) seemed to be more involved in a social network "without any friendships or antipathies" than their hearing peers, and they were scored lower in social competence. Antia and colleagues (2011) commented that it is difficult to compare outcomes in these studies when the students' backgrounds, such as their hearing status, educational settings, and support services, are so diverse. For example, in the Wauters and Knoors study, DHH students were individually integrated in a regular school with sign interpretation services, while DHH students from other studies did not report such services. Therefore, future studies need to isolate those background variables, such as degree of hearing loss or services rendered specifically to the educational settings, as they might impact DHH students' development of a sense of "membership" in the class/school community and hence their social integration. Sometimes, it is not deafness per se, but certain environmental factors that result in differences in the psychosocial adjustments of deaf students (Polat, 2003).

In sum, there are doubtless many factors that directly or indirectly impact social integration between DHH and hearing students in mainstream settings. The current migration of many DHH students with different degrees of hearing loss from special to mainstream settings potentially instills a change of the existing "ecosystem" of the school environment, also affecting hearing students' perceptions toward deafness and DHH students' special education needs.

## PSYCHOSOCIAL ADJUSTMENT OF DHH STUDENTS

An important factor influencing successful social integration is the psychosocial adjustment of individuals, which can be further analyzed into variables including self-perception (e.g., self-esteem, social-identity, acculturation and attitudes toward deafness), social relationships with others, and perceived abilities of establishing and sustaining peer relationships (e.g., social skills, social competence, and sense of loneliness) in the school community. These variables have been proposed to be important factors influencing social integration between DHH and hearing students in particular (e.g., Antia et al., 2002; Leigh et al., 2009).

Because over 95% of DHH students are born to hearing parents, it is natural that they initially identify themselves with the hearing culture, and attempt to submerse themselves in the mainstream hearing community. Education in a mainstream setting that emphasizes oral-aural communication during childhood and adolescence may lead DHH students to think that it is important for them to "fit in" as much as possible in the hearing world—to the extent that they "discount or devalue deafness and people who are deaf" (Punch & Hyde, 2010, p. 489). Hence, deaf adolescents, whether in segregated or mainstream settings, tend to have lower levels of self-perceived social acceptance, fewer close friendships with hearing peers, and lower ego strength when compared to their hearing peers (Van Gent, Goedhart, Knoors, Westenberg, & Treffers, 2012). Many of them may end up with marginalized identities, holding a confused or negative attitude toward their deafness (McKee, 2008). Studies by Bat-Chava (2000) and Leigh and colleagues (2009) using a self-rating technique found that deaf adolescents with a bicultural identity tend to have better self-esteem and more positive attitudes toward deafness and deaf people (see also Hintermair, 2008). Here, we argue that a co-enrollment setting with sign bilingualism supports the development of bicultural identity by DHH students.

Acceptance of one's hearing loss is a fundamental and highly salient trait underlying the self-identity of a DHH person (Rutman, 1989). It is important to examine DHH children's attitudes toward their own deafness, regardless of whether they are positive or negative (Schroedel & Schiff, 1972) because it is a good predictor of self-esteem (Yiu, 1999, 2005). It also affects DHH students' perceptions of social acceptance in a mainstream setting (Saur et al., 1986). In sum, for social integration to be successful, social acceptance of hearing students toward DHH students and, at the same time, DHH students' positive attitudes toward their own deafness are crucial, as both parties need to meet at some level of mutual understanding before they can utilize their internal capacities—perception and attitudes—to support each other's study and play in an environment.

## ATTITUDES OF HEARING STUDENTS TOWARD DHH STUDENTS

When a school environment encourages a positive attitude toward DHH students and deafness, it stands a good chance of integrating DHH students into the school/class community more readily (Cambra, 2002; Saur et al., 1986). A study conducted in Taiwan found that gender, grade, and the frequency of social interactions were the significant factors affecting hearing students' attitudes toward DHH students (Lee, 2002). Cambra (2002) found that although DHH students in mainstream settings in Spain were generally accepted by their hearing peers, they were negatively perceived as not working as hard, and some hearing students thought they would be better placed in a special school. In other words, the DHH students were not considered as peers who could study with the hearing students. Nevertheless, when the educational environment is one of co-enrollment, the hearing students seem to demonstrate better social acceptance toward DHH peers (Pérez Martin, Valmaseda Balanzategui, & Morgan, Chapter 15 of this volume; Hermans, De Klerk, Wauters, & Knoors, Chapter 16 of this volume). Taken together, these results suggest that the educational setting may directly or indirectly impact how hearing students perceive DHH students and their social integration.

## CO-ENROLLMENT IN DEAF EDUCATION

Educational placements of DHH students around the world involve an array of educational settings, from special school environments, resource centers, or separate classes within mainstream environments to fully integrated mainstream settings. Within mainstream settings, co-enrollment recently emerged as an alternative school placement option for DHH students. Co-enrollment invites both DHH and hearing students to study in the same class, co-taught by a regular teacher and a teacher fluent in signed language. It distinguishes itself from a conventional mainstream setting by having (1) a sizable number of deaf enrollments per class, ideally in equal numbers but it may maintain a 1:3 or 1:4 ratio in some programs; (2) dual language input—signed language and spoken language—in the classroom to support the learning and communication of both DHH and hearing students; and (3) co-teaching and co-learning practices by the teachers and the students, deaf and hearing alike; and above all (4) the overall philosophy of accommodation to create inclusive classroom conditions to facilitate education between DHH and hearing students. This last feature differs from conventional mainstream education, where DHH students must make adjustment to "fit into" the hearing majority classroom.

Beginning with sporadic efforts to develop co-enrollment in deaf education, such as the Tripod Program set up in the United States in the 1990s (Kirchner, 1994), this approach to educating DHH students in mainstream settings has appeared in an increasing number of countries, exploring the potential benefits for the academic as well as social integration of DHH students and hearing students (see Tang, Lam, & Yiu, Chapter 13 of this volume, for countries adopting this approach). Certainly, unique circumstances surrounding the environments of co-enrollment education do not justify uniformity in program practices. For instance, the signing teacher may be a hearing teacher for the deaf fluent in signing, a sign interpreter, or a deaf paraprofessional expert in signed language. The extent of sign language support in classroom teaching also may vary from full-fledged sign language coverage of all school subjects to partial support for a few. The signing systems adopted also may vary from a natural sign language to visual communication systems such as cued speech or manually coded spoken language, simultaneous communication, or a combination of all these strategies. The language(s) implemented will depend on the educational philosophies and practices adopted, the availability and qualifications of deaf teachers, and the signing proficiency of hearing teachers of the deaf.

## Language of Co-enrollment Education: Some Theoretical Considerations

Depending on the co-enrollment program, a signed language or a manually coded spoken language may be used in partnership with spoken language as the medium of instruction (see Bowen, 2008; Hermans, De Klerk, Wauters, & Knoors, Chapter 16 of this volume; Jiménez-Sánchez & Antia, 1999; Kirchner, 1994, 2004; Kreimeyer, Crooke, Drye, Egbert, & Klein, 2000; Tang, Lam, & Yiu, Chapter 13 of this volume; Wauters & Knoors, 2008). When co-enrollment involves a deaf teacher co-teaching with a regular hearing teacher in class, this deaf teacher functions as a signed language specialist and a deaf role model for the students, deaf or hearing (Jiménez Sánchez & Antia, 1999; Tang, Lam, & Yiu, Chapter 13 of this volume). Bowen (2008) found that hearing students in a co-enrollment setting also acquire signed language and use it for social interactions with their DHH peers. When both the DHH and hearing students adopt a signed language or an oral language as two common languages for mutual communication, the barriers to social integration created by oral language deficiencies will thus be removed.

Seen in this light, co-enrollment can be categorized as an enrichment form of bilingual education that ensures the continuous development of dual language, that is, a signed language and a spoken language, oral and written, among DHH and hearing students in the educational setting (see Baker, 2011). Specifically, hearing students may learn about signed language and Deaf cultures, and DHH students may immerse themselves in a rich environment for spoken language input from hearing students and teachers, as well as signed language input from deaf teachers and their DHH peers. It indirectly encourages DHH and hearing students to partner with each other in the education process, as well as social integration between the two groups of participants (Antia & Kreimeyer, 1996; Antia & Metz, Chapter 17 of this volume; Kirchner, 1994, 2004; Kreimeyer and colleagues, 2000).

### Self-perception of DHH Students in a Co-enrollment Setting

DHH students with a bilingual-bicultural identity may perceive themselves to be "members" of both Deaf and hearing communities (Bat-Chava, 2000). This process to some extent bears resemblance to findings from oral bilingual education, in which the coexistence of both the minority and majority languages as the medium of instruction successfully facilitates intercultural appreciation and social integration of the language minority and language majority students. In the case of co-enrollment in deaf education, by creating a natural school environment that supports bimodal bilingual acquisition and encourages respect for the coexistence of both signed and spoken languages, the school ethos is instilled with mutual acceptance and understanding of both hearing and Deaf cultures (Bowen, 2008; Kirchner, 1994, 2004).

### Previous Research on Co-enrollment

Research findings regarding the social benefits of co-enrollment programming are promising, though limited. So far, the social benefits can be grouped into (1) psychosocial adjustment of DHH students, (2) attitudes and perceptions of hearing students, and (3) social relationships between DHH and hearing students (see Antia & Metz, Chapter 17 of this volume). In sum, the studies suggest that co-enrollment has potential for supporting not only DHH but also hearing students' development of an embracing attitude toward linguistic diversities and deafness in school, laying the foundation for a sense of partnership in language, educational, and psychosocial development in the school environment.

## THE SIGN BILINGUALISM AND CO-ENROLLMENT PROGRAM

### A Brief History of Hong Kong Deaf Education

Deaf education in Hong Kong was mainly conducted in special school settings from the 1930s to the 1970s (Sze, Lo, Lo, & Chu, 2012). However, the 1977 White Paper of the Hong Kong government "Integrating the Disabled into the Community" changed the landscape dramatically (Hong Kong Government, 1977). In Hong Kong today, more and more DHH students with mild to profound hearing losses are enrolled in mainstream settings and are educated under an "oral-only" approach without any exposure to Hong Kong Sign Language (HKSL). Further, the concept of sign bilingualism has never taken root at the deaf schools in the territory. A recent statement by the United Nations Committee on the Rights of Persons with Disabilities stresses that it "takes note of the difficult situation of persons with hearing impairments in accessing information due to lack of official recognition of the significance of sign language by Hong Kong, China" (United Nations, 2012, p. 10).

In fact, as early as 2006, when research on the linguistics of HKSL and sign language acquisition was in progress, the private Sign Bilingualism and Co-enrollment Program (SLCO Program) was established. The program aims to initiate evidence-based practices in deaf education by introducing an option that combines theories of sign bilingualism and co-enrollment to balance the preponderance of the oral-only approach to deaf education in Hong Kong. In this program, the ratios of DHH and hearing students in a class of each grade vary from about 1:3 to 1:4. About 80% of the lessons for the major subjects are co-taught by a regular hearing teacher and a deaf teacher fluent in HKSL. The remaining 20% of the lessons, for subjects like general studies and English offered at the senior grades, are taught collaboratively by two hearing teachers fluent in HKSL. The SLCO Program had progressed from kindergarten to primary 6 at the time of the study.

### Evaluation of Social Acceptance Between DHH and Hearing Students

Sixteen DHH students from primary 4 to primary 6 participated in the current evaluation. All of them were enrolled in the SLCO Program from primary 1 onward, and thus had 4 to 6 years of SLCO experiences. The majority of them had severe or profound hearing loss; others were hard of hearing with a mild or moderately severe loss. Their ages ranged from 9;7 to 14;1. Seven of them received cochlear implants at an average age of 2;10 (ranging from 1;11 to 5;9), and 8 others wore hearing aids. Except for two DHH students who were born to deaf parents, all had hearing parents and started to learn HKSL late, after age 4. The study also included primary 4 to 6 hearing students, 224 from regular classes and 65 from three co-enrollment classes. There have been transfers of hearing students in and out of the co-enrollment classes over the years; of the 65 hearing students in the co-enrollment classes, 44 had full SLCO experience from primary 1, and 21 of them had been transferred into the co-enrollment classes in the interim. Thus the hearing students had 2–5 years of SLCO experiences.

Three measures were adapted from the previous studies to examine social acceptance using peer ratings, hearing students' attitudes toward DHH students, and DHH students' attitudes toward deafness. We suggest that these factors may interact with one another in bringing about social integration between DHH and hearing students in a co-enrollment setting.

*Peer Ratings*

Following Nunes and colleagues (2001) and Wauters and Knoors (2008), peer ratings were used in this study to investigate social acceptance between DHH and hearing students. Both DHH and hearing students in the co-enrollment classes were asked to rate whether they liked to play or study with their classmates based on a visual scale of three faces—happy, neutral, and sad. Face counts well as mean scores were tabulated for each student in order to compare their peer ratings in "study" and "play" conditions.

*Attitudinal Measures*

Two attitudinal measures, Attitudes Toward Deafness Scale (i.e., ATDS) and Hearing Peers' Attitudes Toward DHH Students Scale (i.e., HPATDS), were used in the study. The DHH students took the ATDS, which was a 24-item measure adapted from Yiu's (1999, 2005) Hearing Attitudes Scale, originally developed for measuring attitudes of DHH adolescents in Hong Kong. The hearing students from both the co-enrollment and regular classes also completed the survey. They were asked to indicate their level of agreement to 36 statements in the scale. Note that HPATDS was adapted from Lee (2002), discussed earlier. Both measures adopted a 5-point Likert scale, implying that the higher the mean scores, the more positive the attitudes are.

All three measures were administered by a team of teachers for the deaf who were fluent in HKSL in order to ensure the DHH students' comprehension of the statements in the questionnaire.

## Peer Ratings in Co-enrollment Classes

In exploring peer ratings of DHH and hearing students, we asked (1) if the DHH and hearing students rated each other positively or not, (2) if there was a difference in the way the DHH students rated DHH or hearing students and the way the hearing students rated hearing or DHH peers; (3) if there were bilateral social relationships between DHH and hearing students, and (4) if the duration of SLCO experiences had an impact on the peer ratings of DHH and hearing students.

As shown in Table 14.1, the co-enrollment classes as a whole displayed quite positive social acceptance both between the DHH and hearing students and within each group. The overall mean ratings in the "play" and "study" conditions of both the DHH and hearing students

Table 14.1 Paired Comparisons for Peer Ratings of DHH Students to Hearing Students in the "Play + Study" Conditions

| DHH Students (N = 16) | | | Hearing Students (N = 65) | | | df | t |
|---|---|---|---|---|---|---|---|
| Types | Mean | SD | Types | Mean | SD | | |
| H-rate-D | 4.531 | 0.708 | H-rate-H | 4.459 | 0.599 | 64 | −0.999 |
| D-by-H | 4.517 | 0.480 | H-by-H | 4.458 | 0.489 | 79 | 0.434 |
| D-rate-D | 5.119 | 0.537 | D-rate-H | 4.553 | 0.330 | 15 | 4.037** |
| D-by-D | 5.119 | 0.633 | H-by-D | 4.546 | 0.600 | 79 | 3.384** |

**$p < 0.01$
*$p < 0.05$

were higher than 4.4 (full score = 6). Some categories like "D-rate-D" (DHH students rating DHH students) and "D-by-D" (DHH students rated by DHH students) even received a mean rating higher than 5.

The patterns of positive, neutral, and negative ratings for "H-by-D" (hearing students rated by DHH students) and "D-by-H" (DHH students rated by hearing students) further confirmed that the peer ratings of the two groups of students were very similar, no matter in the "study" or "play" conditions (see Figures 14.1 and 14.2). Negative ratings in both groups were fewer than 10%, far below the positive ratings or the neutral ratings, that is, many of the ratings indicated that students were either neutral or positively inclined toward each other. Statistical analysis performed independently on the DHH and the hearing groups confirmed that there were significantly more positive

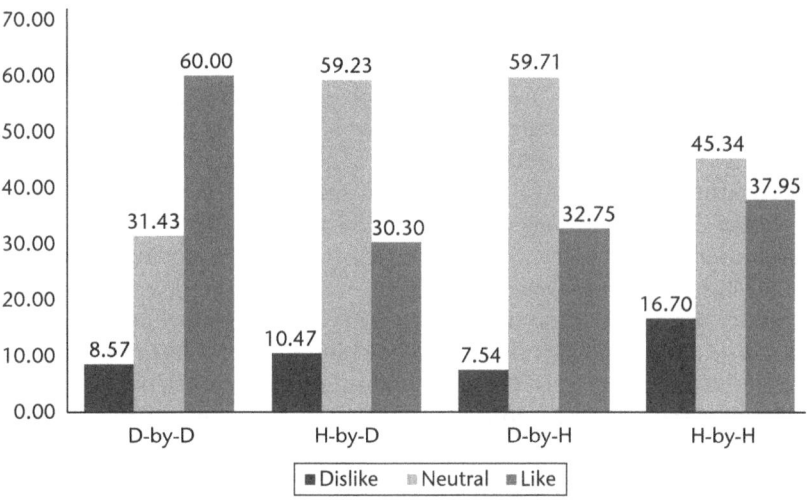

Figure 14.1 Percentages of counts of peer ratings in the "play" condition.

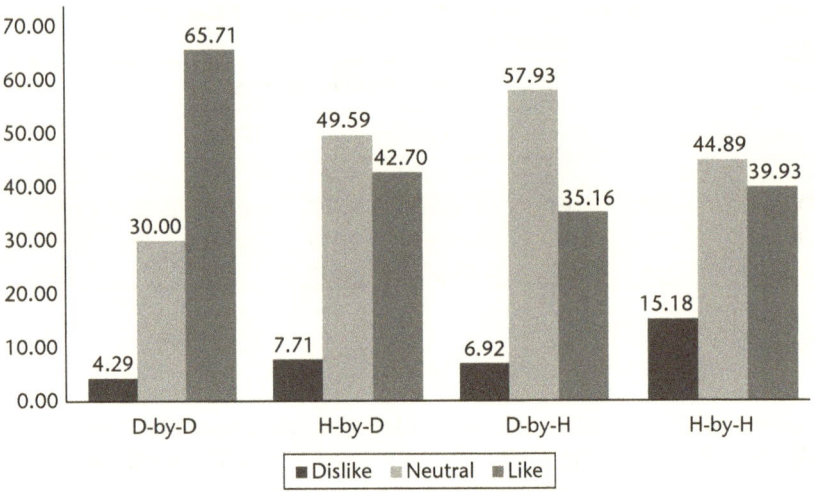

Figure 14.2 Percentages of counts of peer ratings in the "study" condition.

counts than negative counts for both groups of students in both "play" and "study" conditions.

Figures 14.1 and 14.2 show not only positive intergroup ratings (i.e., "D-by-H" and "H-by-D") but also an even higher intragroup rating among the DHH students themselves (i.e., "D-by-D") when compared with the hearing group (i.e., "H-by-H"), in both "play" and "study" conditions. This suggests a stronger sense of mutual support among the DHH students of the program, probably due to the critical mass of DHH students in the co-enrollment setting.

To further investigate whether hearing status was a factor affecting their rating preferences, we examined the ratings of the hearing students and the DHH students independently. Regarding the hearing students, results showed no significant difference between "H-rate-D" (hearing students rating DHH students) and "H-rate-H" (hearing students rating hearing students) (see Table 14.2). A similar observation was found between the mean ratings of "H-by-H" (hearing students rated by hearing students) and "D-by-H" (DHH students rated by hearing students), suggesting that there was no difference in the positive ratings rendered to either the DHH or the hearing students of the co-enrollment classes. In short, the hearing students did not give preferential judgments to either their hearing or DHH peers in the co-enrollment setting.

Similar statistical procedures were performed for the DHH students. Significant differences were found for "D-rate-D" (DHH students rating DHH students) over "D-rate-H" (DHH students rating hearing students), as well as "D-by-D" (i.e., DHH students rated by DHH students) over "D-by-H" (DHH students rated by hearing students). These

Table 14.2 Mean Scores of Attitudes Toward Deafness Scale (ATDS) (N = 16, Cronbach's Alpha = 0.934)

| Factors | Item | M | SD | Item-total correlation | Factor loading |
|---|---|---|---|---|---|
| Factor 1: Acceptance of Deaf Identity (ADI) (7 items) | *I think people are annoyed when I ask them to repeat what they say. | 3.688 | 1.401 | 0.554 | 0.690 |
| | *I don't want to tell people I have hearing loss. | 3.938 | 1.340 | 0.893 | 0.805 |
| | *I don't like people to keep asking me about my hearing loss problems. | 3.813 | 1.328 | 0.853 | 0.845 |
| | *When people ask me if I have hearing loss, I don't want to answer them. | 3.813 | 1.328 | 0.848 | 0.858 |
| | I know how to deal with my hearing problem. | 4.000 | 1.366 | 0.818 | 0.813 |
| | *People make fun of me because of my hearing loss. | 4.125 | 1.258 | 0.765 | 0.921 |
| | I'm happy to answer people's questions about my hearing loss. | 3.938 | 1.340 | 0.802 | 0.916 |
| | Total ADI | 3.902 | 1.181 | | |
| Factor 2: Reactions to Worries and Frustrations (RW/F) (4 items) | *I can't get good exam grades because I have hearing loss. | 3.875 | 1.088 | 0.839 | 0.692 |
| | *I avoid talking to other people because I have hearing loss. | 4.000 | 1.211 | 0.725 | 0.701 |
| | *I don't want to study hard because I have hearing loss. | 4.375 | 0.957 | 0.709 | 0.893 |
| | Although I have hearing loss, I still get good exam grades. | 4.188 | 1.223 | 0.641 | 0.851 |
| | Total RW/F | 4.109 | 1.004 | | |
| Factor 3: Optimism re Coping (OpC) (4 items) | Although I have hearing loss, I can still take part in the activities I love. | 4.813 | 0.403 | 0.259 | 0.926 |
| | Although I have hearing loss, I can still live happily. | 4.688 | 0.602 | 0.709 | 0.627 |
| | Although I have hearing loss, I can still have a lot of friends. | 4.813 | 0.403 | 0.259 | 0.926 |
| | Although I have hearing loss, I still have confidence in myself. | 4.625 | 0.619 | 0.642 | 0.631 |
| | Total OpC | 4.734 | 0.442 | | |
| Factor 4: Readiness for Social Contact (RSC) (3 items) | *I don't want to go out because of my hearing loss. | 4.563 | 0.629 | 0.201 | 0.842 |
| | *I avoid mixing with people because of my hearing loss. | 4.125 | 1.025 | 0.423 | 0.807 |
| | *I don't want to go out with my family because of my hearing loss. | 4.563 | 0.512 | 0.420 | 0.906 |
| | Total RSC | | 4.417 | 0.638 | |
| Total ATDS | | 4.219 | 0.729 | | |

*For items involving negative statements, the scores given by the DHH students were reversed from 5 to 1, 4 to 2, and so forth.

results echoed the earlier observation that DHH students gave higher ratings to their DHH peers than their hearing peers, a clear indication of mutual acceptance among the DHH students in a co-enrollment environment.

Summing up, probably because DHH students constitute a minority group in the school community, they tend to identify themselves with each other more readily and to interact with each other more frequently, hence leading to a higher rating given to DHH students by DHH students than that given by DHH students to hearing students. However, there were no indications that they were less (or more) socially accepted in the co-enrollment classroom when compared with their hearing counterparts.

To investigate whether DHH students developed bilateral social relationships with their DHH and hearing peers, we examined the positive peer ratings (i.e., a happy face) received and given by the 16 DHH students. For this purpose, the same sets of students must be involved for admission to this bilateral social relationship (i.e., A rated B positively and B also rated A positively). In the "study" condition, all of them had bilateral positive ratings with their peers, 11 with both DHH and hearing, and 2 with DHH and 3 with hearing only. In the "play" condition, again 11 had bilateral positive ratings with both DHH and hearing peers, and 3 with DHH and 1 with hearing students only. One DHH student, while ranked third from the top on counts of being rated bilaterally (i.e., quite popular with both DHH and hearing students) in the "study" condition, had no bilateral positive ratings in the "play" condition. However, 9 students (5 DHH and 4 hearing) did rate her positively in the "play" condition, even though those relationships were not "bilateral" according to our criterion. Overall, a great majority of DHH students had established bilateral social relationships with their peers, DHH and/or hearing, probably helping them to avoid a sense of loneliness even though they were studying in a mainstream environment (see Hintermair, Chapter 7 of this volume).

No significant correlations were found between years of SLCO experience and the mean total ratings of "D-by-D" in either condition. In contrast, significant correlations were found with the mean total ratings of "D-by-H" and the years of SLCO experience. Further statistical analysis showed that years of SLCO experience had a significant effect on the mean ratings of DHH students rendered by their hearing peers, especially between the primary 4 and primary 6 students. To conclude, DHH students with longer duration of the SLCO experiences demonstrated a higher degree of social acceptance by their hearing peers.

### DHH Students' Attitudes toward Deafness (ATDS)

Item-total reliability and factor analysis of ATDS scores left 18 items intact to form a scale, and we identified four factors that explained

87% of the total variance (see Table 14.2). The factors that appeared to hold among ATDS items were (1) Acceptance of Deaf Identity (ADI), reflecting DHH students' willingness to accept or disclose their deaf identity and related difficulties to others; (2) Reactions to Worries and Frustrations (RW/F), reflecting DHH students' feelings about the frustrations and worries caused by deafness, which may prevent them from engaging in activities that they like or achieving their goals; (3) Optimism related to Coping (OpC), reflecting DHH students' ability to cope with their deafness; and (4) Readiness for Social Contact (RSC), relating to DHH students' acceptance or reluctance to maintain social contact with others.

Overall, the deaf students held quite high positive attitudes toward their deafness (ATDS overall mean = 4.2 out of 5). Comparing the mean scores of the factors identified for ATDS, we found that OpC obtained the highest overall mean (M = 4.7) and ADI the lowest (M = 3.9). While the OpC means stayed consistently high from primary 4 to 6, ADI showed a gradual improvement from primary 4 (M = 3.1) to primary 6 (M = 4.3). It thus seems that although the DHH students in the co-enrollment classes had quite positive and optimistic attitudes toward their hearing loss, accepting their deaf identities took time.

### Hearing Peers' Attitudes toward DHH Students (HPATDS)

Item-total reliability and factor analysis of HPATDS scores left 28 items to form a scale, and we identified four factors (see Table 14.3). They were (1) Positive Actions (PA), relating to the caring and supportive responses of hearing students toward their DHH peers; (2) Negative Reactions and Perception (NA/P), relating to the hearing students' negative perceptions and behaviors toward their DHH peers; (3) Positive Perception (PP), reflecting hearing students' perceptions of the personalities and behaviors of their DHH peers; and (4) Tolerance to Communication Difficulties (TCD), reflecting hearing students' reactions to the possible difficulties they perceive when communicating with DHH students, in signed or oral language.

Overall, the HPATDS scores mean of all 289 hearing students was 3.8 out of 5. Among the 4 factors identified, Positive Actions (PA) received the highest mean scores (M = 4.02). The next highest was PP (M = 3.96). However, the mean scores of TCD were slightly lower (M = 3.1), but we observed an increase from primary 4 (M = 2.9, 91 students) to primary 6 (M = 3.4, 99 students). In other words, the hearing students had quite positive perceptions of their DHH peers and were ready to render positive actions, care, and support, but for them to understand and accept the communication difficulties facing DHH peers took time.

Does a relationship exist between the hearing students' attitudes toward their DHH peers and the duration of SLCO experiences? The 74 hearing students from the co-enrollment classes with SLCO

**Table 14.3** Hearing Peers' Attitudes Toward DHH Students Scale (HPATDS) (N = 289, Cronbach's Alpha = 0.948)

| Factors | Items | M | SD | Item-total correlation | Factor loading |
|---|---|---|---|---|---|
| Factor 1: Positive Actions (PA) (9 items) | If DHH classmates ask me about homework, I'm happy to explain it to them. | 4.142 | 0.844 | 0.641 | 0.581 |
| | If someone laughs at DHH classmates, I will stand by them. | 3.609 | 0.929 | 0.503 | 0.608 |
| | I am willing to lend my notebooks or stationery to DHH classmates. | 4.308 | 0.837 | 0.680 | 0.586 |
| | We should help DHH classmates because they have hearing difficulties. | 4.308 | 0.816 | 0.655 | 0.658 |
| | I am willing to sit next to DHH classmates and have lessons together. | 3.931 | 1.022 | 0.712 | 0.718 |
| | I am willing to work on a project with DHH classmates. | 4.048 | 0.953 | 0.730 | 0.796 |
| | If I do not understand what DHH classmates say, I will patiently use other ways to understand them. | 4.080 | 0.915 | 0.622 | 0.745 |
| | If I have good toys, I will share them with DHH classmates. | 3.917 | 0.890 | 0.704 | 0.756 |
| | I am willing to play with DHH classmates. | 3.855 | 0.979 | 0.604 | 0.575 |
| | Total PA | 4.022 | 0.697 | | |
| Factor 2: Negative Reactions and Perception (NA/P) (9 items) | *I think DHH classmates have a bad temper. | 3.450 | 1.127 | 0.626 | 0.585 |
| | *I will not do homework with DHH classmates. | 3.626 | 1.105 | 0.638 | 0.730 |
| | *If I have DHH classmates, I will not introduce them to other classmates. | 3.547 | 1.142 | 0.432 | 0.673 |
| | *If DHH classmates have difficulties, I will not help them. | 3.934 | 1.027 | 0.590 | 0.711 |
| | *I will not lend my stationery to DHH classmates. | 4.021 | 1.051 | 0.713 | 0.764 |
| | *I don't want to group with DHH classmates in group activities. | 3.858 | 1.095 | 0.733 | 0.692 |
| | *When I meet DHH classmates in the school playground, I will not greet them. | 3.730 | 1.126 | 0.685 | 0.665 |

*(continued)*

Table 14.3 Continued

| Factors | Items | M | SD | Item-total correlation | Factor loading |
|---|---|---|---|---|---|
| | *If DHH classmates are sitting beside me, I will feel uncomfortable. | 3.841 | 1.088 | 0.639 | 0.690 |
| | *I think DHH classmates are impolite. | 3.751 | 1.112 | 0.640 | 0.643 |
| | Total NA/P | 3.751 | 0.832 | | |
| Factor 3: Positive Perception (PP) (5 items) | I think DHH classmates are kind. | 4.190 | 0.867 | 0.582 | 0.655 |
| | I think DHH classmates are easy to get along with. | 3.654 | 0.953 | 0.561 | 0.487 |
| | I think DHH classmates are capable of helping others. | 4.045 | 0.826 | 0.552 | 0.683 |
| | I think DHH classmates are serious and hard-working. | 3.952 | 0.919 | 0.523 | 0.796 |
| | I think DHH classmates are keen to serve. | 3.941 | 0.905 | 0.620 | 0.415 |
| | Total PP | 3.956 | 0.696 | | |
| Factor 4: Tolerance to Communication Difficulties (TCD) (5 items) | *I think DHH classmates do not speak clearly. | 2.830 | 1.078 | 0.573 | 0.622 |
| | *I don't want to speak to DHH classmates. | 3.626 | 1.067 | 0.669 | 0.513 |
| | *I think DHH classmates often misunderstand or do not understand what people say to them. | 3.097 | 1.033 | 0.465 | 0.680 |
| | *I do not like people communicating with me in sign language. | 3.187 | 1.175 | 0.620 | 0.475 |
| | *I find it hard to comprehend what DHH classmates say. | 2.851 | 1.100 | 0.492 | 0.779 |
| | Total TCD | 3.118 | 0.817 | | |
| Total HPATDS | | 3.761 | 0.647 | | |

*For items involving negative statements, the scores given by the DHH students were reversed from 5 to 1, 4 to 2, and so forth.

experiences from 1 to 6 years (average being 4.2 years) were found to have significantly more positive attitudes toward their DHH peers than those 215 students who had no SLCO experiences. Therefore, the impact of SLCO experiences was clear on cultivating a positive culture toward deafness and DHH students.

Do relationships exist among the DHH students' backgrounds, the peer ratings of DHH and hearing students, the hearing students' attitudes toward the DHH students, and the DHH students' attitudes toward their own deafness? Correlation analyses with the 16 DHH students found no relationships existing between the DHH students' peer rating categories (i.e., "D-rate-H," "D-rate-D," "D-by-H," "D-by-D") and the ages at which they started using hearing aids or cochlear implants or the year of learning sign language. In addition, the degree of hearing loss was correlated only with "D-rate-H," but negatively. In other words, the poorer the hearing level of the DHH students, the more positively they rated their hearing peers. Last, a significant correlation obtained between the duration of SLCO experiences and "D-by-H" only, meaning that the longer the DHH students were enrolled in the SLCO Program, the more positive ratings they received from their hearing peers.

To investigate issues associated with DHH students' language abilities, correlation analyses were conducted between the different peer rating categories of DHH students and their language scores, including their speech perception abilities based on the Cantonese Lexical Neighborhood Test (Yuen, Ng, Luk, Chan, Chan, Kwok, & Tong, 2008), oral language skills in Cantonese based on the subscale "Cantonese Grammar" of the Hong Kong Cantonese Oral Language Assessment Scale (T'sou, Lee, Tung, Chan, Man, & To, 2006), knowledge of written Chinese based on the Assessment of Chinese Grammatical Knowledge (see Tang, Lam, & Yiu, Chapter 13 of this volume), and sign language skills based on the Hong Kong Sign Language Elicitation Tool (ref. Tang, Lam, & Yiu, Chapter 13 of this volume). It turned out that only signed language skills had a significant positive relationship with the ratings of deaf students given by their hearing peers ("D-by-H"); this relationship was more prominent in the "study" condition.

The findings reported thus far contrast with those reported in earlier studies that stronger oral language abilities lead to a higher opportunity for developing a positive social relationship of oral DHH students when studying in mainstream settings (Most, 2007; Most, Ingber, & Heled-Ariam, 2011). Here, neither spoken language performance nor speech perception had a significant impact on peer ratings in the co-enrollment setting, but DHH students with good signing skills received more positive ratings from their hearing peers. Though further evidence is required, the findings may be accounted for as follows: (1) hearing students understand their DHH peers better through sign language, so they like DHH peers with better signing skills; (2) they like signed language and they admire DHH students with better signing skills; and (3) the presence of a deaf teacher and the use of signed language in the classroom may indirectly raise the status of signed language (as a formal medium of instruction) and thus the positive attitudes toward DHH peers. In sum, it seems that hearing students did not find signed language a challenge but ascribed it with a set of positive values with which they judged their DHH peers.

### Students' Attitudes toward Deafness and Social Acceptance

Among DHH students, correlation analyses showed that the overall ATDS mean positively correlated with the DHH students' peer rating in categories "D-rate-D" and "D-by-H" only, but not in other categories. This implies that the more positive attitudes the DHH students had toward their own deafness, the higher they rated the other DHH students and, at the same time, the more positive ratings they received from their hearing peers. This is further confirmed by a more fine-grained analysis in which we found that the factor ADI correlated significantly with "D-rate-D," "D-by-H," and "D-by-D," and RW/F with "D-by-H" but not others. In other words, positive deaf identity and readiness to face worries and frustrations that arise from deafness are essential ingredients for achieving positive social acceptance among DHH students as well as between the DHH and hearing students.

Considering hearing students' attitudes toward DHH peers and social acceptance, results indicated that there was a significantly positive correlation between the overall HPATDS mean with the hearing students' peer rating category "H-by-D" only, implying that the more positive the hearing students' attitudes toward the DHH students were, the more positively the DHH students rated them. Further analyses found a significantly positive relationship existing only between Negative Actions and Perception, and between Tolerance of Communication Difficulty and "H-by-D." The latter was also associated with "H-rate-D." Taken as a whole, the more ready the hearing students were in rejecting the negative actions and perceptions, or the more tolerant they were toward communication difficulties, the higher the ratings they received from or rendered to their DHH peers.

## PUTTING IT ALL TOGETHER

To recapitulate, our examination of social acceptance within a sign bilingual co-enrollment setting revealed quite positive social outcomes for both DHH and hearing students. There is evidence that the DHH and hearing students were teaming up with each other in "study" and "play" conditions; at the same time, there was "in-group" support among the DHH students. Duration of SLCO experiences with hearing students had a positive effect on nurturing mutual understanding and positive attitudes toward the DHH students, who reciprocated by positive ratings toward their hearing peers. Unlike earlier findings based on oral DHH students in the mainstream environment (Most, 2007; Most et al., 2011), spoken language abilities in the SLCO Program are not a determining factor affecting the integration of DHH students; rather, it is signed language and a positive attitude toward one's own deafness that seem to support the development of social acceptance between DHH and hearing students. Adopting a positive attitude toward one's own deafness, as Saur and colleagues (1986) observed, is a crucial ingredient for social acceptance, promoting DHH students' development of a sense of membership in the school/class community.

The positive outcomes of the SLCO Program are encouragingly suggestive of the possibility of mainstream school placements of DHH if the environment is supported by sign bilingualism and co-enrollment (see Marschark, Knoors, & Tang, Chapter 18 of this volume). To account for these findings, we would argue that certain principles and practices subsumed under this learning environment contribute to the positive social integration of DHH and hearing students in the current study, providing the essential ingredients for nurturing social membership of a specific type of school/class community with which they positively associate themselves.

To nurture social integration, in addition to facilitating social acceptance between DHH and hearing students, it is equally important to identify means of bolstering the psychosocial well-being of DHH students. DHH students need social-emotional support to develop a positive attitude toward their own deafness, thus equipping them with a state of mind that is conducive to constructing positive social relationships with others. DHH students, especially those born to hearing parents, may sense a lack of support due to communication barriers and a distinct sense of "self" compared with their peers. It appears helpful for them to be in an environment in which they feel they have an affinity to certain characteristics of the community. These characteristics can be the existing values of the school/class community; however, new values can also be derived that are uniquely shared by both the DHH and hearing students. We believe that it is being sign bilinguals that bonds the DHH and hearing students together, reducing the sense of "otherness" in the mainstream setting.

Collaborative teaching and co-learning practices, the very essence of co-enrollment, create many opportunities for classroom/social interactions between the DHH and hearing students, through which perceptions of attitudes toward deafness and values for social integration are identified and evaluated (see Hermans, De Klerk, Wauters, & Knoors, Chapter 16 of this volume). Adult models, both deaf and hearing, who have accepting attitudes toward each other as co-teachers may foster the values of social interactions and collaborative attitudes for the DHH and hearing students.

Co-learning activities engage students and require them to learn how to negotiate learning outcomes among themselves in either signed language or spoken language, depending on their language abilities as well as language preferences. This may help nurture peer relationships and ultimately group membership (see Antia et al., 2002). Therefore, a mainstream setting that involves sign interpreters is no guarantee for social integration, because it deprives DHH as well as hearing students of opportunities for building social relationships with each other through constant direct interactions and co-construction of a communicative and meaningful classroom discourse. Both groups of students, especially the DHH ones, need such interactions to acquire higher order thinking skills through information elicitation, negotiation, and organization, as well as to develop knowledge of the use of language in communicative contexts.

The high frequency of social interactions between and among the DHH and hearing students in the SLCO Program environment may have led to the observed positive attitudes toward DHH students by hearing students. Note that there was a correlation between the DHH ratings by their hearing peers ("D-by-H") and the DHH students' scores for attitudes toward their own deafness (ATDS), corroborating the observations of Yiu (1999, 2005) that DHH students' attitudes toward deafness are strongly associated with self-esteem. Bat-Chava (2000) also observed that DHH students with bicultural identities had a more positive self-esteem and attitudes toward deafness.

Adopting sign bilingualism in a co-enrollment setting is another important factor for two reasons. First, as we noted earlier, instead of nurturing only DHH students to be sign bilingual, the SLCO Program also supports the hearing students in becoming sign bilingual, thus removing social as well as communication barriers to social integration among DHH and hearing students in the mainstream environment. Second, equipped with knowledge of two languages, DHH students may access communication or the curriculum not only with their DHH peers or deaf teachers, but also with their hearing peers or hearing teachers, in speech or HKSL. As Baker (1996, p. 4), put it, "[the] language of the classroom requires more complex grammatical structures, more technical vocabulary, more abstract use of language often with far less paralinguistic support." Being sign bilingual supports DHH students in facing this daunting task in the classroom learning condition.

To ascribe equal social significance to both HKSL and spoken language development not only for DHH but also for hearing students, classroom/instructional procedures have been devised to support both DHH and hearing students to access communication via either language. Therefore, there is plentiful linguistic input and output opportunities for bilingual acquisition of both DHH and hearing students in the school environment. Tang, Lam, and Yiu (Chapter 13 of this volume) argue that DHH students enrolled early in a co-enrollment environment are best classified as either simultaneous or sequential bimodal bilinguals. Such a setting, with its associated pedagogical practices, reflects an enrichment form of bilingual education benefiting both DHH and hearing students (Baker, 1996, 2011). Also, it secures transmission of HKSL by the "senior" deaf members of the school/class to the junior ones.

Seen in this light, the introduction of sign bilingualism into a co-enrollment setting is not for a "transitional" purpose of supporting DHH students' progression from signed to spoken language development, but for maintaining bimodal bilingual development in the school setting for both DHH and hearing students, with the understanding that there may be ups and downs in terms of their developmental trajectory, as is typical of bilingual development. At least in this environment, the choice of language for communication is determined by the students themselves on the basis of their sign bilingual proficiency at any given point of their development, or on their own assessment of the sociolinguistic variables involved in a communicative situation such as the role and relationship of the language users or the formality of the situation (cf. Hymes's, 1972, "ethnography of speaking").

Spoken language in mainstream settings is usually the only medium in deaf-hearing communication. Therefore, insufficient spoken language or low speech intelligibility can prevent DHH students from developing social relationships with their hearing peers or participating in classroom discussions (Most, 2007). Interestingly, as reported here, neither speech perception nor oral language abilities in the co-enrollment setting are determining factors affecting the ratings of DHH students by their hearing peers. Rather, it is signed language proficiency of DHH students that supports the development of social acceptance between DHH and hearing students, especially in the "study" condition. This reflects that adding a signed language to build the bilingual repertoire for the students, DHH or hearing, compensates for DHH students' speech deficiencies in deaf-hearing communication.

Another factor underlying the social success of co-enrollment is the critical mass of DHH students in that setting. Previous studies on social integration expressed concern over the feelings of "loneliness" among the DHH students. Adopting a sign bilingual and co-enrollment approach, deliberate attempts were made to create a community of DHH students within a larger community of hearing students, where the two communities were connected by sign bilingualism. Alleviating the pressure of access to communication through promoting bimodal bilingual acquisition of both DHH and hearing students, we observed the emergence of a sign bilingual community of DHH and hearing participants within a larger hearing school community. It seems that as the DHH and hearing students came to socially accept each other as members of this unique community, little difference was found in their ratings toward each other. In other words, DHH students in this co-enrollment setting were not restricted to developing social relationships with hearing friends and vice versa; but the critical mass of DHH students in this setting also enabled them to develop affiliation with their DHH peers, in both study and at play.

Finally, we believe that the presence of a deaf teacher, which is quite enticing to young DHH and hearing learners alike, is an important feature in co-enrollment. Jiménez-Sánchez and Antia (1999, p. 223) emphasized the positive impact of team and collaborative models between professionals on DHH and hearing students. In a co-enrollment setting, when deaf teachers are an integral part of a school community and are centrally involved in team-teaching practices, "the most viable benefits was the access of all children to all communication in the classroom where differences were not degraded but viewed as valuable and respected." While hearing teachers are spoken language models, inclusion of a deaf adult in class who assumes the role of teacher is not solely for bringing sign language into the classroom, but also for setting up that teacher as a model and a link to the Deaf community. This has already been found to be effective in previous studies in supporting the development of positive Deaf identities or bicultural identities of DHH students (see Antia et al., 2002; Bat-Chava, 2000; Jiménez-Sánchez & Antia, 1999; Kirchner, 1994, 2004). Deaf teachers also help DHH and hearing students not only to learn in class, but also to "pick up" a new language. Through these practices, the hearing students can achieve an understanding and a positive attitude toward deafness and deaf people. The accepting attitude of the hearing teachers is demonstrated through their team teaching and interacting with deaf teachers, helping students learn about deaf-hearing inclusion and the value of collaboration. These values may be transmitted to the students during co-learning activities, another pedagogical requirement of co-enrollment.

In a study investigating the social acceptance of African American children in mainstream schools, Jackson, Barth, Powell, and Lochman (2006) clearly indicated that both the involvement of an African American teacher and the increase in the proportion of African American children in class are significant factors supporting social integration of those children in mainstream settings. Similarly, the sizable existence of DHH students, as well as a team of deaf teachers, may also have an equivalent impact on social acceptance between DHH and hearing students in the SLCO Program, though further research is definitely necessary to verify the validity of this claim.

In conclusion, there have been few studies that attempt to associate peer ratings, which we assume to reflect social acceptance, with attitudes of DHH students toward their own deafness and attitudes toward DHH students by hearing students, although such a relationship has long been recognized by researchers (Schroedel & Schiff, 1972). In this study, we have at least shown that relationships existed between the peer ratings and attitudes of DHH toward their deafness as well as hearing students toward deafness or deaf persons.

The creation of a sign bilingual and co-enrollment environment, originally set out to accommodate the pedagogical needs of DHH students in their education, turned out to support the DHH and hearing students' positive development of social acceptance toward each other. We argue that being able to access languages bimodally and to be centrally involved in classroom/school activities that require constant interactions and negotiation via two languages, the DHH and hearing participants have plenty of opportunities for learning and appreciating each other's group characteristics. Therefore, co-enrollment is a form of education that builds on children's existing linguistic and intellectual resources and provides an educational environment that continues to enrich their bilingual development. As approximately two-thirds of the world is bilingual, the co-enrollment setting supported by sign bilingualism has the advantages of preserving the development of signed languages while at the same time supporting the expansion of the population of bilinguals. As Baker (2011, p. 2) noted, "while deaf people may consider themselves a language minority, as bilinguals they are in the majority of the world."

## ACKNOWLEDGMENTS

The authors would like to acknowledge the generous funding support of The Hong Kong Jockey Club Charities Trust for the project "Jockey Club Sign Bilingualism and Co-enrollment in Deaf Education Programme" (2006–2014). Special thanks also go to Professor Cheung Shu Fai, University of Macau, for his advice on the validation procedures for the measures used in the study, and to David Lam and Lucia Chow for their support in conducting this study.

## REFERENCES

Andersson, G., Olsson, E., Rydell, A. M., & Larsen, H. C. (2000). Social competence and behavioural problems in children with hearing impairment. *International Journal of Audiology, 39*(2), 88–92.

Antia, S. D. (1982). Social interaction of partially mainstreamed hearing-impaired children. *American Annals of the Deaf, 127*(1), 18–25.

Antia, S. D., Jones, P., Luckner, J., Kreimeyer, K. H., & Reed, S. (2011). Social outcomes of students who are deaf and hard of hearing in general education classrooms. *Exceptional Children, 77*(4), 489–504.

Antia, S. D., & Kreimeyer, K. H. (1996). Social interaction and acceptance of deaf or hard-of-hearing children and their peers: A comparison of social-skills and familiarity-based interventions. *Volta Review, 98*(4), 157–181.

Antia, S. D., & Kreimeyer, K. H. (1997). The generalization and maintenance of the peer social behaviors of young children who are deaf or hard of hearing. *Language, Speech, and Hearing Services in Schools, 28*(1), 59.

Antia, S. D., & Stinson, M. S. (1999). Some conclusions on the education of deaf and hard-of-hearing students in inclusive settings. *Journal of Deaf Studies and Deaf Education, 4*, 246–248.

Antia, S. D., Stinson, M. S., & Gaustad, M. G. (2002). Developing membership in the education of deaf and hard-of-hearing students in inclusive settings. *Journal of Deaf Studies and Deaf Education, 7*(3), 214–229.

Arnold, D., & Tremblay, A. (1979). Interaction of deaf and hearing preschool children. *Journal of Communication Disorders, 12*(3), 245–251.

Baker, C. (1996). Education for bilingualism: Key themes and issues. In P. Knight & R. Swanwick (Eds.), *Bilingualism and the education of deaf children: Advances in practice* (pp. 1–17). Leeds, UK: ADEDC.

Baker, C. (2011). *Foundations of bilingual education and bilingualism* (5th ed.) Bristol, UK: Multilingual Matters.

Bat-Chava, Y. (2000). Diversity of deaf identities. *American Annals of the Deaf, 145*(5), 420–428.

Bowen, S. K. (2008). Coenrollment for students who are deaf or hard of hearing: Friendship patterns and social interactions. *American Annals of the Deaf, 153*(3), 285–293.

Bunch, G. (1994). An interpretation of full inclusion. *American Annals of the Deaf, 139*(2), 150–152.

Cambra, C. (2002). Acceptance of deaf students by hearing students in regular classrooms. *American Annals of the Deaf, 147*(1), 38–45.

Dammeyer, J. (2010). Psychosocial development in a Danish population of children with cochlear implants and deaf and hard-of-hearing children. *Journal of Deaf Studies and Deaf Education, 15*(1), 50–58.

Grosjean, F. (2010). Bilingualism, biculturalism, and deafness. *International Journal of Bilingual Education and Bilingualism, 13*(2), 133–145.

Hintermair, M. (2008). Self-esteem and satisfaction with life of deaf and hard-of-hearing people: A resource-oriented approach to identity work. *Journal of Deaf Studies and Deaf Education, 13*(2), 278–300.

Hong Kong Government. (1977). *White paper: Integrating disabled into the community: A united effort*. Hong Kong: Hong Kong Government Printer.

Hymes, D. (1972). On communicative competence. In J. B. Pride & J. Holmes (Eds.), *Sociolinguistics* (pp. 269–85). Harmondsworth, UK: Penguin.

Jackson, M. F., Barth, J. M., Powell, N., & Lochman, J. E. (2006). Classroom contextual effects of race on children's peer nominations. *Child Development, 77*(5), 1325–1337.

Jiménez-Sánchez, C., & Antia, S. (1999). Team-teaching in an integrated classroom: Perceptions of deaf and hearing teachers. *Journal of Deaf Studies and Deaf Education, 4*(3), 215–224.

Keating, E., & Mirus, G. (2003). American sign language in virtual space: Interactions between deaf users of computer-mediated video communication and the impact of technology on language practices. *Language in Society, 32*(5), 693–714.

Kirchner, C. J. (1994). Co-enrollment as an inclusion model. *American Annals of the Deaf, 139*(2), 163–164.

Kirchner, C. J. (2004). Co-enrollment. In D. Power & G. Leigh (Eds.), *Educating deaf students: Global perspectives* (p. 161). Washington, DC: Gallaudet University Press.

Kluwin, T. N., Stinson, M. S., & Colarossi, G. M. (2002). Social processes and outcomes of in-school contact between deaf and hearing peers. *Journal of Deaf Studies and Deaf Education, 7*(3), 200–213.

Kreimeyer, K. H., Crooke, P., Drye, C., Egbert, V., & Klein, B. (2000). Academic and social benefits of a co-enrollment model of inclusive education for deaf and hard-of-hearing children. *Journal of Deaf Studies and Deaf Education, 5*(2), 174–185.

Lee, Yu-Chin. (2002). *Research on Eastern Taiwan elementary students' attitudes towards and interaction methods with hearing impaired peers.* Unpublished Master's thesis. National Hualien Teachers College.

Leigh, I. W., Maxwell-McCaw, D., Bat-Chava, Y., & Christiansen, J. B. (2009). Correlates of psychosocial adjustment in deaf adolescents with and without cochlear implants: A preliminary investigation. *Journal of Deaf Studies and Deaf Education, 14*(2), 244–259.

Mckee, R. L. (2008). The construction of deaf children as marginal bilinguals in the mainstream. *International Journal of Bilingual Education and Bilingualism, 11*(5), 519–540.

Most, T. (2007). Speech intelligibility, loneliness, and sense of coherence among deaf and hard-of-hearing children in individual inclusion and group inclusion. *Journal of Deaf Studies and Deaf Education, 12*(4), 495–503.

Most, T., Ingber, S., & Heled-Ariam, E. (2011). Social competence, sense of loneliness, and speech intelligibility of young children with hearing loss in individual inclusion and group inclusion. *Journal of Deaf Studies and Deaf Education, 17*, 259–272.

Nunes, T., Pretzlik, U., & Olsson, J. (2001). Deaf children's social relationships in mainstream schools. *Deafness & Education International, 3*(3), 123–136.

Padden, C., & Ramsey, C. (2000). American Sign Language and reading ability in deaf children. In C. Chamberlain, J. Morford, & R. Mayberry (Eds.), *Language acquisition by eye* (vol. 1, pp. 65–89). Mahwah, NJ: Lawrence Erlbaum Associates.

Plaza-Pust, C., & López, E. M. (2008). Sign bilingualism: Language development, interaction and maintenance in sign language contact situation. In C. Plaza-Pust & E. Morales-López (Eds.), *Sign bilingualism* (pp. 333–379). Amsterdam, Netherlands: John Benjamns Publishing.

Polat, F. (2003). Factors affecting psychosocial adjustment of deaf students. *Journal of Deaf Studies and Deaf Education, 8*(3), 325–339.

Punch, R., & Hyde, M. (2010). Children with cochlear implants in Australia: Educational settings, supports, and outcomes. *Journal of Deaf Studies and Deaf Education, 15*(4), 405–421.

Rutman, D. (1989). The impact and experience of adventitious deafness. *American Annals of the Deaf, 134*(5), 305–311.

Saur, R. E., Layne, C. A., Hurley, E. A., & Opton, K. (1986). Dimensions of mainstreaming. *American Annals of the Deaf, 131*(5), 325–330.

Schroedel, J. G., & Schiff, W. (1972). Attitudes towards deafness among several deaf and hearing populations. *Rehabilitation Psychology, 19*(2), 59.

Spencer, P. E., & Marschark, M. (2010). *Evidence-based practice in educating deaf and hard-of-hearing students.* New York, NY: Oxford University Press.

Stinson, M. S., & Antia, S. D. (1999). Considerations in educating deaf and hard-of-hearing students in inclusive settings. *Journal of Deaf Studies and Deaf Education, 4*(3), 163–175.

Sze, F., Lo, C., Lo, L., & Chu, K. (2012). Early deaf education in Hong Kong and its relation with the origin of Hong Kong Sign Language, *Educational Journal, 39, 1–2,* 139–156.

T'sou, B., Lee, T., Tung, P., Chan, A., Man, Y., & To, C. (2006). *Hong Kong Cantonese oral language assessment scale.* Hong Kong: City University of Hong Kong Press.

Tvingstedt, A. L. (1995). Classroom interaction and the social situation of hard-of-hearing pupils in regular classes. In A. Weisel, (Ed.), *Proceedings of the 18th International Congress on Education of the Deaf—1995.* Tel-Aviv, Israel: Ramot Publications, Tel Aviv University.

van Gent, T., Goedhart, A. W., Knoors, H. E., Westenberg, P. M., & Treffers, P. D. (2012). Self-concept and ego development in deaf adolescents: A comparative study. *Journal of Deaf Studies and Deaf Education, 17*(3), 333–351.

United Nations. (2005). *Building peaceful social relationship by, for and with people.* Retrieved on August 30, 2013, from http://www.un.org/esa/socdev/sib/peacedialogue/ soc_integration.htm.

United Nations. (2006). *Convention on the rights of persons with disabilities.* United Nations. Retrieved on June 1, 2013, from http://www.un.org/disabilities/convention/ conventionfull.shtml.

United Nations. (2012). *Committee on the rights of persons with disabilities: Concluding observations on initial report of China, adopted by the committee at its eighth session* (17–28 September 2012). Retrieved on August 30, 2013, from http://legco.gov.hk/yr12-13/english/panels/ca/papers/cacb2-119-1-e.pdf.

Wauters, L. N., & Knoors, H. (2008). Social integration of deaf children in inclusive settings. *Journal of Deaf Studies and Deaf Education, 13*(1), 21–36.

Yiu, K-M. (1999). *Self-concept of hearing impaired students integrated in regular classes: Its relationships to severity of hearing impairment and attitudes towards their disabilities.* Unpublished Bachelor's dissertation, University of Hong Kong.

Yiu, K-M. (2005, July). *Self-concept of hearing impaired students—integrated in regular classes: Its relationships to severity of hearing impairment and attitude towards their disabilities.* Paper presented at the 20th International Congress on the Education of the Deaf, Maastricht, The Netherlands.

Yuen, K. C. P., Ng, I. H. Y., Luk, B. P. K., Chan, S. K. W., Chan, S. C. S., Kwok, I. C. L., & Tong, M. C. F. (2008). The development of Cantonese Lexical Neighborhood Test: A pilot study. *International Journal of Pediatric Otorhinolaryngology, 72*(7), 1121–1129.

# 15

# Sign Bilingual and Co-enrollment Education for Children with Cochlear Implants in Madrid, Spain

Mar Pérez Martin, Marian Valmaseda Balanzategui, and Gary Morgan

**PROLOGUE**

The authors combine expertise in education and developmental psychology and have come together to report on the latest findings from bilingual school approaches used in Madrid, Spain. It can be the case that researchers and educationalists have different objectives. Researchers set out to test hypotheses or advance theories, while educationalists are primarily concerned with the everyday experience of children in the classroom in order to improve educational outcomes. We think it is important that both sets of professionals work more in tandem. In this chapter, we will first describe the historical and social background of how bilingual sign education evolved in Spain and the content of the bilingual program used in Madrid schools. We then report on the results of a longitudinal study of the language development of children with a cochlear implant (CI) in these schools. Finally, we conclude with some discussion of the present challenges and implications of our work.

**HOW DID WE ARRIVE AT SIGN BILINGUAL EDUCATION IN MADRID?**

In order to understand current bilingual education practices, it is important to consider social and legal changes toward disability and linguistic minority groups over the past three decades in Spain. Until 1985, deaf children were educated in residential special schools. The experience was one based on rehabilitation, strong moralism, and a parallel or reduced version of the mainstream curriculum. From 1985 onward, this changed to an integration policy for all children with disabilities, including deafness. This policy move was backed up with a significant investment in funding and personnel, which had major educational and social impacts. The government's department of education developed a legal framework and started ambitious plans for teacher training. For deaf children, this integration policy had some special characteristics. Some schools were selected as special mainstream sites for deaf children to attend where there were two objectives: (1) the focusing of teaching resources (materials and personnel) in these schools and (2) the grouping together of deaf children with hearing children to promote social interaction and to avoid social isolation.

At this juncture it was decided that forms of communication other than oral language should be used in the classrooms. Two of these were signed Spanish and cued speech. From this point onward, we witnessed a closer collaboration between the educational administration and the Deaf community in the elaboration of materials in sign language and the training of teachers. Although the Deaf community was critical of the integration policy that existed, it was through these programs that Deaf adults became experts in the eyes of the teaching profession with respect to Spanish Sign Language (LSE) and sign language training. Paradoxically, training professionals in signed Spanish enabled hearing teachers to come into contact with the Deaf community and LSE. Also, Deaf adults collaborated with the educational administration in the development of training materials (MEC, 1989, 1993). Signed Spanish became a usual way of communicating between hearing parents, teachers, and deaf children. Cued speech was also adapted to Spanish (Torres, 1988) and was promoted as a way to improve the creation of phonological representations for words and then reading (Alegria & Leybaert, 1987; Leybaert & Alegría, 2002).

However, within a few years it became evident that it was extremely difficult for hearing teachers to implement visual communication systematically in a classroom of 20 hearing children and only 2 deaf children. In practice, visual communication through signed Spanish and/or cued speech was being used in separate groups in the classroom or in special situations by speech and language therapists (SALTs). Deaf children were in classrooms where spoken language was available, but was not in fact accessible, with the result that educational integration was not meeting their academic needs or the principles of normalization (Diaz-Estébanez & Valmaseda, 1995).

These changes occurred alongside other events: bilingual education was growing and results were emerging from schools in northern Europe (Lewis, 1995), the first LSE publications emerged (Rodríguez, 1992), and an international conference was held in Salamanca on sign language research (Ahlgren, Bergman, & Brennan, 1994). The Spanish Deaf community held large meetings during those years and discussions of the role of sign language in society, Deaf culture, and linguistic recognition were made public. At this point, it is crucial to emphasize the role of the schools in restructuring themselves toward a different model of education. This included the incorporation of LSE into teaching practices and the initiation of joint education of deaf and hearing students. This was in response to demands from parents for a better education for their deaf children. The changes toward educational bilingual models and toward the creation of contexts of co-enrollment were initiated, mainly, by opening the doors of deaf schools to hearing pupils (Apansce, 1998; cf., Antia & Metz, Hermans, De Klerk, Wauters, & Knoors, Chapter 16). There was a redefinition of the schools, as the same buildings that were used previously by deaf children now housed units for co-enrollment of hearing and deaf pupils together, which generated a more diverse and rich educational context. In Spain, therefore, co-enrollment and bilingual education were closely related from the beginning (Alonso, Rodriguez, & Echeita, 2009). The Spanish experience from the outset had some special characteristics compared with other countries:

1. Rather than waiting for a child's sign language development to progress before introducing the spoken or written version of Spanish, both sign language and spoken language, as a form of simultaneous bilingualism, were present in the classroom from the onset of a child's education.
2. It was considered crucial that deaf children had good early contact with peers and adult fluent users of both spoken and signed languages.
3. There was no official recognition of the sign language (this would not happen until 2007), nor was there a body of linguistic or psycholinguistic research on LSE until much later.
4. As the first bilingual schools started incorporating LSE, the number of deaf children receiving cochlear implants was growing, and educational practices needed to take this into account. Bilingual education and CI were closely related from the beginning.

The sign bilingual education that is seen today in Spain is not the direct result of government policymaking but instead has been created bottom-up, from schools and the Deaf community. Without formal support, standard guidelines, or frameworks, and with the laissez-faire attitude of the educational administration, the first bilingual education experiments were quite difficult (Morales-López, 2008). In Spain, only two educational modalities are regulated: mainstreaming and special education. Mainstreaming is the most widespread. Typically this is where one or two deaf pupils join an ordinary classroom in an environment of oral communication, and they receive support from teachers for children with special educational needs and from speech therapists. Officially, bilingual education is regulated legally (LEY 27/2007). This law, applicable nationally, stipulates that "the educational administrations will offer bilingual educational models, which will be of free choice for the deaf, hearing-impaired and deaf-blind students or their parents or legal representatives." However, in practice, there has been no application of this law in any of the 17 autonomous communities in Spain. It is not clear how many schools label themselves bilingual (Muñoz- Baell et al., 2011). Often, if sign language is used at all, even minimally, it is termed a sign bilingual school. Morales-López (2008), looking at only Madrid and Barcelona, described the bilingual education situation as continuing to be driven by bottom-up policies rather than any official positions, resulting in a kind of invisible policy of deaf education.

## BILINGUAL SCHOOLS IN THE MADRID REGION

In this section we describe the educational practices in four schools in the Madrid community. The aim is to describe in detail what we are doing and what this educational experience involves. As in the rest of the country, deaf and hard-of-hearing children in Madrid are schooled primarily in mainstream classrooms. This usually happens in a typical school without specific resources for deafness, or in a more specialized mainstream school with some preference for hearing impairment, where there are one or two deaf children per classroom. From the existing four special schools for the deaf in Madrid, three of them moved toward bilingual education and then, slowly, toward co-enrollment education (15–20 hearing and 5–6 deaf children per classroom). The four schools continue to run special units. They have, therefore, acquired a double identity or status: integration and special education. In order to place a deaf or hard-of-hearing child in special education or in an integrated setting, a statutory assessment and a statement are required. The assessment is carried out by a team composed of various professionals, such as educational psychologists, speech and language theapists, audiologists, and deaf professionals, but the parents must agree to this assessment before it can take place. Bilingual/co-enrollment education does not exist as an official option, but in practice it is considered under the integration choice.

The total deaf child population in Madrid at the time of writing was 597. The proportion of children going to the four bilingual co-enrollment schools is 24% (n = 141), out of which 53% have cochlear implants (see Table 15.1) There are also 65 pupils in these schools who have additional disabilities or social disadvantages and who attend the special units but may also share some activities with the rest of the students. This shows the high degree of diversity in terms of student backgrounds in the schools.

### Curriculum Organization in the Bilingual Schools

Of the four schools that appear in Table 15.1, Piruetas covers the 0–3-year-old period and is the only one that has been using a sign

Table 15.1 Names of Schools and Census 2013

| Name of school | Beginning year as a bilingual-co-enrollment school | 0–3 years (Infant school) | 3–6 years (Preschool) | 6–12 years (Primary) | Total | With cochlear implants |
|---|---|---|---|---|---|---|
| Piruetas | 1999 | 6 | – | – | 6 | 2 |
| Sol | 2000 | – | 18 | 43 | 61 | 35 |
| Ponce | 2004 | – | 13 | 33 | 46 | 21 |
| Gaudem | 2008 | 1 | 10 | 17 | 28 | 17 |
| Total | | 7 | 41 | 93 | 141 | 75 |

bilingual and co-enrollment philosophy since its inception in 1999. The Sol, Ponce, and Gaudem schools offer infant school (age 3–6 years), primary school (age 6–12 years), and special education (age 6–16 years). As described in the earlier section, it is important to recognize that when these schools were first set up they were schools for deaf children, so when the move to co-enrollment occurred they "opened their doors" to hearing children. This meant that the expertise in the schools was already high, as they focused on deaf children from the outset (see descriptions in Alonso et al., 2009; Las Heras, 1999; Sanjuán & Pérez, 2005). In the practical organization of the schools there is a close relationship between the decisions made concerning "special education" and "co-enrollment." In this way, management of the children is closely coordinated, taking into consideration these two factors. As we outlined earlier, the approach of deaf education adopted in these schools is quite different from that of other countries. When all children in these schools enter the infant stage of their education (0–6 years), they receive bilingual input directly and in a co-enrolled context. At the end of this period they are evaluated by a team of psychologists and language specialists and, in agreement with the family, future educational paths are planned for them (e.g., continue in a bilingual and co-enrollment setting or move to another type of educational setting).

In each bilingual and co-enrollment classroom there are 5–6 deaf children and 15–20 hearing peers with two hearing co-teachers. Deaf and hearing children share not only the physical space but also the curriculum and the language of instruction—in other words the everyday life of the classroom. Having other deaf and hearing peers in the classroom enables children to develop their own identity.

### What Do the Schools Teach?

All the children (deaf and hearing) receive the same content but each school has to develop their own curriculum, taking into account their own learning objectives and how these are taught in both sign and spoken language. It is worth noting that although ideologically it is held that LSE has the same status as Spanish, officially no such recognition exists in the curriculum. The infant stage of education (0–6 years) is split into two age groups (0–3 and 3–6 years). This period of educational programming is optional in Spain, but we have found that most parents do in fact send their children to schools at this age and especially so when their children are deaf. It is an invaluable period, as the schools can work with parents of the children from an early age on communication and the use of hearing aids/CIs. From 0–3 years the curriculum does not include content subjects but instead "fields of experience" (e.g., a special focus on language development). In the second stage (3–6 years) the curriculum is organized around content areas. One of the main subjects is "Communication and Representation," which normally would focus on spoken language; however, in the bilingual schools, signed and spoken language are included because for some deaf children LSE is their main mode of communication.

In primary school (6–12 years) the subjects are more diverse, including science, art, mathematics, physical education, and foreign languages. Here the focus for teachers is on how to deliver this curriculum in both spoken and signed language in the same classroom. This means deciding what subjects are taught by which language(s). In all the primary school years, LSE is considered to be a communication and educational tool, but it has also become a new curriculum area. In order to teach LSE to children, the authors collaborated with the National Center for Deaf People in Spain to develop a teaching guide (CNSE, 2006). The LSE curriculum includes learning objectives, content, and evaluation criteria adapted to suit the different levels of skill of the hearing and deaf children. As with other aspects related to sign language in schools, while LSE is officially recognized, this curriculum is not universally adopted. In the next section we will attempt to explain what we mean by the term "curriculum for all," which is a difficult concept, as we have different levels and two languages.

### How Do the Schools Teach? Methodological Issues in Increasing Participation and Breaking Down Barriers

Though each of the four schools has its own methodological approach, they all share the ideology of inclusive education. Inclusive education, which is included in international guidelines (UNESCO, 2005) as well as in the national laws of Spain, refers to a philosophy of educating all students together in regular or general education settings, regardless of the presence or absence of disabilities. The philosophy and policies supporting it assume that methods and services will be used to provide for the varied learning needs of individual students. Inclusive education is a broad term that refers to a transformational process that promotes an educational system aiming to deliver quality education and that may be adapted to support learners with diverse needs. We follow the inclusive educational practices as discussed in the literature (Ainscow, Booth, & Dyson, 2006; Dyson & Millward, 2000; Echeita, 2006), which see learning potentials as not determined solely by personal conditions (e.g., deafness, family, or types of aid) but also by the learning contexts where pupils are. The teacher's responsibility is to remove barriers to communication and to enable all children to learn (Alonso & Echeita, 2006).

Traditionally in Spain, teachers use the same textbook with all the children in a classroom. This practice implies that there is homogeneity in the learners, which some researchers consider a myth (Pujolas, 2008). Classrooms are full of different children, including deaf children, and such a composition means diversity. If we add two languages and two teachers working together, a great amount of time must be devoted to organizing the teaching. Each of the schools in this study developed its own teaching methods, but they all aim to remove barriers to learning and to promote maximum participation by deaf children in the classroom.

The main changes that the schools introduced focused on accessibility and diversity. When looking at deaf children in a bilingual classroom shared with other hearing children, two main issues must be addressed. The first issue is what barriers exist for the child's participation, and this most commonly concerns language ability. The second issue is barriers to effective learning, and this most commonly concerns the teaching practices in the classroom.

*Accessibility*

Having two languages means that all the children can access the curriculum, but this does not mean that both languages are in use all the time in every situation. Simultaneous and constant use of both languages is in fact a misconception in discussions of sign bilingualism. Centers develop linguistic plans that define how each language is used in anticipation of which children are involved in each of the activities. This means that a great deal of time is needed for planning. For example, in the infant school after the second term, when the main meeting time of the whole school or "general assembly" is already part of the learned daily routines, conversations or questions about "Who is here today?" or "Who has not come?" could be delivered in spoken language. In primary school, there may be three deaf children with a CI and two deaf children without a CI working together in the same classroom. The teachers must decide whether the general instructions from the teacher include Spanish and LSE. When activities takes place in a small group, some children with a CI will be working only in spoken Spanish; other groups that include children without a CI will be using LSE. There are thus moments when both languages are present for everybody (e.g., in large group activities) and other moments when only one language is adopted.

How is the accessibility of both languages ensured? With spoken and written Spanish, appropriate equipment (e.g., sound field frequency-modulated systems) and systems such as visual phonics (Juarez, 1985) or cued speech are used. This practice is based on evidence from language development and reading (Alegria & Dominguez, 2009; Dominguez, Rodriguez, & Alonso, 2011; Leybaert, Bayard, Huyse, & Colin, 2012; Santana, Torres, & García, 2003).

We attempt to give LSE the same status as Spanish at the centers. Accessibility of LSE means that we have hearing co-tutors who are fluent signers and deaf staff working together. The signing co-tutor takes responsibility for the use of LSE in all activities (except those where we have plans for using spoken language in isolation). This could be in general assemblies, classroom zones concentrating on mathematics, symbolic play, literacy, and investigation projects (Pérez, Herrero, & Pérez, 2008). Access for all children is thus guaranteed by two co-tutors in the classroom all of the time. Each teacher works in different zones and with different languages following the bilingual principle "one person—one language" where a single person is identified with a single language (Barron-Hauwaert, 2004; Saunders, 1988). This interaction stimulates conversations, hypothesis testing, and exchanges of opinions where the students engage in negotiating the content of classroom discussions (Ruiz, 2000). This means that children are learning language by practically interacting with each other, which resembles the natural processes of language acquisition. This practice means that teachers must pay attention to what activities they are using to promote language learning. The activities should encourage meaningful and real communication and interaction, where children learn how to use either LSE or Spanish to perform these functions (Hymes, 1972).

*Diversity*

While diversity in learners and the possibility of multiple intelligences exist (Gardner, 1983), it is also crucial to accept the fact that all children, deaf and hearing, may bring different learning strategies to the classroom. The methodology used is based on the ideas of Piagetian constructivism and cooperative learning (Johnson, Johnson, & Holubec, 1993; Kagan, 1992). This approach allows us to break down the structure of a conventional classroom and use activities that all children can take part in, as these activities may have several levels of difficulty and ways of solving similar problems (UDL—Universal Design for Learning Center for Applied Special Technology [CAST] 1990).

The topics taught are often chosen by children themselves (termed research projects) and are used to induce the children to elaborate on their language and thinking. Each activity, however, has to have different levels so that all children can be accommodated. An example of this is our work zones. Imagine four zones (mathematics, art, Spanish, and LSE). In each zone there are five children (deaf and hearing) with a variety of activities planned by the teacher. For mathematics, for instance, which may be more diverse in terms of the children's abilities, more varied activities can be planned for the week. We see bilingualism as a continuum (Pearson, 2009) in which each child is encouraged to achieve his or her maximum potential in both languages. As such, the planning of both languages to be used is not the same across all activities and contexts; instead, it needs to be planned depending on the skills of each child in each classroom group. During each school year the co-tutors plan which language will be used in which zones, based on the profiles of children in the classroom. Because there are two teachers, each can look after his or her own zone and language.

By following this type of social and cooperative learning, we see that both deaf and hearing children can access the same curriculum. The added benefits of this approach for deaf and hearing children are mutual: hearing children acquire signs, and deaf children feel part of the wider group. Both groups learn to respect the intrinsic differences of people in their class.

### Specific Subject Areas for Deaf Children

The way we have organized the classroom practices means that all children can both participate and learn; however, this is not sufficient on its own to ensure that a deaf child improves comprehension and production of spoken and written Spanish. Our intervention is based on what we term "linguistic planning." Each of the four bilingual schools in Madrid therefore develops linguistic planning unique to the deaf children in their schools, which can vary between schools, but activities may include spoken language sessions (using cued speech, signed Spanish and visual/manual phonics), written language workshops, extended activities focusing on meta-phonology, or speech and language therapy for improving auditory discriminations.

With respect to written Spanish, we place a great emphasis on early exposure to different types of written texts (newspapers, underground tickets, narrative and expository text, etc.). In our work on written language development, we focus on the constructivist approach (Ferreiro & Teberosky, 1979) and use established psycholinguistic models of reading (Alegría 2003) to guide interventions for deaf children's meta-phonological awareness. The constructivist perspective for reading and writing places priority on the meaning and function of what children are reading. Following this principle, we encourage children to think about what it means "to read and write." An example of how we integrate both approaches—constructivist and psycholinguistic—is in order here. Using the idea of a menu, we ask the children to read or write about what they will be eating that day (providing meanings and functions of reading); then we work on their metalinguistic skills, focusing the child on segmenting words. In this last aspect we use visual phonics, cued speech, and a sequence of tasks: counting, identifying, omitting or adding syllables and phonemes (Dominguez, Rodriguez, & Alonso, 2011).

Additionally, all the deaf children in our schools also receive oral language intervention outside the bilingual schools.

**People Involved in the Work**

We could not carry out all of the previous types of activities without the appropriate team of professionals in place. These include deaf LSE specialists, two co-tutors per class, SALTs, and interpreters.

*Deaf LSE Specialists*

Deaf LSE specialists are trained in LSE teaching, and some are also qualified teachers or infant educators. Across the four schools we have 14 of these professionals, and they are contracted staff to the school. While this aspect of schools has existed for several years, it is only very recently that a job description has been put forward by the educational administration that includes teaching LSE to deaf pupils, teaching LSE and deaf awareness to hearing pupils, teaching/training of LSE and visual communication for families, training teachers in communication and visual strategies for effective learning, and finally promoting Deaf cultural activities to the wider school staff.

*Co-tutors*

Each classroom has two hearing co-tutors who act as language reference points for the children. They are always in the classroom, except when specialist provision is happening (e.g., English or music classes). One uses LSE and the other Spanish to communicate with the children as well as to teach. Normally they have a background in SALT or LSE. They share the same status in the classroom, which facilitates extremely close collaboration in teaching and planning. Both co-tutors plan the subject area (mathematics, science, etc.) together, as well as teaching them. This means that the signing teachers are not interpreters, nor are they interpreters for each other; instead, each teacher is teaching according to the level of the children in the group.

*SALTs*

Speech and language therapists (SALTs) are common figures in mainstream schools with deaf children as well as in the bilingual schools. Their responsibility is to guarantee the spoken and listening stimulation required for children's speech and literacy development. Again, they have a close collaboration with co-tutors.

*Interpreters*

In infant and primary levels, interpreters work only with the deaf and hearing adult staff in internal meetings or in contact with families. In secondary education and beyond, they take a more active role in the classrooms.

Up to this point, we have described the bilingual schools in order for the reader to be able to visualize the activities, organization, and staff. However, we also have to recognize that there is a hidden curriculum that is more difficult to describe in words. What we mean by this is that our schools need to constantly work on enabling children to develop and maintain a sense of competence and positive self-image (Power & Grez, 2011). With the details of the educational framework, curriculum content, and practices explained, we move to some description of the evaluations we have carried out.

## AN INVESTIGATION INTO THE OUTCOMES OF BILINGUAL EDUCATION IN MADRID

From other chapters in this volume (e.g., Marschark & Lee, Chapter 9; Walker & Tomblin, Chapter 6), it will be clear that a systematic review of the impacts of sign bilingualism on deaf children's development is sorely needed in order to anticipate future practices, especially with the widely adopted practice of early cochlear implantation. With this in mind, we have been carrying out several projects investigating spoken, sign language and socio-emotional development in children with a cochlear implant in sign bilingual schools. In this section we describe this work in the context of wider research in the same area.

In recent years, most deaf children (even those with deaf parents) are receiving an early cochlear implant. As Knoors and Marchark (2012) have described, this widespread practice in other countries has influenced the popularity of sign language in educational settings and has greatly increased the amount of research into spoken language development in deaf children (Geers et al., 2011; Manrique et al., 2006; Niparko et al., 2010). However, there are very few studies of early spoken/sign language development in deaf children in bilingual schools. Swedish researchers (Preisler Ahlström & Tvingstedt, 1997, 2005) found that the early language modality most preferred by deaf children with cochlear implants was sign language, and that this reduced over time but continued to be used in situations where complex language was required. They reported that children with better levels of language had elevated scores in both modalities. Wiefferink, Spaai, Uilenburg, and Vermeij (2008), examining Flemish and Dutch children, found better spoken language development (intelligibility, receptive and productive vocabulary) in the spoken monolingual than bilingual contexts. Complexity of sign language syntax, measured through the mean number of morphemes per utterance (MLU), did not progress in these Dutch bilingual children. According to the authors, this might be explained by the fact that the children were exposed at home to more spoken language than to sign language (see Walker & Tomblin, Chapter 6 of this volume). Jiménez, Pino, and Herruzo (2009) pointed out that the advantages and disadvantages of bilingual education for deaf children with cochlear implants depend on what specific areas of language are being evaluated. In addition to having few studies on this topic, those that were cited fail to define precisely what type of bilingual education is being studied.

As described earlier, the schools where the current study is based are sign bilingual and co-enrollment, meaning that both deaf and hearing children are taught in Spanish and LSE by native users of both languages. In terms of bilingual development, the children in the four Madrid schools have all the necessary conditions to engender good outcomes. What have we observed? During the school years 2010–2012, we evaluated 17 children aged 0–6 years on their language and social-emotional skills. While this sample is small, it represents the entire group receiving bilingual education in these schools (at the time point the study started) who had no additional disabilities; their parents used Spanish or LSE, and all were implanted before 2 years of age (12 unilateral, 4 bilateral, and 1 a trunk implant). The advantage of the sample was that they had arrived in these schools from an early age and not after several years of attendance at other types of schools, which is often the situation with deaf children who come into a sign language environment because other interventions have failed. We were interested in both vocabulary and grammar in both LSE and Spanish, but because the age of the children varied, we were unable to test all children on all of the same tests. We also carried out preliminary investigations into their social-emotional development. We illustrate in Table 15.2 the sets of assessments carried out and the number of children tested; Table 15.3 shows the specific test that each child took.

We first present results on Spanish and LSE separately, then combined. (For more detailed results, see Pérez, Valmaseda, De la Fuente, Montero, Mostaert, 2013; Mostaert, 2012).

### Spoken Spanish Skills

*Audition*

We used the parent questionnaire Little Ears (MED-EL) to obtain information about the children's auditory behavior 2 years after cochlear implantation. From 11 children tested, 10 had auditory development above their hearing age, with one exception (the child with a trunk implant).

**Table 15.2 Assessment Tools and Number of DHH Children Tested**

| Areas evaluated for Spanish | Test (number of children tested) | Norms available? | Areas evaluated for LSE | Test (number of children tested) | Norms available? |
|---|---|---|---|---|---|
| Audition | Little Ears (11) | Yes (0–24 hearing age) | | | |
| Receptive vocabulary | Peabody (11) | Yes (from 2;6) | Receptive vocabulary | LSE inventory (13;8 at two time points) | No |
| Expressive vocabulary | CDI (12) K-Bit (11) | Yes (8–36 months) Yes (from 4 years) | Expressive vocabulary | LSE inventory | No |
| Receptive grammar | CEG (11) | Yes (from 4 years) | Receptive grammar | LSE grammar test (13;9 at two time points) | No |
| Social-emotional evaluations | PSA (17) | Yes, French norms (2.5–6 years) | | | |

*Spoken Spanish*

Spanish vocabulary and grammar were assessed with four tests determined by the child's chronological and hearing age. The spoken Spanish CDI (López-Ornat et al., 2005) was used for vocabulary for children between 8 and 30 months. Thal, Desjardin, and Eisenberg (2007) demonstrated that this test was appropriate for deaf children up to hearing age 36 months. We also used the Spanish version of the PPTV-III Peabody (Dunn, 2006) for vocabulary after 30 months. For children older than 4 years we used the K-Bit (Spanish version: Cordero & Calonge, 2000) but only for expressive vocabulary. For Spanish grammar we used the CEG (Mendoza, Carballo, Muñoz, & Fresneda, 2005), which is suitable for children between 4 and 11 years.

Children tested on the Spanish CDI for expressive vocabulary (n = 12) had a mean percentile score appropriate for their hearing age (mean percentile 65). However, there was variability: in 8 of 12 of these children, their vocabulary scores were above their hearing age equivalents; 2 were at this level and 2 were below. Thus, these children have vocabulary development in Spanish between their chronological

Table 15.3 Details of Which Test Each Child Took

| Test/Children | Little Ears | CDI LO | Peabody | k-BIT | CEG | Inventory LSE | Grammar Test LSE | PSA |
|---|---|---|---|---|---|---|---|---|
| N 1 | 1 | | 1 | 1 | 1 | 1 | 1–2 | 1 |
| N 2 | 1 | 1–2 | 1 | | | 1–2 | 1 | 1 |
| N 3 | | 1–2 | 1 | 1 | | 1–2 | 1 | 1 |
| N 4 | 1 | 1–2 | 1 | 1 | 1 | 1–2 | | 1 |
| N 5 | 1 | 1–2 | | | | 1–2 | | 1 |
| N 6 | 1 | 1–2 | 1 | 1 | 1 | 1–2 | | 1 |
| N 7 | | | 1 | 1 | 1 | | 1–2 | 1 |
| N 8 | | | 1 | 1 | 1 | | 1–2 | 1 |
| N 9 | 1 | 1 | 1 | 1 | 1 | | 1–2 | 1 |
| N 10 | 1 | 1–2 | 1 | 1 | | 1–2 | 1 | 1 |
| N 11 | 1 | 1 | 1 | 1 | | 1 | 1–2 | 1 |
| N 12 | | 1 | 1 | 1 | 1 | 1 | 1–2 | 1 |
| N 13 | | | 1 | 1 | 1 | | 1–2 | 1 |
| N 14 | 1 | | 1 | 1 | 1 | 1–2 | | 1 |
| N 15 | 1 | 1 | 1 | 1 | 1 | 1 | 1–2 | 1 |
| N 16 | 1 | 1 | 1 | 1 | 1 | 1 | 1–2 | 1 |
| N 17 | | | 1 | 1 | 1–2 | 1–2 | 1 | 1 |
| Totals | 11 | 12 (6 at two time points) | 11 were tested on these 3 tests | | | 13 (8 at two time points) | 13 (9 at two time points) | 17 |

1 = 1st assessment; 2 = 2nd assessment after 12 months

and hearing ages (similar results are reported in Duchesne, Sutton, Bergeron, & Trudeau, 2010).

Older children (n = 11) were tested on comprehensive and expressive vocabulary using the PPVT and K-Bit (n = 11). The scores were within the normative range (see Table 15.4) with slightly higher scores in expressive vocabulary, similar to Geers et al. (2009) and Duchesne, Sutton, and Bergeron, (2009). This pattern is atypical, as hearing children's receptive vocabulary normally surpasses their expressive vocabulary. The reverse trend has also been reported in previous research with deaf children (Moeller, 2000). It also seems to be the case in children who received CI early. These results might be related to what Geers and colleagues (2009) pointed out, regarding language teaching strategies that put emphasis on naming. The same 11 children were also tested on Spanish grammar with the CEG. We see in Table 15.4 that mean scores, compared with chronological age norms, are within normal percentile ranges (percentiles 16–85) but are in the lower ranges and have a great deal of variability: across 11 children tested, 5 performed at chronological age, 2 at hearing age, and the other 4 below hearing age. These

Table 15.4 Performance of 11 DHH Children in Vocabulary and Receptive Grammar in Spanish

| Vocabulary | | | | Grammar | |
|---|---|---|---|---|---|
| Receptive | | Expressive | | Receptive | |
| CA | HA | CA | HA | CA | HA |
| M: 18.47 | M: 60.46 | M: 37.09 | M: 65.96 | M: 16.73 | M: 29.44 |
| SD (23.25) | SD (37.88) | SD (33.80) | SD (34.00) | SD (22.28) | SD (31.65) |

M = mean; SD = standard deviation; CA = chrolological age; HA = hearing age

results, while positive, support the findings that grammar is the most difficult part of the spoken language to be mastered by deaf children (Inscoe, Odell, Archbold, & Nikolopoulos, 2009), even in deaf children with early implants and in early sign bilingual environments.

We followed up the children at a second time point, allowing us to investigate whether this developmental trajectory was maintained. In 6 children we were able to test spoken Spanish 12 months later with the CDI. All the children made significant gains over time, with high percentiles for hearing age during two time periods (71.5 at Time 1 and 61.5 at Time 2). In 9 older children tested 12 months later with the Peadbody and K-Bit (the CDI was not age appropriate), there was the same positive trajectory. Scores were within the normal chronological age range at both time points, but again expressive vocabulary was better than receptive.

## Spanish Sign Language (LSE) Skills

As in many other counties, there are no standardized assessments of sign language in Spain. One of the objectives of our work has been to develop such methods. In the following results, therefore, we report raw scores instead of norms. The Inventory of LSE vocabulary has been developed based on existing CDIs for ASL (Anderson & Reilly, 2002), BSL (Woolfe, Herman, Roy, & Woll, 2010) and spoken Spanish (López Ornat et al., 2005).[1] To evaluate LSE grammar we also piloted an adapted BSL receptive skills test for LSE (Herman, Holmes, & Woll, 1999), which is aimed at children aged 3–11 years.

Here we report LSE vocabulary development over two time periods (12 months apart) for 8 children aged 23–42 months (7 with hearing parents). The sample had between 15 and 24 months of exposure to LSE. We found a significant development in LSE across time periods and, contrary to the spoken Spanish tests reported previously, better receptive than expressive scores (see Figure 15.1).

It appears that when the language is fully accessible, assessments reveal typical developmental processes, and that comprehension precedes production. However, in line with the evaluation of Spanish,

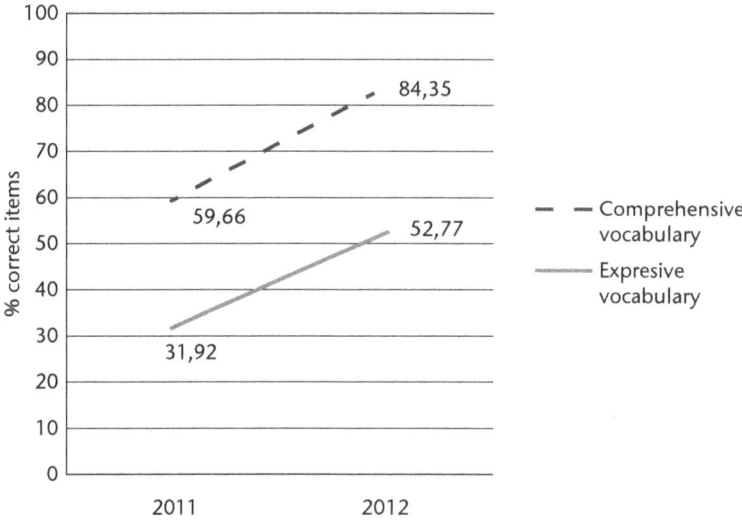

**Figure 15.1** Percentage of LSE vocabulary in 8 children.

there was a good deal of variability among the children. As an approximate indicator of how fast they are acquiring LSE, we compared the deaf children with hearing and deaf parents' sign exposure age (how long they have been learning LSE) to the native signer scores reported for BSL. While this cannot be an exact comparison, we observed that the 3 native signers have an equivalent lexical development to their BSL native signing peers, and positively the 7 non-native LSE learners have vocabulary scores above their sign exposure age. Thus we observed a similar LSE vocabulary development, as that described for their Spanish: some variability but scores between the age of exposure and chronological ages.

For LSE grammar we used the pilot LSE receptive skills test with 9 children over a 12-month period. At the first assessment the children had mean age 5;1 and mean exposure time to LSE of 3;6. Contrary to Wiefferink and colleagues (2008), who did not observe progress in the children's syntax in bilingual contexts, we observed a statistically significant development ($p < .01$) of LSE grammar over the two time periods tested (see Table 15.5). Therefore, although these children are not acquiring LSE from their parents but from the school, they have a good developmental trajectory of the language in both comprehension and production.

### Comparison Between the LSE and Spanish

Next we carried out some more comparative analyses of the development of Spanish and LSE. Studies on simultaneous bilingualism in

Table 15.5 LSE Receptive Skills Test in 9 Children

| % Correct items | |
| --- | --- |
| Time 1 | Time 2 |
| M: 54.72 | M: 67.22 |
| SD (17.96) | SD (12.40) |

M = mean; SD = standard deviation

hearing children indicate that if exposure to two languages has a rich and proportional input in quantity and quality, and if both languages to which they are exposed have the same status, both languages will develop in a balanced way. In the case of the children in our schools, things are somewhat different, as most of the children have hearing parents who do not sign well and the children do not get their first exposure to LSE until after 2 years of age. Also, the status of LSE is not the same as that of Spanish. Even with these differences, we are interested in whether deaf children with early CI and LSE exposure will develop in similar ways to children exposed to two spoken languages.

In our assessments of vocabulary in Spanish and LSE, we observe both LSE and Spanish expressive vocabulary develop side by side. It is not the case that exposure to LSE negatively affects the growth of Spanish vocabulary. Similar results are reported for deaf children in the United Kingdom (Woll, 2013). In Figure 15.2 we saw data from 6 children for two time points with 12 months apart. The mean chronological age at the first time point was 2;8, and mean age of initial exposure (the mean age at which children initiated this contact) to LSE and Spanish was 1;7. While the two languages make significant gains over time, there is a shift across time periods in the vocabulary levels. First LSE is dominant, but this changes to Spanish in the second assessment. We believe this is due to the educational context in which the children are learning (see Figure 15.2).

Several researchers note that evaluating language in bilinguals can sometimes disfavor these children if *conceptual* vocabulary is not considered (Pearson, 1998; Oller, 2005; see Rinaldi, Caselli, Onofrio, & Volterra, Chapter 3 of this volume). Typically, bilingual children in each of their two languages initially produce less vocabulary than their monolingual peers, so it is advisable to combine scores for the two languages. Combined scores represent the child's total conceptual vocabulary where some concepts are presented in both (doublets) while others only in one language (singletons). Therefore, we combined singletons and doublets in a sample of 11 children (8 DoH and 3 DoD). In Figure 15.3 we see the children assessed, ordered from left to right according to hearing age and age of exposure to LSE.

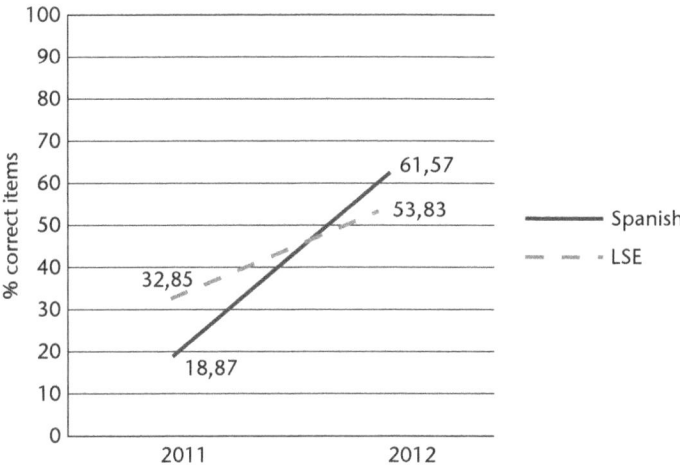

Figure 15.2 Development of Spanish and LSE in 6 children with CI.

In general, as mean scores, there are no differences in lexical size between Spanish and LSE, but conceptual vocabulary is larger in all children, even in the 3 native signers. In the same figure we see that children with less hearing age in months have greater LSE; however, this dominance shifts to spoken Spanish at 24 months hearing age, as described previously. This shift occurs also in native signers but not in the one child with the trunk implant (N6).

### Social-Emotional Skills

We carried out some preliminary assessments of social-emotional skills using the Profil Socio-Affectif (PSA) in the French adaptation (Dumas et al., 1997). Previously, this measure was used as a screening instrument by Virole, Bounnot, and Sánchez (2003) with children who had received a CI, and also in Spain by Silvestre (2008) in a follow-up with 54 deaf children with and without CI. Virole and colleagues (2003) reported that 58% of children had normal development, 13% had major difficulties, and 47% had at least one difficulty across the different scales. The test is an 80-item teacher/caregiver rating scale that assesses social competence, affective expression, and adjustment. We used it to describe the children's behavior but also to focus the attention of teachers and parents not only on language but on the child's adaptation to and functioning within his or her environment. The test gives teachers the child's profile of strengths and weaknesses, and indicates which are the focus areas for intervention. Scores between 38 and 63 are in the normal range; scores below 37 represent difficulties. Though the results must be taken with certain caution (since French norms of the test were used), test scores in two global scales (social competence

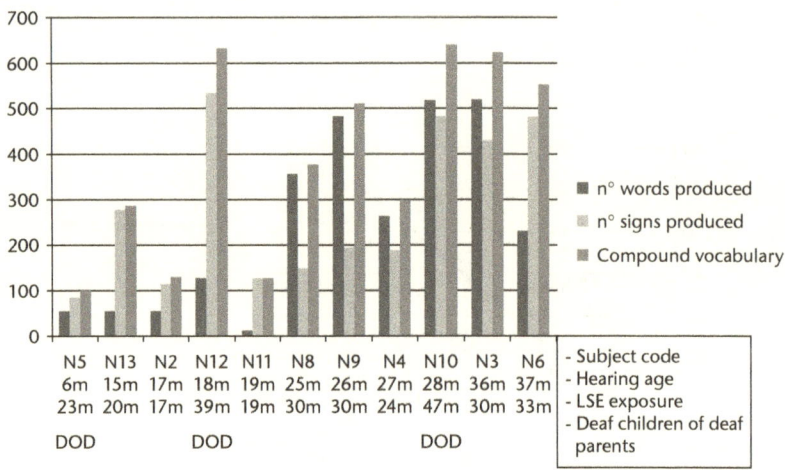

Figure 15.3 Number of signs, words, and conceptual vocabulary in each subject.

and general adaptation) reveal that the 17 children evaluated had good social-emotional development (the means for general adaptation was 53; for social competence, 51 points; and only one child presented difficulties, scoring 38 and 35 points, respectively; see Figure 15.4).

Thus we can conclude in this section that the children we evaluated are well adapted and able to deal with the social-emotional demands of their environment well enough. There is an interaction between social-emotional development and bilingualism. As soon as the children begin school at around 2 years of age, they are able to access LSE, and using signs can establish important early interaction with other children and with deaf and hearing adults. Virole and colleagues (2003) also noted that an early cochlear implant provokes a perceived certainty in hearing parents that early language can be heard and developed, which can lower anxiety and facilitate more natural interaction in the family

## CONCLUSIONS AND FUTURE DIRECTIONS

### Bilingualism

In our assessments we can see good development of language, even within normal ranges; however, this is coupled with much variability between children and also between aspects of language evaluated. What can this tell us about the type of context that a bilingual school offers a deaf child? With the arrival of early cochlear implants and early exposure to LSE, the children in our schools have the best possibilities of achieving the highest levels of competency of both languages possible. We observe that children develop abilities in both languages

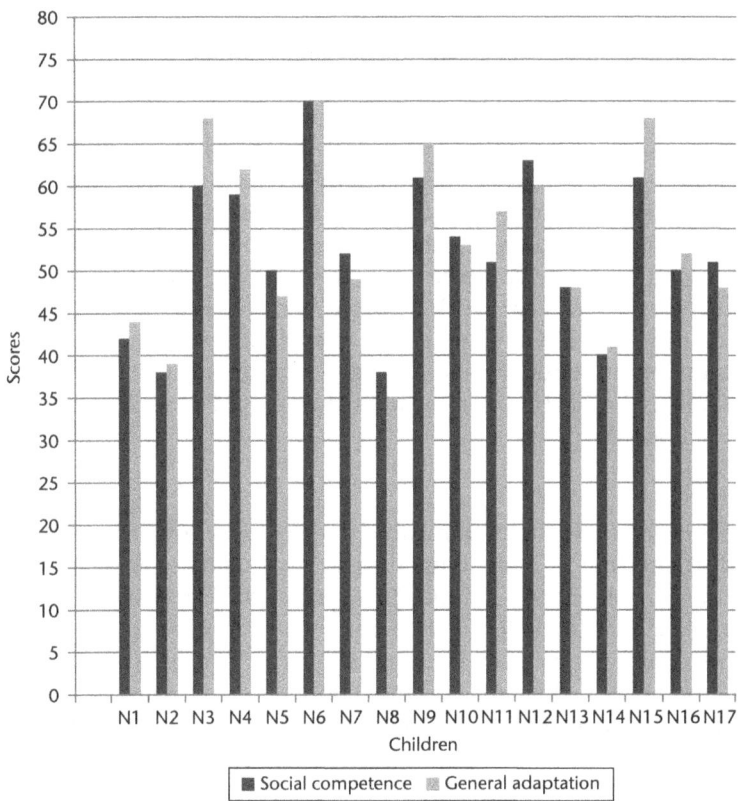

**Figure 15.4** Scores of 17 CI children in the PSA task.

between their chronological and hearing ages. This implies that on a positive note the children are where we expect them to be, but it also gives us some idea of the distance needed to travel in order for the child to be at the level comparable with his or her hearing-age peers and for the types of tasks the teacher is asking the child to understand and master.

Initially, we observed a preference for LSE over Spanish, which at 2 years after implantation began to invert. This early sign preference is probably due to the greater accessibility that deaf children have to the visual modality early on. Early sign exposure means that children and parents/professionals are not losing valuable time, waiting for the cochlear implant to be functional or auditory stimulation to become interpretable; instead, concepts are developing and crucial communicative skills are being honed. Once the implant begins to facilitate spoken language development, the child already understands the referential nature of language, the need to pay attention to interlocutors when they are speaking and to use the pragmatic inferences they have acquired previously via LSE. This "sign language bootstrapping" is very important in early and rich bilingual environments. In our schools the majority of conversations that children are hearing and the opportunities to acquire Spanish are multiple and varied, but crucially this is not the only option. If the quality of the input from the implant is temporarily suboptimal for technical reasons, interaction and education can continue. The advantage of our bilingual centers, needs also to be monitored, as it could be possible that the oral language environment is neglected. Our work concentrates on keeping both quantity and quality of the two languages at an optimal level. This implies that bilingual environments must ensure good acoustic conditions, create a culture of respecting conversation turns, and maintain the use of technical aids.

**Variability**

Vocabulary development is relatively better developed than grammar for deaf children in our bilingual sample, as well as for deaf children educated in other monolingual "oral" schools (Duchesne et al., 2009; Geers, Nicholas, & Sedey, 2003; Geers et al., 2009; Inscoe et al., 2009). Spanish grammar is difficult to hear, lip-read and produce, with important grammatical elements and function words appearing at the end of words and sentences as temporally brief phonetic material. These elements are also typically difficult for hearing bilingual learners in their second language (Paradis, Genesee, & Crago, 2011). This implies that sign bilingual schools should make grammar development a main area of development through explicit activities.

While we can control many of the factors that affect individuals' development, there remains variability, perhaps stemming from natural differences in the child's development, functioning of the cochlear implant, social differences between the families, and possibly educational differences between schools. Variability tells us that we need to incorporate careful observation of progress and put in place early and targeted interventions before chronic delays appear. Persistent delays are a possible sign of language impairments (Hawker et al., 2008; Mason et al., 2010; Monfort, 2006). The key to early interventions is flexibility in the educational responses for each child. This continues to be a major challenge for the success for the bilingual schools.

**Future Challenges**

Bilingualism in sign language and spoken language is a delicate balance. The medical perspective is a powerful one in the lives of deaf children. Most parents today go ahead with early cochlear implants with the strong desire that their children become fluent speakers. Professionals working with deaf children also put great emphasis on spoken language skills. For many years there has been a debate for one modality over the other, with signing considered a failure in many schools. We must move on from this impoverished argument. It is time to consider that whatever linguistic skills a child can obtain (mono/bi/trilingual), these are all valuable and will be appropriate at different points in a child's development. Changes to Madrid schooling policies are affecting how we think about sign bilingual education. The wider educational establishment is aiming for children to be early learners of English. This policy has also been introduced into schools where deaf children are educated, meaning that 30% of the school curriculum is in English. This will greatly affect the planned, careful balance of spoken language(s) and LSE, as well as affecting the involvement of parents (mostly non-English speakers) in deaf education. In general it is necessary that the bilingual centers have more integration and guidance from the policymakers, including legal support.

## Moving Forward

In writing this chapter we were faced with several issues relevant to the general problem of a lack of evidence-based practice in deaf children's bilingual education (Knoors & Marschark, 2012). We were faced with different starting points and ways of thinking about deaf children. We had to find a consensus for writing about both research and practice. This was not without challenges and involved much discussion about how research and educational practice could link up more. It also involved some translation of thinking between the two paradigms for researching development: language development and classroom learning. In much published research on deaf children where the focus is language and cognitive development, many researchers use a cognitive or psycholinguistic framework to pose questions and do research. This means that professionals in education, while working within frameworks that stem from the work of pedagogical researchers, such as those that use models and theoretical processes of learning and teaching, are not familiar with the large amount of psychology of deafness research that has been carried out (e.g., Marschark & Hauser, 2008). Therefore there is a distance between what researchers do and how educational professionals carry out their work in isolation from each other (see Knoors & Marschark, 2014).

One area that is very much in need of further investigation concerns the actual learning processes that occur in the classrooms of deaf children in bilingual schools. If more researchers were able to tackle these questions in collaboration with educational professionals we would have more meeting points. A model already exists for this type of collaboration in the field of reading research. Cognitive science researchers have moved their focus from psycholinguistic models of reading to also look at the classroom practices that promote reading in children

(Sanchez et al., 2010; Snowling & Hulme, 2008). The process of translation and searching for bridges might be a reflection of the gap that some researchers and educationalists feel exists. We have to work together more in order to arrive at realistic objectives and relevant findings of research, but this does not happen automatically. Part of the current absence of research evidence on bilingual educational for deaf children may be a reflection of the difficulties in getting different groups of professionals speaking together in mutually understandable and even bilingual ways.

## ACKNOWLEDGMENTS

The research of Gary Morgan was supported by a grant from the Economic and Social Research Council of Great Britain (RES-620-28-6001): Deafness Cognition and Language Research Centre.

## NOTE

[1] This inventory will be standardized by the University of Sevilla in a research project financed by the Junta de Andalucía (Reference: SEJ-7417).

## REFERENCES

Ahlgren, I., Bergman, B., & Brennan, M. (Eds). (1994). Perspectives on sign language usage. *Papers from the Fifth International Symposium on Sign Language Research*. Durham, NC: ISLA.

Ainscow, M., Booth, T., & Dyson, A. (2006). *Improving schools, developing inclusion*. New York, NY: Routledge.

Alegría, J. (2003). Deafness and reading. In T. Nunes & P. Bryant (Eds.), *Handbook of children´s literacy* (pp. 459–489). Dordrecht, Netherlands: Kluwer Academic.

Alegría, J. (2006). Por un enfoque psicolingüístico del aprendizaje de la lectura y sus dificultades—20 años después [Support for a psycholinguistic approach to reading acquisition and reading difficulties—twenty years later]. *Infancia y Aprendizaje*, 29(1), 79–94.

Alegría, J., & Leybaert, J. (1987). *Adquisición de la lectura en el niño sordo* [Reading acquisition in the deaf child]. Madrid, Spain: CNREE Ministerio de Educación y Ciencia.

Alegría, J., & Domínguez, A. B. (2009). Los alumnos sordos y la lengua escrita [Deaf students and written language]. *Revista Latinoamericana de Educación Inclusiva*, 3(1), 95–111.

Alonso, P., & Echeita, G. (2006). Barreras para el aprendizaje y la participación de los alumnos sordos [Barriers for learning and participation of deaf children]. In V. Acosta (Coord.), *La sordera desde la diversidad cultural y lingüística* (pp. 141–154). Barcelona, Spain: Massón.

Alonso, P., Rodríguez, P., & Echeita, G. (2009). El proceso de un centro específico de sordos hacia una educación más inclusiva: Colegio Gaudem Madrid [The process of a specific center for the deaf toward a more inclusive education: Gaudem School Madrid]. *Rinace*, 3(1), 167–187.

Anderson, D., & Reilly, J. (2002). The MacArthur Communicative Development Inventory: Normative data for American Sign Language. *Journal of Deaf Studies and Deaf Education, 7*(2), 83–119.
APANSCE. (1998). *Experiencias bilingües en la educación del niño sordo.* Barcelona, Spain: Ediciones Mayo.
Barron-Hauwaer, S. (2004). *The one parent–one language approach.* Clevedon, UK: Multilingual Matters.
Booth, T., & Ainscow, M. (2011). *Index for inclusion: Developing learning and participation in schools* (3rd ed.). Manchester, UK: CSIE.
CNSE. (2006). *Propuestas curriculares orientativas de la Lengua de Signos Española para las Etapas Educativas de Infantil, Primaria y Secundaria Obligatoria.* Madrid, Spain: CNSE.
Cordero, A., & Calonge, I. (2000). *Adaptación española del K-Bit.* Madrid, Spain: TEA.
Díaz-Estébanez, E., & Valmaseda, M. (1995). En el camino hacia una educación de calidad para los alumnos y alumnas sordos [On the path to quality education for deaf students]. *Infancia y Aprendizaje, 60*–70, 45–61.
Dominguez, A. B., Rodriguez, P., & Alonso, P. (2011). Cómo facilitar el aprendizaje de la lectura de niños sordos: Importancia de las habilidades fonológicas [How to facilitate reading acquisition in deaf children: The role of phonological skills]. *Revista de Educación, 356,* 353–375.
Duchesne, L., Sutton, A., & Bergeron, F. (2009). Language achievement in children who received cochlear implants between 1 and 2 years of age: Group trends and individual patterns. *Journal of Deaf Studies and Deaf Education, 14,* 465–486.
Duchesne, L., Sutton, A., Bergeron, F., & Trudeau, F. (2010). Le développment lexical précoce des enants porteurs dún implant cochleaire. *Canadian Journal of Speech-Language Pathology and Audiology, 34*(2), 132–145.
Dunn, L. L. M., Dunn, L. M., & Arribas, D. (2006). *PPVT-III Test de vocabulario en imágenes.* Adaptación española. Madrid, Spain: TEA.
Dyson, A., & Millward, A. (2000). *School and special needs: Issues of innovation and inclusion.* London, UK: Paul Chapman.
Echeita, G. (2006). *Educación para la inclusión o educación sin exclusiones.* Madrid, Spain: Nancea.
Ferreiro, E., & Teberosky, A. (1979). *Los sistemas de escritura en el desarrollo del niño.* Buenos Aires, Argentina: Siglo XXI.
Gardner, H. (1983). *Frames of mind: The theory of multiple inteligences.* New York, NY: Basic Books.
Geers, A., Nicholas J. G., Sedey, A. L. (2003). Language skills of children with early cochlear implantation. *Ear and Hearing, 24*(1), 46–58.
Geers, A., Moog, J., Biedenstein, J., Brenner, C. & Hayes, H. (2009). Spoken language scores of children using cochlear implants compared to hearing age-mates at school entry. *Journal of Deaf Studies and Deaf Education, 14*(3), 371–385.
Geers, A. N., Strube, M. J., Tobey, E. A., Pisoni, D. B., & Moog, J. S. (2011). Epilogue: Factors contributing to long-term outcomes of cochlear implantation in early childhood. *Ear and Hearing, 32*(1), 84–92.
Hawker, K., Ramirez-Inscoe, J., Bishop, D., Twomey, T., O'Donoghue, G. M., & Moore, D. R. (2008). Disproportionate language impairment in children using cochlear implants. *Ear and Hearing, 29*(3), 467–471.

Herman, R., Holmes, S., & Woll, B. (1999). *Assessing BSL development: Receptive Skills Test*. Coleford, UK: Forest Books.

Hymes, D. (1972). *On communicative competence*. In J. B. Pride & J. Holmes (Eds.), *Sociolinguistics*. Harmondsworth, UK: Penguin.

Inscoe, J. R., Odell, A., Archbold, S., & Nikolopoulos, T. (2009). Expressive spoken language development in deaf children with cochlear implants who are beginning formal education. *Deafness and Education International*, 11(1), 39–55.

Jiménez, M. S., Pino, M. J. & Herruzo, J. (2009). A comparative study of speech development between deaf children with cochlear implants who have been educated with spoken or spoken + sign language. *International Journal of Pediatric Otorhinolaryngology*, 73, 109–114.

Johnson, D. W., Johnson, R. T., & Holubec, E. J. (1993). *Cooperation in the classroom* (6th ed.). Edina, MN: Interaction Book Company.

Juarez, A. (1985). Ayudas visuales a la lectura labial. In M. Monfort (Ed.), *Los trastornos de la Comunicación en el niño*. Madrid, Spain: CEPE.

Kagan, S. (1992). *Cooperative learning*. San Juan Capistrano, CA: Resources for Teachers.

Knoors, H., & Marschark, M. (2012). Language planning for the 21st century: Revisiting bilingual language policy for deaf children. *Journal of Deaf Studies and Deaf Education*, 17, 291–305.

Knoors, H., & Marschark, M. (2014). *Teaching deaf learners: Psychological and developmental foundations*. New York, NY: Oxford University Press.

Las Heras, T. (1999). La educación de las alumnas y alumnos sordos. *Aula de Innovación educativa*, 83–84, 13–14.

LEY 27/2007, de 23 de octubre, por la que se reconocen las lenguas de signos españolas y se regulan los medios a la comunicación oral de las personas sordas, con discapacidad auditiva y sordociegas. *BOE (Boletín Oficial del Estado)*, 255.

Leybaert, J., & Alegría, J. (2002). The role of cued speech in language development of deaf children. In M. Marschark & P. E. Spencer (Eds.), *Handbook of deaf studies, language and education* (pp. 261–274). New York, NY: Oxford University Press.

Leybaert, J., Bayard, C., Huyse, A., & Colin, C. (2012). Perception multi-modale de la parole chez l'implanté cochléaire. L'implant cochélaire chez le jeune enfant: langage, parole et cognition (multi-modal speech perception in the case of cochlear implants. CI in young children: language, speech and cognition). *Rééducation orthophonique*, 252, 33–53.

Lewis, W. (1995). *Bilingual teaching of deaf children in Denmark: Description of a project (1982–1992)*. Aalborg, Denmark: Doveskolernes Materialcenter.

López-Ornat, S, Gallego, C., Gallo, P., Karousou, A., Mariscal, S. & Martínez, M. (2005). *Inventarios de Desarrollo Comunicativo MacArthur: Manual técnico & cuadernillo*. Madrid, Spain: Ediciones TEA.

Manrique, M., Ramos, A., Morera, C., Cenjor, C., Lavilla, M. J., Boleas, M. S., & Cervera-Paz, F. J. (2006). Evaluación del IC como técnica de tratamiento de la hipoacusia profunda en pacientes pre y post locutivos [Analysis of cochlear implant as a treatment technique for profound hearing loss in pre and post-locutive patients]. *Acta Otorrinolaringologica Española*, 57, 2–23.

Mason, K., Rowley, K., Marshall, C. R., Atkinson, J. R., Herman, R., Woll, W., & Morgan, G. (2010). Identifying specific language impairment in deaf children acquiring British Sign Language: Implications for theory and practice. *British Journal of Developmental Psychology, 28*, 33–49.

MEC. (1989). *Introducción a la comunicación bimodal* [Introduction to signed communication]. Madrid, Spain: CNREE-Centro Nacional de Recursos para la Educación Especial. Serie Formación. Ministerio de Educación y Ciencia.

MEC. (1993). *Cómo organizar un curso de lengua de signos* [How to organize a course on sign language]. Madrid, Spain: CNREE-Centro Nacional de Recursos para la Educación Especial. Serie Formación. Ministerio de Educación y Ciencia.

Mendoza, E., Carballo, G., Muñoz, J., & Fresneda, M. D. (2005). *CEG: Test de comprensión de estructuras gramaticales*. Madrid, Spain: TEA Ediciones.

Moeller, M. P. (2000). Early intervention and language development in children who are deaf or hard of hearing. Online version: http://pediatrics.aappublications.org/content/106/3/e43.full.html.

Monfort, M. (2006). Dysphasie et surdité. In C. Hage, B. Charlier, & J. Leybaert (Eds.), *Competences cognitives, lingüistiques et sociales de l'enfant sourd. Pistes dévaluation* (pp. 150–164). Bruxelles, Belgium: Editions Mardaga.

Morales-López, E. (2008). Sign bilingualism in Spanish deaf education. In C. Paza-Pust & E. Morales-López (Eds.), *Sign bilingualism: Language development, interaction, and maintenance in sign language contact situations* (pp. 223–276). Philadelphia; Amsterdam: John Benjamins Publishing.

Mostaert, S. (2012). *Desarrollo de la lengua oral y de la lengua de signos española en niños con implante coclear precoz y escolarizados en centros bilingües (Sign and spoken language development in children with early CI and in bilingual schools)*. Trabajo de fin de master [unpublished Master's thesis]. Universidad Autónoma de Madrid. Director: Ignacio Montero.

Muñoz-Baell, I., Alvarez Dardet, C., Ruiz, M. T., Ferrero-Lago, E., & Aroca Fernandez, E. (2011). Understanding deaf bilingual education from the inside: A SWOT analysis. *International Journal of Inclusive Education, 15*(9), 865–889.

Niparko, J. K, Tobey, E. A., Thal, D. J., Eisenberg, L. S., Wang, N., Quittner, A. L., & Fink, N. D. (2010). Spoken language development in children following cochlear implantation. *JAMA, 303*(15), 1498–1506.

Oller, K. (2005). The distributed characteristic in bilingual learning. In J. Cohen, K. T. McAlister, K. Rolstad, & J. MacSwan (Eds.), *Proceedings of the Fourth International Symposium on Bilingualism*. Somerville, MA: Cascadilla Press.

Paradis, J., Genesee, F., & Crago, M. B. (2011). *Dual language development and disorders: A handbook on bilingualism and second language learning* (2nd ed.) Baltimore, MD: Brookes.

Pearson, B. Z. (1998). Assessing lexical development in bilingual babies and toddlers. *The International Journal of Bilingualism, 2*, 347–372.

Pearson, B. Z. (2009). Children with two languages. In E. Bavin (Ed.), *Handbook of child language* (pp. 379–398). Cambridge, UK: Cambridge University Press

Pérez, M., Herrero, E., & Pérez, M. (2008). La asamblea con niños sordos y oyentes: Un espacio para compartir [Assembly with deaf and hearing children: A space to share]. Universidad Pontificia de Salamanca. *Papeles Salmantinos de Educación, 11*, 267–298.

Pérez, M., Valmaseda, M., De la Fuente, B., Montero, I., & Mostaert, S. (2013). Desarrollo del vocabulario temprano en niños con implante coclear escolarizados en centros con bilingüismo oral-signado [Early vocabulary development in deaf children with cochlear implants educated in oral signed bilingual schools in Madrid]. *Revista de Logopedia, Foniatría y Audiología*.

Power, D., & Grez L. (2011). Currículum: Cultural and comunicative contexts. In M. Marscharck (Ed.), *The Oxford handbook of deaf studies, language and education* (2nd ed., vol. 1). New York, NY: Oxford University Press.

Preisler, G., Ahlström, M., & Tvingstedt, A. L. (1997). The development of communication and language in deaf preschool with cochlear implant. *International Journal of Pediatric Otorhinolaryngology, 41*, 263–272.

Preisler, G., Tvingstedt, A. L., & Ahlstrom, M. (2005). Interviews with deaf children about their experiences using cochlear implants. *American Annals of the Deaf, 150*(3), 260–267.

Pujolas P. (2008). *El aprendizaje cooperativo* [Cooperative learning]. Barcelona, Spain: Graó.

Rodríguez González, M. A. (1992). *Lenguaje de signos* [Sign language]. Madrid, Spain: CNSE.

Ruiz, U. (2000). *Didáctica de la segunda lengua en educación infantil y primaria*. Madrid, Spain: Síntesis Educación.

Sanchez, E., García, R., & Rosales, J. (2010). *La lectura en el aula: Qué se hace, qué se debe hacer y qué se puede hacer*. Barcelona, Spain: Graó.

Sanjuan, M., & Pérez García, M. (2005). Proyecto de integración "inclusiva" de niños sordos en educación infantil (A inclusive educational Project in deaf children in infant schools). *Monografías para el debate, 1*, 47–57. Universidad Pontificia de Comillas.

Santana, R. Torres, S., & García, J. (2003). The role of cued speech in the development of Spanish prepositions. *American Annals of the Deaf, 148*(4), 323–332.

Saunders, G. (1988). *Bilingual children: From birth to teens*. Clevedon; Avon; Philadelphia: Bilingual Matters.

Snowling, M. J., & Hulme, C. (2008). Reading intervention for children with language learning impairments. In C. F. Norbury, J. B. Tomblin, & D. V. M. Bishop, (Eds.), *Understanding developmental language disorders: From theory to practice* (pp. 175–188). Hove; Sussex: Psychology Press.

Thal, D., Desjardin, J. L., & Eisenberg, L. S. (2007). Validity of the MacArthur-Bates Communicative Development Inventories for measuring language abilities in children with cochlear implants. *American Journal of Speech-Language Pathology, 16*(1), 54–64.

Torres, S. (1988). *La palabra complementada* [Cued speech]. Madrid, Spain: CEPE.

UNESCO. (2005). *Guidelines for inclusión: Ensuring access to education for all*. París, France: UNESCO. http://unesco.org/educacion/inclusive.

Wiefferink, C. H., Spaai, G. W., Uilenburg, N., & Vermeij, B. (2008). Influence of linguistic environment on children's language development: Flemish versus Dutch children. *Deafness and Education International, 10*(4), 226–243.

Woll. B. (2013). Sign language and spoken language development in young children: Measuring vocabulary by means of the CDI. In L. Meurant, A. Sinte, M. Van Herreweghe, & M. Vermeerbergen (Eds.), *Sign language research, uses and practices: Crossing views on theoretical and applied sign language linguistics.* Berlin, Germany: deGruyter Mouton & Ishara Press.

Woolfe, T. Herman, R., Roy, P., & Woll, B. (2010). Early vocabulary development in deaf native signers: A British Sign Language adaptation of the communicative development inventories. *Journal of Child Psychology and Psychiatry, 51*(3), 322–331.

# 16

# The Twinschool

## *A Co-enrollment Program in the Netherlands*

Daan Hermans, Annet de Klerk, Loes Wauters,
and Harry Knoors

Special education programs have always been a prominent part of the educational system in the Netherlands. In comparison to other countries in Europe, many children with hearing disabilities, visual disabilities, specific language impairments, learning disabilities, or behavioral problems are enrolled in special schools (Pijl, 1997; Smeets, 2007). In 2006, this amounted to approximately 4.1% of the children between 4 and 11 years old. Although this percentage is comparable to the percentages in Northern European countries like Belgium and Germany, the average percentage across all European countries is considerably lower (2.0%). As pointed out by Smeets (2007), countries with a high proportion of children in special schools or separate educational programs traditionally have shared the view that children need guidance from specialist professionals in separate programs to fulfill their cognitive and social possibilities. Such beliefs are generally deeply rooted in society and are not very open to change (Herzberg, 1994).

This view on the appropriate educational environment for children with special needs in general, and deaf and hard-of-hearing (DHH) children in particular, was firmly supported by government policies until the beginning of the twenty-first century. Bilingual-bicultural education programs were implemented in the Netherlands in special schools for DHH children starting from the early 1990s. For several years, we have been witnessing a considerable change in policy with respect to the appropriate educational environment for children with special needs, now increasingly favoring a policy of inclusion. This change in view has been backed up by several changes in the legal system in the Netherlands. "Leerling Gebonden Financiering" (Student-related Financing) became operative in 2003; "Passend Onderwijs" (Appropriate Education) was introduced in 2012 and will be operative in August 2014. "Passend Onderwijs" means that children with disabilities have a legal right to an appropriate educational placement, either in mainstream schools or in special schools (with support).

In other words, the policy on the least restrictive educational environment, also for DHH children, has changed in the Netherlands in the last two decades.

Quite interestingly, during the same period, professionals in the field of deafness have been confronted with several changes that have already had a profound impact on the development of many DHH children. A national newborn hearing screening program was implemented in the Netherlands between 2000 and 2005, with two major implications. First, early detection of children's hearing loss has resulted in an earlier start of intervention programs for DHH children. Second, as pointed out by Knoors and Marschark (2012), national newborn hearing screening programs have not only led to an increase in the number of deaf children who receive cochlear implants, but also to a decrease of the age of implantation. Although the impact of both factors is by no means a guarantee for an optimal language and cognitive development of DHH children, it seems very safe to conclude that it has led to major improvements in the hearing skills and speech abilities of many DHH children (Dettman & Dowell, 2010; Hammer, 2010; Verbist, 2010; see Walker & Tomblin, Chapter 6 of this volume). Improvement of speech abilities and hearing skills may lead to better prospects for the successful inclusion of DHH children in mainstream education.

The improved prospects of DHH children and, especially, the change in policy in the Netherlands will lead to an increase in the proportion of DHH children enrolled in mainstream schools. And as the number of children who enroll in mainstream programs grows, educational programs like co-enrollment programs become an increasingly more interesting option. Such programs can effectively combine the advantages of programs in special and mainstream education (Kreimeyer, Crooke, Drye, Egbert, & Klein, 2000).

There have been only very few co-enrollment programs with DHH and hearing children. But to the extent that experiences with these programs have been evaluated and described, evaluations tend to be quite positive (Bowen, 2008; Kreimeyer et al., 2000). One of the best-known co-enrollment programs for DHH children is the TRIPOD program in Burbank, California, established in 1982 (now called Foothill Selpa). In the TRIPOD program the educational environment is changed (and not the curriculum, which is often the case when DHH children are mainstreamed) by introducing an extra teacher of the deaf in the regular classroom, by reducing the number of hearing children to include DHH children, and by the use of signs in a total communication (TC) environment. Though it is not described in published reports on this program, total communication generally includes spoken language, Sign Supported English, and American Sign Language. The two teachers in the TRIPOD program use a team-teaching model.

Kirchner (1994), the founder of the TRIPOD program, reported that teachers indicated that DHH children were meeting age-appropriate academic and social expectations. Nevertheless, Kirchner also mentioned that full inclusion becomes difficult when DHH children cannot meet the requirements of the academic work. So it seems that not *all* children are meeting age-appropriate academic expectations and that some children (partly) follow an individual program at their own pace. This can lead to a "special" position of those DHH children in the classroom. Teachers also indicated that it is an advantage to have two teachers to plan, share ideas, and help each other, but the combination of the two teachers requires careful attention. The published reports on the TRIPOD program give no further information about this last issue, but the communication skills of the teachers, their will and motivation to cooperate, the flexibility of their personalities, and their personal stance toward each other (DHH and hearing) may play a role in the relationship between the two teachers.

In a survey, the majority of parents were positive about this co-enrollment program. They mentioned that they observed a growth in the social-emotional development of their child and an increase in the mixed friendships of DHH and hearing children (Kirchner, 1994). However, systematic investigations of the school achievements and social-emotional development of DHH children and hearing children in the TRIPOD program seem to be absent.

Another example of a co-enrollment program described in the literature is the program in Tucson, Arizona. This program is conceptually based upon the TRIPOD program (Kreimeyer et al., 2000; see Antia & Metz, Chapter 17 of this volume). The aim of the Arizona program is to create an inclusive environment in which DHH children communicate comfortably with hearing children and show growth in their educational development. This program has classrooms with DHH children and hearing children of various ages and grade levels. The co-enrollment classrooms are taught by two teachers, a mainstream education teacher and a certified teacher of the deaf, both of whom stay with the same class for several years. A signing teaching assistant supports instruction. Although the signing skills of the certified teachers of the deaf are not described extensively, the teacher of the deaf described in the Kreimeyer et al. (2000) study had interpreter-level signing skills. The regular classroom teachers often acquire signing skills on the job. To illustrate, Kreimeyer et al. (2000) reported that one of the mainstream teachers supported her speech with signs approximately 80% of the time after two years. As the role of the two teachers within the classroom has not been described extensively, it remains unclear which form of co-teaching actually is used in this program.

Direct interaction between DHH children and hearing children is one of the key objectives in the Arizona program. For that purpose, hearing children are stimulated to acquire signing skills through a diversity of activities in and outside the classroom. To further stimulate signing interaction, a considerable proportion of the instruction in the classroom takes place in small groups consisting of hearing and DHH children. Furthermore, hearing children are also trained in visual attention-getting strategies. Interestingly, teachers reported that 50–60% of the conversations in and outside the classroom between hearing and DHH children occurred in sign without voice.

Data from the research of the first three years of the Arizona program are positive. The amount of interaction between DHH and hearing children, one of the main objectives of the program, grew steadily during the first 3 years of the program. The stimulation of hearing children's signing skills in and outside the classroom has presumably contributed considerably to this increase in interaction between DHH and hearing children in and outside the classroom. Furthermore, the academic achievements of the DHH children tended to be better in comparison to the academic achievements of DHH children in different educational settings (mainstream education, special schools), especially with respect to reading comprehension. Importantly, Kreimeyer and colleagues (2000) specifically mention that the success of their co-enrollment program can be attributed to the commitment to the idea of inclusive education of the parents and professionals involved. They also note that a successful co-enrollment program requires an intensive collaboration of all participants (children, parents, and professionals).

In 2004, Talent, a school for the deaf and part of Royal Dutch Kentalis, and one mainstream school in the south of the Netherlands started a co-enrollment program called "the Twinschool." This co-enrollment program is predominantly based upon principles of the TRIPOD co-enrollment program. The program is called The Twinschool because two existing schools, one special school and one mainstream school situated on the same premises, started an intensive cooperation. Groups of DHH children entered the mainstream school, along with a teacher of the deaf, a deaf sign language teacher, and a speech therapist.

In this chapter the Twinschool program first will be described. Subsequently, we will focus on the description of the results of a 6-year evaluation that was initiated in 2004.

## THE TWINSCHOOL PROGRAM

Before 2004, Royal Dutch Kentalis had a long and strong tradition of integrating DHH children into mainstream schools. This concept of integration implied that the educational program of the mainstream school was not sufficiently attuned to children with special needs; additional assistance was necessary. The child had to adapt himself or herself to the program, for instance, by having extra individual training outside the classroom by specialists from outside the school (Knoors, 2004). Since the start of the twenty-first century, Kentalis began to embrace the idea of inclusion rather than integration. Inclusion means that the educational program is tailored to the needs of the children in a classroom. Regardless of whether children have a disability or not, all children in the classroom are included in social and educational activities.

In 2003 Kentalis was looking for opportunities to start a structural collaboration with mainstream education in order to realize a linguistically rich environment for DHH children incorporating spoken and written Dutch, Sign Supported Dutch, and Sign Language of the Netherlands (SLN). Such an opportunity came in 2004, and the Twinschool was born.

### Aims and Potential Benefits of Co-enrollment

The aim of the Twinschool co-enrollment program is to combine the strengths of the two systems, special and mainstream education. For the DHH children, this means specialized education by a trained teacher of the deaf, (additional) instruction in sign language or Sign Supported Dutch, and attention for identity/Deaf culture in the curriculum. The mainstream classroom also can offer DHH children a larger social group with more possibilities for interaction with peers. Another strength is the faster pace of instruction in mainstream education. In special schools there is a tendency to elaborate on instruction because many DHH children have difficulties in comprehending the curriculum content. Teachers in special schools tend to focus on the DHH children in the classroom who need the most support for learning or the regulation of their behavior. To illustrate, one of the teachers in a special school for deaf children recently indicated that her language use, the content of the instruction, and the pace of the instruction was attuned to the DHH children in the classroom with the lowest level of language proficiency and cognitive skills. In contrast, in mainstream education, in general, teachers have a faster pace of instruction and will continue their instruction despite the fact that not all children fully grasp the content immediately. They have the task of delivering a certain amount of curriculum during a school year, and this "forces" them to keep their pace. DHH children may profit from this faster pace of instruction in the co-enrollment classrooms. Another positive aspect in mainstream education is the independence of children. Due to the fact that classrooms in schools for the deaf are rather small (approximately 6 to 12 children), teachers tend to help children more often than is necessary. This may result in "learned helplessness" of DHH children. Just because of the fact that there are more children in a mainstream classroom, children are forced to become more independent of their teacher(s).

Hearing children in the classroom may benefit from the presence of the teacher of special education who is specialized in communication, language, and reading. Children who need extra instruction can do so in a small group or benefit from extra attention during lessons in the classroom. Because advantages were expected for both groups of children, it was clear from the start of the program that the two teachers involved (from mainstream and special education) should be committed to and responsible for teaching all children, DHH and hearing.

**Demographics of the Twinschool**

This co-enrollment program has combined groups of DHH and hearing children. On average there are 25 to 30 children in a classroom. Between 2004 and 2012, three groups of DHH children have been enrolled. The first group of four DHH children started in grade 2 (2004) and left primary education (grade 6) in 2009. The second group of seven DHH children started in kindergarten (2006) and are currently (2013) in grade 5. The third group of four DHH children started in grade 2 (2008) and are now in grade 6 (2013). No DHH children repeated a class.

In all, 18 DHH children (14 deaf and 4 hard of hearing), have been enrolled in the Twinschool; all deaf children had cochlear implants. The DHH children first were placed in a special school with a bilingual education program. The age at which children enrolled in the Twinschool varied considerably. Two groups of children started in grade 2, whereas one group started in K-1. Furthermore, three DHH children (no. 8, 9, and 18) made the transition from the special school to the Twinschool one or more years after the whole group started.

As shown in Table 16.1, seven children left the Twinschool before they finished primary education and subsequently enrolled in secondary schools. Four of them left for a mainstream school near their homes. Their parents preferred that their children went to a school close to their home mainly to facilitate social contacts in the neighborhood. Three others went back to the special school for the deaf. These children appeared to have additional needs that could not be addressed adequately in the Twinschool. These children, who had behavioral or learning problems, were thought to be better off being taught in a smaller group in a special school. For children with learning problems, it may be more appropriate to be in a smaller group at the special school, where the learning content is delivered in a more adapted pace and more tuned to their needs. For children with severe behavioral problems, the environment of the mainstream school can be too hectic and stressful. The environment at the special school with a more structured program and smaller groups could then be a better place for these children. This is not to say that a co-enrollment program, by definition, is not an appropriate place for DHH children with extra needs. This depends on the context of the mainstream school. This particular school is a school that attracts hearing children from higher socioeconomic backgrounds. Most children have above average learning possibilities. The gap in learning and

Table 16.1 Characteristics of the DHH Children at the Twinschool

| Group | Gender | HS | CI | Entry | Exit |
|---|---|---|---|---|---|
| Group 1 | | | | | |
| 1 | Male | HoH | – | Grade 2 | Grade 6 |
| 2 | Male | Deaf | Yes | Grade 2 | Grade 6 |
| 3 | Male | Deaf | Yes | Grade 2 | Grade 5 (high. school) |
| 4 | Female | Deaf | Yes | Grade 2 | Grade 3 (spec. school) |
| Group 2 | | | | | |
| 5 | Female | Deaf | Yes | K1 | K2 (main. school) |
| 6 | Female | Deaf | Yes | K1 | Grade 2 (main. school) |
| 7 | Female | Deaf | Yes | K1 | Grade 2 (main. school) |
| 8 | Female | Deaf | Yes | K1 | – |
| 9 | Female | HoH | – | Grade 5 | – |
| 10 | Female | HoH | – | Grade 3 | – |
| 11 | Male | Deaf | Yes | K1 | Grade 4 (spec. school) |
| 12 | Male | Deaf | Yes | K1 | Grade 2 (main. school) |
| 13 | Male | Deaf | Yes | K1 | – |
| Group 3 | | | | | |
| 14 | Male | Deaf | Yes | Grade 2 | – |
| 15 | Female | HoH | – | Grade 2 | – |
| 16 | Female | Deaf | – | Grade 2 | – |
| 17 | Female | Deaf | Yes | Grade 2 | Grade 3 (spec. school) |
| 18 | Male | Deaf | Yes | Grade 3 | – |

social development between hearing and DHH children in this situation can become relatively large because of the background of most hearing children.

The selection of the children who enrolled in the Twinschool depended upon several factors. A multidisciplinary team of professionals at the school for the deaf assessed the development of the DHH children. They advised concerning the most appropriate/least restricted learning environment for the children: the school for the deaf because of the intensive support or the Twinschool because of the rich multilingual and social environment. Most of the children had average or above average nonverbal intelligence. The possibilities of the children to access this environment (communication, language, and curriculum content) were important parameters in the decision for the placement. Another important issue was the number of hearing children already present in the classroom. Some classes were literally full, and there was no possibility of adding DHH children to these groups. The mainstream school in which the Twinschool program was realized was and is a rather popular school and has to deal with waiting lists to place children.

## Language Proficiency of the DHH Children at Entry into the Program

All DHH children who have been enrolled during the past years have had considerable access to spoken Dutch and have been able to communicate with their hearing classmates without the help of an interpreter. The skills of the children in spoken Dutch before or briefly after they enrolled at the Twinschool are shown in Table 16.2.

Note that the spoken language skills of the children in group 1 and group 3 were assessed through four subtests of the TAK-R (Verhoeven & Vermeer, 2001), whereas the skills of most of the children in group 2 were assessed through the administration of the Reynell test for language comprehension (Van Eldik et al., 1995) and the Schlichting test for language production (Schlichting et al., 1998).

As shown in Table 16.2, the language delays of the DHH children were quite large, and the variability in the children's scores was high. On average, however, their proficiency in spoken Dutch is high in comparison to deaf peers from special schools.

Table 16.2 Language Proficiency in Spoken Dutch (in Standard Deviations) of the DHH Children upon Entry in the Twinschool

|   | Receptive Vocabulary | Receptive Grammar | Expressive Vocabulary | Expressive Grammar |
|---|---|---|---|---|
| Group 1 | | | | |
| 1 | <-3.00 | -1.57 | -1.57 | -0.95 |
| 2 | <-3.00 | <-3.00 | <-3.00 | -1.95 |
| 3 | <-3.00 | -2.91 | -2.91 | -1.62 |
| 4 | -2.91 | -2.91 | <-3.00 | <-3.00 |
| Group 2 | | | | |
| 1 | n.a. | -1.50 | -1.50 | -1.30 |
| 2 | n.a. | -1.30 | -1.50 | -1.50 |
| 3 | n.a. | -0.90 | -1.40 | -1.70 |
| 4 | n.a. | -2.30 | -1.60 | -2.50 |
| 5 | n.a. | -2.20 | <-3.00 | -1.60 |
| 6 | -1.64 | -1.53 | <-3.00 | n.a. |
| 7 | n.a. | -1.10 | -1.30 | -0.90 |
| 8 | n.a. | -0.80 | -0.90 | -0.90 |
| 9 | n.a. | -0.70 | -1.10 | -1.60 |
| Group 3 | | | | |
| 1 | -1.94 | -1.36 | n.a. | -1.36 |
| 2 | -2.24 | -1.26 | -1.26 | -1.78 |
| 3 | <-3.00 | <-3.00 | n.a. | <-3.00 |
| 4 | <-3.00 | <-3.00 | n.a. | -2.30 |
| 5 | -0.80 | <-3.00 | n.a. | <-3.00 |

(n.a. = no data available)

The children's proficiency in SLN was assessed prior to their enrollment in the Twinschool. Most of the children scored well above average on tests assessing their proficiency with respect to the phonology, the vocabulary, and the grammar of SLN (Hermans, Knoors, & Verhoeven, 2007, 2009). To illustrate, 69%, 87%, and 94% of the children's scores with respect to the phonology, the vocabulary, and the grammar of Sign Language of the Netherlands were above average (Hermans et al., 2007, 2009). In other words, most of the children in the Twinschool were relatively proficient in both Sign Language of the Netherlands and spoken Dutch.

**Educational System of the Twinschool**

The team of instructors consists of two teachers, one from the mainstream school and one teacher of the deaf. The number of hours that the teacher of the deaf is present varies as a function of the number of DHH children in the classroom. To provide a full-time teacher of the deaf, financially, approximately 7 to 10 DHH children are needed in a classroom. For example, with four DHH children in a classroom the teacher of the deaf is present for two days or four half days a week. So in reality the teacher of the deaf is often present on a part-time basis.

The two teachers use a flexible system of co-teaching. This co-teaching has been based on the model of Clarke and DeNuzzo (2003). They distinguish six approaches of co-teaching: (1) one teach, one observe, (2) one teach, one drift, (3) station teaching, (4) parallel teaching, (5) alternative teaching, (6) team teaching. In general, the teachers plan all their teaching activities in advance so that they know who is responsible for each activity. In practice, this means that one of the two teachers can teach the whole group and the other teacher gives extra support/instruction to specific children, hearing or DHH. It can also mean that one teacher works inside the classroom with a group of mixed children and the other teacher works with a group of mixed children in a different classroom to give them extra, intensive instruction. In team teaching, both teachers are in front of the classroom and they deliver the curriculum content together by having a dialogue about the content of the lesson. This works very well for a modeling activity. Station teaching gives the possibility to deliver different curriculum content attuned to the needs of a smaller group. Observing can give information about, for example, social relations in the classroom. When one teacher is teaching, there is time for the other to observe.

A deaf sign language teacher and a speech therapist are also part of the team. The deaf sign language teacher is present at the Twinschool for two and a half hours a week. He teaches SLN as a subject to the DHH children and delivers pre-teaching for reading lessons and lessons with a more complex content like geography and history. He also discusses issues about Deaf identity (being deaf in a hearing world) and Deaf culture, such as Deaf history and poetry. These activities take place in the small group of DHH children. The sign language teacher also teaches the whole class some sign language and discusses issues that are related to Deaf culture. The speech therapist supports the speech and spoken language development of the DHH children in individual sessions. Sometimes she or he advises the teacher about the language development of a hearing child.

**Team of Support**

The teachers of the Twinschool are supported by two supervisors, one from each school. Together with the teachers, they monitor the development of the children and support the teachers to optimize the program for individual children. They discuss issues concerning access to instruction, curriculum goals, and social emotional support. From the start of the Twinschool program, a support structure was created for the development of the program. A board of advisors consists of parents and principals of both schools and the project leader. A project group consists of supervisors, teachers, sign language teachers, and speech therapists. This group discusses the organization and content of the program and meets on a regular basis.

**Language Policy in the Twinschool**

Central within the language policy of the Twinschool is the concept that the instruction should be accessible to all DHH children and all hearing children in the classroom. As we described earlier, the DHH children in the Twinschool, as a group, can be characterized as DHH children who are relatively proficient in SLN and in spoken Dutch in comparison to deaf peers in special schools. More important, the variability in DHH children's skills in spoken Dutch and SLN is quite high. This variability makes it difficult to implement a "one size fits all" language policy in the Twinschool. The choice and implementation of the language policy are further complicated by the rather unpredictable development of DHH children in the Twinschool in spoken Dutch and SLN, the view of the parents of the DHH children regarding the appropriate educational environment of their children, and financial constraints (again, the provision of a full-time teacher of the deaf requires 7 to 10 DHH children). In other words, providing optimal access to instruction for the whole group of DHH children is easier said than done, and it requires a dynamic and pragmatic stance rather than a theoretical one.

Most mainstream education teachers in the co-enrollment program use spoken Dutch as the language of instruction in the classroom. Some mainstream teachers also use (some) signs that they have learned during the past years (e.g., Kreimeyer et al., 2000). Both the mainstream teacher and the teacher of the deaf use an FM system.

When teaching the whole class or teaching a group of DHH and hearing children, the language of instruction of the teacher of the deaf is Sign Supported Dutch, as the hearing children are generally not proficient in SLN. However, when the teacher of the deaf works with the DHH in smaller groups or individually, SLN is often used as the language of instruction. Some of the teachers of the deaf involved in the program have interpreter-level skills in SLN. However, this is not (yet) the case for all teachers involved in the Twinschool.

Due to financial restrictions, the teacher of the deaf is present for two days or four half days a week when there are four DHH children in a classroom. For the past year, there has been the possibility of providing an SLN interpreter in the classroom when the teacher of the deaf is not present. Although the role of the interpreter is clearly different from the role of the teacher of the deaf, she or he will at least increase DHH children's access to the instruction.

## THE EVALUATION

Although there are several co-enrollment programs for DHH children throughout the world, there is little documented evidence concerning the advantages and disadvantages for DHH and hearing children (for a summary of the available data, see Metz, 2011). In addition, the co-enrollment program in the Netherlands cannot easily be compared with existing co-enrollment programs elsewhere. To illustrate, the Twinschool constitutes cooperation between a mainstream school and a special school for DHH children. This is in contrast with other co-enrollment programs, like the TRIPOD program in Burbank, California, and the Jockey Club Sign Bilingualism and Co-enrollment in Deaf Education Program in Hongkong (see Yiu & Tang, Chapter 14 of this volume), where DHH children are included groupwise but no school for the deaf is involved.

As Kentalis had no prior experience with co-enrollment programs for DHH children, a 6-year research study was set up from the start of the program in 2004. The research study focused on (1) the social position of DHH children within the Twinschool, (2) the advantages or disadvantages for DHH and hearing children with respect to their achievements in reading comprehension, mathematics, and spelling, (3) the DHH children's skills in spoken Dutch and Sign Language of the Netherlands, and (4) the perceptions of children and parents on the Twinschool.

### The Social Position of DHH Children

Stinson and Antia (1999) define social integration as the ability to interact with, make friends with, and be accepted by peers. The social position of children in the classroom has a crucial impact on children's well-being, both in the short and long term (e.g., Shaffer, 2005). Social integration, being accepted by classmates and having friends, is often assumed to be one of the major challenges for DHH children in inclusive settings.

Nevertheless, the empirical evidence does not unambiguously support the assumption that the social position of DHH children in mainstream schools is problematic. Some studies have revealed that DHH children in mainstream education often have few friends, have less interaction with hearing peers, and are more often rejected or neglected than their hearing peers. In addition, some of these studies have shown that DHH children often feel isolated and lonely (Kluwin, Stinson, & Colarossi, 2002; Musselman, Mootilal, & MacKay, 1996; Stinson & Antia, 1999; Stinson & Kluwin, 2003). Other studies have found more positive results regarding DHH children's social position in mainstreams schools (Antia et al., 2011; Wauters & Knoors, 2008; Wolters, Knoors, Cillessen, & Verhoeven, 2011).

For DHH children in co-enrollment programs, the social position seems to be more positive (Bowen, 2008; Metz, 2011). Theoretically, co-enrollment programs provide the opportunity of intensive contact between DHH children and their hearing peers in an environment where they are not the only DHH child (Antia & Kreimeyer, 2003; Kirchner, 1994). Although DHH and hearing children have been found to interact more with peers with the same hearing status (Kluwin et al., 2002), interaction between DHH and hearing peers increased during the co-enrollment program studied by Kreimeyer and colleagues (2000). DHH children in co-enrollment programs do not feel lonely or isolated, do not have lower self-esteem, and do not differ from their hearing peers in how much their peers like them (Bowen, 2008; Kluwin, 1999; Nunes, Pretzlik, & Olsson, 2001), although Nunes and colleagues (2001) found DHH children to be neglected more often than their hearing peers and to have fewer friends in the classroom.

When the Twinschool was initiated in 2004, we assumed that the co-enrollment program would strengthen DHH children's social position and therefore would increase DHH children's well-being at school. This assumption was not only supported by the available evidence or experiences in other co-enrollment programs for DHH children, but also from results of various studies on the impact of classroom composition regarding children's race and gender on their social position (Graham & Cohen; 1997; Hallinnan & Texeira, 1987; Jackson, Barth, Powell, & Lochman, 2006; Singleton & Asher, 1979). Those studies have revealed that children generally have a strong social preference for children with the same gender and for children from the same race. Interestingly, children's social preference for children from the same gender is larger than their social preference for children from the same race (Graham & Cohen, 1997).

In other words, the classroom composition in terms of the gender and race characteristics of the children can strongly affect a child's social position. Consistent with this conclusion, Jackson and colleagues (2006) found that minority children's social position improved as the number of minority children in the class increased. Similarly, we assumed that DHH children would also have this in-group social bias, a preference for children with same hearing status, and that increasing the number of DHH children in a classroom will generally strengthen DHH children's social position.

There may, of course, be a downside to DHH children being co-enrolled in a mainstream school. As the number of DHH children increases, the DHH children may more strongly form a subgroup within the class, which may affect DHH children's social position negatively as they may receive more negative nominations from their hearing classmates (negative out-group biases). This assumption is consistent with the results reported by Durkin and colleagues (2012), who found that peer aggression experienced by minority children increased as the percentages of minority children in a class increased. It is unclear to what extent the positive effects of in-group biases are eliminated by the negative effects of out-group biases.

In the evaluation of the Twinschool program, we assessed the social position of DHH children through the administration of two sociometric tasks and the administration of a questionnaire to the hearing classmates of DHH children in the co-enrollment program and the hearing classmates of DHH children who are individually enrolled in mainstream education. The sociometric tasks were administered to 16 DHH children in the Twinschool and their 96 hearing classmates each year from the start of the evaluation. In the first sociometric task, the peer rating task, children received a booklet with the names or photographs of their classmates. On the right side of each name/photograph was a visual scale, consisting of three faces (a happy face, a neutral face, and a sad face). For each classmate, children were instructed to choose the face corresponding to how much they liked to play with him or her by drawing a circle around that face. In the second sociometric task, the peer nomination task, children were asked to name the three classmates they liked the most and three classmates they liked the least.

Table 16.3 summarizes the main findings of this study. Averaged across all test administrations, DHH children received a slightly lower score in the peer rating task, significantly less positive nominations, and significantly more negative nominations than their hearing classmates.

As we pointed out above, we assumed that DHH children in the Twinschool could find support in the presence of DHH classmates. To verify that assumption, we analyzed the data in the sociometric tasks as a function of the match or mismatch in gender and hearing status between the child who gave and the child who received the judgment. As shown in Table 16.3, DHH and hearing children showed a preference for children with the same gender and hearing status in the

Table 16.3 Results of the Peer Rating and Peer Nomination Task (in z-scores)

|  | Peer rating | Positive peer nominations | Negative peer nominations |
|---|---|---|---|
| Overall | | | |
| DHH | −.14 | −.14 | .17 |
| Hearing | .03 | .02 | −.03 |
| DHH children | | | |
| Match gender and hearing status | .36 | .91 | −.04 |
| Match gender, mismatch hearing status | −.03 | −.14 | .16 |
| Mismatch gender, match hearing status | −.01 | .16 | .37 |
| Mismatch gender and hearing status | −.46 | −.35 | .21 |
| Hearing children | | | |
| Match gender and hearing status | .24 | .34 | −.08 |
| Match gender, mismatch hearing status | .08 | .01 | −.11 |
| Mismatch gender, match hearing status | −.13 | −.21 | −.02 |
| Mismatch gender and hearing status | −.23 | −.26 | .06 |

analyses of the scores in peer rating tasks and the percentages of positive nominations in the peer nomination task. To illustrate, DHH children received the highest ratings in the peer rating tasks from DHH children with the same gender and hearing status (z-score .36). They obtained significantly lower ratings from DHH children with a different gender (z-score −.01) and from hearing children with the same gender (z-score −.03). And they received the lowest rating from hearing children with a different gender (z-score −.46). The same pattern was obtained in the analysis of the percentages of positive nominations, but not in the analysis of the percentages of negative nominations. Furthermore, hearing children showed the same preference for children with the same gender and hearing status.

Overall, the data suggest that, as a group, the social position of DHH children is slightly less positive in comparison to their hearing classmates. This finding is not surprising, given the larger proportion of hearing children in the class, in addition to the preference of hearing and DHH children for children with the same hearing status. This preference of DHH and hearing children for children with the same hearing status is consistent with studies that have shown the impact of classroom composition (e.g., gender and race) on the social position of children. The results suggest that DHH children do find support in the presence of DHH classmates.

As noted above, the downside of this support is that DHH children who are co-enrolled in mainstream schools more clearly form a separate group within the class. This, in turn, may negatively affect the judgments they receive from hearing classmates and may affect their social position. The current sociometric study does not warrant any conclusion concerning this issue. However, during the evaluation we also investigated the attitudes of hearing children toward the mainstreaming of DHH children. We administered a questionnaire by Cambra (2002) to the hearing classmates of DHH children in the Twinschool and the hearing classmates of seven individually enrolled children in mainstream schools. Overall, we found no difference between the attitudes of hearing classmates of DHH children at the Twinschool and the hearing classmates of DHH children individually enrolled in mainstream education. If anything, the hearing classmates' attitude toward DHH children in the Twinschool was somewhat more positive.

One of the final issues concerning the social status of DHH children that we would like to touch upon in this chapter is the impact of the hearing status of their teacher. Bellmore and colleagues (2007) found that the social status of minority children improves when their teacher is from the same minority group than when their teacher is from the majority group at that particular school. The co-teaching team consists of two hearing teachers. If the results of the study by Bellmore and colleagues (2007) can be generalized to DHH children, this may imply that the presence of a DHH teacher would strengthen a DHH child's social position.

In short, we found that the social position of DHH children in the Twinschool was slightly less positive in comparison to their hearing classmates. We also found that DHH children in the Twinschool can and do find support in the presence of DHH children in the same class. In a series of interviews, several DHH children indicated that they really appreciated the presence of DHH classmates. Although this finding supports the underlying assumptions of the Twinschool program, it still remains unclear how the co-enrollment concept affects children's contacts with hearing classmates.

**School Achievements**

*Hearing Children*

When the Twinschool was initiated, several parents of hearing children raised concerns about the impact of the co-enrollment class on the school achievements of their child. More specifically, they were worried that the presence of DHH children in the classroom would slow down the pace of instruction and therefore negatively affect their child's development (see also Metz, 2011). Although the available evidence seems to refute this claim (Metz, 2011), we decided to assess the impact of the Twinschool on the school achievements of the hearing children.

Achievement data for reading comprehension, mathematics, and spelling were collected using national achievement tests (CITO tests) for the hearing children in the Twinschool classes (n = 62) and the hearing children in classes without DHH children at the same school (n = 74) for hearing children from grade 3 to grade 6 (group 1), grade 1 to grade 5 (group 2), or grade 2 to grade 6 (group 3). The data of hearing children were included if achievement data were available for each year. The data of 34 children were excluded from these analyses. These children either enrolled in the school after 5 years (n = 24), left school (n = 6), changed from the Twinschool class to the parallel class or vice versa (n = 2), or no achievement data were available (n = 2).

In the Netherlands, nearly all mainstream schools administer the CITO tests to their children throughout primary education. For all tests, the scores of the children can be placed in one of five categories corresponding to equal percentile intervals: category I (percentile 81–100), category II (percentile 61–80), category III (percentile 41–60), category IV (percentile 21–40), or category V (percentile 1–20). Table 16.4 depicts the distribution of the hearing children in the Twinschool and the parallel classes across the five categories over the 4-year period (group 1) or 5-year period (group 2 and group 3).

As shown in Table 16.4, the hearing children in the Twinschool generally perform above average. To illustrate, for reading comprehension, between 39 and 47 percent of the children scored in the highest category, which is well above the national average of 20 percent. This was confirmed by a series of analyses that revealed that, averaged across all years, the scores of the hearing children in the Twinschool and parallel classes were not equally distributed across the five categories for reading comprehension, mathematics, and spelling.

Furthermore, at the start of the Twinschool, there was no difference between the distribution of the scores across the five categories between the children in the Twinschool classes and the parallel classes for reading comprehension, mathematics, and spelling, and the distribution of the scores in both classes remained the same in the subsequent years.

In other words, these analyses demonstrated that hearing children in the Twinschool and parallel classes perform well above the national average in reading comprehension, mathematics, and spelling. The co-enrollment system does not seem to positively or negatively affect hearing children's acquisition of reading comprehension, mathematics, and spelling.

*DHH Children*

The achievements of DHH children at school generally fall behind the achievements of their hearing peers (Karchmer & Mitchell, 2003; Powers, Gregory, & Thoutenhoofd, 1990). A recent study on the achievement data of DHH children in special schools in the Netherlands indicated that, on average, DHH children are 2 to 3 years behind their hearing peers in mathematics, spelling and reading comprehension at the end of primary education (Hermans, 2010).

A comparison between the achievements of DHH children in the Twinschool and the achievements of DHH children in special schools

**Table 16.4 Distribution of the Scores on Reading Comprehension, Mathematics, and Spelling for Hearing Children in the Twinschool Classes and Parallel Classes across the Five Categories (I = percentile 81–100, II = percentile 61–80, III = percentile 41–60, IV = percentile 21–40, V = percentile 1–20) over Five Years**

| Subject | | | Year 1 | Year 2 | Year 3 | Year 4 | Year 5 |
|---|---|---|---|---|---|---|---|
| Reading comprehension | Twinschool | I | 43.7 | 45.5 | 38.6 | 42.3 | 47.2 |
| | | II | 16.8 | 27.7 | 16.6 | 19.1 | 19.4 |
| | | III | 18.9 | 16.8 | 28.2 | 10.9 | 22.4 |
| | | IV | 14.5 | 6.2 | 13.7 | 19.4 | 3.2 |
| | | V | 6.1 | 3.8 | 2.9 | 8.3 | 7.8 |
| | Parallel class | I | 36.1 | 33.0 | 21.2 | 38.2 | 38.2 |
| | | II | 25.8 | 27.8 | 27.7 | 15.4 | 25.5 |
| | | III | 20.4 | 15.1 | 27.7 | 19.3 | 19.3 |
| | | IV | 14.6 | 13.4 | 10.6 | 21.0 | 1.9 |
| | | V | 3.1 | 10.7 | 12.8 | 6.1 | 15.1 |
| Mathematics | Twinschool | I | 41.8 | 46.2 | 39.2 | 47.2 | 46.6 |
| | | II | 28.9 | 24.7 | 32.1 | 33.4 | 24.7 |
| | | III | 19.4 | 11.4 | 17.9 | 14.3 | 22.1 |
| | | IV | 6.5 | 17.1 | 9.5 | 1.3 | 3.3 |
| | | V | 3.4 | 0.6 | 1.3 | 3.8 | 3.3 |
| | Parallel class | I | 45.4 | 40.1 | 36.2 | 48.7 | 43.4 |
| | | II | 25.2 | 26.8 | 27.2 | 32.2 | 25.3 |
| | | III | 20.2 | 11.4 | 16.4 | 7.9 | 20.1 |
| | | IV | 9.2 | 13.7 | 9.4 | 9.4 | 9.4 |
| | | V | 0.0 | 8.0 | 10.8 | 1.8 | 1.8 |
| Spelling | Twinschool | I | 41.8 | 31.9 | 21.5 | 17.1 | 18.7 |
| | | II | 24.6 | 30.5 | 20.4 | 29.6 | 30.6 |
| | | III | 22.4 | 10.6 | 26.1 | 29.6 | 30.6 |
| | | IV | 7.3 | 21.2 | 17.3 | 17.1 | 13.7 |
| | | V | 3.9 | 5.8 | 14.7 | 6.6 | 6.4 |
| | Parallel class | I | 42.2 | 33.7 | 10.6 | 20.7 | 32.6 |
| | | II | 21.8 | 23.0 | 23.1 | 20.7 | 12.8 |
| | | III | 20.5 | 16.2 | 10.6 | 19.2 | 18.6 |
| | | IV | 13.2 | 14.1 | 25.4 | 19.2 | 21.2 |
| | | V | 2.3 | 13.0 | 30.3 | 20.2 | 14.8 |

remains problematic, as the DHH children who enroll in the Twinschool do not constitute a random sample of the group of DHH children (see section on demographics of the Twinschool). Furthermore, as the number of DHH children in the Twinschool is rather small for such analyses and a relatively large number of children either went back to the special school (n = 3) or enrolled individually in a mainstream school (n = 4), the results of the DHH children will be presented descriptively.

Table 16.5 Distribution of the Scores on Reading Comprehension, Mathematics, and Spelling of Hearing and DHH Children in the Twinschool Classes across the Five Categories (I = percentile 81–100, II = percentile 61–80, III = percentile 41–60, IV = percentile 21–40, V = percentile 1–20) over Five Years

| Subject | | | Year 1 | Year 2 | Year 3 | Year 4 | Year 5 |
|---|---|---|---|---|---|---|---|
| Reading comprehension | Hearing | I | 43.7 | 45.5 | 38.6 | 42.3 | 47.2 |
| | | II | 16.8 | 27.7 | 16.6 | 19.1 | 19.4 |
| | | III | 18.9 | 16.8 | 28.2 | 10.9 | 22.4 |
| | | IV | 14.5 | 6.2 | 13.7 | 19.4 | 3.2 |
| | | V | 6.1 | 3.8 | 2.9 | 8.3 | 7.8 |
| | DHH | I | 0.0 | 0.0 | 0.0 | 10.0 | 12.5 |
| | | II | 6.8 | 12.7 | 0.0 | 0.0 | 0.0 |
| | | III | 13.6 | 20.0 | 20.0 | 10.0 | 12.5 |
| | | IV | 43.2 | 40.0 | 40.0 | 30.0 | 37.5 |
| | | V | 36.4 | 27.3 | 40.0 | 50.0 | 37.5 |
| Mathematics | Hearing | I | 41.8 | 46.2 | 39.2 | 47.2 | 46.6 |
| | | II | 28.9 | 24.7 | 32.1 | 33.4 | 24.7 |
| | | III | 19.4 | 11.4 | 17.9 | 14.3 | 22.1 |
| | | IV | 6.5 | 17.1 | 9.5 | 1.3 | 3.3 |
| | | V | 3.4 | 0.6 | 1.3 | 3.8 | 3.3 |
| | DHH | I | 11.2 | 20.5 | 22.4 | 22.2 | 28.6 |
| | | II | 11.2 | 4.5 | 16.8 | 5.6 | 0.0 |
| | | III | 22.4 | 11.2 | 5.6 | 22.2 | 14.3 |
| | | IV | 32.8 | 11.2 | 32.8 | 32.8 | 0.0 |
| | | V | 22.4 | 52.6 | 22.4 | 17.2 | 57.1 |
| Spelling | Hearing | I | 41.8 | 31.9 | 21.5 | 17.1 | 18.7 |
| | | II | 24.6 | 30.5 | 20.4 | 29.6 | 30.6 |
| | | III | 22.4 | 10.6 | 26.1 | 29.6 | 30.6 |
| | | IV | 7.3 | 21.2 | 17.3 | 17.1 | 13.7 |
| | | V | 3.9 | 5.8 | 14.7 | 6.6 | 6.4 |
| | DHH | I | 13.4 | 18.1 | 10.6 | 0.0 | 0.0 |
| | | II | 7.2 | 12.2 | 10.6 | 16.8 | 25.0 |
| | | III | 19.5 | 0.0 | 22.2 | 16.8 | 25.0 |
| | | IV | 26.6 | 28.7 | 28.3 | 44.2 | 25.0 |
| | | V | 33.3 | 41.0 | 28.3 | 22.2 | 25.0 |

Table 16.5 depicts the results of the DHH children in relation to the results of their hearing classmates. On average, DHH children score well below the average achievements of their hearing classmates in all subjects. The gap between hearing and DHH children's achievements is quite large. To illustrate, whereas from 55% to 73% of the scores of hearing children on reading comprehension are in the two highest categories, 67% to 80% of the DHH children's scores are in the lowest two

categories. In other words, the scores of the average hearing child in the Twinschool are much better than the scores of the average DHH child in the Twinschool. It is difficult, if not impossible, to determine how DHH children's school achievements are positively or negatively affected by the Twinschool. Nevertheless, teachers indicated in a series of interviews that they thought that the pace of instruction in the Twinschool and the high expectations that are set for DHH and hearing children must have affected DHH children's school achievements positively.

Two important points need to be stressed here. First, some of the DHH children perform well above average on particular subjects. To illustrate, between 22% and 39% of the scores of DHH children on mathematics are in the two highest categories. Second, scores in the lowest ranges are common in most mainstream schools, and teachers generally have to adapt their lessons according to the abilities of the children in their class. In other words, differentiation by the teacher is the rule rather than the exception in most primary schools. Even though hearing children at this school perform well above the national average in all school subjects, there are also a number of children whose scores are in the lower categories. Although this implies that teachers must adjust their instruction in order to provide appropriate instruction for all children, the advantage of the Twinschool in comparison to mainstream schools is clearly that there are two teachers in the classroom for a considerable proportion of the time. This will obviously facilitate the differentiation that is required to provide appropriate instruction for all children in the class.

**Language Proficiency**

*Spoken Dutch*

When the DHH children enrolled at the Twinschool, all of them had significant delays in the acquisition of most domains in spoken Dutch (see Table 16.2). However, their delays were generally less severe in comparison to the delays of DHH peers from bilingual education programs, as access to and proficiency in spoken Dutch was one of the criteria on the basis of which they were selected to enroll in the Twinschool.

To investigate how DHH children developed their spoken language skills in the Twinschool, receptive vocabulary skills were assessed by administering the PPVT to 12 DHH children in group 2 and group 3 and their hearing classmates 1 year and 2 years after they enrolled at the Twinschool. The mean vocabulary score (in standard deviations) of DHH children 1 year after they had enrolled in the Twinschool was −1.69 standard deviations and −0.97 standard deviations 2 years after they had enrolled, a growth that turned out to be significant. Apparently, the Twinschool program facilitates the acquisition of the vocabulary of spoken Dutch. Assessment of the DHH children's skills in different domains of spoken Dutch (e.g., productive vocabulary, grammar) takes place every year. However, the specific tests involved are often not the same in consecutive years, which makes it difficult to monitor the children's progress from a scientific point of view. Therefore, it remains unclear to what extent this finding in the domain of receptive vocabulary can be generalized to other domains of spoken Dutch (productive vocabulary, grammar).

On average, the scores of their hearing classmates were significantly higher (respectively, 0.42 and 0.49 standard deviations) than the scores of the DHH children in both years. In other words, the receptive vocabulary scores in spoken Dutch of the DHH children remained behind in comparison to their hearing classmates. Nevertheless, the growth in DHH children's receptive vocabulary scores was surprisingly positive.

*Sign Language of the Netherlands*

Most of the DHH children were proficient in Sign Language of the Netherlands before they enrolled in the Twinschool. To illustrate, respectively 69%, 87%, and 94% of the children's scores on tests assessing their proficiency with respect to the phonology, the vocabulary, and the grammar of Sign Language of the Netherlands were above average (Hermans et al., 2007, 2009). Thus, the DHH children at the Twinschool were highly proficient in SLN when they left the bilingual education program at the special school and enrolled in the Twinschool. This particular profile, DHH children being proficient in SLN and written/spoken language, has frequently been observed (Hermans, Ormel, & Knoors, 2010; Hermans, Ormel, Knoors, & Verhoeven, 2008; Niederberger, 2008).

In a questionnaire administered in the first year of the evaluation of the Twinschool, many of the parents of the DHH children at the co-enrollment program indicated that they regarded SLN as a vital part of their child's educational program. To investigate how the DHH children's skills in SLN developed at the Twinschool, the SLN tests were administered to the children 2 years after they enrolled at the Twinschool. Quite remarkably, the children's scores tended to remain above average, even though the input they received in SLN decreased. Respectively 81%, 87%, and 81% of the children scored above average on tests assessing their proficiency with respect to the phonology, the vocabulary, and the grammar of Sign Language of the Netherlands. In sum, the proficiency in SLN of the DHH children was above average when they enrolled in the Twinschool and remained so 2 years after they enrolled.

## Children's and Parents' Perceptions of the Twinschool

*Children's Perceptions of the Twinschool*

In the Netherlands, children's perceptions of and experiences at school are commonly used to assess and improve the quality of educational programs. The "Zelf Evaluatie Basis Onderwijs" (Self-Evaluation Primary Education) developed by Hendriks and Bosker (2003) is one example of such an instrument. Castelijns (2006) stated the following about students' perceptions:

> If one talks with students and is sincerely interested in their views about what school means to them, one will soon notice that they have outspoken, remarkably well articulated views. When students talk about school they prove to possess sharp observation skills and balanced ways of expression. Even more so, the views that students share provide schools with valuable and applicable information. (p. 5, our translation)

In other words, children's perceptions can provide schools with valuable information about the quality of their educational programs.

To investigate children's perceptions of the Twinschool, we administered the "Zelf Evaluatie Basis Onderwijs" (ZEBO) questionnaire during the evaluation. This questionnaire consists of 70 statements (e.g., "I think that we have to work really hard at school"), which are divided into seven major topics: (1) Achievement pressure, (2) Teacher support, (3) Didactics, (4) Peer relationships, (5) Task adaptation, (6) Time for task, and (7) Classroom climate. For each statement, children have to indicate whether or not that statement is "true" (3 points), "a bit true" (2 points), or "not true" (1 point). The results from the scale "Peer relationships" will not be discussed here, as this scale was investigated in more depth in the sociometric studies.

For the purpose of the evaluation of the Twinschool, the ZEBO was administered to 16 DHH children and 59 hearing children in the Twinschool classes. Furthermore, with respect to the second scale (Teacher support), both teachers were judged by the children.

The results are shown in Table 16.6. With respect to achievement pressure, DHH children experienced significantly more achievement pressure than their hearing classmates. More specifically, DHH children experienced more negative feedback from their teacher than their hearing classmates did.

The support that children received from their teacher, both in terms of the teacher-student relationship and support in terms of the frequency of explanation, pace of helping a child, and mood of the teacher, was judged significantly lower by DHH children in comparison to hearing children. Quite remarkably, DHH children judged both dimensions of teacher support to be similar for the teacher from the special school and the teacher from the mainstream school. The same finding was observed for hearing children. No differences were found between the judgments of DHH and hearing children on the scales "Didactics," "Task adaptation," "Time for task," and "Classroom climate" (level of quietness and management skills of the teachers).

Table 16.6 The Scores of the Hearing and DHH Children in the Twinschool Classes across the Different (Sub)Scales of the "Zelf Evaluatie Basis Onderwijs"

| Scale | DHH | Hearing |
|---|---|---|
| 1. Achievement pressure* | 2.55 | 2.38 |
| Achievement pressure felt by the child | 2.41 | 2.34 |
| Positive encouragement by teacher | 2.67 | 2.65 |
| Negatively judging quality of work by teacher | 2.50 | 2.00 |
| 2. Teacher-student relationship/Teacher support* | 2.36 | 2.59 |
| Teacher-student relationship | 2.34 | 2.52 |
| Teacher support | 2.38 | 2.63 |
| 3. Didactics | 2.33 | 2.30 |
| Structuring of lessons | 2.26 | 2.14 |
| Effectiveness of explanation | 2.44 | 2.52 |
| 4. Task adaptation | 1.69 | 1.91 |
| The difficulty level of classroom tasks | 1.80 | 1.82 |
| The challenge of classroom tasks | 1.43 | 2.13 |
| 5. Time for task | 2.24 | 2.28 |
| 6. Classroom climate | 1.97 | 2.04 |
| Level of quietness | 2.03 | 2.15 |
| Management skills of teachers | 1.93 | 1.95 |

(*differences between DHH and hearing children significant at p <.05)

Overall, the DHH children were quite positive about the Twinschool. But in comparison to their hearing classmates, they indicated to a greater extent that they felt their work was judged negatively by the teachers. Furthermore, they judged the support they received from their teacher, both in terms of relationship and the instructional support they received, more negatively. Quite remarkably, we have also observed this in special schools (see Hermans, Wauters, De Klerk, & Knoors, Chapter 11 of this volume). The absence of a difference on the scale "Didactics" is, in our view, crucial as it suggests that DHH children feel they have access to the instruction provided by their teachers.

*Parents' Perceptions of the Twinschool*

Parents' involvement at school is a variable that is known to affect children's achievements at school (Fan & Chen, 2001). In their model of parental involvement at school, Kohl, Lengua, and McMahon (2000) emphasize that parental endorsement of the school's policy and educational system is a vital part of parents' involvement. Negative parental perceptions of the school's policy and educational system will affect their involvement at school.

As we pointed out earlier, some of the parents (of hearing children) expressed their concerns regarding the Twinschool. More specifically, they were concerned that the presence of a group of DHH children would negatively affect their child's development. When the Twinschool started, the parents of hearing and DHH children were informed about the program in considerable detail. However, parents of hearing children were given no choice on whether or not their hearing child was placed in one of the Twinschool classes. As a consequence, some of them initially expressed their concerns and hesitations. For the parents of the DHH children, the Twinschool was one of the educational options for their child.

In order to assess the perceptions of parents, a questionnaire was developed and administered to all parents of the children in the Twinschool classes in 2008 (group 1 [grade 5] and group 2 [year-2 kindergarten]) and 2010 (group 2 [grade 2] and group 3 [grade 3]). The questionnaires administered to the parents of DHH and hearing children were not identical (see Table 16.7). The questionnaire consisted of 12 statements ("I am satisfied with the education given to my child") that had to be judged on a 3-point scale ("agree" [2 points], "partly agree" [1 point], or "disagree" [0 points]). Thus, the scores on each statement can vary between 0 (negative perception) and 2 (positive perception). Six additional questions were asked of the parents of DHH children. We will report the major findings of this questionnaire, averaged across both administrations. We will not discuss general questions concerning the parents' view on their child's well-being and parents' view on their child's contact with DHH and hearing classmates.

Overall, the parents of DHH and hearing children were very positive about the Twinschool (question 6). They responded positively on statements regarding the education that their child received (questions 1 and 4) and the information they had received, for instance, through newsletters and informative meetings at school (question 2). Parents of hearing children also indicated that they thought that the presence of a group of DHH children in the classes was a valuable experience for their child, whereas parents of DHH children were similarly content with their child's experience in mainstream education (question 5). Parents of hearing children were the least positive on the statement "If I had to choose now, I would place my child in the Twinschool," in contrast to the parents of DHH children. All of the parents of DHH children indicated that they thought there were advantages of the Twinschool both in relation to special schools and to mainstream schools in which their child would be individually enrolled. However, a few of these parents also indicated that there were disadvantages of the Twinschool, especially compared to other mainstream schools. This disadvantage is related to the fact that their child still could not go to a school near home.

Table 16.7 The Response of the Parents on the Questionnaire

| Statements | Hearing | DHH | Average |
|---|---|---|---|
| I am satisfied with the education my child receives. | 1.87 | 1.92 | 1.89 |
| I am satisfied with the information I have received about the Twinschool. | 1.86 | 2.00 | 1.89 |
| If I had to choose (hearing) / choose again (deaf), I would place my child in the Twinschool. | 1.56 | 1.92 | 1.63 |
| I think the co-teaching system stimulates my child's development. | 1.81 | 2.00 | 1.85 |
| My child has acquired more knowledge about (a) deafness and deaf children (parents of hearing children) (b) hearing children (parents of deaf children). My child's knowledge about our society has increased. I appreciate that. | 1.97 | 1.92 | 1.96 |
| In general, I am satisfied with the Twinschool. | 1.95 | 1.92 | 1.94 |
| I think there are a lot of advantages of the Twinschool in relation to special schools. | – | 2.00 | – |
| I think there are a lot of disadvantages of the Twinschool in relation to special schools. | – | 0.16 | – |
| I think there are a lot of advantages of the Twinschool in relation to mainstream schools. | – | 2.00 | – |
| I think there are a lot of disadvantages of the Twinschool in relation to mainstream schools. | – | 0.50 | – |

This was also the main reason that four parents decided to enroll their child in a mainstream school near home (see section on demographics).

## SUMMARY AND CONCLUDING REMARKS

In this chapter, we have described the Twinschool co-enrollment program that started in 2004 in the south of the Netherlands. The Twinschool constitutes cooperation between a special school for deaf children and a mainstream school. Through 2013, 18 DHH children had enrolled in the Twinschool. The evaluation of the program revealed that DHH children do find support in the presence of DHH classmates. It is nevertheless unclear how this, either positively or negatively, affects their social contacts with hearing children. It is important to note that the Twinschool is not situated near the DHH children's homes. This complicates the contacts with hearing and DHH classmates after school, and is one of the major reasons that the parents of four DHH children decided to enroll their child individually in a mainstream school near home.

The evaluation further revealed that the school achievements of hearing children were not positively or negatively affected by the Twinschool program. The hearing children in this mainstream school generally perform well above the national average of children in the Netherlands. The absence of either a positive or negative effect of the Twinschool on hearing children's school achievements may be due to the generally high level of achievement at this school. Hearing children with lower levels of achievement may profit more from the co-teaching system in the Twinschool.

The Twinschool does seem to have a positive effect on DHH children's acquisition of spoken Dutch. Their scores on the PPVT improved considerably over two years. The speech therapists of the DHH children confirmed this finding from their evaluations. They were often surprised by the progress that DHH children made on the acquisition of the vocabulary and grammar of spoken Dutch, although we can only partly support this impression through standardized language assessment tests. Although there was a decrease in the SLN that DHH children received in the Twinschool, their language proficiency in SLN remained above average in comparison to deaf peers.

Finally, the DHH and hearing children and their parents had a positive view of the Twinschool. Although DHH children's judgment on the instruction they received was in some respects a bit more negative in comparison to their hearing classmates, DHH children, overall, were positive on the instruction they received. In addition, parents of DHH and hearing children were positive about the Twinschool.

Many questions concerning the impact of the Twinschool on DHH children's development remain difficult, if not impossible, to answer. The group of DHH children cannot easily be compared with their DHH peers in special schools or with DHH peers who are individually enrolled in mainstream schools. Although we are very aware of this particular restriction, to us the evaluation demonstrates that a co-enrollment program is a very attractive and interesting educational program for DHH children that we will explore in more depth in the future.

## REFERENCES

Antia, S. D., Jones, P., Luckner, J., Kreimeyer, K. H., & Reed, S. (2011). Social outcomes of students who are deaf and hard of hearing in general education classrooms. *Journal of Exceptional Children, 77,* 489–504.

Antia, S. D., & Kreimeyer, K. H. (2003). Peer interactions of deaf and hard-of-hearing children. In M. Marschark & P. E. Spencer (Eds.), *Oxford handbook of deaf studies, language, and education* (pp. 164–176). New York, NY: Oxford University Press.

Bellmore, A. D., Nishina, A., Witkow, M. R., Graham, S., & Juvonen, J. (2007). The influence of classroom ethnic composition on same- and other-ethnicity peer nominations in middle school. *Social Development, 16,* 720–740.

Bowen, S. K. (2008). Co-enrollment for students who are deaf or hard of hearing: Friendship patterns and social interactions. *American Annals of the Deaf, 153,* 285–293.

Cambra, C. (2002). Acceptance of deaf students by hearing students in regular classrooms. *American Annals of the Deaf, 147*, 38–43.

Castelijns, J. (1996). *Beelden van bekwaamheid: Een onderzoek naar de implementatie en effecten van het programma Responsieve instructie voor leerkrachten in groep 1 en 2 van de basisschool* [Images of competence: A study into the implementation and effects of the program Responsive instruction for teachers in kindergarten]. Doctoral dissertation, University of Utrecht, the Netherlands.

Clarke, A., & DeNuzzo, D. (2003). *Co-teaching in inclusive classrooms: Practical practice.* Paper presented at the International Conference on Inclusion, the Netherlands.

Dettman, S., & Dowell, R. (2010). Language acquisition and critical periods for children using cochlear implants. The demands of writing and the deaf writer. In M. Marschark & P. E. Spencer (Eds.), *The Oxford handbook of deaf studies, language and education* (vol. 2, pp. 331–342). New York, NY: Oxford University Press.

Durkin, K., Hunter, S., Levin, K. A., Bergin, D., Heim, D., & Howe, C. (2012). Discriminatory peer aggression among children as a function of minority status and group proportion in school context. *European Journal of Social Psychology, 42*, 243–251.

Fan, X., & Chen, M. (2001). Parental involvement and students' academic achievement: A meta-analysis. *Educational Psychology Review, 13*, 1–22.

Graham, J. A., & Cohen, R. (1997). Race and sex as factors in children's sociometric ratings and friendship choices. *Social Development, 6*, 355–372.

Hallinan, M. T., & Teixeira, R. A. (1987). Students' interracial friendships: Individual characteristics, structural effects, and racial differences. *American Journal of Education, 95*, 563–583.

Hammer, A. (2010). *The acquisition of verbal morphology in cochlear-implanted and specific language impaired children.* Doctoral dissertation, Leiden University. LOT Dissertation Series, 255. Retrieved from http://www.lotpublications.nl.

Hendriks, M. A., & Bosker, R. (2003). *ZEBO instrument voor zelfevaluatie in het basisonderwijs: Handleiding bij een geautomatiseerd hulpmiddel voor kwaliteitszorg in basisscholen* [ZEBO, instrumentation for self-evaluation in primary education: Manual to the computerized instrumentation for quality care in primary education]. Enschede, Netherlands: Twente University Press.

Hermans, D. (2010). *Projectverslag inventarisatie schoolprestaties Kentalis-scholen* [Project report inventory school achievement Kentalis-schools]. *Internal report*, Sint-Michielsgestel, the Netherlands.

Hermans, D., Knoors, H., & Verhoeven, L. (2007). *Testbatterij Nederlandse Gebarentaal* [Proficiency Test Sign Language of the Netherlands]. Nijmegen, The Netherlands: Radboud University Nijmegen, Expertisecentrum Atypische Communicatie.

Hermans, D., Knoors, H., & Verhoeven, L. (2009). Assessment of sign language development: The case of deaf children in the Netherlands. *Journal of Deaf Studies and Deaf Education, 15*, 107–119.

Hermans, D., Ormel, E., & Knoors, H. (2010). On the relation between the signing and reading skills of deaf bilinguals. *International Journal of Bilingual Education and Bilingualism, 13*, 187–199.

Hermans, D., Knoors, H., Ormel, E., & Verhoeven, L. (2008). The relationship between the reading and signing skills of deaf children in bilingual education programs. *Journal of Deaf Studies and Deaf Education, 13*, 518–530.

Herzberg, B. (1994). Community service and critical teaching. *College Composition and Communication, 45,* 307–319.

Jackson, M. F., Barth, J. M., Powell, N., & Lochman, J. E. (2006). Classroom contextual effects of race on children's peer nominations. *Child Development, 77,* 1325–1337.

Karchmer, M., & Mitchell, R. E. (2003). Demographic and achievement characteristics of deaf and hard-of-hearing students. In M. Marschark & P. E. Spencer (Eds.), *Oxford handbook of deaf studies, language, and education* (pp. 21–37). New York, NY: Oxford University Press.

Kirchner, C. J. (1994). Co-enrollment as an inclusion model. *American Annals of the Deaf, 139,* 163–164.

Kluwin, T. N. (1999). Co-teaching deaf and hearing students: Research on social integration. *American Annals of the Deaf, 144,* 339–344.

Kluwin, T. N., Stinson, M. S., & Colarossi, G. M. (2002). Social processes and outcomes of in-school contact between deaf and hearing peers. *Journal of Deaf Studies and Deaf Education, 7,* 200–213.

Knoors, H. (2004). Regulier basisonderwijs voor dove kinderen: een lonkend perspectief? [Mainstream education for deaf children: an attractive perspective?]. *Tijdschrift voor Orthopedagogiek, 43*(10), 395–410.

Knoors, H., & Marschark, M. (2012). Language planning for the 21st century: Revisiting bilingual language policy for deaf children. *Journal of Deaf Studies and Deaf Education, 17,* 291–305.

Kohl, G. O., Lengua, L. J., & McMahon, R. J. (2000). Parent involvement in school conceptualizing multiple dimensions and their relations with family and demographic risk factors. *Journal of School Psychology, 38*(6), 501–523.

Kreimeyer, K. H., Crooke, P., Drye, C., Egbert, V., & Klein, B. (2000). Academic and social benefits of a co-enrollment model of inclusive education for deaf and hard-of-hearing children. *Journal of Deaf Studies and Deaf Education, 5,* 174–185.

Metz, K. (2011). *The status of the evidence of co-enrollment as a successful model of inclusion for students who are deaf or hard of hearing.* Paper presented at the conference of the Association of College Educators—Deaf & Hard of Hearing, Fort Worth, TX.

Musselman, C., Mootilal, A., & MacKay, S. (1996). The social adjustment of deaf adolescents in segregated, partially integrated, and mainstreamed settings. *Journal of Deaf Studies and Deaf Education, 1,* 52–63.

Niederberger, N. (2008). Does the knowledge of a natural sign language facilitate Deaf children's learning to read and write? Insights from French Sign Language and written French data. In C. Plaza Pust & E. Moralez-Lopez (Eds.), *Sign bilingualism: Language development, interaction, and maintenance in sign language contact situations* (pp. 39–50). Amsterdam; Philadelphia: John Benjamins Publishing.

Nunes, T., Pretzlik, U., & Olsson, J. (2001). Deaf children's social relationships in mainstream schools. *Deafness and Education International, 3,* 123–136.

Pijl, Y. J. (1997). *Twintig jaar groei van het speciaal onderwijs* [Twenty years of growth in special education]. De Lier, Netherlands: Academisch Boekencentrum.

Powers, S., Gregory, S., & Thoutenhoofd, E. D. (1999). The educational achievements of deaf children: A literature review executive summary. *Deafness and Education International, 1,* 1–9.

Schlichting, J. E. P. T., Van Eldik, M. C. M., Lutje Spelberg, H. C., Van der Meulen, S. J., & Van der Meulen, B. F. (1998). *Schlichting Test voor Taalproductie: Handleiding* [Schlichting Test for Language production: Manual]. Lisse, Netherlands: Swets & Zeitlinger.

Shaffer, D. R. (2005). *Social and personality development*. Belmont, CA: Wadsworth.

Singleton, L. C., & Asher, S. R. (1979). Racial integration and children's peer preferences: An investigation of developmental and cohort differences. *Child Development, 50*, 936–941.

Smeets, E. (2007). *Speciaal of apart: Onderzoek naar de omvang van het speciaal onderwijs in Nederland en ander Europese landen* [Special or different: Research into the size of special education in the Netherlands and other European countries]. Nijmegen, Netherlands: ITS.

Stinson, M. S., & Antia, S. D. (1999). Considerations in educating deaf and hard-of-hearing students in inclusive settings. *Journal of Deaf Studies and Deaf Education, 4*, 163–175.

Stinson, M. S., & Kluwin, T. N. (2003). Educational consequences of alternative school placements. In M. Marschark & M. E. Spencer (Eds.), *Oxford handbook of deaf studies, language, and education* (pp. 52–64). New York, NY: Oxford University Press.

Van Eldik, M. C. M., Schlichting, J. E. P. T., Lutje Spelberg, H. C., Van der Meulen, B. F., & van der Meulen, S. J. (1995). *Reynell Test voor taalbegrip, RTT* [Reynell Test for Language Comprehension]. Lisse, Netherlands: Swets.

Verbist, A. (2010). *The acquisition of personal pronouns in cochlear implanted children*. Doctoral dissertation, Leiden University. LOT Dissertation Series, 242. Retrieved from http://www.lotpublications.nl.

Verhoeven, A., & Vermeer, A. (2001). *Taaltoets Alle Kinderen* [Language Test for All Children]. Arnhem: Citogroep.

Wauters, L., & Knoors, H. (2008). Social integration of deaf children in inclusive settings. *Journal of Deaf Studies and Deaf Education, 28*, 1–16.

Wolters, N., Knoors, H., Cillessen, A. H. N., & Verhoeven, L. (2011). Predicting acceptance and popularity in early adolescents as a function of hearing status, educational setting, and gender. *Research in Developmental Disabilities, 32*, 2553–2565.

# 17

# Co-enrollment in the United States

## *A Critical Analysis of Benefits and Challenges*

Shirin Antia and Kelly K. Metz

Co-enrollment for deaf and hard-of-hearing (DHH) students was a model described by Kirchner (1994) as a solution to the difficulties that arose when these students were educated with their hearing peers in general education classrooms. The purpose of co-enrollment models was to change the learning environment for DHH students by providing them full access to both the general education curriculum as well as to DHH and hearing peers. Co-enrollment classrooms are characterized by three key components: (1) the classroom contains a critical mass of DHH students, (2) the class is team-taught by a general education teacher and a teacher of DHH students, and (3) both sign and spoken languages are used in the classroom.

This chapter will describe the rationale for co-enrollment programs, the benefits expected, the academic, social, and communication outcomes of students enrolled in these programs in the United States, and the challenges encountered when implementing this model. Co-enrollment programs have also been started outside the United States, and research on two of these programs is addressed by Tang, Lam, and Yiu (Chapter 13 of this volume) and Hermans, De Klerk, Wauters, and Knoors (Chapter 16 of this volume).

## HISTORY AND PHILOSOPHY

A co-enrollment program for DHH students was started in 1982 under the direction of Carl J. Kirchner, in Burbank Unified School District in California. Kirchner (1994) proposed co-enrollment as an alternative inclusion model with a group of DHH students integrated into a general education classroom, co-taught by a general education teacher and a teacher of DHH students, as opposed to one student in a classroom of hearing staff and students, with fragmented support services from a variety of professionals. Kirchner highlighted the benefit to DHH students of having access to the general education curriculum without losing access to a DHH peer group. Kirchner's description of the program sparked interest in the co-enrollment model, leading to the establishment of other co-enrollment programs.

The intent of co-enrollment is to seek equality for DHH and hearing students, not by pursuing a "separate but equal" strategy, but rather by ensuring that all students have equal access, academically and socially, to the school and classroom community. A key aspect of a co-enrollment program is the presence of a critical mass of DHH students who are integral members of the classroom. In this respect, the co-enrollment classroom differs from the typical mainstreamed classroom. Although most DHH students are educated in general education classrooms in public schools (Gallaudet Research Institute, 2011), these classrooms are likely to enroll only a single DHH student. Co-enrollment must also be distinguished from the "cluster" model of group inclusion. Guralnick (2001) describes the cluster model as occurring when a group of students with special needs are "grafted" onto a general education classroom (p. 10). The special education teacher often accompanies the students into the classroom, but does not necessarily share responsibility for curriculum delivery. Another model of group inclusion is "reverse mainstreaming," in which a group of hearing students, often accompanied by a general education teacher, joins a classroom of students who are DHH. In both the cluster model and the reverse mainstreaming model the DHH and hearing students and their respective teachers are not members of the classroom; instead, they are often seen as visitors.

A difference between traditional models of inclusion and the co-enrollment model is the philosophical difference between being a visitor and a member of a classroom. When DHH students are treated as visitors to a classroom, it is assumed that their needs are sufficiently different from those of all other students, and therefore are best met by specialized professionals, be they speech-language pathologists, audiologists, or teachers of DHH students (Antia, Stinson, & Gaustad, 2002). The visiting students need to be qualified to enter the general education classroom either by virtue of their academic achievement, their ability to access the general education teachers' instruction, or their ability to participate in the classroom. Although special accommodations occur to allow the DHH students access to classroom communication and academic content, differences between the DHH students and the other hearing students are emphasized. As a consequence, the DHH student can feel uncomfortably singled out. The teacher or interpreter who accompanies these students is also considered a visitor, and may be expected to follow the directions of the general education teacher or to primarily interact with the DHH students. In contrast, the co-enrollment classroom extends membership to all students. When DHH students make up a large proportion of the class and are seen as members of the classroom, the presence of a hearing loss is no longer the salient characteristic that singles them out. The DHH students' communication, education, and social needs are part of the classroom culture and practice, as are the communication, educational, and social needs of the other students. In addition, all students have access to same-age DHH and hearing peers.

Co-teaching by a general education teacher and a teacher of DHH students is also a critical component of the co-enrollment classroom. Co-teaching is defined as the partnering of two teachers, typically a general educator and a specialist, for the purpose of collaboratively delivering instruction to a group of students with a wide variety of educational needs (Friend, Cook, Hurley-Chamberlain, & Shamberger, 2010). The two teachers are equally responsible for the instruction and education of all students, and both have equal status in the classroom (Morocco & Aguilar, 2002). Both teachers are expected to have "ownership" of the students and the curriculum and to jointly plan and deliver instruction. Both teachers take an active role in evaluating the performance of each student in the classroom (Luckner, 1999). While co-teaching is team teaching, co-teaching differs from classic descriptions of team teaching in that the two teachers have different areas of expertise that complement one another.

While co-enrollment classrooms can include many different kinds of students needing special education, a unique feature of co-enrollment classrooms that include DHH students is attention to language and communication accessibility. Because all instruction is expected to be accessible to all students, the classrooms are often bilingual, that is, teachers and students are expected to learn and use signed and spoken language, although sign language interpreters may be used as needed (Bowen, 2008). Hearing students are also offered specific sign language instruction (Kreimeyer, Crooke, Drye, Egbert, & Klein, 2000). Although there is a growing interest in co-enrollment, there are only a few studies of co-enrollment programs in the United States. The studies reviewed in this chapter are outlined in Table 17.1.

### Benefits of Co-enrollment

Several studies have focused on the perceptions of stakeholders as to the benefits of co-enrollment. Luckner (1999) interviewed the teachers, parents, students, and administrators of a recently opened co-enrollment program. Jimenez-Sanchez and Antia (1999) interviewed three teams of teachers who were currently team teaching or had team taught in a co-enrollment program. Metz and Spolsky (2013) surveyed teachers, interpreters, and support personnel of a well-established co-enrollment program.

### Benefits to Students

One of the major benefits was high academic expectation for all students. Luckner (1999) noted that a major academic benefit noted by

Table 17.1 Research Studies on Co-enrollment programs in the United States

| Author(s) | Participants | Kind of data collected |
|---|---|---|
| Bowen (2008) | DHH and hearing students in two 3rd–4th grade classrooms (one co-enrolled) | Social acceptance; sign language proficiency; student interviews |
| Jimenez-Sanchez and Antia (1999) | Five teams of teachers in co-enrolled classroom | Teacher interviews |
| Kluwin (1999) | DHH students in grades 4–8 who had been in co-enrolled classrooms; random sample of hearing students | Self-concept; loneliness; perceptions of classroom environment |
| Kreimeyer, Crooke, Drye, Egbert and Klein (2000) | DHH and hearing students in a co-enrolled classroom grades 3–5; Teachers | Academic achievement; social interaction; teacher interviews. |
| Luckner (1999) | Teachers, administrators, parents, DHH and hearing students involved with co-enrollment program grades 1–4 | Stakeholder and student interviews; classroom observations |
| McCain and Antia (2005) | DHH and hearing students in co-enrolled classroom grades 3–5 | Academic achievement; classroom participation; social skills |
| Metz and Spolsky (2013) | Teachers and support staff involved with co-enrolled classroom grades K–5 | Survey |

both teachers and parents was that the DHH students were exposed to the regular academic curriculum, thus enabling them to learn age-appropriate content taught by a general education teacher skilled in delivering grade-level curriculum. The teachers interviewed by Jimenez-Sanchez and Antia (1999) thought of the DHH and hearing students as equally academically capable; hearing loss was not seen as a limiting factor in any area of development. Teachers in these classrooms expected all students to be attentive, to complete their homework, and to learn and use appropriate study skills. When asked specifically about the level of academic engagement (attention, participation, and time on task) of DHH students compared to their hearing classmates, educators perceived the DHH students as being as engaged as their hearing peers (Metz & Spolsky, 2013).

Another benefit was the ability of co-enrollment to enhance appreciation of diversity, and to develop empathy and acceptance of special needs among students (Metz & Spolsky, 2013). For the DHH students, the opportunity to learn how to interact and function in a hearing world was seen as a benefit, while the hearing students learned that DHH students are capable and able to learn in a manner similar to themselves (Jimenez-Sanchez & Antia, 1999).

All students benefited from having access to DHH and hearing peers. The presence of hearing peers and the use of oral language as one of the languages in the classroom provided a context and motivation for the use of spoken language by the DHH students. The hearing students benefited from the opportunity to learn a second language within a bilingual environment (Metz & Spolsky, 2013). As the hearing students improved in their use of sign language, the communication barrier between DHH and hearing peers was reduced, thus promoting social interaction and friendship between DHH and hearing students (Kreimeyer et al., 2000). A benefit not mentioned by other researchers is the routine use of amplification technology in the co-enrollment classroom. Because amplification technology is in use all day every day in the classroom, the use of these devices is not seen as a stigmatizing characteristic for the DHH students.

Co-enrollment creates a sense of community and connection for all the students. In the classrooms studied by Luckner (1999) and Kreimeyer et al. (2000), students received special services within the classroom rather than being pulled out. One teacher in Luckner's study reported being pleased that the DHH students were present all the time and therefore did not miss any classroom social or academic activities; they were therefore more likely to be seen as class members rather than visitors.

**Benefits to Teachers**

The co-teaching approach resulted in professional growth for all the teachers involved, as well as the opportunity to share responsibilities and receive support from one another. The presence of two teachers in the classroom lowered the student-teacher ratio, and also allowed for more individualized attention to each student. The most significant cited benefit for educators was that of skill expansion through working together. For instance, the teachers of DHH were able to deepen their knowledge of the general education curriculum and learn large-group classroom management techniques from general educators, while general educators expanded their skills in implementing differentiated instruction and use of varied strategies (Jimenez-Sanchez & Antia, 1999; Luckner, 1999; Metz & Spolsky, 2013).

**Outcomes**

Because one of the goals of co-enrollment programs is to provide access to grade level curriculum and content to DHH students, it is important to examine whether the DHH students are able to achieve academically at a level commensurate with their peers (DHH and hearing) and whether they make adequate academic progress. Additionally, DHH students in the co-enrollment program have a group of DHH peers; thus researchers hypothesize that these students will not experience the loneliness and isolation that may occur when a student is the only DHH student in the local public school. The presence of hearing peers as models may also provide some social advantages (Levine & Antia, 1997).

**Academic Outcomes**

Luckner (1999) conducted a qualitative study of two elementary co-enrollment classrooms. The DHH students in these classrooms had previously received instruction primarily from a teacher of DHH for all or part of the school day. Luckner interviewed teachers, administrators, randomly selected DHH and hearing students, and their parents. He asked questions about the academic and social aspects of the co-enrollment approach and the use of sign language in the classroom. In addition, he conducted observations of the classrooms to obtain information about the learning environment, student learning, and teacher-student interactions. The results of the interviews showed that in the co-enrollment classrooms the DHH students were exposed to content information appropriate to their grade level. They were held to the same standards as other students and learned appropriate study skills and behaviors. Comments taken from the interviews indicated that parents and administrators believed that the DHH students benefited by becoming independent learners who were accountable for their own learning, rather than being dependent on teachers and tutors.

Kreimeyer, Crooke, Drye, Egbert, and Klein (2000) studied an elementary co-enrollment program during the first three years of inception. The co-enrollment classroom was a multi-age class for grades 2/3/4 during the first year of the study, and grades 3/4/5 for the second and third years of the study. The student participants included between 7 and 8 DHH students and between 17 and 23 hearing students. The classroom was taught by two experienced teachers: one general education teacher and one certified teacher of DHH, with support from a speech language pathologist and sign language interpreters. Academic achievement data were collected in Years 2 and 3. The researchers obtained the Stanford 9 Achievement Test scores for the DHH students for the two consecutive years and compared their scores to the norms for the general population, and to the norms for DHH students (Gallaudet Research Institute, 1996). The results indicated that there were no significant differences in Years 2 or 3 in reading vocabulary scores between the co-enrollment DHH students and the hearing grade-level norms; nor were there significant differences between the co-enrolled students and the DHH norms. In reading comprehension, however, the co-enrolled students scored significantly higher than the DHH norms, but significantly lower than the hearing grade-level norms.

In mathematics problem-solving and procedures, the DHH co-enrolled students performed similarly to the DHH norms. In Year 3 the DHH co-enrolled students performed similarly to the grade level norms, but in Year 2 they obtained significantly lower scores. The results for the hearing co-enrolled students showed that they achieved at grade level in reading and math for both years. See Table 17.2 for a chart depicting these results.

The academic outcomes reported by Kreimeyer et al. (2000) therefore are somewhat mixed. The DHH co-enrolled students did as well or better than the DHH norming group in all areas, but, unlike their hearing classmates, were not performing at grade level in reading comprehension or in math. It should be remembered that the DHH students had been in co-enrollment programs for only 3 years; prior to this time they had been in a self-contained classroom for DHH students taught by a teacher of DHH. Luckner (1999) mentions that in such a context the DHH students are unlikely to receive grade-level curriculum or to follow a sequenced plan of study. It is possible that the DHH co-enrolled students were not able to make sufficient academic progress to meet the grade level norms within this initial 3-year period. It is also possible that the expectations of equal academic achievement of DHH and hearing students may not be reached as long as their early communication and educational environments are not comparable.

A second study of the same co-enrollment program was conducted by McCain and Antia (2005) four years later, when the program had been in existence for 7 years. Achievement data were once again collected from the grade 3/4/5 classroom. Eighteen hearing and 10 DHH students participated in the study; 5 of the DHH students were "typical" students, while 5 had additional identified attention, learning, or cognitive disabilities. The authors examined two kinds of academic

Table 17.2 Co-enrolled Student Performance on Stanford 9 Achievement Subtests

| SAT 9 Subtest | DHH students Compared to Hearing Norms | DHH students Compared to DHH Norms |
|---|---|---|
| Reading vocabulary | No significant difference | No significant difference |
| Reading comprehension | Below norms | Above norms |
| Mathematical problem-solving | No significant difference for year 3, but below norms for year 2 | No significant difference |
| Mathematical procedures | No significant difference for year 3, but below norms for year 2 | No significant difference |

*Note:* This table portrays results described by Kreimeyer et al. (2000).

outcomes: teacher-rated academic status and standardized test achievement scores.

To obtain teacher ratings of students' academic status, the two teachers (one a general educator, the other the teacher of DHH) completed a standardized academic competence rating scale on all participating students. Items on the scale included teachers' perceptions of students' reading and math performance compared to peers and to expectations for the specific grade level, motivation, and overall academic performance. There were no significant differences in the teacher ratings between the hearing and the typical DHH students, but the DHH students' scores tended to be in the low-average range, while the hearing students' scores tended to be in the average range. The DHH students with disabilities scored significantly lower than their peers, both DHH and hearing.

The authors examined the academic progress made by the students over the previous 3-year period by examining their scores on the Stanford Achievement Test (Harcourt Brace, 1997) in reading and math. Achievement scores were only available for the typical DHH students, and, because of the small numbers, only a descriptive analysis was conducted. In the area of reading, some of the DHH students showed decreased scores between grades 3 and 4, but maintained or increased scores between grades 4 and 5. Nevertheless, the gap between the DHH students and their hearing classmates in the co-enrollment program increased every year. In math, the DHH students either maintained or increased their scores relative to the hearing norms each year. Although a gap remained between their scores and those of their hearing classmates, the gap was not as wide as in reading.

Although the DHH students were not at grade level in their reading and math achievement, they all received scores above the 50th percentile when compared to DHH norms (Gallaudet Research Institute, 1996). Thus, the DHH students benefited academically from the co-enrollment program; however, the achievement gap between them and their hearing classmates continued to exist.

While co-enrollment appears to benefit DHH students academically, the small number of students and the availability of academic achievement scores from only one co-enrollment program suggest that more research is needed on the extent of the academic benefit. We need data from DHH students during their middle school years to know if early gains are maintained and whether the achievement gap is narrowed. Co-enrollment is, of course, not the magic bullet solving all academic issues of DHH students. While the DHH students made progress, their progress, at least as shown by McCain and Antia (2005), was slower than their hearing peers. Neither Kreimeyer et al. (2000) nor McCain and Antia (2005) were able to compare the co-enrollment DHH students to students in other educational placements. Research on other

DHH students in general education classrooms (Antia, Jones, Reed, & Kreimeyer, 2009) who are not in co-enrollment classrooms and do not get full-time co-teaching support from a teacher of DHH also make one year's gain in one year's time. The research also does not rule out other influences on students' progress. For example, the parents of these DHH students had to make an active choice to place their child in the co-enrollment program. Such a choice may indicate that parents are highly involved in their child's education, perhaps leading to higher academic expectations and resulting academic benefits.

**Social Outcomes**

Researchers interested in social outcomes of co-enrollment classrooms have examined peer social interaction, social acceptance, and social competence. Kreimeyer et al. (2000) observed the peer social interaction of DHH students in the co-enrollment classroom and during lunch. Baseline data on peer interaction were collected on five DHH students starting at the beginning of the school year when the co-enrollment program was initiated. The researchers continued to collect data on interaction with both hearing and DHH peers throughout the school year, in both the classroom and the lunchroom. Interaction with hearing peers was minimal when co-enrollment started. After the first week of school, the teachers created opportunities within the co-enrollment classroom for the hearing students to learn sign language and for the DHH and hearing students to participate jointly in small group activities. Over the course of the academic year, all five DHH students increased their interaction with hearing peers in the classroom. Increases were also seen in interaction with hearing peers in the lunchroom, showing that interaction between hearing and DHH peers generalized beyond the classroom.

Social interaction is a necessary, but not sufficient, condition for friendship and social acceptance. Although positive peer interaction is desirable, it is also necessary to examine social acceptance within the co-enrollment classroom. Acceptance refers to the degree to which peers like a child (Bierman, 2004). Bowen (2008) examined social acceptance patterns of DHH students in a co-enrollment grade 3 and 4 classroom. She hypothesized that DHH students would be more accepted by their hearing peers within the co-enrollment classroom than by hearing peers in a traditional classroom that included no DHH students. The co-enrollment classroom consisted of 24 hearing students and 5 DHH students, some of whom had been in a co-enrollment classroom since first grade. The traditional classroom consisted of 23 hearing students. Participating students each nominated three peers (from either classroom) in response to eight positive and eight negative social situations. Students were also interviewed to probe their attitudes and acceptance of deafness. There were no differences in the social rankings of the

DHH and the hearing students in the co-enrollment classroom, indicating that all students were equally accepted. The pattern of nominations by hearing students in the two classrooms appeared to be quite different. Hearing students in the co-enrollment classroom made both positive and negative nominations of DHH peers, while hearing students in the traditional classroom made mostly negative nominations. Thus, in the co-enrollment classroom, hearing peers expressed both likes and dislikes toward DHH peers, similar to the manner in which they might rate their hearing peers.

Another way of examining the social effects of co-enrollment is to obtain information on specific social skills and behaviors from teachers and from the students themselves. McCain and Antia (2005), in their study of the co-enrollment 4/5/6 classroom, gave a standardized social skills questionnaire to students and teachers. They found no significant differences on either self-rated or teacher-rated social behavior between DHH students without disabilities and their hearing peers; however, the self and teacher ratings of the DHH students with disabilities were significantly lower than those of the DHH students without disabilities. Thus, although typical DHH students had no specific social difficulties in the co-enrollment classroom, DHH students with disabilities continued to have social problems.

Kluwin (1999) examined the long-term effects of co-enrollment on loneliness and self-concept of fourth to eighth grade DHH students who had experienced co-enrollment prior to third grade. He administered self-report scales that measured loneliness and self-concept, as well as an inventory that examined classroom social characteristics including friction, cohesiveness, satisfaction, difficulty, and competitiveness. He found that there were no differences between the DHH and hearing students on any aspect of self-concept including school status, popularity, happiness, or satisfaction. Nor were there any differences in loneliness. The DHH students had significantly higher classroom satisfaction scores than their hearing classmates.

Because researchers have reported similar results from three different programs, the data on social outcomes of co-enrollment are more definitive than the data on academic outcomes. Within co-enrollment classrooms DHH students interact with hearing peers, are accepted by them, and develop appropriate social skills. There appear to be no social differences between elementary-age hearing and typical DHH students, and the positive effects of co-enrollment appear to continue through until eighth grade.

*Communication Outcomes*

Communication is the biggest barrier when trying to teach DHH and hearing students together. In the co-enrollment classroom, spoken and sign language are both used. We hypothesize that a reason for the success of co-enrollment is the ability of the teachers and students to communicate directly with one another because of opportunities to learn and use both languages fluently. The ability of both DHH and hearing students to communicate comfortably within the classroom should also contribute to equal levels of classroom participation.

*Signed Communication*

Sign language learning in the co-enrollment classrooms is not left to chance. Kreimeyer et al. (2000) described a "Drop Everything and Sign" daily period when all students used sign or non-vocal communication. The hearing students were also taught sign language as part of the classroom center activities; during sign language instruction, the DHH students acted as sign mentors for their hearing peers. In the co-enrollment classroom described by Luckner (1999), the predominance of small group instruction and active learning provided all students with opportunities to interact, and therefore learn sign and spoken language. Bowen (2008) reported that all hearing students at the school received two 45-minute sign classes each week. Because the use of both languages is critical to success of co-enrollment programs, researchers have been interested in documenting sign language use by students and teachers.

Informal anecdotes recounted by Luckner (1999) and experienced by the first author (and a volume editor) indicate that visitors to co-enrollment classrooms were not immediately able to differentiate DHH from hearing students on the basis of communication mode. Many hearing students signed fluently, while several DHH students used spoken English. Teachers reported that sign conversations between DHH and hearing students occurred about 50% of the time in the classroom (Kreimeyer et al., 2000). General education teachers also started to sign, using simultaneous communication during instruction and interaction with all students. By the beginning of the third year of co-enrollment programming, Kreimeyer et al. (2000) reported that the general educator was using sign independently about 80% of the time.

More formal measurement of sign language learning also yielded positive results. Bowen (2008) evaluated the sign language abilities of hearing students in the co-enrollment and the traditional classroom (with no DHH students). All students received sign language instruction for 45 minutes, twice a week, but students in the co-enrollment classroom had more opportunity to use expressive and receptive sign. She videotaped a one-on-one interview with each student, asking them to use as much sign as they could during the interview. A deaf adult then assessed students' expressive sign language use on a 5-point Likert scale. Bowen reported that the co-enrolled students scored significantly higher (3.0 on the 5 point scale) than the students in the traditional classroom (2.0–2.5 on the 5 point scale). She also reported a significant positive relationship between number of years in a co-enrollment classroom and student signing skill.

*Classroom Participation*

Because teacher-student communication and student-student communication are primary means of learning in classrooms, the ability to communicate with teachers and peers is a major component of academic success. Students who have difficulty communicating may choose not to participate in classroom activities, which, in turn, affects their learning and their academic achievement (Long, Stinson, & Braeges, 1991). Unfortunately, in many general education classrooms, barriers exist that diminish DHH students' classroom participation. These barriers include rapid rates of discussion, turn taking, and change of topics; the high number of speakers involved in discussions; and more than one student talking at a time (Saur, Layne, Hurley, & Opton, 1986). When students and teachers are speaking, classroom noise levels make comprehension difficult, especially for those DHH students who use spoken language. When an interpreter enters the communication equation, the lag time between the spoken and signed message may prevent DHH students from answering questions in a timely manner (Stinson & Liu, 1999; Stinson, Liu, Saur, & Long, 1996). The difficulties of classroom participation may affect students' engagement in classroom tasks. Students who feel that they are understood by teachers and peers also report being more actively involved in school learning (Long et al., 1991).

One way of examining student classroom participation and engagement is through perceptions of communication ease within the classroom. In a co-enrollment classroom where teachers and students are learning and using sign language, and also are aware of the DHH students' visual and auditory communication needs, we would expect all students to fully participate in classroom communication and for communication barriers to be minimized. McCain and Antia (2005) administered the Classroom Participation Questionnaire (CPQ) (Antia, Sabers, & Stinson, 2007) to all students in the co-enrollment classroom that they studied. The CPQ measures student perceptions of their communication with teachers and peers as well as their attitudes toward the classroom (Antia et al., 2007). The four subscales include:

- Communication with teachers: for example, I understand my teachers.
- Communication with students: for example, other students understand me.
- Positive affect towards the classroom: for example, I feel good about how I communicate in class.
- Negative affect toward the classroom: for example, I feel unhappy in group discussions in class.

Students rate each item on a four-point scale. The authors found that the hearing students scored highest on teacher and student communication and positive affect, and lowest on negative affect. The typical DHH student scores were not significantly different from those of their hearing classmates. The DHH students with additional disabilities scored significantly worse than their hearing peers on all four scales. Even though there were no statistically significant differences between the hearing and the typical DHH students, the DHH students' scores were consistently slightly below those of the hearing students. This might indicate that, although classroom participation is not a major difficulty for these students, there remains room for improvement. These are data from one classroom, so classroom-specific procedures could influence the communication participation scores. Observation studies of communication within the classroom, especially during academic activities, and documentation of student engagement are needed before making definitive conclusions about classroom participation within co-enrollment classrooms.

## CHALLENGES OF CO-ENROLLMENT

Interviews and surveys of stakeholders in the co-enrollment setting provide information about the challenges of implementing this model. The challenges have typically centered on the time and skills needed for co-teaching, the commitment required from all stakeholders to make the program successful, and the ability of teachers and students to acquire sign language skills. The following challenges are gleaned from the results of interviews conducted with teachers, parents, and administrators by Luckner (1999), Kreimeyer et al. (2000), Jimenez-Sanchez and Antia (1999), and also a survey given to all co-enrollment teachers and staff by Metz and Spolsky (2013).

The ability to team requires strong problem-solving and interpersonal communication skills on the part of the teachers. Teachers need to trust one another; therefore teams should be compatible in their teaching philosophy. In addition, teachers need to be able to give up some autonomy. Teachers who have difficulty sharing control of the classroom may not be able to work successfully in a team. Within the co-enrollment classrooms, teachers must perceive each other as equals with complementary skills. In some school climates, special educators are seen as supports to the general classroom teacher. In such a climate, equality of teams would be difficult to achieve. Time was frequently mentioned as a challenge for the teachers. Team teaching takes additional work and planning time from the teachers. Teachers had to find the time to plan lessons, to decide each teacher's role during the teaching day, and to have explicit discussions about every aspect of instruction such as pace, evaluations, accommodations, and materials.

All teachers had to learn new skills and to rethink their ideas about the abilities and needs of their students. A teacher of DHH interviewed by Kreimeyer et al. (2000) mentioned that it was difficult, but necessary, to give up assumptions that she had learned during her teacher preparation program. Specifically, she had to revise assumptions about the need to teach DHH students only in small groups, the need for simplified material and content, and the inability of hearing students to learn to communicate in sign.

Learning to sign was the skill that was often mentioned as a challenge for both adults and students. Although sign language interpreters are often present in the classroom to ensure that all communication is accessible to all students at all times, the adults surveyed by Metz and Spolsky (2013) mentioned that communication in the co-enrollment classroom could sometimes be frustrating. Although the general education teachers made efforts to learn sign, Luckner (1999) noted that the time involved in becoming fluent was a problem, and prevented the general education teachers from interacting with the DHH students.

**QUALITY OF THE EVIDENCE**

Although the results reported in this chapter indicate that co-enrolled students have positive academic and social outcomes, it is important also to examine the quality of the research done on co-enrollment programs, particularly as special educators increasingly focus on evidence-based practices. Metz accordingly undertook to evaluate the research studies on co-enrollment using the *Practice Studies Manual* developed by the Council for Exceptional Children (CEC) (Council for Exceptional Children, 2008). The manual provides guidelines for systematically analyzing the quality of evidence of educational practices and interventions. It also contains rubrics for evaluating the quality of experimental, single subject, correlational, and qualitative research. The rubrics are used to evaluate each study based on the appropriate design for the given research questions, the implementation quality, and the effect of the target practice. Metz and a colleague independently used these rubrics to evaluate the published research that focused on co-enrollment outcomes. We provide a brief summary of the analysis here.

The studies evaluated included Bowen (2008), Jimenez-Sanchez and Antia (1999), Kreimeyer et al. (2000), Kluwin (1999), Luckner (1999), and McCain and Antia (2005). Each of these studies examined some aspect of the outcomes of co-enrollment as a placement option for DHH students. The study by Kreimeyer et al. was a mixed method study; therefore each part of the study was evaluated using the appropriate rubric for the given research design. This included use of the qualitative research rubric for examining the reported results of observations and interviews, the experimental rubric for examining the analysis of achievement test scores, and the single-subject rubric for examining the results of the study that examined social interaction. The studies by Luckner (1999) and Jimenez-Sanchez and Antia (1999) were both qualitative studies relying on interviews and observation and thus were examined using the qualitative research rubric. The studies by Bowen, Kluwin, and McCain and Antia were quasi-experimental studies and thus were examined using the experimental research rubric.

The research studies shared several strengths. Each author clearly stated the research questions or a purpose for conducting the study and chose an appropriate design for addressing the research questions. The analysis of the quasi-experimental studies showed that social and academic data were collected using valid and reliable instruments. These studies did not include a true control or comparison group, which limits the conclusions that can be drawn about the effects of co-enrollment on outcomes. Because placement in co-enrollment programs is not random, it is possible that positive outcomes are due to the characteristics of students and families who choose to attend these programs rather than characteristics of the co-enrolled program itself.

Kreimeyer et al. (2000) used a single-subject design to examine the effect of co-enrollment on frequency of interaction between DHH students and their peers. The strengths of this study included detailed and reliable observations, the stability of the baseline, sufficient data points that show an increasing trend, and a generalization component. Single-subject studies should include either a staggered multiple baseline or a reversal to baseline (ABA) to show experimental control. Unfortunately, Kreimeyer et al. (2000) used an AB design, which is a comparatively weak design that does not allow the researcher to rule out the influence of variables other than the co-enrollment program on the results.

The qualitative research studies (Jimenez-Sanchez & Antia 1999; Kreimeyer et al., 2000; Luckner, 1999) were well conducted and showed that all major stakeholders, including teachers, parents, and administrators, had positive perceptions about co-enrollment. While qualitative studies are very important, they do not examine cause and effect relationships; thus these studies cannot be used to determine whether co-enrollment programs provide benefits over and above other kinds of programs.

A major weakness of each of these studies was that none of the authors provided any kind of essential elements checklist for co-enrollment programming, thus making it difficult for future researchers to compare various co-enrollment programs or to determine the fidelity of the co-enrollment intervention. Merely identifying a program as co-enrollment does not define the characteristics of the program and therefore limits comparability between programs. An initial checklist

Table 17.3 Co-enrollment Fidelity of Implementation Checklist

| Characteristics of the Co-enrollment Classroom | Check if evident | Comments |
|---|---|---|
| The class consists of a critical mass of deaf and hard of hearing students (e.g., 20–50%), with the remainder of the class being typical hearing students. | | |
| Class is co-taught by a general education teacher and a teacher of DHH students. Co-teachers have equal responsibility for instructing all students enrolled in the class. | | |
| Qualified sign language interpreters are available as necessary for all classes. | | |
| Instruction in how to use a sign language interpreter is provided to all staff and students, school-wide. | | |
| Sign language instruction is provided for teachers and students, in the co-enrollment program as well as for the school community. | | |
| Both speech and sign language are valued and used in the classroom. | | |
| All students have necessary visual and auditory support or accommodations to fully access classroom instruction. | | |

that can be used by researchers and practitioners when planning or implementing a co-enrollment program is included in Table 17.3.

Despite some problems, each of these US studies was moderately well implemented. Based on this evaluation, co-enrollment appears to be a promising practice; however, there has not yet been enough research to consider it an evidence-based practice. Future research needs to compare the academic and social outcomes of co-enrollment with other kinds of placement, to examine results from additional co-enrollment programs, to describe the co-enrollment programs carefully, and finally to examine the long-term benefits of co-enrollment.

## CONCLUSIONS

In order for a co-enrollment program to be successful, several elements need to be in place. All stakeholders need to be committed to the idea that DHH and hearing students are capable of learning together and interacting with each other. Teaching teams need to have compatible philosophies of education and classroom management styles and designated time for planning and collaboration. Finally, both teachers should be equally responsible for all students in the class.

We end with these comments from co-enrollment staff surveyed by Metz and Splosky (2013):

> I have taught in a variety of settings, and the co-enrollment setting solves some social isolation issues along with challenging each Deaf student to achieve the same academic standards as their hearing peers.
> 
> –Teacher of DHH

> When the program is well run and managed, it benefits both hearing and DHH students. They become a single class and community.
> 
> –Support personnel

## REFERENCES

Antia, S. D., Jones, P. B., Reed, S., & Kreimeyer, K. H. (2009). Academic status and progress of deaf and hard-of-hearing students in general education classrooms. *Journal of Deaf Studies and Deaf Education, 14,* 293–311.

Antia, S. D., Sabers, D., & Stinson, M. S. (2007). Validity and reliability of the Classroom Participation Questionnaire with deaf and hard of hearing students in public schools. *Journal of Deaf Studies and Deaf Education, 12,* 158–171.

Antia, S. D., Stinson, M. S., & Gaustad, M. G. (2002). Developing membership in the education of deaf and hard of hearing students in inclusive settings. *Journal of Deaf Studies and Deaf Education, 7,* 214–229.

Bierman, K. L. (2004). *Peer rejection: Developmental processes and intervention strategies.* New York, NY: The Guilford Press.

Bowen, S. (2008). Coenrollment for students who are Deaf or Hard of Hearing: Friendship patterns and social interactions. *American Annals of the Deaf, 153,* 285–293.

Council for Exceptional Children (2008). *Classifying the state of evidence for special education professional practices: CEC practice study manual.* Arlington, VA: Council for Exceptional Children.

Friend, M., Cook, L., Hurley-Chamberlain, D., & Shamberger, C. (2010). Co-teaching: An illustration of the complexity of collaboration in special education. *Journal of Educational and Psychological Consultation, 20,* 9–27.

Gallaudet Research Institute. (1996). *Stanford Achievement Test Series, 9th edition, Form S, Norms Booklet for Deaf and Hard of Hearing Students.* Washington, DC: Gallaudet University.

Gallaudet Research Institute. (2011). *Regional and national summary report of data from the 2009–2010 Annual Survey of Deaf and Hard of Hearing children and Youth.* Washington DC: GRI, Gallaudet University.

Guralnick, M. (2001). A framework for change in early childhood inclusion. In M. J. Guralnick (Ed.), *Early childhood inclusion: Focus on change* (pp. 3–35). Baltimore, MD: Paul H. Brookes.

Harcourt Brace. (1997). *Stanford Achievement Test Series, 9th edition.* Technical data report. San Antonio, TX.

Jimenez-Sanchez, C., & Antia, S. D. (1999). Team teaching in an integrated classroom: Perceptions of deaf and hearing teachers. *Journal of Deaf Studies and Deaf Education, 4*, 215–224.

Kirchner, C. J. (1994). Co-enrollment as an inclusion model. *American Annals of the Deaf, 139*(2), 163–164.

Kluwin, T. N. (1999). Coteaching deaf and hearing students: Research on social integration. *American Annals of the Deaf, 144*(4), 339–344.

Kreimeyer, K. H., Crooke, P., Drye, C., Egbert, V., & Klein, B. (2000). Academic and social benefits of a coenrollment model of inclusive education for deaf and hard-of-hearing children. *Journal of Deaf Studies and Deaf Education, 5*, 174–185.

Levine, L. M., & Antia, S. D. (1997). The effect of partner hearing status on social and cognitive play. *Journal of Early Intervention, 21*, 21–35.

Long, G., Stinson, M. S., & Braeges, J. (1991). Students' perception of communication ease and engagement: How they relate to academic success. *American Annals of the Deaf, 136*, 414–421.

Luckner, J. (1999). An examination of two coteaching classrooms. *American Annals of the Deaf, 144*, 24–34.

McCain, K., & Antia, S. D. (2005). Academic and social status of hearing, deaf, and hard-of-hearing students participating in a co-enrolled classroom. *Communication Disorders Quarterly, 27*, 20–32.

Metz, K. K., & Spolsky, S. (2013). *Co-enrollment as a placement option for deaf and hard-of-hearing children: Benefits, challenges, and caveats.* Paper presented at the Association of College Educators Deaf/Hard of Hearing, Santa Fe, New Mexico.

Morocco, C. C., & Aguilar, C. M. (2002). Coteaching for content understanding: A schoolwide model. *Journal of Educational and Psychological Consultation, 13*, 315–347.

Saur, R. E., Layne, C. A., Hurley, E. A., & Opton, K. (1986). Dimensions of mainstreaming. *American Annals of the Deaf, 131*, 325–330.

Stinson, M. S., & Liu, Y. (1999). Participation of deaf and hard of hearing students in classes with hearing students. *Journal of Deaf Studies and Deaf Education, 4*, 191–202.

Stinson, M. S., Liu, Y., Saur, R. E., & Long, G. (1996). Deaf college students' perceptions of communication in mainstream classes. *Journal of Deaf Studies and Deaf Education, 1*, 40–51.

# Epilogue

# 18

# Perspectives on Bilingualism and Bilingual Education for Deaf Learners

Marc Marschark, Harry Knoors, and Gladys Tang

Writing the concluding chapter of an edited book has advantages and disadvantages. One advantage, of course, is that having read the various contributions multiple times, we have the opportunity to bring together their common threads while noting theoretical and empirical differences. One disadvantage is that having read the various contributions multiple times, we have the challenge of bringing together their common threads while accommodating their theoretical and empirical differences. Some of the more obvious differences among the contributors, at least in this volume, are the result of their diverse disciplinary backgrounds, including linguistics, (deaf) education, psychology, child development, and others. Anyone familiar with deaf education also will understand that in a group of contributors of this size, beyond personal and professional interests in the various facets of deaf studies, language, and education, there are also going to be philosophical differences with regard to raising and educating deaf children and the language(s) involved in doing so. Our goal in this chapter therefore is to bring all of these perspectives and findings together, if not into a set of unequivocal, mutually agreeable conclusions, at least into a coherent whole that moves us forward in both research and practice.

In part because of the international and interdisciplinary nature of this book's contributors, there is both overlap and disjunction among the various chapters. Certainly (or perhaps we should say hopefully), no one would expect that any one of the editors would be familiar with all of the literature cited in all of the chapters. Not only is some important work described here for the first time, but the mix of both contributors and editors is such that, from the outset, we have never expected a high degree of homogeneity. Indeed, we see this mix as the greatest strength of this volume, but it also presents challenges beyond simply writing the chapter. One issue, noted in the first chapter, is that while there is a new *méthode du jour* in deaf education every few years, the desire(s) for change and those changes that actually occur frequently are associated with sensitive interpersonal and cultural topics. A related issue, also associated with the vantage point of the near-end of this volume, is recognition that not everyone involved in this project has shared common definitions or understandings of some of the issues. If there were the opportunity for everyone to go back, having read all of the chapters, no doubt there would be many additions (resisting that is difficult even for us!), different ways of saying things, and added nuances in the interpretations of new and existing findings. As it is, however, the responsibility lies with us to describe where we have been, where we are, and where we are going. To a large extent, the first of these, where we have been, has been described in the introductory chapter. That chapter expressed our view that the future of bilingual deaf education is in danger. In large measure, this is a result of questions about its theoretical foundations and the limited evidence base with regard to its outcomes. Both of these issues have been addressed in various chapters of this volume, and we will address them further here. Looking ahead, the important questions are going to focus on the effectiveness of various versions of bilingual education in different domains and for different learners. Before considering the theoretical and empirical issues, however, it is important to ensure a common understanding of the topic of discussion.

## OF DEFINITIONS, PERSPECTIVES, AND REAL OR PERCEIVED BOUNDARIES

At various levels, all three of us are involved in deaf education, bilingual deaf education, and co-enrollment programs for deaf and hard-of-hearing (DHH) students. That does not mean that we are involved in the same ways or even that we understand these activities and terms in the same way. For example, being involved in educating deaf students bilingually, meaning both in sign language and the written/spoken vernacular, is not the same as being involved in explicitly designed bilingual deaf education. So let us articulate our understanding and use of the terms used throughout this chapter on the basis of international consensus. Our hope is that providing this small bit of clarity will help to avoid the kinds of confusion that all too often have prevented DHH students and their parents from having full access to educational information and opportunities.

### Bilingual Deaf Education

As should be apparent from the previous paragraph as well as various chapters in this volume, "bilingual education for DHH students" may be a bit of a misnomer. Within the field, it generally refers to the use of (at least) two modes of communication in the classroom, one of them involving the sign language and one involving the written/spoken language of the local community. Even this simple description masks greater complexities. For the moment, we will leave aside the fact that in many, if not most, countries, children have more than two written/spoken languages. This is especially pronounced in Europe, Asia, and Africa, and most often lacking in English-speaking countries, but there are further complexities. Most notable in this volume is the situation encountered by deaf children in Hong Kong, described by Tang, Lam, and Yiu in Chapter 13, most of whom are exposed to Cantonese as the primary spoken language, Mandarin as the primary written language, English, and (if they are lucky) Hong Kong Sign Language.

Across bilingual deaf education programs, the motivation and thus the character of those programs vary considerably. For example, several programs in the United States that refer to themselves as bilingual are explicitly ASL-first programs, with written/spoken English seen as secondary. In some cases, the motivation for such program design is cultural, in the belief that acquiring a sign language as an L1 allows deaf children to develop identities as Deaf individuals and members of the Deaf community (even if at least 95% of deaf children have hearing parents; see Hintermair, Chapter 7 of this volume). In other cases, the motivation is based on the assumption that children need to be fluent in an L1 before acquiring an L2, a belief apparently held primarily in English-speaking countries. Programs in other countries advocate bilingual education in a more balanced sense. Hermans, Wauters, De Klerk, and Knoors (Chapter 11 of this volume), for example, indicate that bilingual education in the Netherlands was introduced initially in order to provide profoundly deaf children with greater access to language, thus enhancing academic outcomes. They point out that in at least some schools for the deaf, there initially was an SLN-first attitude on the assumption that sign language generally could provide DHH children with greater access to instruction than written/spoken Dutch. The lack of evidence in that regard and contrary evidence from work with older students (e.g., Borgna, Convertino, Marschark, Morrison, & Rizzolo, 2011; Marschark and colleagues, 2009) have led to both Sign Language of the Netherlands (SLN) and spoken and written Dutch being equally emphasized in some cases and grouping students for instruction in their stronger language (SLN or spoken Dutch) in others. Swanwick, Hendar, Dammeyer, Kristoffersen, Salter, and Simonsen (Chapter 12 of this volume) similarly point out that models of bilingual programming in Nordic countries and the United Kingdom vary considerably, while earlier emphases on sign language-first have waned.

### Simultaneous Communication and Total Communication

It is important to note at this juncture that even programs that describe themselves as using "sign language" frequently do not exclusively use the linguistically codified natural sign language of the local Deaf community. In some cases, educational settings make use of simultaneous communication (often referred to as sign-supported speech outside the United States) or manually coded versions of the vernacular to a greater or lesser extent (see, for example, Hermans, De Klerk, Wauters, & Knoors, Chapter 16 of this volume; Marschark, Sapere, Convertino, & Pelz, 2008).

Simultaneous communication and sign-supported speech should not be confused with total communication (or TC). The total communication philosophy with regard to deaf education emerged in the 1960s and was named by Roy Holcomb, a prominent Deaf American. Total communication originally was called the Total Approach, indicating the notion that instructional approaches with deaf children have to be flexible, eclectic, and child-centered (T. Holcomb, personal communication, September 2, 2013; see Holcomb, 2013). In particular, TC originally emphasized using whatever communication method(s) worked for a child, instead of imposing the restriction of spoken language only. This included a shift in classroom communication policy from teacher-centered to child-centered, with family members playing a central role in supporting deaf children in their education. Holcomb argued that a total communication environment, ensuring fully accessible communication through sign language, is critical in providing deaf children with access to incidental learning and fully integrating deaf children into their families.

Perhaps because so many deaf children in the United States grew up with several alternative forms of communication, and sometimes used them with different people in different situations, as adults they frequently are less concerned than others about the label "American Sign Language" (ASL). But the issue of the sign languages and sign systems used in deaf education becomes more complex when members of Deaf communities use such modified sign systems. When observed being used among deaf individuals, both native signers and non-native signers alike, this situation is sometimes described in terms of registers. In any case, the frequency with which "sign language" is defined as whatever it is that deaf (or Deaf) individuals use suggests that the ambiguity (if not the confusion) is going to be with us for some time, both in deaf education and in society at large.

The extent to which bilingual programs for DHH students utilize or encourage spoken language in addition to the written vernacular also varies widely. As Swanwick, Hendar, Dammeyer, Kristoffersen, Salter, and Simonsen (Chapter 12 of this volume) emphasize, one reason for the decreasing popularity of bilingual deaf education in some countries has been the explicit "marginalization" of spoken language, at least from the perspective of hearing parents. We do not believe that this necessarily reflects naïveté, ignorance, or prejudice on the part of those parents, at least today. Rather, as several authors have made explicit (e.g., Knoors & Marschark, 2012; Swanwick, Hendar, Dammeyer, Kristoffersen, Salter, and Simonsen, Chapter 12 of this volume; Walker & Tomlin, Chapter 6 of this volume), the current trend to a return to spoken language in deaf education in some countries is a reflection of the fact that it is potentially more available to many deaf children than ever before. This is not simply a matter of early interventionists or educational programs somehow forcing deaf children into an oral channel (although that certainly happens). Rather, new technologies such as digital hearing aids and cochlear implants, as well as earlier hearing loss diagnosis and intervention, and new interventions plus educational methodologies have offered a greater breadth of opportunities (Wauters & De Klerk, Chapter 10 of this volume).

### Bilingual and Bicultural Deaf Education

For the present, we will use the term "bilingual deaf education" as referring to the use of both a signed language/sign system and the written/spoken vernacular in educating DHH youth, recognizing that in both cases these refer to continua rather than to opposite poles of a single continuum. At this point, however, we should add a brief note about bilingual-*bicultural* deaf education. We noted in the introductory chapter that in today's society, bilingualism typically also involves being associated with two cultures. In the case of deaf education, there is broad consensus in the field that DHH children benefit from being exposed to deaf adults as models, be they parents, teachers, or paraprofessionals (see Tang, Lam, & Yiu, Chapter 13 of this volume). Whether or not those individuals are members of the Deaf community and whether or not DHH students are explicitly exposed to information about the history and functioning of the Deaf community (e.g., Holcomb, 2013), about Deaf individuals who have contributed to society at large (e.g., Lang & Meath-Lang, 1995), or about contemporary Deaf art and theater (e.g., Padden & Humphries, 2005), the impact of bicultural programming on DHH children does not appear to have been investigated (see Marschark & Lee, Chapter 9 of this volume).

Interactions among DHH and hearing students do appear to have a positive impact on both groups (e.g., Hintermair, Chapter 7 of this volume; Yiu & Tang, Chapter 14 of this volume; Pérez Martin, Valmaseda Balanzategui, & Morgan, Chapter 15 of this volume), but Deaf acculturation is quite another matter (e.g., Maxwell-McCaw & Zea, 2011). The extent to which exposure to deaf models and/or Deaf culture and the Deaf community significantly affects DHH children's language, social-emotional functioning, achievement, or other domains is well worthy of investigation, whether or not it occurs in the context of bilingual-bicultural educational programming.

## Bilingual Deaf Education Settings

Variation in the continua of educational placements for DHH students around the world clearly indicates that bilingual education does not have to occur in any particular setting. Schools and programs for deaf students currently range from those that utilize only spoken/written language to those that utilize only sign language as the language of instruction, depending on the latter to provide a bridge to literacy in the vernacular. The extent to which this bridging actually occurs is still a matter of debate, as the chapters by Holzinger and Fellinger (Chapter 5 of this volume) and Tang, Lam, and Yiu (Chapter 13 of this volume) attest. Regardless of whether a particular bilingual curriculum is followed in a school for the deaf, a self-contained classroom in a regular (or mainstream) school, or a mainstream classroom is likely to have an impact on outcomes across the various domains addressed in this volume (e.g., language, cognition, social-emotional functioning, academic outcomes). This does not mean that all versions of bilingual education will yield the same results, or that any particular version will work in all settings with all students. Attempts in the existing literature to generalize too broadly across such variables may lead parents, educators, and others down various garden paths of optimism or pessimism.

## Bilingualism in Co-enrollment Settings

One bright light on the educational horizon is co-enrollment programming. Chapters in the present volume, taken together, provide perhaps the best summary of the current state of the art with regard to co-enrollment, a topic we will address in greater depth later. With regard to terminology, it is important to recognize that even "co-enrollment" has various nuances in different countries. At present, we are only aware of slightly more than a handful of such programs (see Tang, Lam, & Yiu, Chapter 13 of this volume) and, as the present chapters indicate, they vary considerably. As described by Antia and Metz (Chapter 17 of this volume), the common philosophy behind co-enrollment programs is the avoidance of both the academic segregation of DHH students and their integration into classes with hearing students without appropriate support services or modification of instructional methods and materials. Rather, it seeks to give DHH learners the best of both educational worlds.

Marschark and Knoors (2012; Knoors & Marschark, 2014, chapter 6) argued that demonstrated cognitive differences between DHH and hearing learners, above and beyond language, necessitate such adjustments if DHH students are to be able to reach their full academic potentials. Co-enrollment programs specifically achieve this goal through the involvement of two teachers, usually in a mainstream setting, one of whom has training and expertise in deaf education. In some programs, that individual is deaf; in others, he or she is a certified teacher of the deaf, but neither should be confused with deaf (or certified hearing) teachers' aides, communication workers, or other paraprofessionals. If, despite its apparent promise, the case for co-enrollment programming has not yet been made, that situation likely reflects the relative youth of the co-enrollment model. The extent to which current evidence offers more definitive support for co-enrollment, as well as charting directions for future research and practice, is the subject of several chapters in this volume and an issue that we will address in a later section of this one.

## ASSESSING THE OUTCOMES OF EDUCATIONAL PROGRAMMING FOR DHH STUDENTS

There is broad agreement across stakeholders involved in educating DHH learners that language is perhaps preeminent in ensuring personal, academic, and career success, even if there also is broad disagreement on how best to support deaf children's attainment of language fluencies and the extent to which various language abilities are related to various outcomes (e.g., Humphries and colleagues, 2012; Knoors & Marschark, 2012). For those interested specifically in language, there are issues associated with the linguistics of signed versus written/spoken languages and their mutual influence; DHH children's pragmatic, social, and academic fluencies in one, two, or more languages in the same or different modalities and how these might influence each other; and the ways in which all of these affect social-emotional functioning, cognitive functioning, and academic outcomes. Frequently, relations among these various domains are considered only in terms of statistical correlations. A number of contributors to this volume, however, emphasize that correlation does not entail causation, even if it frequently implies it. At the same time, the recognized heterogeneity among DHH learners relative to their hearing peers, as well as their small numbers in all but a few educational settings, means that arguments based on parametric statistical significance and longitudinal data are difficult to come by. Strong and broad generalizations nonetheless are frequently made in the literature, and rarely is there the opportunity offered by a collection such as this one to draw conclusions from a body of reviews and findings that are "all present." In an admittedly brief attempt to do so, let us deal with several of these issues in turn.

The following sections should not be taken to be exhaustive reviews of the extant literature or even of the chapters in this volume. For that, we leave readers to consult the various contributors themselves. Rather, our goal here is to point out some of the key conclusions that can be drawn from the evidence base at this point, as well as pointing out some that should not be drawn, even if they frequently are. In what follows, we first consider outcomes related to bilingual deaf education, followed by those related to co-enrollment. As noted earlier, these two

## Cognitive-Academic Outcomes Related to Bilingual Education

### Cognition and Bilingual Education

Chapters in this volume by Ormel and Giezen (Chapter 4), by Mineiro, Nunes, Moita, Silva, and Castro-Caldas (Chapter 8), and by Marschark and Lee (Chapter 9) have described several advantages and, to a much lesser extent, some disadvantages apparently bestowed by bilingualism among DHH individuals in the cognitive domain. However, broad agreement is still lacking regarding causal and outcome cognitive factors associated with bilingualism and bilingual deaf education. Also unclear is the nature of interactions among those factors and how they might be influenced by others considered later.

Holzinger and Fellinger (Chapter 5 of this volume) noted that neurolinguistic studies have demonstrated that early access to a second language (L2) is a better predictor of L2 outcomes than the level of skills in a child's first language (L1). This finding contrasts with claims made by some interested in bilingual deaf education that children first need to be fluent in their L1 before attempting to acquire an L2. The strong form of such a claim is clearly disputed by the competent bilingual and multilingual children throughout the world, but there are varieties of interesting and potentially important theoretical and practical implications of such studies. Mineiro, Nunes, Moita, Silva, and Castro-Caldas (Chapter 8 of this volume), for example, describe findings indicating that the grammatical categories of an individual's two languages remain distinct even when acquired at different ages, perhaps one reason for findings by Mayberry and Lock (2003) and others suggesting that late learners of a language will rarely if ever demonstrate the grammatical fluencies of the native language learner (but see later). Mineiro and colleagues argue that the critical factor for the "convergence" of knowledge and abilities of L1 and L2 at several levels is the individual's degree of proficiency in the two languages. They take this as evidence in support of convergence at the level of brain structure, while Ormel and Giezen (Chapter 4 of this volume) focus on convergence at the cognitive-linguistic level, with both sets of investigators focusing on word and syntactic processing. Mineiro and colleagues argue that similar convergence does not occur with regard to semantic processing, perhaps because of different organization in the brain. Marschark, Convertino, McEvoy, and Masteller (2004) demonstrated differences in semantic organization between deaf and hearing students in terms of inter-item associative structure and associative strength, but the language backgrounds and developmental histories of those (college) students were not examined.

Both the neurolinguistic data offered by Mineiro and colleagues and evidence of cross-linguistic facilitation offered by Ormel and Giezen argue for the potential importance of children acquiring their two (or more) languages at the same time (but see Cormier, Schembri, Vinson, & Orfanidou, 2012), although empirical elaborations of causal and correlational connections among semantic memory, language acquisition, and language use remain to be made at several levels. One possibility suggested by Mineiro and colleagues is that differences in implicit and explicit language knowledge could explain the different neural activation seen in early and late bilinguals, because procedural memory and declarative memory might not be located in the same regions of the brain. That suggestion is consistent with evidence indicating that L2 acquisition is faster in adult (late) bilinguals than child (early) bilinguals because they can use language to learn language (DeKeyser & Larson-Hall, 2005). It also is consistent with Ormel and Giezen's linking of cross-language interactions and the fact that L2 acquisition is related to children's fluencies in each of their languages, at least among spoken language bilinguals. They noted that bilingualism among hearing individuals affects non-linguistic cognitive abilities as well as language-related abilities, so the control mechanisms necessary for selectively activating or suppressing one language or the other appear to provide bilinguals with more generally flexible executive functioning. The possible neuropsychological interaction of bilingual education with executive functioning and self-esteem, both of which have their loci in prefrontal cortex, is just one of many tantalizing areas awaiting investigation.

Ormel and Giezen (Chapter 4 of this volume) provide a review of research on executive functioning in spoken language (i.e., unimodal) bilinguals. They note that studies into bimodal bilingualism have resulted in conflicting findings, and it is too soon to tell whether the cognitive advantages that are observed among adult bimodal bilinguals will be found in children. Together with Holzinger and Fellinger (Chapter 5 of this volume), they argue that cognitive as well as language correlates of bilingualism are likely to depend on the age of acquisition of both of the child's languages (see also Walker & Tomblin, Chapter 6 of this volume). Indeed, the lack of early fluency in their L1 by many, if not most, deaf children creates difficulties not only for acquisition of their L2, but for their continuing L1 development, cognitive development, social development, and academic achievement. Meanwhile, when the written/spoken vernacular is the L2, literacy and other academic activities within that language obviously are going to be better the earlier that L2 is acquired (e.g., Kovelman, Baker, & Petitto, 2008). At this point, however, the influence on cognitive development of age of acquisition for either L1 or L2 remains largely unexplored. Ormel and Giezen point out that factors such as length of L2 exposure and the setting in which the L2 is acquired are likely to affect both language and cognitive growth, and we would add that the same is likely true for L1. In the case of DHH children, the confounding of age of acquisition with the modalities of L1 and L2 (perhaps as well as the order by modality interaction) makes the situation even more complex but no less in need of investigation.

*Academic Outcomes and Bilingual Education*

If research into the extent to which bilingual deaf education is associated with cognitive development is just beginning, its impact on academic outcomes has been the subject of a number of studies, even if they have yielded varying and sometimes contradictory answers. Factors already mentioned with regard to both L1 and L2, such as age of acquisition, L1 and L2 attainment, simultaneous versus successive acquisition, and the setting(s) of acquisition (i.e., school and/or home) clearly are involved and remain to be disentangled. Simple correlations, for example, between a child's sign language or spoken language skills and his or her reading achievement do not address the issue of what or whether some form of bilingual education will be better than any other for particular children (Marschark & Lee, Chapter 9 of this volume). However, they do enable us to understand that knowledge and skills of languages are interconnected—relationships that educators might want to tap in supporting deaf children's language and academic development.

Only rarely considered in the above mix are the specific teaching methods used and the extent to which they match the cognitive strengths and needs of deaf students. As Wauters and De Klerk (Chapter 10 of this volume) noted, the increased access to and use of spoken language with the increasing prevalence of digital hearing aids and cochlear implants has provided some enhancement in academic achievement by DHH students. As is also the case with bilingual education, however, it has not fully closed the gaps between them and hearing children (see Walker & Tomblin, Chapter 6 of this volume, with regard to language outcomes). Although some studies have found younger children with cochlear implants more likely to be reading at grade level (e.g., Archbold and colleagues, 2008; Geers, Tobey, Moog, & Brenner, 2008; but see Nitrouer, Caldwell, Lowenstein, Tarr, & Holloman, 2012), the same investigators and others have found them to be lagging behind hearing peers when they reach later grades. In large measure, this situation may be related to the fact that deaf children with and without cochlear implants appear to lag behind hearing peers in the same cognitive domains (e.g., Pisoni, Conway, Kronenberger, Henning, & Anaya, 2010) and simply may be cognitively different from their hearing peers in some similar ways (Marschark & Knoors, 2012).

For DHH learners with and without cochlear implants, we would expect that greater access to instruction through the use of sign language would prove facilitative, although results are mixed (e.g., Marschark, Leigh, and colleagues, 2006). If cognitive differences between deaf and hearing students account for some of their academic underachievement, simply providing instruction in a different (or two) language(s) is not going to provide a complete remedy. However, providing sign language to students with cochlear implants (either as an L1 or an L2) may support reading in the vernacular, even if the notion remains unpopular among many proponents of pediatric cochlear implantation (see Holzinger & Fellinger, Chapter 5 of this volume; Knoors & Marschark, 2012; Marschark & Lee, Chapter 9 of this volume; Walker & Tomblin, Chapter 6 of this volume).

Stinson and Kluwin (2011), in reviewing the available literature on school placement, concluded that whether DHH student are enrolled in regular classrooms or schools or programs for the deaf accounts for less than 5% of the variability in academic outcomes. Although regular versus special school placement is not synonymous with a dichotomy of spoken versus sign language, their finding suggests that, overall, which language is used in instruction may be less important than how we teach DHH students (Knoors & Marschark, 2014). That is, different DHH students will be more or less comfortable with, have a greater or lesser preference for, and learn more or less (whether or not they are aware of it) from instruction in sign language or spoken language. In either case, the goal of the teacher is to provide rich instructional contexts to support learning, recognizing the differing background knowledge and cognitive abilities of their DHH students. Wauters and De Klerk (Chapter 10 of this volume) address this issue specifically with regard to reading, emphasizing not only ways in which skilled teachers of the deaf integrate new information with what their students already know, but also providing them with the cognitive tools to be able to do so themselves.

This emphasis on metacognition is consistent with the existing literature indicating that DHH students lag behind hearing peers in executive functioning related to learning in school, often failing to utilize knowledge they have, to transfer skills across contexts, or to judge accurately how much they understand or are learning (Borgna and colleagues, 2011; Hauser, Lukomski, & Hillman, 2008). Ultimately, it may be that individual students' acquisition and utilization of these cognitive functions will be faster or deployed more flexibly and effectively if instruction is in a signed language or a spoken language. To date, however, the case for these possibilities has not been made. Nor has the case been made that one language or the other is necessarily better for any particular area of instruction (including reading) for all DHH students. Rather, just as sign language made its way into the classroom because exclusively oral instruction for DHH students was not generally successful, we need to be cognizant of the fact that exclusively signed instruction for DHH students may not be entirely successful.

Holzinger and Fellinger (Chapter 5 of this volume) examined the relationship between sign language and reading, seeking to evaluate the frequent claim that the observed correlation between DHH students' sign language skills and reading is a causal one. They concluded that despite the positive correlation between these two domains, the existing empirical findings are contradictory, and the link might be the result of the confluence of a variety of intrinsic and extrinsic factors. Together with Wauters and De Klerk (Chapter 10 of this volume), they suggest that reading among DHH students who use sign language is supported by their greater access to instruction and knowledge of the world and not only to language qua language. For students with good speech perception skills, instruction in spoken language might provide the same advantages. In fact, Holzinger and Fellinger found that in one of their samples, reading comprehension was negatively related to sign language skill, whereas it was positively related to knowledge of German vocabulary and grammar and skills in spoken German. In their other sample, sign language skill was positively related to reading. They concluded only that automatic transfer of language skills from L1 to L2 should not be assumed. Together with findings reported in other chapters of this volume (e.g., Tang, Lam, & Yiu, Chapter 13 of this volume), their results suggest that transfer of L1 sign language skills to written language can happen when effective, early access to signing results in high proficiency. The extent to which extensive exposure later can yield similar effects remains unclear (see, for example, Cormier and colleagues, 2012). History leads us to similar conclusions with regard to spoken language and reading among DHH students, and yet battles continue to rage about which mode is (near) universally better. As a number of contributors to this volume note, the key is early, effective access to an L1 and high proficiency in that language, whatever its modality.

DHH children's proficiencies in L1 and L2 are an important issue for research as well as to children's development. As noted earlier, longitudinal studies and relatively large samples (of both children and language) are necessary if we are to fully understand the foundations and consequences of bilingual education (e.g., Tang, Lam, & Yiu, Chapter 13 of this volume), but such studies are hard to come by, as the population of school-age DHH students tends to be small. Nover, Andrews, Baker, Everhart, and Bradford (2002) and Lange, Lane-Outlaw, Lange, and Sherwood (2013), however, reported on academic outcomes in groups of DHH students who had been enrolled in one bilingual education model (in different schools) over several years (see Marschark & Lee, Chapter 9 of this volume). Nover and colleagues found that after at least 3 years in the program, reading comprehension levels were significantly above the available norms for DHH children, although they were not as high as a sample of same-aged children in a total communication program who took the same standardized assessment in the same year (Knoors & Marschark, 2014, chapter 5). Lange and colleagues reported that after at least 4 years in their program, 41% of the children were reading at or above the normative national average (including both hearing and DHH children), and 55% percent of children were at or above average in mathematics. However, DHH students with lower levels of achievement were excluded from the study, so the generality of their findings may be limited. While concluding that their bilingual model was largely successful, Lange and colleagues therefore cautioned against assuming that it or any other model of deaf education would be appropriate for all DHH children. The academic outcomes of some DHH children clearly can benefit from bilingual education, given appropriate environments at home and at school, including strong foundations in an L1. Still to be determined are the methods and materials that allow that to happen.

*Pedagogy and Bilingual Education*

Stinson and Kluwin (2011) suggested that with little evidence that school placement or student characteristics could explain the majority of variance in the academic achievement among DHH learners, we should look to instruction and teacher variables for more potent predictors. More recently, Knoors and Marschark (2014) made a similar argument, suggesting that neither school placement nor the language of instruction were sufficient to account for the achievement (or underachievement) of DHH students. Their emphasis on the match between teaching methods and students' strengths and needs, social-emotional functioning in the classroom, and teacher characteristics was echoed in the findings of Hermans, Wauters, De Klerk, and Knoors (Chapter 11 of this volume) with regard to quality of instruction. They reported that when DHH children were taught material in their preferred and non-preferred language modalities, there was essentially no difference in performance, while they scored significantly below hearing peers in both. Similar results were reported by Marschark, Sapere, Convertino, and Seewagen (2005) and Marschark and colleagues (2008) in studies involving DHH college students in a bilingual education environment. Hermans, Wauters, and colleagues suggested that one possible explanation for their own results was that the DHH students' sign language skills were not sufficient to benefit fully from the signed material. Marschark and colleagues' consistent findings that DHH college students' sign language skills did not predict their learning from signed instruction (with no ceiling effects) are consistent with that interpretation. At the same time, both groups of investigators have emphasized the considerable heterogeneity among DHH students in content knowledge as well as language and cognitive abilities, all of which combine to making classroom instruction difficult.

Several investigators have emphasized the role of classroom dynamics in education at large and with regard to special education in particular (Bergin & Bergin, 2009; see Knoors & Marschark, 2014, chapter 7, for a review). Beyond issues such as curriculum planning and classroom management that are covered in teacher training programs, teacher-student relationships are emerging as a particularly important topic for both practical and research purposes. As Hermans, Wauters, De Klerk, and Knoors (Chapter 11 of this volume) point out, stronger student-teacher relationships are associated with greater student motivation, which, in turn, is linked to students' attending more to instruction and learning more from it. In addition to replicating previous findings of DHH students being less satisfied with relationships with their teachers, in this case in a bilingual setting, Hermans, Wauters, and colleagues found DHH students less satisfied with their teachers' classroom management skills (e.g., effectiveness of explanations, time on task). They concluded that the quality of instruction in bilingual schools, or at least DHH students' perception of it, is rather less than is generally expected from such settings.

Taken together, the findings described in this and the previous two sections indicate that as was true with oral education, mainstreaming, and other modifications to deaf education, bringing sign language into the classroom (resulting in bilingual education) is not going to resolve all the challenges faced by DHH students. Those students show increasing diversity as a result of more varied speech perception via assistive listening devices, varied exposure to forms of signed communication during early intervention, and neurological, psychological, or physical impediments to learning. Simple exposure to language resulting in low to moderate fluencies is not going to lead to the cognitive and academic language proficiencies that allow DHH children to reach their full potential. A broader perspective and broader interventions may well be necessary, and we therefore now turn to another area associated with bilingual education that has rather more clear-cut evidence: social-emotional functioning.

## Social Outcomes Related to Bilingual Education

Perhaps the most consistent positive findings from bilingual education, including co-enrollment, come from studies of social-emotional functioning, identity, and well-being (e.g., Bagga-Gupta, 2004; Dammeyer, 2010). Bilingual settings have the opportunity to provide DHH children with foundations for healthy social-emotional growth, access to rich social communication, diverse social experiences with similar adults and peers, and the opportunity to develop cultural affiliations. Hintermair (Chapter 7 of this volume), for example, reported that the use of sign language among young DHH children is associated with the quality of parent-child communication and children's global assessment of their self-worth. His findings indicated that early parent-child communication in particular is an important contributor to DHH children's feelings of well-being and quality of life, independent of its modality (Calderon & Greenberg, 2011). As a result, Hintermair concluded that bilingual settings are more likely to support DHH students' social-emotional growth than settings that utilize only spoken language (see Yiu & Tang, Chapter 14 of this volume). As earlier studies had shown, the emotional availability of parents (and now teachers) is a key element for normal attachment and social-emotional development, and such availability is unlikely when children and their parents do not share an effective channel of communication (Marschark, 1993, chapter 3).

Additional findings with regard to social functioning associated with bilingual deaf education are discussed later, with regard to co-enrollment settings. An interesting aspect of research in this area, however, is the lack of it in North America. While investigators in other countries have approached bilingual deaf education with questions across academic, linguistic, and social domains, North American investigators largely have maintained a tight focus on literacy, with far less attention to either linguistic or social outcomes. Davidson, Lillo-Martin, and Pichler (2014), however, examined the spoken English skills of two groups of 4- to 8-year-olds. One group consisted of deaf children born to deaf parents who had both cochlear implants and exposure to ASL input since birth. They were compared to a group of hearing children, also born to deaf parents, who were similarly ASL-English bilingual. Their results indicated that the two groups had comparable English language skills, leading to the conclusion that early exposure to sign language does not interfere with the acquisition of spoken language and may even support it. Whether the lack of other studies of this sort or any considering social development reflects a cultural divide or the relative youth of bilingual education in North America, the lack of broader empirical support (or interest in gaining it) for bilingual deaf education in American classrooms clearly has contributed to the continuing popularity of "oral" programming, despite its less than stellar history. Let us therefore turn to an important topic about which there is less interest among American researchers: specific language-related outcomes of bilingual deaf education.

### How Does Bilingual Education Affect Bilingualism?

The issue of how bilingual education affects language growth is more complex than it might appear at first glance. First, we have already noted that outside co-enrollment settings, studies relevant to the issue have focused primarily on increasing abilities with regard to the written vernacular rather than the signed vernacular. In that regard, some of the findings might be considered as relevant to the acquisition of literacy as to language per se. Second, as we indicated earlier, the nature of bilingual instruction varies widely over bilingual deaf education settings, from "pure" natural sign language to simultaneous communication. It thus may be difficult to sort out the factors contributing to gains in language and literacy, an issue that could be as important to those who object to simultaneous communication as it is to those who find it useful in the classroom (see Marschark and colleagues, 2008).

An early (American) study by Andrews (1988) demonstrated that extensive practice with fingerspelling over a 9-month period gave DHH kindergarteners a significant advantage over a comparison group in their ability to label words with their ASL signs. More recently, several Dutch studies have demonstrated related findings. Wauters, Knoors, Vervloed, and Aarnoutse (2001), for example, found that DHH primary school children recognized more Dutch words that they had learned via both signs and spoken words than those learned only through spoken words. Mollink, Hermans, and Knoors (2008) obtained similar results in a study of younger hard-of-hearing children. Wiefferink, Spaai, Uilenburg, Vermeij, and De Raeve (2008), in contrast, found that in small groups of preschoolers with cochlear implants, Flemish children who used sign-supported speech in school and speech at home showed greater expressive and receptive spoken language skills than Dutch children who attended a bilingual program and whose parents used sign language and speech at home. Importantly, the Dutch children were diagnosed considerably later, and they and their parents received only half the amount of hours of early intervention compared to their Flemish counterparts. The investigators suggested that parents' initial use of sign-supported speech with children with implants would allow effective communication early on, while waiting to determine the extent to which their children would be able to rely exclusively on spoken language.

Rinaldi, Caselli, Onofrio, and Volterra (Chapter 3 of this volume) present data from Italy, where some deaf parents as well as hearing parents use spoken language rather than sign language with their DHH children. Italian bilingual education typically involves teaching assistants competent in Italian Sign Language (LIS) providing limited language support in the classroom in LIS, Signed Italian, or Sign-Supported Italian. Rinaldi and colleagues examined DHH children's competencies in both LIS and Italian, a rare kind of research (but see Tang, Lam, & Yiu, Chapter 13 of this volume). Most generally, those children whose deaf or hearing parents were most accepting of their hearing losses showed greater language abilities. The investigators ascribed that advantage to parents' active participation in their children's education, encouraging their autonomy, and fostering bilingual and bicultural awareness. Finding that the children's combined skills in both LIS and Italian were comparable to the language skills found in Italian-speaking children led them to conclude that "[t]his kind of bilingualism could allow deaf children and adults to move between one culture and language and the other, depending on the different contexts and the different people involved," seemingly the ideal outcome from bilingual deaf education.

Despite the apparent success of simultaneous communication and sign-supported speech with regard to classroom learning (see Marschark & Lee, Chapter 9 of this volume), Plaza-Pust (Chapter 2 of this volume) argues that it was lack of success in the total communication movement rather than in spoken language–only programming that was largely responsible to the turn to bilingual deaf education. With Hermans, Wauters, De Klerk, and Knoors (Chapter 11 of this volume), she noted the role of bimodal communication in classroom communication, rather than primarily as a means of acquiring the written/spoken vernacular. In that context, she voiced support for the importance of prolonged exposure to, if not immersion in, sign language early on as a necessary part of a "global" linguistic-educational effort if children are to become proficient in language and succeed in personal and academic domains. The results of her work and others' indicate that early, effective access to language is essential if children are to become fluent, particularly in the grammar of a language, be it L1 or L2 (see Mayberry, 2010; Plaza-Pust, 2000). Most research concerning DHH children in bilingual programs, however, has included children (of hearing parents) exposed to sign language later, perhaps resulting in the underestimation of bilingualism outcomes.

Plaza-Pust (Chapter 2 of this volume) notes that language acquisition occurs within the gestalt of development—cognitive and social as well as linguistic. Indeed, the larger context of development has broad impact on language acquisition from vocabulary and the organization of lexical knowledge to the ways in which grammar and discourse structure map onto the world and the interactions of metalinguistic and metacognitive functioning in formal and informal learning environments. Marschark and Hauser (2012, chapter 2) described this situation as the interactive and cumulative nature of development, as language, learning, and experience in the world are constantly influencing each other in "top-down" and "bottom-up" ways, just as in the case of reading: what children know (implicitly and explicitly) influences not only what they learn but how they learn it. For that reason, they argued that narrow research foci in specific domains such as language, cognition, or social functioning are insufficient to explain the academic challenges of DHH learners.

Such limited perspectives also have the potential to mislead or even derail efforts to improve linguistic, cognitive, social, and academic outcomes for deaf learners. What is needed is an educational philosophy that accommodates the large individual differences among DHH learners, as well as those between them and their hearing peers. This usually will require accommodations or modification of the learning environment and instructional methods to match the special strengths and needs of DHH students. In others, it may necessitate teaching DHH students new learning and problem-solving strategies that are flexible enough for functioning in broader educational settings and the everyday world. One context in which all of this may be possible is the co-enrollment program. Co-enrollment classrooms certainly are not typical of mainstream classrooms, but they also differ significantly from separate schools and programs for DHH students, even if they are explicitly designed for them.

## CO-ENROLLMENT PROGRAMS FOR DHH AND HEARING STUDENTS

Co-enrollment programs, like bilingual programming, have had slightly different motivations in different countries. Pérez Martin, Valmaseda Balanzategui, and Morgan (Chapter 15 of this volume) explain that such programming in Spain was aimed at reducing DHH students' continuing underachievement in both regular schools and schools for the deaf. In the Netherlands, the goal was to create a viable alternative for individual mainstreaming, taking advantage of its benefits while preserving some of the advantages of schools for the deaf (Hermans, Wauters, De Klerk, and Knoors, Chapter 11 of this volume). As described earlier, co-enrollment programming also varies widely. What those programs have in common is the presence of a critical mass of DHH students being educated in a regular school with hearing peers. By virtue of being embedded within a mainstream classroom, DHH students in a co-enrollment program receive grade-level appropriate instruction in curricula (Luckner, 1999; Tang, Lam, & Yiu, Chapter 13 of this volume; Pérez Martin, Valmaseda Balanzategui, and Morgan, Chapter 15 of this volume) and, at least in principle, are held to the same expectations as hearing peers.

We noted earlier that co-enrollment classrooms involve two teachers, one of whom, either deaf or hearing, usually is either a specialist in education of the deaf (as in the United States) or a deaf individual trained "on the job" (as in Hong Kong). Several chapters in the present volume, and Hermans, De Klerk, Wauters, and Knoors (Chapter 16) in particular, provide information concerning collaborations and communication between teachers and co-enrollment classrooms. Classes in most co-enrollment programs are taught in both sign language and the written/spoken vernacular, but this is not a definitional necessity. There is no reason that a co-enrollment program could not involve spoken language instruction only for DHH students rather than being a bilingual setting. For that reason, this and the following sections consider co-enrollment programming and its outcomes separately from the earlier discussion of bilingual deaf education.

Hermans, de Klerk, Wauters, and Knoors (Chapter 16 of this volume) described six different approaches to the co-teaching that can occur in co-enrollment programs. What they all have in common is that the two teachers coordinate their activities so that they complement rather than repeat each other. Other programs, such as that described by Tang, Lam, & Yiu (Chapter 13 of this volume) and Yiu and Tang (Chapter 14 of this volume) always include a Deaf teacher, who sometimes teaches the same materials simultaneously. At other times, one teacher takes up the major role of teaching and the other assists. To date, there is no evidence that any particular form of co-teaching or co-enrollment programming is necessarily better than any other. Presumably, the precise form of any particular program will depend on the country, context, and students involved. At the same time, the co-enrollment programs represented in this volume all appear to include recognition of the need for flexibility, rather than being driven by a philosophically determined instructional model. As should be apparent to readers of previous chapters, supporters of those programs do have very specific ideas about the nature of the language instruction and language environments in them. By way of putting language issues into the larger context of co-enrollment programming for DHH learners, let us briefly consider the same topic areas we considered for bilingual education. As in the previous sections, these are intended to be representative but not exhaustive, and we refer readers to the earlier chapters for more complete discussion.

## Cognitive and Academic Outcomes Related to Co-enrollment Programming

As far as we are aware, there have not yet been studies conducted on possible cognitive consequences of hearing children being educated in co-enrollment classrooms. Perhaps the closest relevant study is one conducted by Capirci, Cattani, Rossini, and Volterra (1998) in which hearing children who learned Italian Sign Language in school were found to demonstrate significant increases in nonverbal working memory and problem-solving. One can imagine that similar findings might be obtained among hearing children in bilingual co-enrollment programs, although the elementary school students in this particular study were not enrolled in the Italian co-enrollment program. More interesting, perhaps, are the potential effects of co-enrollment programming on DHH students who would be exposed to the learning and problem-solving strategies of their hearing classmates through group activities.

If we do not yet have research directly related to cognitive outcomes for DHH students in co-enrollment programs, there is an emerging body of literature concerning their academic outcomes. In perhaps the first study in that regard, Kreimeyer, Crooke, Drye, Egbert, and Klein (2000) provided in-depth description of the first 3 years of co-enrollment program in the United States (see Antia & Metz, Chapter 17 of this volume). DHH students represented one-quarter to one-third of the students in the elementary school classrooms. On the Stanford Achievement Test (SAT) reading comprehension subtest over 2 years, the DHH students' scores were significantly higher than the DHH norms, but significantly lower than the hearing norms. There were no significant differences between the reading vocabulary scores of DHH students and either the DHH or the hearing norms. The SAT at that time included two mathematics subtests, problem-solving and procedures; overall, the DHH students' performance did not differ from the DHH norms. Antia and Metz (Chapter 17 of this volume) suggest that the mixed Kreimeyer and colleagues results may have been the result of the DHH students' having been in the co-enrollment program for only 3 years. They noted, however, that those students previously had been taught by a teacher of the deaf in a self-contained classroom, which presumably would have involved bilingual programming.

A follow-up study of the US program conducted by McCain and Antia (2005) 7 years after the program had been created found an increasing gap between DHH and hearing students' scores on the SAT reading comprehension subtest. The DHH students made gains in their mathematics subtests scores relative to their hearing peers but still lagged behind them. Still, the authors noted that DHH students in the co-enrollment program outpaced DHH peers in other academic settings according to the SAT DHH norms. Although Hermans, de Klerk, Wauters, and Knoors (Chapter 16 of this volume) did not have test scores available for a similar comparison, they reported that teachers in their co-enrollment program felt that the pace of instruction, coupled with high expectations for all students, was positively associated with the DHH children's academic outcomes. Hermans and colleagues noted in particular that the DHH children's receptive vocabulary scores in their studies were "surprisingly positive," although they still lagged behind those of hearing children. In one of the few reports of academic effects on hearing students in co-enrollment programs, they also reported that co-enrollment did not appear to have either positive or negative effects on hearing children's performance, an important finding for those parents of hearing children who initially were concerned that having DHH children in the classroom might slow their own child's academic growth. Marschark and colleagues (2008) reached a similar conclusion with regard to the use of simultaneous communication in mixed college classrooms of DHH and hearing students.

In short, there is not yet any strong evidence to indicate that co-enrollment programs have any generalized positive (or negative) effects on DHH students' academic achievement or cognitive growth. Results thus far are promising but mixed, perhaps because most programs are quite young. On the other hand, we have already noted that the existing co-enrollment programs all largely are aimed at providing DHH children with instruction in accessible language and a social context that encourages integration with hearing peers. In both of those domains, somewhat more evidence is available.

## Social Outcomes Related to Co-enrollment Programming

An important aspect of the co-enrollment model is the goal of engendering mutual understanding and respect between DHH students and their hearing classmates through their sharing of everyday activities in the classroom (Pérez Martin, Valmaseda Balanzategui, and Morgan, Chapter 15 of this volume). In the US program described by Kreimeyer and colleagues (2000) and Antia and Metz (Chapter 17 of this volume), hearing as well as DHH students may use sign language, and at times it is difficult to know which students are which. Pérez Martin and colleagues suggested that hearing students' learning to sign helps to create a more homogenous learning environment. They found that mutual acceptance of individual differences among the children in their co-enrollment program increased over time, although there was considerable variability. Whether because of increased ease of communication (Antia, Sabers, & Stinson, 2007) or simply getting to know each other as individuals, Kreimeyer and colleagues noted increasing social interactions over time between DHH and hearing students inside and outside the classroom. McCain and Antia's (2005) study of the same program with slightly older children found comparable social behavior ratings for hearing students and DHH students, at least for those who did not have disabilities. Both self- and teacher ratings of social behavior of DHH students with disabilities were significantly lower than those of the DHH students without disabilities. As yet, it does not appear that co-enrollment programs have dealt with this issue, but it is one that continues to create social and academic difficulties in classrooms for the relatively large proportion of DHH children who have multiple disabilities (see Knoors & Marschark, 2014, chapter 7).

Better social relationships between DHH and hearing students also were reported by Kluwin (1999), Bowen (2008), and Wauters and Knoors (2008) in their studies of social functioning in co-enrollment programs. Bowen found that in a primary school classroom, DHH and the hearing students were equally accepted by each other (Yiu & Tang, Chapter 14 of this volume), a finding not obtained in a comparison regular classroom. Among older students who had been in co-enrollment classrooms before third grade, Kluwin found DHH and hearing students to be comparable in terms of their self-concepts with regard to happiness and social standing. Hermans, De Klerk, Wauters, and Knoors (Chapter 16 of this volume), however, suggested that co-enrollment classrooms might not always encourage greater social inclusion of

DHH students. With greater numbers of DHH students, they may be more likely to create their own subgroup, potentially creating greater separation from hearing peers. Further, Hintermair (Chapter 7 of this volume) found that DHH children who spent more time with hearing peers evidenced lower self-esteem with regard to social as well as academic functioning. As in previous studies involving regular classrooms, Hermans, De Klerk, and colleagues found that DHH and hearing students in their co-enrollment program preferred to interact with peers of the same hearing status. They also reported no real differences in the attitudes of hearing students toward DHH peers as a function of being in co-enrollment or regular classrooms, but there was a trend toward those in the co-enrollment setting feeling more positive toward their DHH classmates.

Yiu and Tang (Chapter 14 of this volume) also evaluated hearing students' attitudes toward DHH peers in a co-enrollment program. When children were asked if they liked to play or study with peers of the opposite hearing status, the very positive ratings that each group gave the other were not significantly different. Interestingly, peer ratings also were associated with the DHH children's own attitudes toward deafness. Although initially intended to address the academic needs of DHH children in the complex, multilingual context of Hong Kong, the Yiu and Tang finding of effective social integration in a setting where DHH children were greatly outnumbered by hearing peers demonstrates the broad parameters within which co-enrollment can be mutually beneficial for both groups. Future research may indicate that successful social integration in the Hong Kong co-enrollment program is influenced to some extent by the greater community orientation of Chinese and other Asian cultures relative to the more Western emphasis on individual achievement (cf. Hintermair, Chapter 7 of this volume). Such a finding would not detract from the growing body of literature on co-enrollment, but would help to more clearly articulate where it might be particularly beneficial for various aspects of development and achievement.

Taken together, these findings suggest that co-enrollment programming may have greater impact on the social-emotional functioning of DHH students than their academic outcomes, at least as far as we can tell at this point. In large measure, their lesser social isolation and feelings of loneliness likely are fueled by a greater understanding and acceptance by hearing peers; studies aimed specifically at the social skills of DHH students in co-enrollment and other programs are only beginning (Yiu & Tang, Chapter 14 of this volume).

Studies of the social integration of deaf children with cochlear implants have shown that the use of spoken language alone is insufficient to ensure their acceptance by hearing peers inside or outside the classroom. Generally, such acceptance is related to the quality of deaf children's speech and hearing, as only those with the best skills in those domains are included in the activities of hearing peers (e.g., Bat-Chava & Deignan, 2001). Similar findings might be expected in co-enrollment programs, with both DHH and hearing students who are better at communicating with each other scoring higher on various measures of social acceptance, and DHH students who find they are better able to participate in class demonstrating more positive social-emotional functioning (Antia and colleagues, 2007). Yiu and Tang (Chapter 14 of this volume) found that DHH students' sign language skills, but not their spoken language skills, were positively associated with hearing peers' social ratings of them. They interpreted that result as reflecting the social benefit of enhanced communication in the co-enrollment classroom. Other social skills and linguistic factors also may have been involved because of the extent to which the setting encourages peer interaction of mutual understanding. At present, however, it appears that there are relatively few studies of the *social language skills* of DHH students (or hearing students) in co-enrollment programs, even if facilitating language growth is sometimes seen as their *raison d'être*. Until further studies are conducted, we will have to extrapolate long-term social as well as academic outcomes from the limited information available on language skills of students in co-enrollment programs.

### How Does Co-enrollment Affect Bilingualism?

In describing the advent of bilingual programming and co-enrollment in Spain, Pérez Martin, Valmaseda Balanzategui, and Morgan (Chapter 15 of this volume) note that the two were intertwined from the beginning in order to ensure that classroom communication for DHH students was not just available, but accessible. Having two languages in the classroom not only makes the curriculum accessible to all students but, as noted in the previous section, serves to enhance social understanding and integration. Pérez Martin and colleagues reported that the planning of school activities and language at the same time has resulted in DHH children making significant gains in their sign language skills, albeit with considerable variability, with greater vocabulary growth than DHH students in other educational settings. In contrast to findings with regard to spoken language, co-enrolled DHH students made greater gains in their receptive than their expressive language scores, and their language dominance slowly shifted from Spanish Sign Language to spoken Spanish (see Wheeler, Archbold, Hardie, & Watson, 2009). Pérez Martin and colleagues concluded "that when the language is fully accessible, assessments reveal typical developmental processes, and comprehension precedes production."

Tang, Lam, and Yiu (Chapter 13 of this volume) focused on the language development of children in their co-enrollment program, particularly in the grammatical development of DHH children acquiring spoken Cantonese, written Mandarin, and Hong Kong Sign Language. Their findings indicted that growth of children's syntactic and morphosyntactic competence in the three languages was interrelated, as development in one appeared to predict development in another, and vice versa, likely because of shared knowledge of language (Mineiro, Nunes, Moita, Silva, & Castro-Caldas, Chapter 8 of this volume). Consistent with the general point made earlier, Tang and colleagues found no negative effects of sign language acquisition on children's development of spoken Cantonese or written Mandarin. Just as Ormel and Giezen (Chapter 4 of this volume) suggested that cross-linguistic transfer at the word level facilitates DHH children's language growth, Tang and colleagues argue that the bilingual if not multilingual exposure of Hong Kong children with the three languages likely encourages cross-linguistic transfer at the grammatical level (but see Holzinger & Fellinger, Chapter 5 of this volume, concerning the importance of timing in acquisition). Together with Plaza-Pust (Chapter 2 of this volume), Hermans, Wauters, De Klerk, and Knoors (Chapter 11 of this volume), and others, they argue that the essential factors are the extent to which children are immersed in a rich and consistent language environment and when.

Even if DHH children in Hong Kong have a more complex language-learning situation than DHH peers in other countries, the characteristics of effective learning environments are undoubtedly the same. Whether the results of Tang and colleagues are function of the co-enrollment program in which they were obtained, the trilingual language situation of DHH children in Hong Kong, social and cognitive factors related to the program, or a combination of other factors (e.g., culture, teaching methods, the central role of deaf teachers) remains to be determined. Together with findings from the other co-enrollment programs described in this volume, however, their findings suggest that language programming that recognizes the diverse language and literacy needs of DHH children is more likely to succeed than programming that unilaterally favors one modality or language over others in the child's environment.

## THE WAY FORWARD

Swanwick, Hendar, Dammeyer, Kristoffersen, Salter, and Simonsen (Chapter 12 of this volume) pointed out that we have much to learn from the communication journeys of families of deaf children who receive cochlear implants. The same no doubt is true of the journeys of the families of DHH children and the children themselves (Sutherland & Young, 2007) who experience bilingual education, co-enrollment, and other forms of educational programming. Too often, however, the stories that are told are either testimonials from parents who have found "the true path" in one educational placement or another or the frustrations of families that have not been able to obtain appropriate placement for their DHH children. One can only wonder about the many positive stories that are untold and whether they reveal specific educational factors, beyond the oft-noted impact of parental involvement, that can help us to understand the factors that contribute to the academic, social, and personal successes of so many DHH students. In particular, it is rare that investigators explore the real-world language mosaic of DHH students, which is not one of lifelong or even school-years-long unimodal or monolingual language (Walker & Tomblin, Chapter 6 of this volume). Certainly there are some DHH learners who are surrounded by hearing family members and hearing peers and who come to sign language later, if ever. There are also some DHH learners who are surrounded by deaf family members and deaf peers who come to spoken language later, if ever. Neither of these groups is likely to be the majority, however, and at some point in their lives, perhaps more often later rather than earlier, we expect that most DHH individuals will want to, need to, or benefit from being bilingual. This is not to be prescriptive; this is to be realistic.

Understanding the myriad factors that contribute to child development and academic achievement has never been easy for educational researchers interested in normally developing hearing children, and the situation is far more complex in the case of DHH children and especially those with special needs. Not surprisingly, the smaller the special population involved, the less research is likely to be devoted to it, just as there are fewer assessment tools appropriate for evaluating their growth. In the case of DHH children, it may be that their unique status in many countries as legally disabled but at the same time potentially members of a linguistic-cultural minority explains the difficulties related to discussions about the language(s) to which they are exposed and the educational setting(s) in which they are placed. For better or worse, the relatively limited time frame of "modern" deaf education, since recognition that sign languages are true languages in the 1960s, means that there are still many research questions to be answered and many more still to be asked.

The research reviewed and new findings presented in this volume are too extensive to be easily summarized, but there are points that we believe are self-evident at this point and some promising developments for further investigation. First, we present several broad conclusions with which we would hope most involved in the raising and educating deaf children would agree:

- Early, effective access to language is essential to the normal development of all children, including those who are deaf and hard of hearing.

- Children who do not have such access early on will find it difficult or impossible to become fluent at a later age.
- Lack of language fluency will impede cognitive and social development as well as academic achievement.
- Judging by the majority of children in the world, bilingual education is not dangerous, confusing, or delaying in the context of development.
- The population of DHH children is more diverse than the population of hearing children, and as a result it is unlikely that there will be a single educational method that will be optimal for them all.
- One consequence of this diversity is that there are DHH children who succeed with spoken language, DHH children who succeed with sign language, and DHH children who succeed with both, but no one route should be expected to for all DHH children.

There are also some ways forward indicated by the research and classroom practice described in the previous chapters. With regard to the foundations of language acquisition, both cognitive and linguistic, Ormel and Giezen and Plaza-Pust provide theoretical insights into cross-linguistic and cross-modal transfer, together with cognitive advantages of bilingualism. These appear to offer a framework for future research and practice that is more appropriate for DHH learners and bilingual bimodalism than is the linguistic interdependence model of Cummins (1981). Holzinger and Fellinger (Chapter 5 of this volume) have demonstrated that DHH children do not necessarily have automatic transfer from a signed L1 to a written/spoken L2. But some DHH learners make that leap successfully, even if we do not fully understand which learners succeed or how they achieve that transfer. There is now considerable evidence that such transfer depends on early, effective access to L1 that provides the learner with the foundations of language at several levels (Holzinger & Fellinger, Chapter 5 of this volume; Tang, Lam, and Yiu, Chapter 13 of this volume; Pérez Martín, Valmaseda Balanzategui, & Morgan, Chapter 15 of this volume). Other factors that support the L1-L2 bridge remain to be explored. Some of these will turn out to lie outside language per se. That is, the evidence described in this volume concerning the cognitive and academic advantages of bilingual deaf education point to its complexity as a function of factors related to individual students (e.g., home environments, prior formal and informal educational experiences, language and cognitive abilities), as well as those related to the academic setting (e.g., the quality of language instruction, sensitivity to individual differences in cognitive abilities, the availability of appropriate support services) (Hermans, Wauters, De Klerk, & Knoors, Chapter 11 of this volume; Marschark &

Lee, Chapter 9 of this volume). Future studies will need to indicate how these factors combine for learners of different ages and circumstances.

It is in the social domain where bilingual education, and co-enrollment in particular, appears most successful. Truly inclusive education, "membership" rather than "visitorship," creates a learning environment in which DHH and hearing peers can gain mutual understanding, engage in educational and purely social interactions, and contribute to children's understanding of interpersonal functioning (Yiu & Tang, Chapter 14 of this volume; Hermans, De Klerk, Wauters, & Knoors, Chapter 16 of this volume; Antia & Metz, Chapter 17 of this volume). With inclusive education increasingly the norm, it also holds promise for positively influencing both cognitive development (e.g., executive functioning) and academic achievement, as DHH and hearing children deal with situations that require flexible problem solving. Co-enrollment settings have the advantage of teachers who are cognizant of the strengths and needs of DHH learners (Knoors & Marschark, 2014, chapter 11) and linguistic environments that can support provide rich and diverse learning opportunities.

In order to implement and fully understand the dynamics of such settings, we need more research conducted in the classroom by those who know education best, the teachers (Wauters & De Klerk, Chapter 10 of this volume; Hermans, de Klerk, Wauters, & Knoors, Chapter 16 of this volume). Studies described in this volume contribute to building an evidence base, but future studies are needed both to increase statistical power (i.e., validity) and to allow us to determine the generality of findings obtained from the limited number of co-enrollment programs currently in existence (i.e., reliability). Comparison groups or multiple baseline studies will be helpful in this regard (e.g., Kreimeyer and colleagues, 2000) given the relatively small populations of students involved and differences in programming. For bilingual education more generally, it is essential that studies consider interactions among language, cognition, achievement, and social functioning, rather than focusing on narrowly early-defined questions in these individual areas. Lack of a more holistic approach to research in the area creates greater likelihood of missing important connections between domains and underestimating the synergism they can create.

Taken together, the chapters of this volume reflect the progress being made by people around the world working to educate DHH students in bilingual and inclusive settings while also conducting research to understand how best to do so. Bilingual education may be no more likely than any other form of deaf education to be a panacea, but it clearly is effective for some students in some settings. Additional study will indicate which students will benefit most, and what points in their educational careers, with what kinds of curricular activities and support services.

Swanwick, Hendar, Dammeyer, Kristoffersen, Salter, and Simonsen (Chapter 12 of this volume) argue that "[a] plural view of languages throughout deaf education (not framed as unique to a bilingual perspective) would bring about changes to our knowledge base of deaf children's languages and cultures and would provoke the development of tools to capture the language demographics of our populations, as well as diverse individual language profiles." The knowledge base obtained from this perspective and related educational, developmental, and linguistic research also would provide better foundations for determining when the educational context needs to change to match the DHH student and when the DHH student needs to change to match the educational context. Only then, as Swanwick and colleagues suggested, would we be able to create appropriate language frameworks that build on the strengths and meet the needs of this diverse population. At the same time, this would allow us to better understand the nuances of language development, social development, cognitive development, and learning of DHH children in the context of their larger family and social environments. We would then be able to better inform parents of the options, timelines, and likely outcomes of the decisions they will need to make as they raise and educate their DHH children. We also could design early intervention programming that supports DHH children's language development, going beyond what is considered "low normal" for hearing peers, and provide appropriate, evidence-based professional development for teachers of DHH students (Hermans, Wauters, de Klerk, & Knoors, Chapter 11 of this volume; Knoors & Marschark, 2014, chapter 12; Wauters & de Klerk, Chapter 10 of this volume). Importantly, all of this pertains to DHH children with as well as without cochlear implants. As Walker and Tomblin (Chapter 6 of this volume) noted, both parents and service providers need to consider a variety of factors, including age at intervention and language and intervention histories in deciding which intervention approach is most appropriate if, indeed, any one is preferable to another.

In this volume and elsewhere, we have good evidence that children in bilingual programs show "normal" language growth, but the comparison groups are usually norms or anecdotal generalizations involving children with unknown language and intervention histories. Studies comparing groups of DHH children with specific or at least known backgrounds are essential to determine who will benefit most from what form of bilingual education or some other language intervention. "What form" is important here for two reasons. First, again, bilingual deaf education programs vary widely, and DHH children have diverse language, cognitive, and social needs that may be better served by one kind of program or another. Second, in all of these domains, evidence offered in this volume by Hintermair, Holzinger and Fellinger, Ormel and Giezen, Plaza-Pust, and others has emphasized that earlier language acquisition is clearly better than later language acquisition. Yet if the critical or sensitive periods for language learning are early on, similar periods for various cognitive and social interventions may not be. In those domains, as well as in various aspects of language learning, there may be zones of proximal development (Vygotsky, 1993) that differ for DHH children relative to hearing age-mates and differences within the population of DHH children depending on their context and the specific language(s) they are learning.

If the preceding suggests that we have any doubts about the importance of bilingual education for DHH children, it is only about the nuances of such programming and not about its core tenets. Although it may not be necessary for all DHH learners, there seems little doubt that various forms of bilingual education and co-enrollment will be beneficial for a large number of DHH learners who vary widely on personal and environmental dimensions. The chapters of this volume demonstrate the viability of those methods as well as outlining specific questions and directions for practice, professional development, and future research. If the product of the various reviews and studies is not as clear as some might have hoped, it is not for lack of trying, but a reflection of reality. Still, as the Chinese proverb warns and encourages us, a journey of 1,000 miles begins with a single step.

## REFERENCES

Andrews, J. F. (1988). Deaf children's acquisition of prereading skills using the reciprocal teaching procedure. *Exceptional Children, 54*, 349–355.

Antia, S. D., Sabers, D., & Stinson, M. S. (2007). Validity and reliability of the Classroom Participation Questionnaire with deaf and hard-of-hearing students in public schools. *Journal of Deaf Studies and Deaf Education, 12*, 158–171.

Archbold, S. M., Harris, M., O'Donoghue, G. M., Nikolopoulos, T. P., White, A., & Richmond, H. L. (2008). Reading abilities after cochlear implantation: The effect of age at implantation on outcomes at five on seven years after implantation. *International Journal of Pediatric Otorhinolaryngology, 72*, 1471–1478.

Bagga-Gupta, S. (2004). *Literacies and deaf education: A theoretical analysis of the international and Swedish literature*. Stockholm: The Swedish National Agency for School Improvement.

Bat-Chava, Y., & Deignan, E. (2001). Peer relationships of children with cochlear implants. *Journal of Deaf Studies and Deaf Education, 6*, 186–199.

Bergin, C., & Bergin, D. (2009). Attachment in the classroom. *Educational Psychological Review, 21*, 141–170.

Borgna, G., Convertino, C., Marschark, M., Morrison, C., & Rizzolo, K. (2011). Enhancing deaf students' learning from sign language and text: Metacognition, modality, and the effectiveness of content scaffolding. *Journal of Deaf Studies and Deaf Education, 16*, 79–100.

Bowen, S. (2008). Coenrollment for students who are deaf or hard of hearing: Friendship patterns and social interactions. *American Annals of the Deaf*, 153, 285–293.

Calderon, R. & Greenberg, M. (2011). Social and emotional development of deaf children: Family, school, and program effects. In M. Marschark & P. E. Spencer (Eds.), *The Oxford handbook of deaf studies, language, and education* (2nd ed., vol. 1, pp. 188–199). New York, NY: Oxford University Press.

Capirci, O., Cattani, A., Rossini, & Volterra, V. (1998). Teaching sign language to hearing children as a possible factor in cognitive enhancement. *Journal of Deaf Studies and Deaf Education*, 3, 135–142.

Cormier, K., Schembri, A., Vinson, D., & Orfanidou, E. (2012). First language acquisition differs from second language acquisition in prelingually deaf signers: Evidence from sensitivity to grammaticality judgement in British Sign Language. *Cognition*, 124(1), 50–65.

Cummins, J. (1981). *Bilingualism and minority language children*. Ontario, Canada: Ontario Institute for Studies in Education.

Dammeyer, J. (2010). Psychosocial development in a Danish population of children with cochlear implants and deaf and hard-of-hearing children. *Journal of Deaf Studies and Deaf Education*, 15, 50–58.

Davidson, K., Lillo-Martin, D., & Pichler, D. C. (2014). Spoken English language development in native signing children with cochlear implants. *Journal of Deaf Studies and Deaf Education*, 19, 238–250.

DeKeyser, R., & Larson-Hall, J. (2005). What does the critical period really mean? In J. F. Kroll & A. B. de Groot (Eds.), *Handbook of bilingualism: Psycholinguistic approaches* (pp. 88–108). New York, NY: Oxford University Press.

Geers, A., Tobey, E., Moog, J., & Brenner, C. (2008). Long-term outcomes of cochlear implantation in the preschool years: From elementary grades to high school. *International Journal of Audiology*, 47(Supplement 2), S21–S30.

Holcomb, T. K. (2013). *An introduction to American deaf culture*. New York, NY: Oxford University Press.

Humphries, T., Kushalnagar, P., Mathur, G., Napoli, D. J., Padden, C., Rathmann, C., & Smith, C. R. (2012). Language acquisition for deaf children: Reducing the harms of zero tolerance to the use of alternative approaches. *Harm Reduction Journal*, 2012, 9–16.

Kluwin, T. N. (1999). Coteaching deaf and hearing students: Research on social integration. *American Annals of the Deaf*, 144, 339–344.

Kovelman, I., Baker, S. A., & Petitto, L. A. (2008). Age of first bilingual language exposure as a new window into bilingual reading development. *Bilingualism: Language and Cognition*, 11, 203–223.

Knoors, H., & Marschark, M. (2012). Language planning for the 21st century: Revisiting bilingual language policy for deaf children. *Journal of Deaf Studies and Deaf Education*, 17, 291–305.

Knoors, H., & Marschark, M. (2014). *Teaching deaf learners: Psychological and developmental foundations*. New York, NY: Oxford University Press.

Kreimeyer, K. H., Crooke, P., Drye, C., Egbert, V., & Klein, B. (2000). Academic and social benefits of a coenrollment model of inclusive education for deaf and hard-of-hearing children. *Journal of Deaf Studies and Deaf Education*, 5, 174–185.

Lang, H. G., & Meath-Lang, B. (1995). *Deaf persons in the arts and sciences: A biographical dictionary*. Westport, CT: Greenwood Press.

Lange, C. M., Lane-Outlaw, S., Lange, W. E., & Sherwood, D. L. (2013). American Sign Language/English bilingual model: A longitudinal study of academic growth. *Journal of Deaf Studies and Deaf Education, 18*, 532–544.

Luckner, J. (1999). An examination of two coteaching classrooms. *American Annals of the Deaf, 144*, 24–34.

Marschark, M. (1993). *Psychological development of deaf children*. New York, NY: Oxford University Press.

Marschark, M., Convertino, C., McEvoy, C., & Masteller, A. (2004). Organization and use of the mental lexicon by deaf and hearing individuals. *American Annals of the Deaf, 149*, 51–61.

Marschark, M., & Hauser, P. C. (2012). *How deaf children learn*. New York, NY: Oxford University Press.

Marschark, M., & Knoors, H. (2012). Educating deaf children: Language, cognition, and learning. *Deafness and Education International, 14*, 137–161.

Marschark, M., Leigh, G., Sapere, P., Burnham, D., Convertino, C., Stinson, M., Knoors, H., Vervloed, M. P. J., & Noble, W. (2006). Benefits of sign language interpreting and text alternatives to classroom learning by deaf students. *Journal of Deaf Studies and Deaf Education, 11*, 421–437.

Marschark, M., Sapere, P., Convertino, C. M., & Pelz, J. (2008). Learning via direct and mediated instruction by deaf students. *Journal of Deaf Studies and Deaf Education, 13*, 446–461.

Marschark, M., Sapere, P., Convertino, C., & Seewagen, R. (2005). Access to postsecondary education through sign language interpreting. *Journal of Deaf Studies and Deaf Education, 10*, 38–50.

Maxwell-McCaw, D., & Zea, M. C. (2011). The Deaf Acculturation Scale (DAS): Development and validation of a 58-item measure. *Journal of Deaf Studies and Deaf Education, 16*, 325–342.

Mayberry, R. I. (2010). Early language acquisition and adult language ability: What sign language reveals about the critical period for language. In M. Marschark & P. Spencer (Eds.), *The Oxford handbook of deaf studies, language, and education* (vol. 2, pp. 281–291). New York, NY: Oxford University Press.

Mayberry, R. I., & Lock, E. (2003). Age constraints on first versus second language acquisition: Evidence for linguistic plasticity and epigenesis. *Brain and Language, 87*, 369–383.

McCain, K., & Antia, S. D. (2005). Academic and social status of hearing, deaf, and hard-of- hearing students participating in a co-enrolled classroom. *Communication Disorders Quarterly, 27*, 20–32.

Mollink, H., Hermans, D., & Knoors, H. (2008). Vocabulary training of spoken words in hard-of-hearing children. *Deafness and Education International, 10*, 80–92.

Nitrouer, S., Caldwell, A., Lowenstein, J., Tarr, E., & Holloman, C. (2012). Emergent literacy in kindergartners with cochlear implants. *Ear and Hearing, 33*, 683–697.

Nover, S., Andrews, J., Baker, S., Everhart, V., & Bradford, M. (2002). *ASL/English Bilingual instruction for deaf students: Evaluation and impact study. Final report* 1997–2002. Retrieved April 2, 2013, from http://www.gallaudet.edu/Documents/year5.pdf.

Padden, C., & Humphries, T. (2005). *Inside Deaf culture*. Cambridge, MA: Harvard University Press.

Pisoni, D. B., Conway, C. M., Kronenberger, W., Henning, S., & Anaya, E. (2010). Executive function, cognitive control and sequence learning in deaf children with cochlear implants. In M. Marschark & P. E. Spencer, *The Oxford handbook of deaf studies, language, and education* (vol. 2, pp. 439–457). New York, NY: Oxford University Press.

Plaza-Pust, C. (2000). *Linguistic theory and adult second language acquisition: On the relation between the lexicon and the syntax.* Frankfurt am Main, Germany: Peter Lang.

Stinson, M. S., & Kluwin, T. N. (2011). Educational consequences of alternative school placements. In M. Marschark & P. Spencer (Eds.), *The Oxford handbook of deaf studies, language, and education* (2nd ed., vol. 1, pp. 47–62). New York, NY: Oxford University Press.

Sutherland, H., & Young, A. M. (2007). "Hate English! Why . . ." Signs and English from deaf children's perception: Results from a preliminary study of deaf children's experience of sign bilingual education. *Deafness and Education International, 9*, 197–213.

Vygotsky, L. S. (1993). *The Collected Works of L. S. Vygotsky, volume 2: The fundamentals of defectology (abnormal psychology and learning disabilities)*, R. W. Rieber and A. S. Carton (Eds.). New York, NY: Plenum Press.

Wauters, L., Knoors, H., Vervloed, M. P. J., & Aarnoutse, C. (2001). Sign facilitation in word recognition. *Journal of Special Education, 35*, 31–40.

Wheeler, A., Archbold, S. M., Hardie, T., & Watson, L. M. (2009). Children with cochlear implants: The communication journey. *Cochlear Implants International, 10*, 41–62.

Wiefferink, C., Spaai, G., Uilenburg, N., Vermeij, B., & De Raeve, L. (2008). Influence of linguistic environment on children's language development: Flemish versus Dutch children. *Deafness and Education International, 10*, 226–243.

# Index

Page numbers followed by f and t refer to figures and tables page numbers respectively.

Academic outcomes. *See also specific types*
   of bilingual education programs, 454–457
      Austrian studies of, 110–125
   of co-enrollment programs, 463–465
      in U.S., 429–432, 430t
   factors predicting, 247–248
   language of instruction on, 275–279, 278t
      child's preference of, grouping by, 276
      Marschark et al. studies of, 275–276
      sign language of the Netherlands *vs.* sign-supported Dutch in, 276–279, 278t
Accessibility, in Madrid sign bilingual and co-enrollment programs, 374–375
Achievement pressure, on quality of instruction, 285–286, 285t
Added-value bilingual education, 215
Age of acquisition, language, 331
   on bimodal bilingual brain, 197–198
   early, for sign language, 214–215
      benefits of, 197–199
   on functional anatomy of brain, 189–190
      with ASL, 189–190
   on language proficiency, 88–91, 93
Alphabetics, 249–250
American Sign Language (ASL). *See also specific programs and topics*
   age of acquisition of, on functional anatomy of brain, 189–190
   proficiency and reading comprehension in, on bimodal bilingual brain, 201
   research on
      early linguistic, impetus for, 313
      on raising and educating deaf children, 313–314
   sign bilingual programming for, 314–317
Aphasia, 187
Arizona program, 398–399

Assessment
   of bilingual deaf education, 2–3
   definition of, 58
   of linguistic skills in preschoolers, 58–61
      code-mixing phenomena on, 59–60
      combination of methods in, 60
      deaf professional presence on, 67–68
      dominant language on, 59
      integrated language assessment for, 67
      reliable and valid tools in, 60
      sign language tests in, 60–61 (*See also specific tests and programs*)
   of psychosocial development, 177
Assessment, outcome, of DHH student bilingual programming, 451–462
   bilingualism in, 459–462
   cognitive-academic outcomes in, 452–458
      academic outcomes in, 454–457
      cognition in, 452–454
      pedagogy in, 457–458
   generalizations on, 451
   language importance in, 451
   learner heterogeneity on, 451
   signed *vs.* written/spoken language linguistics in, 451
   social outcomes in, 458–459
Assistive listening devices. *See also specific types*
   on bilingualism in classroom, 214
   on Northern European sign language bilingual education, 296–298
   speech discrimination with, on reading comprehension, 105–106, 110, 121, 122, 125, 126, 128
Attitudes toward deafness, in Hong Kong co-enrollment program
   peer ratings of, 352–354, 353t
   of students
      DHH, 353t, 354–355
      social acceptance and, 359

Attitudes toward DHH students, of hearing peers' in Hong Kong co-enrollment program, 346, 355–358, 356t–357t
Auditory cortex. *See also* Bilingual brain; Bimodal bilingual brain
cross-modal reorganization of, 195
Auditory-oral communication, 138–139
Auditory-oral communication, *vs.* total communication
with cochlear implants, 143–147 (*See also under* Cochlear implants, communication mode on language development with)
with hearing aids, 140–143
early studies on, 140
Geers and Moog later adolescence studies on, 142–143
Geers and Schick on, 141–142
Greenberg, Calderon, and Kusché on, 140–141
Geers, Moog, and Schick on, 141
Auditory sensory-modality deprivation, on bimodal bilingual brain, 195–196
Austria, studies of academic outcomes of bilingual programs in, 110–125. *See also under* Reading comprehension, sign language and
Automaticity, improving, in reading instruction, 260, 260f
Automatic transfer, of sign language skills as L1 to L2 literacy, 102, 103, 124, 125–128. *See also* Reading comprehension, sign language and

Balanced bilingualism, 218
Behaviorally oriented approaches, to instruction, 279
Behavioral problems, 161–163
Belgium, Dutch-speaking, cochlear implants on language development in, 135, 136–137
Bicultural affiliation, for psychosocial development, 178
Bicultural deaf education, 449
Bilingual acquisition
co-enrollment on, 331
simultaneous or sequential, 332–333

Bilingual-bicultural education, 215
Bilingual-bicultural programming, 215–216
with cochlear implants, 135–138
research on, 135
Bilingual brain, 190–195
age of L2 acquisition on, 192–194
bilingual switching areas in, 191
caudate nucleus in, 191
cognitive benefits of, 218–220
executive control processes in, 192
gray matter density and performance in, 192
language knowledge in, implicit *vs.* explicit, 195
language organization in, functional, 194–195
language processing in, dual-language, 190–191
language proficiency and brain architecture/processing in, 194
language task schemas in, 191–192
plasticity of, 190, 192
Bilingual deaf education, 1–16. *See also specific types and topics*
bilingualism and, 4–5
context and philosophy of, 2–3
definitions and boundaries of, 446–447, 449
evaluation of, 2–3
foundations of, 3–7
bilingualism and bilingual education in, 4–5
Deaf people as cultural and linguistic minority in, 5–6
results of oral Deaf education in, 6–7
sign language research in, 3–4
history of, recent, 1
implementation of, controversy in, 1
issues in, 9–16
bilingual education and, 10–11
cochlear implants in, 10, 12, 64–66, 92
Cummins's Linguistic Interdependence model in, 11, 24, 25–28
globalization in, 10–11
hearing parents in, 12–13
research on, lack of, 10, 13–15
rich learning environments in, 12–13, 93

meaning of, 213–214
in the Netherlands, 9, 272–273
    quality of instruction in, 272–273
objectives and programming in, 7–9
parallel bilingual education in, 8–9
in Scandinavia, 7, 8
school setting in, 9
second language in, 8–9
settings for, 450
Bilingual education, 10–11
on reading comprehension, 223
Bilingualism. *See also* Sign bilingualism; *specific topics*
advantages of, 75
balanced, among deaf children, 218
bilingual education on, 459–462
as brain exercise, 75
in classroom (*See* Classroom, bilingualism in)
co-enrollment programs on, 467–468 (*See also* Co-enrollment programs)
in deaf students, 2
definition of, 94
on reading comprehension, 226
Bilingual language acquisition in deaf learners, 28–41
critical period effects in, 29–30, 89–90
sign language development in, 30–35
    challenges to sign language learners in, 30–31
    in children of hearing non-signing parents, 31
    developmental trajectories in, 30
    in French-speaking Switzerland (Niederberger, Tuller et al.), 31–32
    in Germany (Plaza-Pust), 35
    referential establishment in, 31
written language development in, 35–41
    attaining target L2 grammar in, 36–41
    attaining writing system in, 35–36
Bilingual switching areas, 191
Bimodal bilingual brain, 195–203
age of acquisition of language on, 197–198
ASL proficiency and reading comprehension in, 201
auditory sensory-modality deprivation on, 195–196
in children of deaf parents, 201

code-blends *vs.* code-switching in, 196–197
cognitive advantages of, 218–219
cross-modal reorganization of auditory cortex in, 195
early sign language acquisition benefits in, 197–199
functional connectivity in, 203
grammatical judgments in, 201–202
neural plasticity in, extra, 196
phonology and reading in, 200–201
reading decoding and visual word form area in, 199–200
signing and reading skills in, 200
vocabulary in, 201
Bimodal bilinguals (bilingualism), 54, 74
cochlear implants on, 10, 12, 92
    longitudinal study of, 64–66
cognitive control in, 86–88
cross-language interaction by, 74–94 (*See also* Cross-language interaction, bimodal bilingual)
educational contexts for, differing, 57–58
in Italy, 55–57
language acquisition in, research on, 317
prevalence of, 227
sign language plus written language in, 235
types of, 74–75
*vs.* unimodal bilingualism, 56
Brain. *See also* Neurobiology, of bilingualism and bimodal bilingualism
bilingual, 190–195 (*See also* Bilingual brain)
bimodal bilingual, 195–203 (*See also* Bimodal bilingual brain)
language areas in, 187–189, 189f
Brain plasticity
in bilingual brain, 190
in bimodal bilingual brain, 196
structural, 192
Broca's area, 187, 188, 189f

Caudate nucleus, in bilingual brain, 191
Chaining, 45
Child development, language, cognition, and emotion in, 154–156

Children of deaf parents, bimodal bilingual brain in, 201
Classroom, bilingualism in, 213–235
  bilingual education for hearing vs. deaf students in, 220
  cognition and, 218–220
  deaf parents as mentors/models for deaf children in, 216–217
  digital hearing aids and cochlear implants on, 214
  future of, 232–235
    bilingualism at home vs. school in, 233–234
    cognitive development/functioning in, 234
    complexity of issue in, 233
    lack of empirical support in, 232–233
    research needs in, 234–235
  L1 to L2 skills transfer in, 217
  learning and school in, 220–226
    bilingualism on reading achievement in, 222–226 (See also Reading comprehension, bilingualism on)
    in Scandinavian deaf education, 220–222
  meaning of bilingual deaf education in, 213–214
  overview of, 214–216
    added-value bilingual education in, 215
    bilingual-bicultural education in, 215
    bilingual-bicultural programming in, 215–216
    early acquisition of sign language in, 214–215
  as safe harbor, 230–232
    on functional aspects of language, 230
    lack of empirical support for, 230–232
    mainstreaming as improved education in, 230–231
  vs. sign language at home in, 216
  sign language on, 214
  simultaneous communication, bimodality, and deaf education in, 227–230
    definition of, 227
    signing and children with cochlear implants in, 228–230
    written/spoken vernacular fluency in, 213–214

Classroom climate, 285t, 286
Classroom communication, 213
Classroom participation, co-enrollment programs on, 435–436
Cochlear implants
  auditory-oral communication vs. total communication with, 143–147
  benefits of, 134
  on bilingual deaf education, 10, 12
  on bilingualism in classroom, 214
  on bimodal bilingualism, 92
    in Italian children, 66
    longitudinal study of, 64–66
  educational settings with, research on, 134
  in Italian children, 58, 66
  on Northern European sign language bilingual education, 296–298
  on reading, 244–245, 454
  sign bilingual co-enrollment with, in Madrid, Spain, 368–390 (See also Co-enrollment programs, sign bilingual with cochlear implants in Madrid)
  signing for children with, 228–230
  sign language instruction with, on academic achievement, 454–455
  social integration of deaf children with, 466–467
  speech discrimination with, on reading comprehension, 105–106, 110, 121, 122, 125, 126, 128
Cochlear implants, communication mode on language development with, 134–148
  auditory-oral approaches in, 138–139
  auditory-oral vs. total communication and, with hearing aids, 140–143
  early studies on, 140
  Geers and Moog later adolescence studies on, 142–143
  Geers and Schick on, 141–142
  Greenberg, Calderon, and Kusché on, 140–141
  Geers, Moog, and Schick on, 141
  auditory-oral vs. total communication in, with cochlear implants, 143–147
  Connor et al. on, 146–147

Dawson et al. on, 144
equivocal research on, 143–144
Geers and Sedey on, 145
Geers et al. on, 144–145
Geers, Spehar, and Sedey on, 146
Hyde and Punch on, 146
Moog and Geers on, 144
prevalence of, 143
Robbins et al. on, 144
technology improvements on, 143
Watson et al. on, 147
bilingual-bicultural approaches in, 135–138
in the Netherlands and Dutch-speaking Belgium, 135, 136–137
in Norway, 135–136, 137
Wie et al. on, 135–136, 137
Wierrerink et al. on, 135, 136–137
deaf education models and, 134–135
evidence-based research on, need for, 148
models of deaf education and, 134–135
total communication approaches in, 139–140
Code-blending, 57, 76
in bimodal bilingual brain, 196–197
in preschoolers, 57, 59
Code-mixing, 59–60, 76
Code-switching
in children, 59
in classroom, 45–46
Co-enrollment programs, 318–319. *See also specific types*
aims and potential benefits of, 400–401
on bilingualism, 467–468
bilingualism in, 450–451
*vs.* cluster inclusion models, 425
cognitive and academic outcomes of, 463–465
co-teaching in, 426, 462–463
in Hong Kong (*See* Hong Kong Sign Bilingualism and Co-enrollment Program)
inclusion in, 174–176
motivations for, 462
origin of, 424
perspectives on, 462–468
social integration in (*See* Social integration, in sign bilingual and co-enrollment environment)

*vs.* traditional inclusion models, 425–426
variations in, 462
Co-enrollment programs, in United States, 424–440
Arizona program, 398–399
benefits of, 426
to students, 426–428
to teachers, 428
challenges of, 436–437
co-teaching in, 426, 462–463
history and philosophy of, 424–426, 427t
origins of, 424
outcomes of, 428–436
academic, 429–432, 430t
classroom participation, 435–436
communication, 433–434
importance of, 428–429
signed, 434–435
social, 432–433
purpose of, 424
research on
quality of evidence on, 437–439, 439t
summary of, 427t
staff comments on, 440
*vs.* traditional inclusion models, 425–426
TRIPOD (Foothill Selpa), 397–398
Co-enrollment programs, sign bilingual education in the Netherlands, 396–420
history of, 396–399
Twinschool program evaluation in, 406–419
focus of, 406
language proficiency in, of sign language of the Netherlands, 415
language proficiency in, of spoken Dutch, 414–415
perceptions of, children's, 415–417, 417t
perceptions of, parents', 417–419, 419t
school achievements in, of DHH children, 411–414, 413t
school achievements in, of hearing children, 410–411, 412t
school achievements in, summary of, 419–420
social position of DHH children in, 406–410, 409t

Co-enrollment programs, sign bilingual education in the Netherlands (*Cont.*)
  Twinschool program in, 399–406
    aims and potential benefits of, 400–401
    demographics of, 401–402, 402t
    educational system of, 404–405
    founding and role of, 399–400
    language policy in, 405–406
    language proficiency of DHH children at entry in, 403–404, 403t
    support team in, 405
Co-enrollment programs, sign bilingual with cochlear implants in Madrid, 368–390
  bilingual schools participating in, 371–378
    curriculum in, 372–373
    curriculum organization in, 371–372
    methodology of, 373–376
    specific subject areas for deaf children in, 376–377
    students, structure, and organization of, 371, 372t
    team members in, 377–378
  conclusions and future directions in, 386–390
    bilingualism in, 386–387
    challenges in, 387–388
    moving forward in, 388–389
    variability in, 387
  history of, 368–371
  outcome study of, 378–386
    assessments and participants in, 379, 380t, 381t
    audition in, 379
    need for, 378–379
    previous studies and, 378–379
    social-emotional skills in, 385–386, 387f
    Spanish sign language skills in, 382–383, 383f, 384t
    Spanish sign language *vs.* Spanish skills in, 383–385, 385f, 386f
    spoken Spanish skills in, 380–382, 382t
  special characteristics of, 370
Cognition. *See also* Brain
  bilingual education on, 452–454
  bilingualism and, 218–220
  in child development, 154–156
  co-enrollment programs on, 463
Cognitive control, bilingualism on, 83–88
  in bimodal bilinguals, 86–88
  in children learning two spoken languages, 85–86
  research on, overview of, 83–84
  in unimodal bilingual adults, 84–85
Cognitive factors, in deaf students' learning, 245–247
  executive function in, 247
  information and learning integration in, 246
  knowledge and knowledge orientation in, 245–246
  memory in, 246–247
  metacognition in, 246
  reading instruction in, 247
Co-learning, 360–361
Collaborative teaching. *See* Co-teaching
Communication. *See also specific types*
  centrality of, 302
  classroom
    on students, 213
    on teachers, 213
  co-enrollment programs on, 433–434
  parent–child, 176
  plurilingualism in, 300–304 (*See also* Plurilingualism, in Northern Europe)
Contact, with other DHH children and adults, 178
Co-teaching
  in co-enrollment programs, 426, 462–463
  in sign bilingual and co-enrollment, 360–361
Co-tutors, 377
Critical mass, of DHH students in sign bilingual and co-enrollment programs, 362–363
Critical period effects, 29–30, 89–90
Critical period hypothesis, 194
Cross-language interaction, bimodal bilingual, 74–94
  age of acquisition and language proficiency in, 88–91, 93
  bilingualism on cognitive control in, 83–88
  in bimodal bilinguals, 86–88

in children learning two spoken
languages, 85–86
research on, 83–84
in unimodal bilingual adults, 84–85
by bimodal bilingual adults, 78–80
bimodal *vs.* unimodal bilinguals in, 74
code-mixing and code-blending in, 76
cross-linguistic transfer and, 76
developmental perspective on, 80–83
in children learning spoken language
and sign language, 81–83, 82f
in children learning two spoken
languages, 80–81
on educational practice, 91–94
family support services and medical
professionals in, 93–94
fundamentals of, 74–75
by unimodal bilingual adults, 76–77
Cross-linguistic transfer, 76
Cross-modal language borrowing, 42–45
Cross-modal language contact
phenomena, 41–46
code-switching in classroom in, 45–46
cross-modal language borrowing in,
42–45
language choice in, 41–42
Cross-modal reorganization, of auditory
cortex, 195
Cummins's Linguistic Interdependence
Model. *See* Linguistic
Interdependence Model
Curriculum, in Madrid sign bilingual and
co-enrollment schools
content of, 372–373
organization of, 371–372
specific subject areas for deaf children
in, 376–377

Deaf, 292
Deaf affiliation, 178
Deaf education. *See also specific types and topics*
bicultural, 449
cochlear implants and, 134–135 (*See also*
Cochlear implants, communication
mode on language development
with)
inclusive, co-enrollment in, 343–345
(*See also* Co-enrollment programs)

models of, 134–135
oral, results of, 6–7
Deaf identities, in psychosocial
development, 178–179
Deaf people, as cultural and linguistic
minority, 5–6
Deaf sign language specialists, 369, 377
Deaf teacher presence, 363
Denmark. *See also* Northern Europe, sign
language bilingual education in
history of bilingual education in, 294–295
inclusion agenda in, 298
teacher training in deaf education in,
302–303
Developmental linguistics, 24
Didactics, in quality of instruction, 285t,
286
Difference, *vs.* deficiency, 153–154
Digital hearing aids. *See* Hearing aids
Directed-reading thinking activity
(DRTA), 253
Direct instruction
on reading instruction, 262, 263f
on student engagement, 280
Diversity, in Madrid sign bilingual and
co-enrollment schools, 375–376
Dominant language, on linguistic skills
assessment in children, 59
Dutch-speaking Belgium, cochlear
implants on language development
in, 135, 136–137

Educational system, in sign bilingual
co-enrollment programs
in Hong Kong, 320–321
in Madrid, Spain, 371–372
in the Netherlands, 404–405
Education, bilingualism in. *See* Classroom,
bilingualism in
Education, deaf
bicultural, 449
bilingual (*See* Bilingual deaf education)
cochlear implants and, 134–135 (*See also*
Cochlear implants, communication
mode on language development
with)
inclusive, co-enrollment in, 343–345
models of, 134–135
oral, results of, 6–7

Emotional problems, 161–163
Emotion, in child development, 154–156
Empowerment perspective, 153
Environments. *See also specific types*
    learning, rich, 12–13, 93
Error-Related Negativity (ERN)-like response, 85
Evaluation. *See* Assessment
Evidence-based education, 3
Executive control processes, in bilingual brain, 192
Executive function, in deaf students' learning, 247
Explaining and maintaining goal, in reading instruction, 262, 263f
Explicit language knowledge, in bilingual brain, 195

Fluency, 250
Fluency instruction, 250–251
Foothill Selpa program, 397–398
French-speaking Switzerland, sign language development in, 31–32
Functional connectivity, in bimodal bilingual brain, 203

Germany, sign language development in, 35
Globalization, 10–11
Goals
    explaining and maintaining, in reading instruction, 262, 263f
    positive, 153
Grammar
    brain processing of, 189
    cross-model linguistic transfer of, between signed language and spoken language, 329–330 (*See also* Co-enrollment programs, sign bilingual education in Hong Kong)
    development of
        attaining target L2 grammar in bilingual language acquisition and, 36–41
        in Hong Kong co-enrollment study, 321–323
        in Madrid sign bilingual and co-enrollment schools, 380–385, 382t, 384t, 388
    judgments on, in bimodal bilingual brain, 201–202
Graphemes, 249
Gray matter density, and performance in bilingual brain, 192

Happy life, psychosocial development for, 152
Hearing aids
    auditory-oral *vs.* total communication with, 140–143
        early studies on, 140
        Geers and Moog later adolescence studies on, 142–143
        Geers and Schick on, 141–142
        Greenberg, Calderon, and Kusché on, 140–141
        Geers, Moog, and Schick on, 141
    on bilingualism in classroom, 214
    on Northern European sign language bilingual education, 296–298
    on reading, 244–245
Hearing parents. *See* Parents, hearing
Hong Kong Sign Bilingualism and Co-enrollment Program, 319–334, 346–359. *See also* Social integration, in sign bilingual and co-enrollment environment
    assessment outcomes in, 324–328, 324t, 327t
    assessment procedures in, 321–323
        CGA-primary and KG (Chinese grammatical knowledge), 323
        HKCOLAS-CG (Cantonese grammar), 321–323
        Hong Kong Sign Language Elicitation Tool, 323
    attitudes toward deafness and social acceptance in, students', 359
    attitudes toward deafness in, DHH students', 353t, 354–355
    attitudes toward DHH students in, hearing peers', 346, 355–358, 356t–357t
    child participants in, 321, 322t
    concluding observations on, 333–334
    *vs.* conventional mainstream setting, 346–347
    goals of, 320
    history of, 348–349

implications of findings of, 328–333
  bilingual acquisition in, 331
  cross-modal, linguistic transfer of grammar between signed language and spoken language in, 329–331
  Cummins's interdependence hypothesis and, 330–331
  for deaf children of hearing parents, 331–332
  early L2 acquisition in, 332
  immersion in an acquisition-rich environment in, 333
  interactions between signed and spoken language in, 329
  scaffolding effect of transferring of linguistic knowledge in, 331
  simultaneous or sequential bilingual acquisition in, 332–333
  timing of language input in, 331
language of co-enrollment education in, 347–348
peer ratings in, 350–354, 351f, 351t, 352f, 353t
previous research on, 348
self-perception of DHH students in, 348
social acceptance between DHH and hearing students in, 349–350
sociolinguistic context of, 320–321
varieties of, 347

Identities
  inclusion and, 171–172
  in psychosocial development, 178–179
Immersion, in acquisition-rich environment, 333
Implicit language knowledge, in bilingual brain, 195
Inclusion, 170–176
  in co-enrollment programs, 174–176, 343–345 (*See also* Co-enrollment programs)
  in Madrid, Spain, 373–374
  identity and, 171–172
  philosophy of, 170–171
  on psychosocial development, 178
  psychosocial risks of, 172–174
Information and learning integration, 246
Instruction. *See* Reading instruction; *specific types*

Interacting systems, in bilingual language development, 23
Interpreters, 378
Italian sign language and spoken language, in preschoolers, 61–66
  bimodal bilingualism and cochlear implants in, longitudinal study of, 64–66
  from deaf *vs.* hearing families, 61–63
  difficulties maintaining bilingualism in, 66
  lexical production assessment and total conceptual vocabulary in, 63–64
Italy
  bilingualism in, 54–58
    educational contexts for, differing, 57–58
    minority language bilingualism in, 55
    official status of, 55
    research on, scarcity of, 66–67
    unimodal and bimodal bilingualism in, 54–57
  cochlear implants in, 58
  language acquisition by bilingual deaf preschoolers in, 54–68 (*See also* Preschoolers, bilingual deaf, language acquisition by)

Knowledge, in deaf students' learning, 245–246
Korthagen model of reading instruction, 255, 255f

L1, as sign *vs.* print language, 223–224
L1 to L2 skills transfer, 217
  automatic, of sign language skills, 102, 103, 124, 125–128 (*See also* Reading comprehension, sign language and)
L2
  age of acquisition of
    on bilingual brain, 192–194
    early, in Hong Kong co-enrollment study, 332
  face-to-face comprehension and expressive proficiency in, interdependence hypothesis on, 103
  literacy in, L1 skills and, 102–104
  as written language, deaf learner acquisition of target grammar in, 36–41

Language. *See also* Sign language; *specific programs and topics*
  acquisition of, bilingual, 23
    by preschoolers, 54–68 (*See also* Preschoolers, bilingual deaf, language acquisition by)
  in bilingual brain
    brain architecture/processing and, 194
    functional organization of, 194–195
    processing of, 190–191 (*See also* Bilingual brain)
  in child development, 154–156
  choice of, 41–42
  cross-modal borrowing of, 42–45
  proficiency in
    age of acquisition on, 88–91, 93
    brain architecture/processing in, 194
    reading comprehension and, 118–121, 119t
Language contact phenomena, 24
Language development and interaction, bilingual, 23–49
  bilingual language acquisition in deaf learners in, 28–41
    critical period effects in, 29–30, 89–90
    sign language development in, 30–35 (*See also* Sign language development)
    written language development in, 35–41 (*See also* Written language development)
  cross-modal language contact phenomena in, 41–46
    code-switching in classroom in, 45–46
    cross-modal language borrowing in, 42–45
    language choice in, 41–42
  external and internal factors in, 23
  interacting systems in, 23
  interdependence hypothesis of, 25–28
  research on, 23–25
    measures in, 24
    overall results of, 24–25
    on pooling linguistic resources, 47
    population in, 24
    qualitative developmental studies in, 48
    review of, 47–48
    theoretical perspectives of, 23–24
    sign bilingualism in, 23
    sign language transcription conventions and, 48–49
Language development, in sign bilingual and co-enrollment programs, 313–334
  co-enrollment programming in, 318–319
  in Hong Kong, 321–328 (*See also* Co-enrollment programs, sign bilingual education in Hong Kong)
    assessment tools for, 321–323, 329–332
    implications of, 328–333
    outcomes of, 324–328, 324t, 327t
  in Madrid, Spain, 379–385, 388 (*See also* Co-enrollment programs, sign bilingual with cochlear implants in Madrid)
    assessments and participants in, 379, 380t, 381t
    Spanish sign language skills in, 382–383, 383f, 384t
    Spanish sign language *vs.* Spanish skills in, 383–385, 385f, 386f
    spoken Spanish skills in, 380–382, 382t
  in the Netherlands, Twinschool program (*See also* Co-enrollment programs, sign bilingual education in the Netherlands)
    at entry, 403–404, 403t
    for sign language of the Netherlands, 415
    for spoken Dutch, 414–415
    research on bimodal bilingual acquisition in, 317
    sign bilingual programming in, 314–317
    sign language in mainstream settings and, 317–318
Language mixing. *See* Code-blending; Code-mixing
Language of instruction, on learning gains, 275–279, 278t
  child's preference of, grouping by, 276
  Marschark et al. studies of, 275–276
  sign language of the Netherlands *vs.* sign-supported Dutch in, 276–279, 278t
Language task schemas, in bilingual brain, 191–192

Learning environments, rich, 12–13, 93
Learning gains. *See* Academic outcomes; *specific types*
Learning integration with information, 246
Left hemisphere, 187–188
Lexical production assessment, total conceptual vocabulary and, 63–64
Linguistic Interdependence Model, 4–5, 11, 24, 25–28, 102, 109, 125, 127
  bilingual deaf education and
    Austrian study on, 110–125 (*See also* Reading comprehension, sign language and)
    previous research on, 103–104
    problems with, 103
    questions about, 102–103
    in signed and spoken language without target L2, 27–28
    in signed and written/spoken language, 102–103
  co-enrollment and, 330–331
  and cross-modal, linguistic transfer of grammar, between signed language and spoken language, 329–331
  in hearing learners, on L2 face-to-face comprehension and expressive proficiency, 103
  in language development and text-based literacy, 27
  limitations of, 28
  performance in both languages in, linkage of, 26–27
  use of, 25–26
Linguistics
  developmental, 24
  pooling resources in, 47
  in preschoolers, 58–61, 67–68 (*See also* Assessment, of linguistic skills in preschoolers)
  transfer of knowledge of, scaffolding effect of, 331
Literacy, print, impediments to, 223
Loneliness, co-enrollment programs on, 433

Madrid sign bilingual and co-enrollment schools, 371–378
  curriculum of, 372–373
  curriculum organization in, 371–372
  methodology of, 373–376
    accessibility in, 374–375
    diversity in, 375–376
    shared inclusive ideology in, 373–374
    *vs.* traditional Spanish education, 374
  personnel in
    co-tutors, 377
    deaf Spanish sign language specialists, 369, 377
    interpreters, 378
    speech and language therapists, 369, 377
  specific subject areas for deaf children in, 376–377
  students, structure, and organization of, general, 371, 372t
Mainstreaming
  co-enrollment sign bilingual education in Hong Kong *vs.*, 346–347
  improved education assumption in, 230–231
  introducing signed language in, 317–318
  poor educational interpreting in, 231
  on reading comprehension, *vs.* special schools, 225–226
Management skills, teacher, 285t, 286
Mathematics, co-enrollment programs on, 430–432, 430t
Memory, in deaf students' learning, 246–247
Metacognition, in deaf students' learning, 246
Minority, cultural and linguistic, deaf people as, 5–6
Minority language bilingualism, 55
Modalities. *See also specific types*
  efficient use of, in reading instruction, 259, 259f
Modeling, in reading instruction, 260–261, 261f

Netherlands
  co-enrollment programs in (*See also* Co-enrollment programs, sign bilingual education in the Netherlands)

Netherlands, the
  bilingual-bicultural policies in, 272, 396–397
  cochlear implants on language development in, 135, 136–137
  co-enrollment programs in, 396–420
  history and development of special education in, 396–399
  quality of education in, 273–274
  quality of instruction in, 9, 272–288 (*See also* Quality of instruction)
Neurobiology, of bilingualism and bimodal bilingualism, 187–204
  bilingual brain in, 190–195 (*See also* Bilingual brain)
  bimodal bilingual brain in, 195–203 (*See also* Bimodal bilingual brain)
  brain, language, and language development in, 187–190
    age of acquisition on functional anatomy in, 189–190
    aphasia in, 187–188
    Broca's area in, 187, 188, 189f
    function over form in, 188–189
    left hemisphere in, 187–188
    semantic and grammatical processing in, 189
    in signed *vs.* spoken language, 187–188
    Wernicke's area in, 187, 188, 189f
Northern Europe, sign language bilingual education in, 292–305
  bilingual movement in, 292–293
  changing language approaches in, 299–300
  current issues in, 296–299
    inclusion agenda in, 298–299
    language, policy, and approach in, 296
    signed *vs.* spoken language education in, 296
    technologies in, potential of, 296–298
  "deaf" in, 292
  direction and future of, concerns about, 293
  history of, 294–295
  looking again at, 293–294
  models for measurement of, 293
  new language model (plurilingualism) in, 300–304

  benefits of, 300–301
  practice implications of, 302
  professional development implications of, 302–304
  research implications of, 301–302
  shifting contexts and practices in, 304–305
  translanguaging in, 293
Norway. *See also* Northern Europe, sign language bilingual education in
  history of bilingual education in, 294–295
  inclusion agenda in, 299
  teacher training in deaf education in, 302

One person–one language, 375
Oral/aural approach, 138–139
Outcome assessment, in DHH student bilingual programming, 451–462. *See also* Assessment, outcome, of DHH student bilingual programming; *specific assessments and programs*

Parallel bilingual education, 8–9
Parent–child communication, 176
Parent–child relationship, 176
Parents, deaf
  bimodal bilingual brain in children of, 201
  as mentors/models for deaf children, 216–217
  reading comprehension in children of, 224–225
Parents, hearing, 12–13
  deaf children of
    co-enrollment on, 331–332
    language skills in, 74–75
    sign language development in, with nonsigning parents, 31
  fast-track sign-language courses for, 93
Pedagogy
  of bilingual education, assessment of, 457–458
  of Madrid sign bilingual and co-enrollment schools
    content of, 372–373
    organization of, 371–372
    specific subject areas for deaf children in, 376–377

Peer ratings, co-enrollment programs on
  in Hong Kong, 350–354, 351f, 351t, 352f, 353t
  in the Netherlands, 406–410, 409t
  in U.S., 432–433
Peer relationships, 285t, 286
Perspectives, 445–473. *See also specific topics*
  challenges in summaries of, 445
  on co-enrollment programs for DHH and hearing students, 462–468
    academic outcomes of, 463–465
    bilingualism in, 467–468
    cognitive outcomes of, 463
    co-teaching in, 462–463
    motivations for, 462
    social outcomes of, 465–467
  on definitions and boundaries, 446–451
    for bilingual and bicultural deaf education, 449
    for bilingual deaf education, 446–447
    for bilingual deaf education settings, 450
    for bilingualism in co-enrollment settings, 450–451
    for simultaneous communication and total communication, 447–449
  on future, 468–473
  key issues in, 445–446
  on outcome assessment in DHH student programming, 451–462 (*See also* Assessment, outcome, of DHH student bilingual programming)
Phonemes, 249
Phonemic awareness instruction, 249–250
Phonology, reading and, in bimodal bilingual brain, 200–201
Plasticity, brain
  in bilingual brain, 190
  extra, in bimodal bilingual brain, 196
  structural, 192
Plaza-Pust, Carolina
  on cross-modal language mixing, 43–45
  on sign language development in Germany, 35, 38–41
Plurilingualism, in Northern Europe, 300–304
  benefits of, 300–301
  practice implications of, 302

professional development implications of, 302–304
  research implications of, 301–302
Positive goals, 153
Preschoolers, bilingual deaf, language acquisition by, 54–68
  difficulties maintaining bilingualism in, 66
  evaluation of linguistic skills in, methods for, 58–61
    code-mixing phenomena on, 59–60
    combination of methods in, 60
    deaf professional presence on, 67–68
    dominant language on, 59
    integrated language assessment for, 67
    reliable and valid tools in, 60
    sign language tests in, 60–61
  future challenges in, 66–68
  Italian sign language and spoken language empirical data in, 61–66
    bimodal bilingualism and cochlear implants in, longitudinal study of, 64–66
    lexical production assessment and total conceptual vocabulary in, 63–64
    preschoolers from deaf *vs.* hearing families in, 61–63
  research on, scarcity of, 66–67
  theoretical issues and Italian situation in, 54–58
    education contexts in, differing, 57–58
    minority language bilingualism in, 55
    unimodal and bimodal bilingualism in, 54, 55–57
Print literacy, impediments to, 223
Psychosocial development
  for happy life, 152
  in sign bilingual and co-enrollment programs, 345–346
  well-being in, co-enrollment on, 360
Psychosocial development, 21st century, 156–179
  bilingual deaf education for well-being in, 176–179, 360
    assessment needs in, 177
    bicultural or Deaf affiliation in, 178

Psychosocial development, 21st century (*Cont.*)
- contact with other DHH children and adults in, 178
- deaf identities in, 178–179
- diversity of children in, 177
- inclusive settings on, 178
- parent–child relationship and communication in, 176
- sign language on socio-emotional behavior in, 177
- changing perspectives on, 153–154
- difference *vs.* deficiency in, 153–154
- early intervention for enhancement of, 163–170
  - children's situation in, 166–168
  - counseling in, 169–170
  - family-centered services in, 168–170
  - fundamentals of, 163
  - parents' situation in, 163–165
- emotional and behavioral problems in, 161–163
- for happy, successful life, 152
- inclusions and future prospects for, 170–176
  - co-enrollment programs in inclusion in, 174–176
  - identity and inclusion in, 171–172
  - philosophy of inclusion in, 170–171
  - psychosocial risks of inclusion in, 172–174
- key factors in skills development in, 152
- language, cognition, and emotion in child development and, 154–156
- quality of life in, 158–161
- self-esteem in, 156–158

Pure oralism, 138–139

Quality of education, 273–274
Quality of instruction, 272–288
- bilingual deaf education in the Netherlands and, 272–273
- DHH *vs.* hearing student achievement in, as realistic, 287–288
- Dutch deaf student achievement in, 274–275
- elements of, 279–280
- language of instruction and learning gains in, 275–279, 278t
  - child's preference of, grouping by, 276
  - Marschark et al. studies of, 275–276
  - sign language of the Netherlands *vs.* sign-supported Dutch in, 276–279, 278t
- quality of education and instruction in, 273–274
- students' perceptions of, 282–287, 285t
  - achievement pressure in, 285–286, 285t
  - aspects studied in, 282–283
  - Castelijns on, 282
  - classroom climate in, 285t, 286
  - didactics of teachers in, 285t, 286
  - management skills in, 285t, 286
  - peer relationships in, 285t, 286
  - teacher-student relationships in, 283, 285–286, 285t, 288
  - time on task in, 281, 285t, 286
  - ZEBO instrument study of, 284–286, 285t
- teacher activities and student engagement in, 279–282, 281t
  - behaviorally oriented approaches to instruction in, 279
  - direct instruction in, 280
  - Dutch study of, 280–282, 281t
Quality of life, 158–161

Reading
- phonology and, in bimodal bilingual brain, 200–201
- variation in activities of, 261–262, 262f
Reading aloud, 260, 261f
Reading comprehension, bilingualism on, 222–226
- bilingual programming outcome studies on, 226
- deaf parents' positive effect on, 224–225
- L1 as sign *vs.* print language in, 223–224
- print literacy in, impediments to, 223
- research on
  - dual language methodology in, 223
  - lack of, 222
  - literature review on, 222–223
- special *vs.* mainstream schools on, 225–226

Reading comprehension, co-enrollment
   programs on, 464
 in U.S., 429–432, 430t
Reading comprehension, sign language
   and, 102–128, 125–128
 Austrian studies of academic outcomes
   in, 110–125
  achievement measures in, 113–116
  achievement measures in, cognitive,
   116
  achievement measures in, German
   language, 114
  achievement measures in, hearing,
   115–116
  achievement measures in, reading,
   113–114
  achievement measures in, sign
   language, 114–115
  methodologies in, 111–113, 112t
  outcomes in, 116–121
  outcomes in, language skills and
   reading comprehension, 118–121,
   119t
  outcomes in, sign language
   vs. spoken language user
   characteristics, 116–118, 117t
  research questions in, 111
  sign language skills and reading
   comprehension, 121–125
  sign language skills and reading
   comprehension, Carthinian sample,
   124–125
  sign language skills and reading
   comprehension, Upper Austrian
   sample, 121–124, 123t
  speech discrimination with assistive
   listening devices on, 105–106, 110,
   121, 122, 125, 126, 128
 automatic transfer of sign language
   skills as L1 to literacy in L2 in, lack
   of, 102, 103, 124, 125–128
 L1 skills and L2 literacy in, 102–104
 sign language proficiency in,
   106–110, 201 (See also Sign
   language proficiency, on reading
   comprehension)
 sign language use in, 104–106
Reading decoding, in bimodal bilingual
   brain, 199–200

Reading instruction improvement,
   242–265
 in bilingual education, issues in,
   242–245
  cochlear implants and hearing aids
   in, 244–245
  lack of improvement in, research on,
   242–243
  link between signing and, 243
  spoken language ability in, 243–244
  universal newborn hearing screening
   on, 244–245
 deaf students' learning in, 247
 deaf students' learning in, cognitive
   factors in, 245–247
  executive function in, 247
  information and learning integration
   in, 246
  knowledge and knowledge
   orientation in, 245–246
  memory in, 246–247
  metacognition in, 246
  reading instruction in, 247
 quality of instruction in, 247–254, 264
  evidence-based research on, 248–249
  factors predicting academic
   achievement in, 247–248
  fluency instruction in, 250–251
  interim conclusion on, 253–254
  phonemic awareness instruction and
   alphabetics in, 249–250
  text comprehension instruction in,
   252–253
  vocabulary instruction in, 251–252
 teacher training and video coaching in,
   254–265
  direct instruction in, 262, 263f
  efficient use of modalities in, 259, 259f
  explaining and maintaining goal in,
   262, 263f
  improving automaticity in, 260, 260f
  Korthagen model of, 255, 255f
  modeling in, 260–261, 261f
  reading aloud in, 260, 261f
  role and value of, 254
  variation in reading activities in,
   261–262, 262f
  video coaching on reading instruction
   in, 255–259, 257t, 258f–263f, 258t

Reading skills. *See also specific types and programs*
  cochlear implants on, 454
  signing and, 243
    in bimodal bilingual brain, 200
Referential establishment, 31
Re-Read-Adapt and Answer-Comprehend (RAAC) intervention, 250
Research. *See also* Assessment; *specific programs and types*
  on bilingual language development and interaction, 23–25
    measures in, 24
    overall results of, 24–25
    on pooling linguistic resources, 47
    population in, 24
    qualitative developmental studies in, 48
    review of, 47–48
    theoretical perspectives of, 23–24
  lack of, 10, 13–15
  large-scale studies in, 15
  on sign language, 3–4

Salamanca Agreement of 1994, 298
Salutogenetic perspective, 153
Sandwiching, 45
Scandinavia. *See also* Northern Europe, sign language bilingual education in; *specific countries*
  bilingual deaf education in, 7, 8, 220–222
  history of bilingual education in, 294–295
School setting, 9. *See also specific types*
  for bilingual deaf education, 450
  with cochlear implants, 134
  co-enrollment (*See* Co-enrollment programs)
  inclusive, 178
  for Italian bimodal bilingual preschoolers, 57–58
Self-concept, co-enrollment programs on, 348, 433
Self-esteem, 156–158
Semantic processing, brain, 189
Sensitive period, for language acquisition, 29–30, 89–90
Sign bilingualism. *See also* Co-enrollment programs; *specific programs*
  adoption of, in sign bilingual and co-enrollment programs, 361–362
  definition of, 23
Sign bilingual programming, 314–317
Signed Reading Fluency Rubric for Deaf Children, 251
Signing and sign language. *See also specific programs and topics*
  age of acquisition of (*See also* Age of acquisition, language)
    early, 214–215
    for children with cochlear implants, 228–230
  development of, 30–35
  digital hearing aids and cochlear implants on role of, 214
  at home, *vs.* bilingualism in classroom, 216
  incorporation of, 7–8
  natural (*See also specific types, countries, and settings*)
    in raising and educating children, 2
  reading skills and, 243
    in bimodal bilingual brain, 200
  research on, 3–4
  on socio-emotional behavior, 177
  transcription conventions for, 48–49
Sign language bilingual education, in Northern Europe. *See* Northern Europe, sign language bilingual education in
Sign language development, 30–35
  challenges to sign language learners in, 30–31
  in children of hearing, non-signing parents, 31
  developmental trajectories in, 30
  in French-speaking Switzerland, 31–32
  in Germany, 35
  in Italian preschoolers, 61–66
    bimodal bilingualism and cochlear implants in, longitudinal study of, 64–66
    from deaf *vs.* hearing families, 61–63
    difficulties maintaining bilingualism in, 66
    lexical production assessment and total conceptual vocabulary in, 63–64

in Madrid sign bilingual and
co-enrollment schools, 382–385,
383f, 384t, 385f, 386f
referential establishment in, 31
Sign language of the Netherlands (SSN),
*vs.* sign-supported Dutch, on
learning gains, 276–279, 278t
Sign language proficiency
co-enrollment progams on
in sign bilingual co-enrollment
programs, 362
in U.S., 434–435
on reading comprehension, 106–110, 201
(*See also* Reading comprehension,
sign language and)
Chamberlain and Mayberry study of,
108–109
confounding factors in research on,
110
Convertino et al. study of, 108
Hermans et al. study of, 108
Hoffmeister study of, 107
Mayberry et al. study of, 106–107
Mayberry study of, 108
Moore and Sweet study of, 106, 108
Padden and Ramsey study of,
107–108
Strong and Prinz study of, 107
summary of research on, 109–110
Sign language specialists, deaf, 369, 377
Sign language tests, for children, 60–61.
*See also specific types*
Sign language use
as human right, 2–3
on reading comprehension, 104–106
Sign-supported Dutch *vs.* sign language
of the Netherlands, on learning
gains, 276–279, 278t
Sign-supported speech, 227
bimodality, bilingual education and,
227–230
Simultaneous bilingual acquisition,
332–333
Simultaneous communication, 139, 227.
*See also* Bimodal bilingual
in classroom, on learning, 227–230
signing with cochlear implants in,
228–230
studies of, 227–228

definitions and boundaries of, 447–449
prevalence of, 227
Social acceptance, co-enrollment
programs on, 466–467
in Hong Kong, 349–350, 359
in U.S., 432–433
Social competence, co-enrollment
programs on, 432–433
Social-emotional skills. *See also*
Psychosocial development, 21st
century
in Madrid sign bilingual and
co-enrollment schools, 385–386,
387f
Social integration, 343
co-enrollment programs on, 465–467
of deaf children with cochlear implants,
466–467
definition of, 406
in DHH children, importance of,
406–407
Social integration, in sign bilingual
and co-enrollment environment,
342–364
attitudes of hearing students toward
DHH students in, 346, 355–358,
356t–357t
bolstering DHH students' psychosocial
well-being in, 360
co-enrollment in, 346–348
*vs.* conventional mainstream setting,
346–347
language of co-enrollment education
in, 347–348
previous research on, 348
self-perception of DHH students in,
348
varieties of, 347
collaborative teaching and co-learning
in, 360–361
critical mass of DHH students in,
362–363
deaf teacher presence in, 363
definition of, 343
equal social significance of sign and
spoken language development in,
361–362
feasibility of, recent developments on,
342

Social integration, in sign bilingual and
    co-enrollment environment (*Cont.*)
  in Hong Kong, 348–359 (*See also*
    Co-enrollment programs, sign
    bilingual education in Hong Kong)
  in inclusive deaf education, 343–345
  in the Netherlands, 406–410.309t
  possibility of, 342
  psychosocial adjustments of DHH
    students in, 345–346
  sign bilingualism adoption in, 361–362
  signed language proficiency in, 362
  social interactions in, high frequency
    of, 361
  social outcomes of, in Hong Kong,
    359–360
Social interaction
  in co-enrollment programs
    high frequency of, 361
    in U.S., 432–433
  importance of, 432
Social position, of children in classroom,
  406–407
Social significance, of equal sign and
  spoken language development,
  361–362
Socio-emotional behavior
  co-enrollment programs on, 465–467
  sign language on, 177
Spanish education, traditional, *vs.* Madrid
  sign bilingual and co-enrollment
  schools, 374
Speech and language therapists, 369, 377
Spoken language skills
  fluency in, 213–214
  in Madrid sign bilingual education
    co-enrollment schools, 383–385,
    385f, 386f
Strength-based perspective, 153
Students' perceptions, of quality of
  instruction, 282–287
  Castelijns on, 282
Successful life, psychosocial development
  for, 152
Sweden. *See also* Northern Europe, sign
  language bilingual education in
  bilingual deaf education in, 7, 8
  history of bilingual education in,
    294–295
  inclusion agenda in, 298
  teacher training in deaf education in,
    303
Switzerland, French-speaking, sign
  language development in, 31–32

Teacher-student relationships, 283,
  285–286, 285t, 288, 458
  importance of, 458
Teacher training, in deaf education
  in Denmark, 302–303
  in Norway, 302
  in Sweden, 303
  in United Kingdom, 303
Teacher training, in reading instruction,
  254–265
  direct instruction in, 262, 263f
  efficient use of modalities in, 259, 259f
  explaining and maintaining goal in,
    262, 263f
  improving automaticity in, 260, 260f
  Korthagen model of, 255, 255f
  modeling in, 260–261, 261f
  reading aloud in, 260, 261f
  role and value of, 254
  variation in reading activities in,
    261–262, 262f
  video coaching on reading instruction
    in, 255–259, 257t, 258f–263f, 258t
Teaching theory, 285t, 286
Text comprehension instruction, 252–253
Time on task, 281, 285t, 286
Total communication, 139–140
  *vs.* auditory-oral communication (*See
    also under* Cochlear implants,
    communication mode on language
    development with)
  with cochlear implants, 143–147
  with hearing aids, 140–143
  definitions and boundaries of, 447–449
Total conceptual vocabulary, lexical
  production assessment and, 63–64
Transcription conventions, sign language,
  48–49
Transfer
  automatic, of sign language skills as L1
    to L2 literacy, 102, 103, 124, 125–128
  cross-linguistic and bimodal bilingual
    cross-language interaction in, 76

of cross-modal grammar, between signed language and spoken language, 329–330 (*See also* Co-enrollment programs, sign bilingual education in Hong Kong)
from L1 to L2, 217
of linguistic knowledge, scaffolding effect of, 331
Translanguaging, 293
TRIPOD program, 397–398
Twinschool program. *See* Co-enrollment programs, sign bilingual education in the Netherlands

Unimodal bilinguals (bilingualism), 54, 74
*vs.* bimodal bilingualism, 56
cognitive control in, 84–85
cross-language interaction by, 76–77
definition of, 94
in Italy, 55–56, 57
studies of
attention control in, 219
transferability of, to bimodal bilinguals, 218
United Kingdom. *See also* Northern Europe, sign language bilingual education in
history of bilingual education in, 295
inclusion agenda in, 299
teacher training in deaf education in, 303
Universal Design for Learning Center for Applied Special Technology (UDL CAST), 375

Universal newborn hearing screening, on reading achievement, 244–245

Video coaching, on reading instruction, 255–264
direct instruction in, 262, 263f
efficient use of modalities in, 259, 259f
explaining and maintaining goal in, 262, 263f
improving automaticity in, 260, 260f
Korthagen model of, 255, 255f
modeling in, 260–261, 261f
reading aloud in, 260, 262f
variation in reading activities in, 261–262, 262f
Visual Phonics, 249–250
Visual word form area, 199
Vocabulary
in bimodal bilingual brain, 201
co-enrollment programs on
in Madrid, Spain, 380–385, 388
in U.S., 429–432, 430t
total conceptual, lexical production assessment and, 63–64
Vocabulary instruction, 251–252

Wernicke's area, 187, 189f
Written language development, 35–41
attaining target L2 grammar in, 36–41
attaining writing system in, 35–36
Written language fluency, 213–214